Patient Teaching Manual 1

Patient Teaching Manual 1

Springhouse Corporation
Springhouse, Pennsylvania

Publisher: Keith Lassner
Editor: Regina Daley Ford
Clinical Editors: Marlene Ciranowicz, RN, BSN, MSN; Cathy Furan, RN, BSN, MSN; Susan Krupnick, RN, MSN, CCRN, CEN, CS; Susan Weiner, RN, MSN; Nina P. Welsh, RN
Drug Information Manager: Larry Neil Gever, RPh, PharmD
Art Director: John Hubbard
Editorial Services Manager: David Moreau
Senior Production Manager: Deborah C. Meiris

The clinical procedures described and recommended in this publication are based on research and consultation with nursing, medical, and legal authorities. To the best of our knowledge, these procedures reflect currently accepted practice; nevertheless, they can't be considered absolute and universal recommendations. For individual application, all recommendations must be considered in light of the patient's clinical condition and, before administration of new or infrequently used drugs, in light of latest package-insert information. The authors and the publisher disclaim responsibility for any adverse effects resulting directly or indirectly from the suggested procedures, from any undetected errors, or from the reader's misunderstanding of the text.

Some of the material in this book was adapted from the following Springhouse series: Nurse's Reference Library, Nursing Now, Nurse's Clinical Library, Nursing Photobook, and New Nursing Skillbook.

TPTM1-010487

Library of Congress Cataloging-in-Publication Data
Main entry under title:

Patient teaching manual.

Includes bibliographies and index.
1. Patient education—Handbooks, manuals, etc.
I. Ford, Regina Daley. II. Springhouse Corporation. [DNLM: 1. Health Promotion—handbooks.
2. Patient Education—handbooks. WY 39 P298]
RT90.P376 1987 610.73'06'99 87-6426
ISBN 0-87434-032-2 (v.1)
ISBN 0-87434-066-7 (v.2)

Contents

Contributors

CLINICAL CONTRIBUTORS

Gloria S. Cheeseman, RN, BA, MA
Director, Educational Resources Department
St. Francis Medical Center
Trenton, N.J.
Foreword

Janice Selekman, DNSc, RN
Associate Professor
Thomas Jefferson University
Philadelphia
Chapter 1—"Principles of Patient Teaching"

CLINICAL CONSULTANTS

Dorothy Brooten, PhD, FAAN
Chairman, Health Care of Women and Childbearing
Family Section
School of Nursing
University of Pennsylvania
Philadelphia

Dorothy Kaye Hummel, RN
Perioperative RN
AMI/Single Day Surgery
Ft. Myers, Fla.

Bonnie Joyce Kaplan, RN, MS
Assistant Director of Nursing, Maternal Child Health
Francis Scott Key Medical Center
Baltimore

Janet Y. Mulligan, RN, MA, CCRN
Cardiac Rehabilitation Nurse
Vital Heart Center
New Port Richey, Fla.

Ruth Rankin, RN
Head Nurse
Sarah Bush Lincoln Health Center
Mattoon, Ill.

Foreword

Patient teaching has not always been a top priority for the health care professions. In the past, such questions as "What is my blood pressure?", "Why am I taking this pill?", or "Why must I have this test?" often met with the response, "Sorry, but you'll have to ask your doctor for that information." Patients were expected to accept much, if not all, of their diagnostic workups and therapeutic regimens on blind faith. Our traditional view of patient education did not require the dissemination of valuable and sometimes vital information to our patients. Gradually, under the impetus of professional and legal demands for nursing accountability, our philosophy regarding "the patient's right to know" has changed. The nursing process now stipulates patient and family education concerning health problems and health maintenance as a major responsibility of the professional nurse.

Today especially—with the "sicker and quicker" phenomenon clearly reflected in hospital discharge policies—patient care frequently devolves upon the patient or on the family. Our goal must be to arm the caregivers with the best and most accurate information available to help them achieve an optimal level of health for the patient.

The Springhouse *Patient Teaching Manuals* were created to help nurses and other health care professionals achieve this goal. These manuals are unique, easy-to-use teaching/learning tools. They permit the nurse to choose from a wide variety of topics and to select from the comprehensive content of each teaching plan the exact level and depth of information needed by her patient. Topics dealt with in the text and patient-teaching aids were selected because they are common, difficult, or otherwise significant teaching problems.

Chapter 1, "Principles of Patient Teaching," provides the nurse with a mini-course in patient teaching. It discusses teaching methods, development and implementation of the teaching plan—even instruction of patients with special needs.

The format of subsequent chapters is consistent. There are five sections in each chapter: Patient-Learner Data Base, Explaining Diagnostic Tests, Explaining Disorders, Explaining Treatments, and Patient-Teaching Aids.

The first section, Patient-Learner Data Base, lists significant areas in which a patient may experience a potential knowledge deficit. Not all data (every risk factor, for example) will apply to each patient. But this comprehensive list tells the nurse those areas which should be questioned so that she can identify those which should be pursued further.

The next three sections, Explaining Diagnostic Tests, Explaining Disorders, and Explaining Treatments, present specific teaching plans that address specific patient problems. For example, in Chapter 2, "Cardiovascular Disorders," the 12-lead EKG, myocardial infarction, and CABG are dealt with in the diagnostic tests, disorders, and treatments sections, respectively.

To maximize the quality and effectiveness of the patient education process, the teaching plan content is directly related to the patient objective. The behavioral objectives from which the nurse and patient should select, and upon which they should agree, appear in the left column on each page. The teaching plan content for each patient objective appears in the right column, directly across from the objective.

To individualize her nursing care plan and to promote patient compliance, the nurse must decide which objectives are relevant to that patient's needs, always bearing in mind that prior knowledge is also an important resource for patient learning. Furthermore, she must select information from the teaching plan content based on her knowledge of the patient's ability and desire to learn.

The final section of each chapter comprises selected patient-teaching aids. These aids were chosen either to supplement or complement the textual material, as judged necessary by professional nurses. While they are numerous, they are not intended to be all-inclusive. Several excellent appendices, a list of selected references, and an extensive index appear at the back of each volume.

The Springhouse *Patient Teaching Manuals* provide health care professionals with the tools needed to fulfill their obligation to educate the patient and the family. These tools—basic educational principles telling *how* to teach and specific patient-teaching plans showing *what* to teach—utilized with consistency and continuity, surely will enhance the credibility of the teacher and the receptivity of the learner.

As a nurse and an educator, I am proud and most pleased that these manuals are available to assist health care professionals with their patient education efforts. They engender an awareness of the importance of patient teaching and challenge health care professionals to provide our patients and their families with the knowledge, attitudes, and skills to be true and valuable partners in the promotion, protection, and enhancement of their own health.

GLORIA S. CHEESEMAN, RN, BA, MA

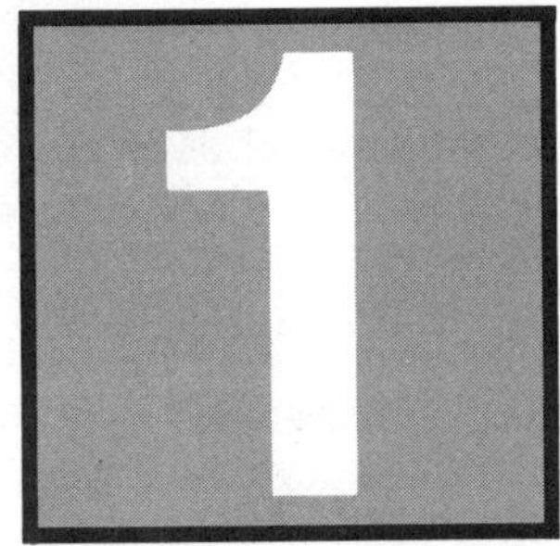

Principles of Patient Teaching

Teaching is an integral component of nursing. To tend only to the physical needs of patients without teaching them to obtain, retain, or regain health is a job half done. While registered nurses and student nurses are expected, and often required, to direct patient teaching, the skill of how to teach patient teaching is often limited in nursing programs. The purpose of this chapter is not only to suggest to the nurse *what* to teach the patient, but also *how* to teach it. We will address such issues as what data the nurse needs before working with a patient, the techniques she can use to aid her teaching, and the variables that interfere with teaching. This chapter will focus on the process of patient teaching.

THE NURSE AS EDUCATOR

Since the turn of the century, nurses have incorporated patient teaching into their professional role. Starting with public health and maternal-child health nurses, the instruction of child care and sanitation measures became the responsibility of the nurse. Lavinia Dock (1858-1956), a pioneer in nursing, emphasized nursing's important role in preventive health care via teaching.

Today, nurses have many opportunities to share their knowledge. This role extends far beyond the treating of acute illness in the hospital setting. While the primary responsibility of nurses is to teach patients the care they need to maintain or regain their health, nurses also inform and support their patients' significant others, especially family members. In addition, nurses promote good public health by working with different groups within society to improve the environment.

While this book focuses on patient teaching, it should be noted that nurses also teach each other by exchanging information, whether during change-of-shift reports or in patient care conferences. This exchange of information promotes continuity of care and, therefore, improves the art of nursing.

Teaching versus learning

Teaching is a collaborative process that involves communication between the nurse and the patient. Its goal is to add to the patient's knowledge base so he can improve or maintain his health and comfort. Teaching can be planned or spontaneous, verbal or nonverbal, individualized or for large groups, affective or cognitive.

Learning is a relatively permanent change in behavior that is inferred from a change in performance or cognitive beliefs occurring as a result of experience. Learning helps the patient to increase his understanding, decrease his anxieties, and alter his health care habits.

Patient teaching and the nursing process

The principles of patient teaching correlate directly with the nursing process. Before any interventions can be planned, assessment must occur and goals must be set. The nursing process involves obtaining a data base, assessing this data base (including identifying a list of needs), writing goals, planning and implementing nursing interventions, and making an evaluation.

This same process is true in patient teaching. Before teaching can occur, the nurse must assess the patient and his environment, identify his needs, write educational objectives, plan and implement a teaching plan, and evaluate the results.

METHODS OF KNOWING/SOURCES OF KNOWLEDGE

Every patient has his own values about health and illness and experiences with the health care system. Before assessing the components of the art of teaching, the nurse must understand the different methods of knowing, because from these sources of knowledge spring the roots of both the nurse's and the patient's belief systems and many of their health care practices.

Magic and the supernatural

Belief in magic and the supernatural as the cause of events is the first method of knowing. This includes carrying good-luck charms, crossing one's fingers for luck, avoiding the number 13, saying "God bless you" after someone sneezes, or knocking on wood. All are attempts to enhance one's safety and health. Since such practices usually cause no harm to a patient who believes in them, they can readily be acknowledged as important in a teaching plan.

Tradition and culture

Knowledge based on *tradition and cultural norms,* including rituals and beliefs without scientific justification, is the second method of knowing. Using herbal teas to treat respiratory or gastrointestinal problems, the hot-cold theory followed by some Hispanic groups, using chicken soup or chest rubs for whatever ails you, or the belief that getting one's feet wet in puddles or sitting in a draft will cause illness are examples of this method. The patient at this stage will often say, "I know it is true just because I know it."

When planning to teach someone whose belief system is founded in tradition and culture, it is important for the nurse to assess whether the beliefs interfere with the proposed treatments or are harmful to the patient. If they are not harmful, an attempt can be made to incorporate these beliefs into the treatment regimen. This provides the patient with a familiar, secure base from which to start learning. Why not include herbal teas as part of the patient's required fluid intake or suggest that the patient's "higher power" would want him to comply with proposed treatments? Building on a base of health beliefs familiar to the patient can decrease his anxieties and increase compliance.

Intuition and personal experience

Intuition or personal experience based on trial and error is involved in the third method of developing a knowledge base. The patient's significant others may say, "I know it will work for you; I can just feel it. It worked for me. Try it." Often, personal success with a specific treatment or pressure from a loved one to try a treatment forms the basis of this knowledge (for example, certain positions or exercises for menstrual cramps, concoctions or practices to bring on sleep, or child-rearing directions from a mother based on what worked for her 25 years earlier). Nurses may also have experiences with health measures unrelated to anything taught in nursing school and untested by the scientific community.

Nurses and patients who believe that unproven health measures can prevent or cure ailments need to assess the validity of these measures. If they pose no danger to the patient, the nurse should enhance the patient's knowledge about such measures (based on scientific fact) by discussing rationales for their use; otherwise, the patient's misperceptions should be corrected. The nurse should give the patient credit for his trial-and-error methods and should help him obtain the most accurate and safest knowledge base.

Authority

A fourth method of knowing is based on trust of those in *authority* or those recognized by society as being influential. It refers, in part, to believing what authorities write or say and personalizing the content. The content may or may not be accurate and empirically supported, but this makes no difference to the believer. Accepting health practices without question is common during childhood. Such comments as "My parents said..." or "My teacher said..." can be expanded to include the teachings of physicians, religious leaders, and Nobel prizewinners. Patients like this are not advocates for themselves; rather, they generalize the teachings of these authority figures and relate them to their own condition and health practices.

Since the nurse is often in a role of authority, the patient will follow her say-so if it is logical, sensitive, and presented in an understandable manner. But how should the nurse respond when another authority figure's advice contradicts the patient's medical needs? Some suggestions include presenting equally authoritative information (preferably in writing) that supports the treatment plan; beginning with a simple, but related, example of cause and effect and then building a solid knowledge base from this situation; and avoiding confronting or insulting the patient's belief model while at the same time reinforcing beliefs that are more focused on health promotion. When the patient states, "The Bible says...," an appropriate nursing response would be, "Yes, but the Bible also states...."

Logical reasoning

Logical reasoning, the fifth source of knowledge, includes inductive and deductive processes. Inductive reasoning is a method of obtaining related facts and then making a generalization about these facts; for example, if taking 500 mg of vitamin C is good, then taking 1,000 mg of vitamin C is even better. While this method of thinking may be fine for vitamin C, it could be fatal for cardiac drugs. The nurse must anticipate the patient's thought processes and address his misconceptions in the teaching plan.

In deductive logic, a specific prediction is derived from a generalized statement; for example, multiple studies have documented that decreasing one's intake of carbohydrates and meat improves cardiovascular status. Anorexics may incorrectly believe this is also true for them. It is important for the nurse to impress each patient with the idea that he is special and unique, and then to explain why certain treatments would or would not be helpful. The teaching plan—like the rest of the nursing care plan—must be individualized to meet the specific needs of each patient. Nurses have always believed in providing an individualized plan of care based on the specific needs of each patient.

Scientific method

The highest level of knowing is obtained via the *scientific method,* which requires observation and testing with a reliable and valid instrument while controlling as many variables as possible. It is logical and objective, with controls that prevent error. This method should be the primary source of knowledge for nurses and should provide the basis of material for the teaching plan.

ASSESSMENT OF THE LEARNER

Factors to assess

A patient's belief system is only one area the nurse must assess before preparing a teaching plan. A second, but related, area requiring assessment is the patient's *knowledge base.* How much does he know about his condition or treatment? How accurate is that knowledge base?

A third area is the patient's *ability to learn:* does he understand easily; does he ask questions; or does his body language indicate confusion of the concepts, content, or sequence of events? Can he follow directions, pay attention, and recall information? Can he hear, see, and communicate? Is he easily distracted, or does he demonstrate other signs of learning problems? Does he understand abstract ideas?

Once the nurse has assessed that a patient *can* learn, she needs to assess if he is *ready to learn.* He might say, "I don't want to know; I can't change at this point in my life." If physical or emotional factors interfere with his readiness to learn, the nurse can attempt to clarify the issues by asking open-ended questions. The nurse must also ask herself, "Does the patient really need to know this material or is it *my* need, as nurse, to teach it to him?"

The nurse must also assess the patient's past *history of compliance.* Simply learning to feed back material verbally will not help him maintain or regain his health; he must put the knowledge into practice.

Assessing the following factors will help the nurse complete her patient data base in preparation for developing a comprehensive teaching plan:

—What is the patient's outlook on life?
—What is his past history with health-related material?
—What is his culture's response to pain and illness?
—What is his educational background?
—What are his fears about his illness or the proposed changes in his life-style?

Factors that interfere with learning

Many factors can alter one's readiness or ability to learn. The first is *anxiety.* It has been well documented that, while mild anxiety enhances learning, severe anxiety can be incapacitating. Patients may verbalize their uneasiness, or the nurse may detect it in their body language. Some causes of anxiety include feeling pressure to perform, feeling a loss of control because of the learning situation or because of the health need that requires this new knowledge base, not wanting to expend the energy necessary to learn, lacking trust in the teacher, and dealing with the financial implications of the new knowledge or health practices on one's lifestyle.

A second factor interfering with learning is *motivation.* In internal motivation, the stimulus and perceived need for change come from the individual himself; in external motivation, the impetus for change comes from significant others. Internally motivated people are more self-directed, and their stimulation for success lasts longer than it does for those who are externally motivated and need repeated reinforcement and praise from others (Redman, 1984).

Motivation is related to *locus of control.* A patient with an internal locus believes that he *can,* if he so desires, change his health by measures he controls. A patient with an external locus believes that his health is controlled by a higher power (God, luck, and/or significant others) and that compliance with treatment would be ineffective. Individuals with such "learned helplessness" feel that they cannot control the outcome of events. Teaching such a patient can be very frustrating for the nurse, for, in addition to presenting needed material, she must also develop and reinforce the idea that the patient can have some control over his condition.

A *lack of trust and honesty* between patient and nurse impedes learning. Providing continuity of care by having a consistent caretaker responsible for the teaching plan can prevent this. In addition, the nurse needs to be prepared, positive, and confident.

The nurse must evaluate the patient's *current physical and emotional status* before attempting teaching. Basic needs must be tended to first. Is the patient hungry or in pain? Is he tired or on drugs that alter his cognitive functioning? Is his mobility limited (this might affect the learning of skills)? Is he lonely or anticipating visitors? Is teaching planned during a time he would rather be with significant others? How much are others pressuring him to perform? What stage of illness is he in? Any of these factors can interfere with learning.

In addition to assessing the patient, the nurse must also evaluate three other factors: the environment, the time factor, and the available resources. *Where* is the teaching/learning to be done? What distractions, such as noise or people, are hindering the patient's ability to concentrate? Is there sufficient privacy? Is there sufficient lighting? Is the room too hot or too cold?

The nurse cannot always control *when* the teaching is to be performed and how much time will be involved. Is one session enough or are many sessions needed? Sessions should be short enough so that patients will have time to absorb the material, both cognitively and psychologically. In some situations, the content to be taught can be presented little by little every time the nurse walks in the room; for example, she can discuss the principles of breathing exercises while setting the patient up for his morning care. Then every time the nurse enters the room that day, she can teach him one new breathing exercise and evaluate his ability to do those already taught. If the nurse does not have enough time to teach the patient adequately or if she does not have a chance to reinforce the material, she should discuss the most important information and provide the remainder of the information in writing.

The final assessment involves exploring the health facility and national organizations for available *educational resources.* A great deal of patient-education material has been developed, and obtaining this material will ease the nurse's teaching role. Clinical specialists are resources for their areas of expertise. The hospital library is often a ready source of ideas and materials. The hospital's continuing education staff may also be able to provide teaching strategies. If a nurse works at a facility affiliated with a nursing school, she can seek help from nursing instructors, who may have access to teaching aids. Also drug and formula companies are often excellent sources of teaching aids, as are national organizations, such as the Cystic Fibrosis Foundation, the American Association of Diabetes Educators, and the American Cancer Society. This material should always be individualized for each patient.

THE TEACHING PLAN

Formulating behavioral objectives

Once the nurse has obtained and interpreted all possible data about the patient and his environment and has identified the problems, needs, or scope of the teaching required, her next step is to identify the patient's long-term and short-term goals by writing behavioral objectives. These objectives will guide the teaching plan and evaluation process.

Behavioral objectives state the change in the patient's behavior expected when "learning" has occurred. Remember that they are *patient* goals, not nursing goals. An effective objective often includes the words, "The patient will...." It is stated in terms of the patient and not the nurse.

To ensure that these objectives are truly patient-oriented, they should be established jointly by the patient and the nurse. Learning is more effective when a patient is motivated to learn, and establishing his own objectives is a reflection of motivation. Defining goals together also decreases the patient's anxiety about learning, since he will have a better idea of what to expect of the nurse and of himself and can have some control over the learning process. This, then, becomes a reflection of the definition of teaching—that of being a collaborative process.

The nurse should ask herself, "What behavioral change do I want to see in this patient? If he only learns one thing from my presentation, what should it be?" Objectives help the nurse focus on the task at hand; they define the expected outcome of the teaching, thereby decreasing the possibility that the patient will be overwhelmed by all available information about the topic.

Behavioral objectives include three major components: the observable behavior and to what degree it will occur; the conditions under which the behavior will be performed; and the criteria to be used to evaluate whether the behavior has been successfully learned. For example: "At the end of the final teaching session about diabetes, the patient will be able to correctly draw up and administer his insulin injection without assistance." In this example, "the end of the final teaching session" indicates *when* the behavior should be learned; the "patient" is *who* will be learning; "drawing up and administering insulin" is *what* will be learned; "correctly" indicates *how* or to what degree the task will be evaluated; and "without assistance" indicates the conditions under which the behavior will be performed.

Behavioral objectives are described in terms of *doing*. In reviewing behavioral objectives, the nurse must ensure that the goal is realistic for the patient and specific to his needs. Can he attain it? Can it be accomplished in the time period specified? What level of cognitive functioning is being addressed, and is it appropriate for the task at hand?

Bloom (1956) developed a system to classify educational objectives for cognitive learning. The stages include knowledge (recalling facts), comprehension (simple understanding), application (applying rules and generalizations to specific situations), analysis (dividing a concept into its parts), synthesis (rearranging the parts into a whole), and evaluation (assessing the value of information).

These stages form a hierarchy, from the easiest cognitive process (rote knowledge) to the most complicated (evaluation). In most situations, patient teaching only involves the first three stages (knowledge, comprehension, and application). However, teaching at any given level can proceed from simple to complex and from concrete to abstract. The nurse should center the objective around an action verb that describes what the patient is expected to accomplish. These verbs are listed in the table on pages 10-11.

While the guidance offered by well-written behavioral objectives usually facilitates learning, a nurse must remain flexible in a teaching situation. She may have to change objectives if the patient's needs change. For example, a patient may verbalize a misconception of something basic to the lesson plan, or the nurse may discover that one part of the teaching plan caused the patient a great deal of confusion and concern.

Writing some behavioral objectives is difficult. First, all learning cannot be anticipated. Also, objectives change as the learning process progresses. The verbs in the table reflect only the cognitive domain (intellectual and problem solving). The descriptors of the psychomotor and affective domains are not as well defined even though the needs of many patients clearly fall into these categories. Nurses should also incorporate these special needs into their teaching plan.

Developing a teaching plan

Once she has written behavioral objectives, the nurse can plan nursing interventions via a teaching plan, which includes the content to be taught and the methods by which it will be presented. Several variables strongly influence the development of a plan: whether teaching will be done one-on-one or in a group; whether material will be presented formally or informally; whether teaching will be performed throughout the shift or at a specific "teaching time"; and how much time is available for teaching. (This is often determined by the institution; for example, how many sessions are available for childbirth education, how many days until a patient is discharged, or how many minutes is a patient willing to stay after a clinic visit?)

An organized and logical teaching plan enhances learning. It is helpful to begin a lesson with content the patient knows and then to progress to new material. *Going from the known to the unknown* decreases

VERBS USED TO DESCRIBE BEHAVIORS OF THE COGNITIVE DOMAIN

Knowledge
(Recalling facts and information)

Accept	Know	Notice	Recognize	Test
Count	Label	Point	Record	Trace
Draw	List	Quote	Reiterate	Underline
Enumerate	Listen	Read	Repeat	Write
Identify	Memorize	Recall	Reproduce	
Indicate	Name	Recite	State	

Comprehension
(Simple understanding of information and ability to draw simple conclusions)

Answer	Contrast	Express	Report
Associate	Define	Inquire	Restate
Classify	Differentiate	Interpret	Review
Compare	Discuss	Locate	Select
Compile	Distinguish	Participate	Tell
Compute	Estimate	Predict	Translate
Consult	Explain	Recognize	

Application
(Applying rules and generalizations to specific problems)

Adopt	Complete	Examine	Schedule	Write
Apply	Decide	Illustrate	Sketch	
Calculate	Demonstrate	Operate	Solve	
Choose	Dramatize	Practice	Use	
Classify	Employ	Present	Utilize	

Analysis
(Breaking down concepts into separate elements and identifying the relationships among them)

Analyze	Construct	Devise	Explain	Realize
Appraise	Contrast	Diagnose	Generalize	Reason
Arrange	Create	Diagram	Infer	Relate
Calculate	Criticize	Discover	Inspect	Solve
Categorize	Debate	Distinguish	Interpret	Summarize
Combine	Detect	Examine	Organize	Support
Compare	Develop	Experiment	Question	Test

Synthesis
(Reassembling elements to create a new idea)

Arrange	Create	Integrate	Plan	Relate
Assemble	Design	Manage	Practice	Set up
Challenge	Determine	Order	Prepare	Transform
Collect	Formulate	Organize	Prescribe	Weigh
Construct	Group	Originate	Propose	

Evaluation
(Assessing the value of materials/ideas)

Appraise	Critique	Evaluate	Rank	Revise
Assess	Determine	Grade	Rate	Score
Assimilate	Establish	Judge	Recommend	Select
Choose	Estimate	Measure	Resolve	Value
Conclude				

anxiety, because the teaching begins on familiar territory. In addition, it helps patients apply information from one setting (past experiences) to their present situation. Starting on comfortable ground reinforces and supports the patient's feelings of having a solid knowledge base. The nurse must ensure that the material is neither too easy nor too hard, so she does not lose the patient's attention or interest.

A second approach involves teaching from *the simple to the complex.* Anatomy, physiology, and pathophysiology involve a language foreign to most patients. Before the nurse can teach them about their myocardial infarction or their beta blockers, she should define the words and approach the concepts simply. Pictures and analogies (if the patient can comprehend these) may help explain normal and abnormal organ functioning. From this simple but solid knowledge base, more complex material can be presented.

The third approach to teaching is to progress from *concrete to abstract* material. Most individuals find it easier to learn new material when they can see, feel, count, hear, or taste it. Since concepts are abstract by nature, they are often difficult to comprehend. Defining the concept of respiratory distress by pointing out the changes it effects, such as increased respiratory rate, wheezing, dusky skin, and retractions, renders it concrete and, therefore, more meaningful.

The final educational concept is that of *multisensory learning.* Perception is necessary for learning. Studies have indicated that a multisensory approach is more effective in learning than a single sensory approach. Some individuals learn better by one approach than another; for example, the pregnant woman listening to a childbirth-preparation lecture experiences only auditory stimulation. This woman may need to *see* a replica of a baby coming through the vaginal canal and *do* the breathing exercises to really understand what will happen during delivery. The nurse needs to plan her teaching so that it involves as many senses as possible.

Additional factors to consider when planning the teaching material include determining what content is most relevant to the patient's condition and needs, prioritizing when performing the teaching role, and avoiding conflict with the patient's culture and past experiences by incorporating his health beliefs into the teaching plan.

Since effective learning requires active participation, the nurse should encourage the patient to participate in each component of the teaching process and should encourage active give-and-take between the teacher and learner. Especially when teaching psychomotor skills, the nurse needs to consider the patient's strength, coordination, and mobility. She must remember that a strong knowledge base enhances the patient's performance of technical skills.

When developing a teaching plan, the nurse can anticipate the patient's fears and concerns and can include questions that decrease the threat of the material with such comments as, "Most new mothers wonder..." or "Many cardiac patients are concerned about...." This type of question reduces the patient's anxiety about the unfamiliar. Being sensitive to psychosocial needs enhances the rapport between the teacher and the learner.

The nurse can use multiple teaching modalities to present material to the patient, including the following:

—*Lecture.* Perhaps the most frequent type of teaching, especially for groups, it is cost effective, uses staff time efficiently, and ensures consistency of material through a structured presentation. However, lectures limit individuality and interpersonal interaction. The nurse should be willing to alter her teaching plan based on the patient's questions and responses. Patients should be involved in the lecture by questions or by challenges to their imagination.

—*Demonstration.* This multisensory presentation involves vision, hearing, and touch, but is limited to very small groups. This method builds skills and is especially effective when a return demonstration is performed by the patient. It is essential for teaching such skills as bathing a baby, walking with crutches, caring for a tracheostomy, and giving insulin injections.

—*Programmed instruction.* This teaching method uses prepared material that is divided into sections or units. The patient must be self-motivated and literate. Working at his own pace, he actively participates in the learning and gets immediate feedback from the source. The nurse does not need to be present, but learning is enhanced if she is involved.

—*Sociodrama.* This group problem-solving technique recreates a real-life situation by having participants act out roles and feelings of the people involved. It helps patients explore feelings and does require planning. It is effective for attitudinal problems.

—*Role-playing.* This teaching technique allows one person to explore alternative behaviors by putting himself in the shoes of another. This is quite effective for siblings or classmates of handicapped patients or of those with chronic disorders.

—*Simulation.* In this teaching method, the nurse and the patient act out a real situation in a mock environment and behavioral processes are replicated. Learning laboratories in nursing programs and cardiopulmonary resuscitation certification programs are multisensory approaches in a nonthreatening environment that make use of simulation. This approach can be effective in teaching techniques that benefit from demonstration; for example, to prepare a patient to give himself an injection by first giving one to an orange.

—*Behavior modification.* This method is very popular with children, smokers, and those with weight problems. It involves operant conditioning with reinforcement. This means that the nurse gives the patient positive reinforcement for a specific behavior, which causes the desired response to occur more frequently and more intensely. Conditioning is a process of learning. A disadvantage of this method is that, when reinforcement slows or stops, so does behavioral change.

—*Contracting.* In this technique, the nurse and the patient agree on behavior(s) needed to achieve a determined goal. This is often effective with adolescents who may wish to have privileges in return for behavioral changes.

—*Audiovisual materials* (pamphlets, films, printed materials, diagrams, models). Patients must be literate in order to use most of the material involved in this teaching method, since most provide only visual information. In order for this method to be effective, the nurse must offer some verbal intervention and must individualize the material.

—*Play.* This teaching technique is commonly used with children in order that they learn about their world.

Medical play is most effective in preparing children for procedures and in helping them deal with their misconceptions and anger after the procedures.

Additional teaching methods include self-monitoring (keeping records, logs, or diaries of an activity), panels or debates, discussion groups, and using a patient's significant other to teach and monitor the patient.

To determine whether to teach patients individually or in groups, the nurse should consider the following factors. Teaching one-on-one is usually more effective, since the nurse can get to know her patient and can alter the teaching plan to meet his needs. The group process, on the other hand, can handle many individuals at once and, therefore, is less costly to run and takes less time than teaching each person separately. While a group can provide peer support in many situations, it can also make sharing feelings about sexuality or other embarrassing material difficult. The privacy and confidentiality of the one-on-one relationship is lost in the group. (This should not be confused with the principles of group therapy.)

While all of these are structured models in which the nurse can initiate the teaching plan, there is one method of patient teaching that the nurse does every minute she is practicing her profession. The nurse is a *role model* to patients, visitors, and other health professionals without ever saying a word or writing a teaching plan. The way she holds and wraps a baby, lifts an object from the floor, washes her hands, and even what she eats influence those around her. Learning often occurs through imitation. The more the patient respects her, the more he will observe and try to emulate her behavior. This teaching can be planned; if the nurse is aware she is being observed by the family, she should be careful about her performance. She can also verbalize *what* she is doing and *why.*

In conclusion, there are multiple teaching modalities. The same material may be taught effectively in many different ways. Or several modalities can often be used together to provide the best learning plan for the patient.

Implementing the teaching plan

When the nurse has the behavioral objectives and teaching plan before her, the process of implementing it is no more difficult than for any other skill in nursing. It requires the nurse to have a *knowledge base* about the material to be taught and the learning process. Since teaching is a form of communication, she must also have *effective communication skills.* Also teaching is easier and more rewarding when the nurse has *self-con-*

fidence about her ability to teach. The first step in self-confidence is taking responsibility for the teaching role.

The ability to engage in quality interaction and to establish a meaningful rapport with patients enhances the teaching/learning situation. In order to make nurse-patient interaction enjoyable, try the following suggestions:

—*Use your voice* to express enthusiasm and concern. If you are bored or scared, your teaching will reflect it. Be enthusiastic!

—*Use short words and sentences.* This makes it easier for the patient to retain your comments.

—*Repeat yourself* in different ways. Repetition enhances learning.

—*Tell the patient what you expect of him* during the session. This promotes a dialogue between the nurse and the patient and allows the patient to feel more comfortable asking questions or expressing concerns.

—*Let the patient teach you.* Allow him to share what he knows about the subject. This builds his self-confidence and makes him feel a part of the learning process. It also gives you an excellent opportunity to identify where to begin the lesson.

—*Provide reinforcement* for learning. Praise him for the knowledge he retains and/or comprehends.

—Allow time and provide routes for the patient to give *continual feedback.* This provides you with the opportunity to identify additional areas of weakness and confusion.

—*Be flexible.* Adjust your objectives, if necessary, based on the feedback you receive from the patient.

—*Take your time,* if possible. Do not rush through the material. Do not make the patient feel you are pushed for time. Everyone learns at a different speed and this cannot always be accounted for in the teaching plan.

—This is a *team effort* between the nurse and the patient. Work *with* the patient; do not just talk *to* him.

—*Make learning pleasant.* Let your personality shine through, and exude optimism.

If teaching is a new experience for the nurse and she feels overwhelmed by all the objectives and planned interventions, she should ask herself, "What one thing do I want this patient to learn today, and what can I do to help him meet this objective?" In addition, she should ask a peer to observe her during her first teaching session so that she can receive feedback. Seeking assistance while practicing the skill of teaching is akin to seeking support when first passing a nasogastric tube or a urinary catheter.

Evaluating the teaching plan

Just as teaching is a part of the nursing role, so too is evaluation an integral component of teaching. Teaching has little worth until its effectiveness is measured. To begin the evaluation process, the nurse should return to the behavioral objectives. What was the main idea/concept to be covered? What behavior did she want to change? The next question she should ask herself is, "How do I evaluate whether the material was learned?"

In nursing school, learning was measured by tests and essays. In a patient-teaching situation, evaluation can be accomplished in a variety of ways: continual feedback from the patient during the teaching session by the patient expressing questions and concerns or by the nurse actually seeking patient responses about the content; patient compliance with the treatment plan, or the extent to which a patient carries out a prescribed treatment plan, indicating a change to the desired behavior; and success in attaining the desired goal.

Both the nurse and the patient should evaluate the teaching/learning. Just because the patient says he understands and does not ask any questions, the nurse cannot assume learning has occurred. The objectives spell out how to evaluate the patient. They tell the nurse what to measure, under what conditions, and to what degree the behavior was to be accomplished. If the teaching program was not successful, the nurse should be willing to admit a lack of success and make a new plan.

Evaluation is the most abused component of the teaching process. The nurse may teach a group of patients and feel that she did a good job. She asks if there are any questions, and no one responds. How does she know she has been successful? How does she know learning has occurred? A checklist of content remembered, a verbal quiz, an ungraded posttest, or a return-demonstration are all methods of inferring whether or not learning has occurred.

Remember: Teaching is never complete until you have evaluated the success of your intervention.

Documenting the teaching process

Before a patient undergoes a surgical procedure, it is the physician's responsibility to inform him of the risks and to have him sign a consent form indicating that he has so been informed. The nurse can also be held liable for not recording that a patient has been taught about health care procedures, especially when that teaching is necessary to maintain or regain health: "The nurse...may be liable for failing to instruct the patient in particulars of care; for example, that a certain medication must be taken with food" (Cushing, 1984, p.

721). Legally, it is best to teach verbally and then to reinforce that teaching with written materials. The nurse should document what she taught, how the patient responded to the teaching, the results of the evaluation of the teaching plan, and the materials that were distributed to the patient.

Documenting patient teaching is important not only in legal issues, but is also an integral factor in the concept of continuity of care. Not all teaching can be done in one session or one shift. By noting in the chart how much of the teaching plan was accomplished and what problems the patient had with the materials, nurses and other health professionals will have an idea of how much the patient knows about his disease and treatments. These health professionals can reinforce the learning already accomplished and clarify any misconceptions. Has the patient indicated to the next shift any confusion about what he was told, or is he already practicing his new skills? Documenting these can assist the nurse responsible for the teaching plan. For patients being taught in a clinic setting, documentation helps the nurse remember what content she taught from week to week for each individual patient.

It is not sufficient to just indicate that the patient was taught about a particular concept. This would indicate that the teaching was not a shared process. Learning occurs in the patient. Only to chart what the nurse did and not to document the patient's response is incomplete.

USING CREATIVITY AND HUMOR IN TEACHING

Creativity is both an art and a science, an active way of thinking and behaving that involves a combination of feelings (subjective input) and knowledge (objective input). The goal of creativity is to improve existing conditions by problem solving. There is no perfect way to teach any particular subject or skill. Since each patient's situation, setting, and time constraints are different, creativity by the nurse becomes essential. How does a nurse teach kidney function in 5 minutes or less? Perhaps comparing the filtration process to that of a tea bag may help the patient associate an unknown mechanism with one he deals with daily.

Creativity and humor are closely linked. In the early days of nursing, humor and any form of self-expression by the nurse was considered inappropriate and unprofessional. However, since humor has been identified as an effective tool in promoting healing and health, it is very appropriate for nurses to express their enjoyment of their professional role via humor. Using analogies or rhymes to remember signs of a disorder may prove very helpful to patients. However, humor and clichés can only be used if the nurse has assessed the patient and is confident that the patient can understand and appreciate this method of presentation. Sarcasm has no place in patient teaching.

TEACHING PATIENTS WITH SPECIAL NEEDS

Those with an altered ability to learn, because of aging, congenital disorders, or pathology and disability require the nurse's special attention when she is developing a teaching plan. She must acknowledge their special needs and alter the proposed teaching mechanisms and content accordingly. Most of these patients have significant others who are interested in obtaining the necessary knowledge base to assist in their loved one's care and in promoting his health. Before planning teaching measures, the nurse must assess the needs and concerns of these significant others. They can be a part of the teaching/learning process, either separately or along with the patient.

Teaching the elderly patient

As the aging process progresses, many individuals find that their central nervous system deteriorates. Visual and auditory capabilities decrease, necessitating the use of prostheses (corrective lenses and hearing aids). Cerebral changes cause a decrease in the speed of processing new stimuli and a decrease in short-term memory. Because of the elderly patient's increased incidence of failing health, he may take multiple medications that may further affect his cognitive abilities. In addition, joints lose their flexibility and his mobility may be limited.

Elderly patients have a wealth of past experience on which to build their new knowledge base. Because they have established patterns of living entrenched in habits, they are often more resistant to change. Many elderly patients are on fixed incomes, and the fear of financial burden as a result of the new treatment or proposed change in their life-style threatens their financial security and increases their anxiety. Depression resulting from the health-related problem may make successful learning even more difficult.

As a nurse, some suggestions you must consider before teaching the elderly patient include the following:

—Check that printed materials have print large enough for the patient to see, especially when directions are involved.

—Speak face-to-face with the patient, and check frequently to make sure he can hear you and understands

the words you are using.
—Discover your patient's daily habits. Avoid making radical changes in his life-style, if possible, and incorporate his daily habits into the teaching plan.
—Give only small amounts of specific information at a time.
—Plan multiple teaching sessions to reinforce material.
—Because of a decrease in short-term memory, repeat information often and show the relationships among the parts of the teaching plan.
—If a skill is involved, multiple return demonstrations will help the patient learn the material.
—Provide verbal reinforcement and rewards to build self-esteem.
—In some situations, group work has been found to improve an elderly patient's problem-solving ability.
—Use reminder aids, such as marking pill containers by the day or hour or making a checklist for exercises when teaching skills.

Teaching children

Teaching plans for children must be extremely flexible and creative. The nurse should consider the child's cognitive level of development, his psychomotor skill level, the amount of trust he has developed with those in his environment, his fears, and his health needs. A great deal of health promotion is taught during the childhood years to assist these young people in developing and obtaining their highest level of wellness.

The nurse needs to assess the child as she would an adult; however, in addition to the factors mentioned earlier in this chapter, she must also assess his development. What is his chronologic age? Are his height, weight, and developmental tasks (fine motor and gross motor skills) appropriate for his age? Is he psychologically and socially (language skills, accountability) age-appropriate? What is the relationship/interaction (trust) between the child and the mother, father, or primary caretaker? What cognitive concepts (time, cause/effect) can the child understand?

Pediatric nurses learn never to assess the child without also evaluating the needs of the parents. What are their anxieties, fears, and needs? Thus, a teaching plan for a child is really two teaching plans: one for the child and one for the parents. For infants, the nurse must teach the parents instead of the child. But for all other age-groups, the child must be involved.

Teaching children involves a completely different perspective than that required to teach adults. Children learn continuously and take in stimuli from all of their senses. Play is the work of children and the method by which they learn about their world. Effective teaching plans incorporate these multiple modalities.

Toddlers (12 months to 3 years)

The toddler's greatest fear is separation from his mother. Therefore, teaching should be done in the presence of the mother, even with the child sitting on her lap. This child's favorite word is "no" and he uses it constantly. However, it is not always related to his intent. If the nurse tells him she is going to change a bandage, he may say "no." The nurse can respond, "I know you don't like this, but we have to keep the area clean." The nurse should be honest about when it will hurt and when it will not. Although the patient may not be able to understand the principles of a dressing change, he will begin to trust her.

The toddler has no concept of time. Because of this, the nurse must teach the toddler while she does the procedure. She can explain the blood pressure cuff as she is about to put it on the child. A toddler cannot delay gratification; therefore, he will not understand N.P.O. status prior to a procedure. Teaching for a toddler is continuous, because everything, such as blood pressure cuffs, stethoscopes, and hospital personnel, is new to him.

Preschoolers (3 to 5 years)

The preschooler fears altered body integrity; for example, he is afraid that he will lose all his blood from a needle stick, thus necessitating the wearing of the magic Band-Aid that uses its sticky ends to hold the skin together and prevent blood loss. He fears any invasion of or treatment to his body.

The preschooler does not understand cause and effect and often has wild fantasies about how his anger or "bad" behavior caused his accident or illness. While the child cannot express these fantasies easily, the nurse must anticipate and respond to them in her teaching plan. Such comments as "You know it's not your fault you got sick" are important in teaching the preschooler.

A preschooler is just beginning to develop a sense of time. He tells time by meals or naps. His attention span is very short, and he learns best when multiple senses are involved. These limitations are important to the teaching plan. A preschooler can be taught immediately before a stressful procedure, but can tolerate preparation for physician's visits and admissions to the hospital at least a week in advance. To tell a child he will be getting an injection in 3 hours will cause him to scream for the next 3 hours. Therefore, wait until 5 minutes before an injection to do the teaching. It is essential, however, to inform the child about the injection and the reasons for it, to tell him when it will hurt and when it will not, and to allow him to assist in choosing a site and putting on the bandage. All of this promotes trust in the health care system.

Prehospitalization visits, in which the child can tour the pediatric unit, play with the toys, see the beds and the way people dress, and then go home, can be very beneficial. Medical play is an effective means of patient teaching with this age-group. Letting a child play physician and nurse, dress up in surgical gowns, gloves, and masks, give injections to dolls, and bandage the nurse's arm can be more educational than a verbal presentation. Teaching these children is often done with the assistance of their dolls; for example, a cast may be put on a child's doll the day before the child is scheduled for orthopedic surgery. (The nurse should make sure she puts on the same type of cast that the child is expected to have.) This not only helps a child prepare for a procedure, but it is also equally effective after a procedure to allow the child to express his anger and any misconceptions.

School-age children (6 to 12 years)

School-age children are concrete thinkers. This is a period of active cognitive growth and the development of multiple concepts. However, they still may have misconceptions about body functions and some cause/effect thinking. These children are curious about their bodies and may ask the nurse questions completely unrelated to their hospital admission or clinic visit. Their fears need to be addressed in the teaching plan, as they still have some "thinking" reminiscent of their preschool days.

School-age children need preparation and explanations for what is happening to them. The nurse must use language appropriate to their cognitive level. Concrete facts should be used to describe a procedure; this is best done with pictures or models of the procedure. The nurse must be careful of the medical terms she uses. She should not refer to the dye injected during a cardiac catheterization, but rather to the medicine injected. She should not tell a child he is going to have his appendix taken out, but rather to have it fixed. Children's imagination may lead to misperceptions about treatments.

These children like to participate in their teaching. The effectiveness of written materials and audiovisual equipment depends on each child's abilities. They respond better with individual teaching, a great deal of positive reinforcement and praise, and affection. As children enter prepuberty, they begin to separate physically from their parents. They usually want their parents present during teaching. This can be helpful to the nurse, as the parents can provide emotional support during the teaching session and later can reinforce the material being taught.

Adolescents (13 to 18 years)

Cognitively, adolescents are in the process of developing abstract thinking and, therefore, can be taught much of the same material as that presented to adults. While many adolescents may like to appear as if they know all about their body, in fact, their knowledge is minimal. A comment by the nurse should ease the teenager's anxiety about admitting ignorance. Ideally, the teenager can view the nurse as someone from whom he can get reliable information about his body so that he is more knowledgeable than his peers.

In addition, adolescents are aware of their changing bodies, and hospitalization may threaten their self-image. For example, an adolescent female was depressed after an appendectomy, and a nursing assessment determined that she was upset because she thought that now she could never have children. Appropriate nursing intervention resolved the misunderstanding and involved explanations about the anatomy and physiology of the appendix and the uterus.

As they become more conscious of their adult bodies, adolescents desire privacy—for their physical self and for their emotional component. Diaries are a great way of helping adolescents express their concerns. Parents may be present during teaching; however, this should be up to the adolescent. Parents can be taught separately, but the confidences shared by the adolescent should be kept confidential.

Adolescents are social beings. Acting like everyone else is important to them, and, therefore, they are hesitant to ask questions and demonstrate their ignorance in front of peers. The decision of whether to teach individually or in a group depends on the individuals involved and on the ability of the nurse to identify the needs of the group members.

Teenagers want to believe that they are not children anymore, and, therefore, it is important to give them an active role in developing the objectives and the teaching plan. Contracts can be effective with adolescents.

As a nurse working with children of all ages, here are some general guidelines you should use in planning and implementing your teaching plans that are different from the guidelines utilized when working with adults:

—Do not ask "yes/no" questions unless you are willing

to accept a "no" answer.
—Give children choices in their treatment.
—Make sure the language you use fits their cognitive development. Do not use a cliché or a medical term without first explaining it.
—Get on an eye level with the child when teaching him. Sit if he is seated. This decreases the anxiety caused by a large, looming figure standing above him telling him what is wrong with his body.
—Be pleasant. Smile. Children of all ages are quick to pick up on adult body language. They can tell when you care and when you do not.
—Many children regress developmentally while hospitalized. You should address teaching measures first to the level to which the patient has regressed and then to his appropriate developmental level.
—Be honest. All people, especially children, need to feel trust in those responsible for their health care.

Teaching the disabled

Disabilities can be developmental or developed, physical or psychological; they can involve cognitive processes or physical ones. The need to learn among the disabled is just as great as among members of the rest of society; however, their ability to learn may be compromised.

When teaching a blind patient, the nurse must use other senses, especially touch and hearing. A tape recording of the directions for a procedure can be very helpful. On the other hand, the deaf patient needs materials in writing (if he can read) and needs to see demonstrations of what is required of him. Visual models can help him learn.

The patient with arthritis needs a variety of teaching aids to assist him in carrying out physical procedures. A portable percussor will make chest percussion easier to manage. The individual with cerebral palsy needs more verbal teaching because of his deficit in motor function.

The illiterate or non-English-speaking patient is a challenge. If the patient can read, a translator can write the directions in his native language. Demonstration and return demonstration will also be helpful. Try to find a significant other who speaks and understands English; then teach them together.

Children and adults with learning disabilities need special assessments of their areas of confusion and the methods by which they can learn most readily. Some cannot read directions, some confuse numbers, and others cannot remember a sequence of events. The teaching plan needs to present alternative approaches to reaching the desired goal.

Should terminally ill patients be taught? The answer is "yes." As long as there are choices to be made, then there is teaching to be done to assist the patient in making an informed decision.

CONCLUSION

"Teachers are eternal learners" (Clark, 1978, p. 9). The more a nurse teaches others, the more she learns herself. The more comfortable the nurse is with herself and the material she presents, the more sensitive she can be to the patient's needs and the more flexible and creative she can be in her teaching plan.

One of the aims of nursing is to encourage patients to be their own advocates and to assume responsibility for their own health care. In order to make healthy choices for themselves, they need information. Nurses must provide much of this.

Not all teaching can be planned. Often nurses' teaching serves to clarify the teaching of others. Nurses may teach indirectly by allowing a patient to express his feelings and to feel more comfortable with his psychological concerns. Nurses teach about the medications they give a patient or the procedures they are doing, such as taking the pulse, every time they have contact with the patient. And, of course, nurses are always a role model to others.

There is no best way to teach. The best technique is one that works best for each individual nurse and for the patient. The art of teaching takes time to develop.

Organizing and evaluating patient teaching

Before your patient can manage his condition, he has a lot to learn. This patient-teaching checklist will help you to organize your teaching sessions. Because the content to be covered is presented as patient objectives, you can also use the checklist as an *evaluation tool* to determine the effectiveness of your teaching, thus saving valuable time.

PATIENT-TEACHING CHECKLIST FOR *Sally Smith—Endometriosis #1*

PATIENT OBJECTIVES	PRE-TEST RESULTS	SESSION I CONTENT	SESSION II CONTENT	POST-TEST RESULTS
Define endometriosis.	Date: 7/7. Patient unaware of definition of endometriosis. She stated her doctor had explained it was "uterine tissue sitting outside the uterus, but still acting like it was in the uterus."	Date: 7/7. Instructed patient on definition of endometriosis. Also, using a chart, instructed the patient on the menstrual cycle.	Date: 7/8. Reviewed the phases of the menstrual cycle with the patient, making sure she understood the mechanics of how endometrial tissue can leave the uterus and attach to other organs.	Date: 7/8. Patient understands the concept of the disease process. Using charts and illustrations of the female anatomy, she went through the menstrual cycle and answered the nurse's questions with intelligent feedback.
Name three possible causes of endometriosis.	Date: 7/7. Patient knew of only one cause: "at time of menstrual period, the pieces of tissue that flow from the womb can attach to other areas of body."	Date: 7/7. Patient was instructed on the three possible causes of endometriosis, using an illustration of the female anatomy.	Date: 7/8. Started the session by answering relevant questions raised by the patient. Reviewed the material from the last session, making sure she understands the concepts.	Date: 7/8. Using role reversal, patient explained to the nurse the three possible causes of endometriosis. The patient accomplished this smoothly, with very little prompting from the nurse.
Explain the two types or forms of endometriosis.	Date: 7/7. Patient totally unaware of the fact that there are two forms.	Date: 7/7. The forms of endometriosis were explained to the patient.	Date: 7/8. Reviewed the concept of two forms of endometriosis.	Date: 7/8. Patient had no trouble answering nurse's questions about this concept. Demonstrates total understanding of concept.

PATIENT-TEACHING CHECKLIST FOR *Sally Smith—Endometriosis #2*

PATIENT OBJECTIVES	PRE-TEST RESULTS	SESSION I CONTENT	SESSION II CONTENT	POST-TEST RESULTS
Describe the five stages of endometriosis.	Date: 7/7. Patient does not know the five stages of disease process. However, she remembered her doctor telling her she "was at Stage II of disease."	Date: 7/8. Using illustrated charts, the five stages of disease were explained to her. She's interested in her stage, and inquired as to whether it could progress to Stages III, IV, V.	Date: 7/9. Once again, went over the five stages of endometriosis. The patient seems very motivated to learn about her disease process.	Date: 7/9. When asked to repeat info back to nurse, the patient did well. She explained the five stages, using medical terminology, and answered the nurse's questions.
Discuss the signs and symptoms of endometriosis.	Date: 7/7. Patient described her symptoms: painful periods and pain a week before her period, which needed very strong medication to give relief; also, some rectal bleeding.	Date: 7/8. Instructed patient on signs and symptoms of endometriosis. Also discussed with her why this pain is different from menstrual cramps.	Date: 7/9. Answered the patient's questions she had from last session. Did not need a review of Session I content.	Date: 7/9. Patient understands signs and symptoms of endometriosis, as illustrated by feedback and her ability to name them for the nurse.
Discuss the differences in signs and symptoms, depending on the site of the ectopic tissue.	Date: 7/7. Patient unaware of the fact that symptoms could differ, depending on where her endometrial tissue has implanted.	Date: 7/8. Using illustrations of female anatomy instructed patient on this concept. Patient had a good number of questions about this.	Date: 7/9. Reviewed material from Session I. Patient appears to understand why different sites of tissue implantation produce the signs and symptoms they do.	Date: 7/9. Patient asked nurse to write down sites with signs and symptoms for her; this was done. Patient understands this concept, but needed prompting from written info to answer the nurse's questions.

PATIENT-TEACHING CHECKLIST FOR Sally Smith — Endometriosis #3				
PATIENT OBJECTIVES	PRE-TEST RESULTS	SESSION I CONTENT	SESSION II CONTENT	POST-TEST RESULTS
Discuss differential diagnosis.	Date: 7/7. Patient knew that a laparoscopy was going to be done to identify the disease process; was unaware of other tests.	Date: 7/8. After conversing with doctor, teaching of this content has been deferred until it is deemed necessary by laparoscopy results.	Date: 7/10. Reinforced info given to patient by her doctor. Discussed the barium enema procedure with the patient.	Date: 7/10. Patient understands that laparoscopy only tells whether she has endometriosis. Patient also understands that barium enema will provide info to doctor about progression of disease.
Discuss treatments for endometriosis.	Date: 7/7. Patient aware of the fact that "certain hormone pills" may be taken to decrease lesion size.	Date: 7/9. Discussed with patient different treatments used for endometriosis, which depend on stage of disease, lesion site, and her desire for future pregnancies. Reinforced info given by doctor.	Date: 7/10. Reviewed Session I material and zeroed in on her specific stage, site of implantation, and treatment.	Date: 7/10. Patient repeated doctor's info for the nurse. Demonstrates a basic understanding of Session I material and understands her particular treatment regimen.
Describe her medication regimen.	Date: 7/10. Patient could not remember name or dosage of her medication.	Date: 7/10. Patient instructed on medication regimen (name, dosage, side effects, and precautions).	Date: 7/11. Reviewed medication regimen. The patient appears to have a grasp of situation.	Date: 7/11 Patient demonstrated her knowledge of medication regimen by explaining it to the nurse.

PATIENT-TEACHING CHECKLIST FOR Sally Smith — Endometriosis #4				
PATIENT OBJECTIVES	PRE-TEST RESULTS	SESSION I CONTENT	SESSION II CONTENT	POST-TEST RESULTS
Explain the importance of routine medical follow-up.	Date: 7/11. Patient told nurse "a yearly exam is important for good health."	Date: 7/11 Discussed with patient importance of an annual pelvic exam and Pap smear for early diagnosis and treatment.	Date: ______	Date: 7/11 Patient understands this concept. Discharged today with a good understanding of her disease process and treatment.
	Date: ______	Date: ______	Date: ______	Date: ______
	Date: ______	Date: ______	Date: ______	Date: ______

A blank sample chart similar to the one above can be found in Appendix C of this manual. You may reproduce the sample chart to use as a tool in organizing and evaluating teaching for your individual patients.

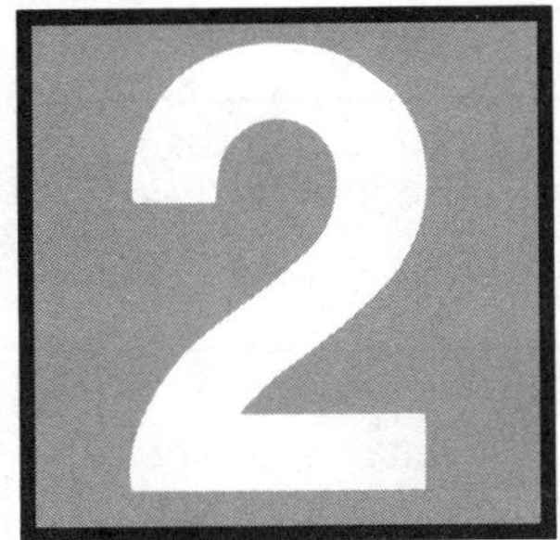

Cardiovascular Disorders

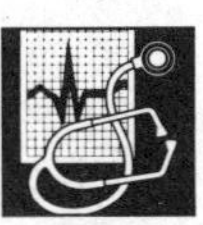

Patient-learner data base*

Areas of potential knowledge deficit
Cardiovascular risk factors
—Smoking
—Overweight, sedentary life-style
—Presence of other chronic diseases (e.g., diabetes)
—Stressful life-style
—Diet high in fat, cholesterol, calories, or salt
—Family history of cardiovascular disease
—Personal history of cardiovascular disease
Anatomy and physiology of the cardiovascular system
Definition of the cardiovascular disease
Causes of the cardiovascular disease
Symptoms associated with the disease
Treatment of the cardiovascular disease
—Diet and exercise
—Medications and treatment
—Stress management
—Guidelines for daily living
Complications of cardiovascular disease

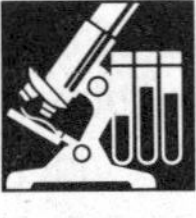

Explaining diagnostic tests

HOLTER MONITORING

Patient objectives	*Teaching plan content*
1 Define Holter monitoring.	Holter monitoring (also called ambulatory electrocardiography) is the continuous recording of the heart's activity as the patient follows his normal routine.

*A general assessment should be done for all patients. For general assessment guidelines, see Chapter 1, Principles of Patient Teaching.

2 State the purpose of Holter monitoring.

The purpose of Holter monitoring is to record the heartbeat over 24 hours to determine how the heart reacts to activity and rest.

3 Describe the procedure used in Holter monitoring.

The procedure involves the following steps:

—Attachment of electrodes to the anterior chest surface (males may be shaved at the site of electrode attachment)

—Attachment of the monitor, which is worn on a belt at the patient's waist, to these electrodes

—Keeping a diary that indicates exact times of activities and symptoms while wearing the monitoring device for 24 hours.

4 Identify experiences to be recorded in the diary.

Experiences to be recorded in the diary include the following:

—Strong emotions

—Medications taken (including nonprescription drugs)

—Such activities as eating, drinking (especially alcohol or caffeinic beverages), moving bowels, urinating, sudden changes in position, sexual activity, exercising, and sleeping

—Any physical symptoms, such as dizziness, headache, pain, or shortness of breath.

5 Discuss patient guidelines for wearing the Holter monitor.

Guidelines for a patient wearing the Holter monitor include the following:

—Do not remove the monitor from its carrying case or meddle with it in any way.

—Do not disconnect the lead wires or electrodes on the chest.

—Do not let the monitor get wet. Do not shower, bathe, or swim with it on.

—Record the times of experiences in the diary, using the clock on the monitor.

—If the light on the monitor flashes on, one of the electrodes on the chest may be loose. Test each one by pressing on the center of it.

—When the 24-hour period is up, return to the hospital with the monitor, and the nurse or technician will remove it. Do not remove it yourself.

—If severe chest pain or shortness of breath occurs, call the physician, and go to the emergency department of a nearby hospital immediately.

12-LEAD ELECTROCARDIOGRAPHY

Patient objectives	*Teaching plan content*
1 Define 12-lead electrocardiography.	Standard 12-lead electrocardiography is the recording of electrical impulses traveling through the heart.
2 State the purpose of 12-lead electrocardiography.	The purpose of 12-lead electrocardiography is to evaluate the heart's function, to determine the presence of abnormal electrical impulses, and to detect heart damage.
3 Explain electrical conduction in the heart.	The heart is a pump with its own built-in generator, called a pacemaker. This is a specialized group of cells located in the upper right portion of the heart. —Each second (approximately), the pacemaker releases an electrical impulse that travels down a pathway of special muscle fibers (the heart's electrical wiring) and spreads throughout the heart. —This impulse stimulates the heart muscle to contract and pump blood through the heart's chambers and out into the rest of the body through the vascular system.
4 Describe the procedure used in 12-lead electrocardiography.	During this procedure, the patient will lie on his back with the skin of his chest, wrists, and ankles exposed. He will feel no pain. —An electrode (a small metal plate) will be attached to each extremity, using rubber tapes and a sticky white paste or a small alcohol pad, which may feel cold. —Six dabs of sticky white paste will be applied to the skin of the left chest wall. —The EKG machine will be turned on and six different leads will be recorded. —One or six additional electrodes (suction cups) will be attached to the chest wall where paste was applied earlier. (If one electrode is used, the electrode will be moved to each place marked with paste.) —Six more leads will be recorded. —All electrodes and paste and/or alcohol pads will then be removed. —The physician will read the recordings to get a total picture of the electrical conduction of the heart. —The patient should know who will perform the test and where and when it will be done. It takes approximately 5 minutes.

5 Explain patient guidelines for 12-lead electrocardiography.	During the procedure the patient should do the following: —Lie flat and relax. —Breathe normally. —Keep his arms and legs still. —Say nothing.

EXERCISE ELECTROCARDIOGRAPHY (Stress test)

Patient objectives	*Teaching plan content*
1 Define exercise electrocardiography.	Exercise electrocardiography records the heart's electrical activity and performance under stress.
2 State the purpose of exercise electrocardiography.	The purpose of exercise electrocardiography is to determine how much stress the heart can take before it needs more oxygen than it can get.
3 Discuss patient guidelines for exercise electrocardiography.	In preparation for exercise electrocardiography, the patient should get a good night's sleep so he can come to the test rested and refreshed. He should not engage in strenuous activity for 12 hours before the test. —The patient should refrain from smoking for 2 hours before the test, if applicable, since nicotine elevates the heart rate. —He should follow these dietary guidelines: • avoid alcohol or caffeine for 2 hours before the test. • eat a light meal at least 2 hours before the test. • avoid milk and milk products on the day of the test. (This precaution helps prevent nausea during the procedure.) —He should ask his physician if he should take his regular medication the morning of the test. —He should wear loose, comfortable clothing for the test (lightweight shorts or slacks, shirt, socks, and rubber-soled shoes, such as sneakers). If the patient is a female, she should wear a bra and a short-sleeved blouse that buttons in the front. This way, she will not have to remove her blouse so that her blood pressure can be measured, chest electrodes applied, and her heart listened to. She should not wear pantyhose.
4 Describe the procedure used in exercise electrocardiography.	Just before the procedure, the physician will complete a medical history, physical examination, and a 12-lead electrocardiogram (EKG). —Then, a series of small electrodes will be firmly taped to the chest. (If the patient is very hairy, some hair may need to be shaved for the electrodes to adhere properly.)

—A blood pressure cuff will be placed on the arm and will remain for the duration of the test.
—Just before the test, the resting blood pressure and pulse rate will be taken and a baseline EKG will be recorded.
—The exercise program is then initiated, using one of three exercises: walking up and down a short series of steps, riding an exercise bicycle, or walking on a treadmill.
—There will be continuous recording of the electrocardiogram and frequent checks on blood pressure while the patient is exercising.
—Resistance may be added to make the exercise more difficult.
—The patient will experience shortness of breath, sweatiness, and a racing heart, which are normal.
—Exercise will be stopped when a predesignated heart rate is reached or signs of fatigue appear.
—EKG and blood pressure monitoring will continue until the readings return to normal; then, the electrodes and blood pressure cuff will be removed.
—The patient should know who will perform the test and where and when it will be done.

5 Name two symptoms to report immediately during exercise electrocardiography.	Chest pain and faintness should be reported immediately. These symptoms are warning signals that the test needs to be stopped.

CARDIAC CATHETERIZATION

Patient objectives	*Teaching plan content*
1 Define cardiac catheterization.	Cardiac catheterization, which permits the physician to inspect the condition of the heart and arteries without performing a surgical procedure, is the insertion of a narrow tube, or catheter, into a blood vessel that leads to the heart. It allows injection of a dye that makes the heart and coronary arteries more visible on X-rays. It also allows withdrawal of blood samples for testing.
2 State the purpose of cardiac catheterization.	The purpose of cardiac catheterization is to determine the condition of the heart and its arteries.
3 Discuss patient guidelines for cardiac catheterization.	Patient guidelines include the following: —The patient must fast after midnight the night before the procedure is scheduled, but he may be permitted fluids. The site where the catheter is to be inserted

will probably be shaved. A consent form must be signed.

—An electrocardiogram (EKG) will be taken the morning of the procedure to determine his heart's current status and to have a standard for later comparisons. Also, before he leaves for the cardiac catheterization laboratory, he will be asked to empty his bladder, since he will not be able to walk to the bathroom once the procedure has begun. He will be given a sedative to help him relax, but will remain awake during the procedure because his cooperation will be needed.

—If the patient has eyeglasses or dentures, he can probably wear them during cardiac catheterization. If he has contact lenses, he may be asked to remove them so he will not be troubled by something getting into his eye during the procedure.

—He will be brought to the laboratory on a stretcher, and family members will be able to accompany him to the elevator or the laboratory door or as far as permitted.

4 Describe the procedure used in cardiac catheterization.

When he arrives at the cardiac catheterization laboratory for the procedure, the patient will be introduced to the staff and told which person to address if he needs any help—for a dry mouth, an itchy nose, and so on. The laboratory staff will talk among themselves during the procedure, but instructions directed to him will be preceded by his name. For example, "Move to the left" is not an instruction for the patient; "Mr. Jones, move to the left" is.

—Then, he will be strapped onto a hard, flat table and covered with sterile sheets. EKG leads will be attached to his body and an intravenous (I.V.) needle inserted. The I.V. is merely a precaution, a way of giving him medication, if necessary.

—Next, the catheter insertion site (usually the back of the knee or the groin) will be scrubbed and a local anesthetic will be injected. After that, he should not feel any pain, though he may feel some pressure as the catheter is inserted.

—The physician first inserts a hollow needle at the site and then passes the catheter through the needle and into a blood vessel that leads to the heart. Sometimes he accomplishes this step on the first try; sometimes a few tries are needed.

—A fluoroscope, which looks like a TV screen, shows the catheter as it is moved slowly toward the heart.

Once the catheter is safely in place, the dye is injected, and X-ray films are made.

—Once the procedure has begun, the lights will be turned down. He can expect to hear loud "thunk" sounds as the X-ray plates are changed. He will also be able to see the fluoroscope and may want to watch what is happening inside him.

—The patient may be asked to move from side to side, or the table may be tilted during the procedure, since the physician needs to view the heart from different angles. He may also be asked to cough or take deep breaths, since these actions help keep the dye moving through the heart and encourage a steady heart rhythm. Also, the physician may have him make bicycling movements with his legs while lying on his back to help determine how well the heart responds to exercise.

—Although cardiac catheterization is not painful, the patient may experience heart palpitations. He can mention these but should not worry, as they are normal. He may also have a hot or dizzy sensation when the dye is injected into the catheter, but this lasts only a few seconds. The greatest discomfort reported by patients undergoing cardiac catheterization is having to lie still during the procedure.

—The patient should know who will perform the test and when it will be done. (If possible, he should visit the laboratory ahead of time.)

—He can expect to be in the cardiac catheterization laboratory for 1 to 4 hours.

5 Discuss what to expect for 8 to 12 hours after cardiac catheterization.

Nurses will be watching him closely for about 8 hours after the procedure. The observation is standard procedure and does not mean that anything is wrong.

—When he returns to the unit, he will be allowed to eat and drink right away if he wishes.

—His pulse and blood pressure, the dressing covering the insertion site, and the area around the site will be checked frequently.

—If he feels any numbness or tingling in the limb where the catheter was inserted or if he sees any blood on the dressing, he should apply pressure and call the nurse immediately.

—He can expect to be allowed out of bed the day after the procedure.

—Until then, *it is urgent that he keep the limb that had*

the catheter in it perfectly straight, to prevent bleeding. As long as he keeps the limb straight, he can lie in any comfortable position; i.e., on his stomach, back, or side.
—While he is in bed, he should wiggle his toes and flex his feet every hour to keep the blood circulating.

PHONOCARDIOGRAPHY

Patient objectives	*Teaching plan content*
1 Define phonocardiography.	Phonocardiography is the graphic recording of heart sounds.
2 State the purpose of phonocardiography.	The purpose of phonocardiography is to obtain a recording of the heart sounds in order to determine the exact timing of abnormal or extra heart sounds.
3 Describe the procedure used in phonocardiography.	During phonocardiography, the patient can expect the following: —First, a skilled technician places one or more small microphones on the patient's chest and secures them with chest straps. Usually, one is placed under the left arm about halfway down the waist—or in this general area—just in front of the underarm, and one is placed on the middle of the breast bone. —Next, the arm and leg leads of an electrocardiogram (EKG) are put in place. —The sounds picked up by the microphones are recorded by a machine that draws a series of waves on a piece of paper at the same time the EKG is being taken. —The physician then compares the sounds the heart makes with the electrical picture obtained from the EKG to determine the problem.
4 Discuss patient guidelines for phonocardiography.	Guidelines for phonocardiography include the following: —During the procedure the technician may ask him to change position, perform isometric (muscle-clenching) exercises, or do certain breathing maneuvers. (The physician can tell a lot about the patient's heart by studying how his heart sounds change when he moves.) —His physician may also have him inhale a gas called amyl nitrite. This gas, which has a slightly sweet odor, may affect the way his heart sounds and provide needed test results. If he feels dizzy or flushed or if he experiences rapid heartbeats for a short time after inhaling the gas, he should not be alarmed, but he should report any unusual sensations to the physician or technician.

ECHOCARDIOGRAPHY

Patient objectives	*Teaching plan content*
1 Define echocardiography.	Echocardiography is a test that uses ultrasonic waves to form a graph or picture of types of tissue in the heart.
2 State the purpose of echocardiography.	The purpose of echocardiography is to evaluate the size, shape, and motion of various heart structures.
3 Describe the procedure used in echocardiography.	During echocardiography, the patient can expect the following: —Conductive jelly will be applied to the patient's chest and a dime-sized transducer will be placed directly over it. —The transducer will send sound waves into the heart and receive them as they bounce back from the tissues. The sound waves are harmless, and the patient will not hear or feel them. —Since pressure will be exerted to keep the transducer in contact with the skin, he may experience some discomfort. —The transducer will be angled to observe different parts of the heart, and the patient may be repositioned on his left side during the procedure. —The test will be performed at bedside or in a laboratory by a specially trained technician. It takes 15 to 30 minutes. —The room may be darkened slightly to aid visualization on the oscilloscope screen (a type of TV screen), and other procedures (electrocardiography and phonocardiography) may be performed simultaneously.
4 Discuss patient guidelines for echocardiography.	Guidelines for echocardiography include the following: —The patient need not restrict food or fluids before the test. —He may be asked to breathe in and out slowly, to hold his breath, or to inhale a gas with a slightly sweet odor (amyl nitrite) while changes in heart function are recorded. —Possible side effects of amyl nitrite are dizziness, flushing, and tachycardia, but such symptoms quickly subside. —The patient must remain still during the test, since movement may distort results.

APEXCARDIOGRAPHY

Patient objectives	*Teaching plan content*
1 Define apexcardiography.	Apexcardiography is the graphic recording of chest movement caused by low-frequency cardiac pulsations.
2 State the purpose of apexcardiography.	The purpose of apexcardiography is to evaluate left ventricular function or to identify heart sounds.
3 Describe the procedure used in apexcardiography.	This procedure is risk-free and painless. —The patient will lie on his left side during the procedure, and electrodes will be attached to his arms and legs for a simultaneous electrocardiogram (EKG). —The transducer will be positioned over the heart and be held in place by an elastic strap. —Recordings will then be taken of low-frequency precordial cardiac pulsations picked up by the transducer, and a simultaneous recording of the heart's electrical activity will be made by the EKG. —When the recordings are completed, the transducer and electrodes will be removed. —The patient should know who will perform the test and where and when it will be done.
4 Discuss patient guidelines for apexcardiography.	Guidelines for apexcardiography include the following: —The patient need not restrict food or fluids prior to the test. —Just before the procedure, he must remove any metallic objects above the sites where the electrodes are to be placed. —He will be instructed to breathe slowly or to hold his breath so that respiratory variations will not distort test results. —He may be asked to do isometric (muscle-clenching) handgrip exercises. —He should not talk or move during the procedure, unless asked to do so.

PULSE WAVE TRACINGS

Patient objectives	*Teaching plan content*
1 Define pulse wave tracings.	Pulse wave tracings graphically record low-frequency vibrations from the jugular vein and carotid artery (two major blood vessels in the neck), which reflect the heart's pulsations during contraction and relaxation.

2 State the purpose of pulse wave tracings.	The purpose of pulse wave tracings is to assess the timing of mechanical events in the cardiac cycle (heart contraction and relaxation).
3 Describe the procedure used in pulse wave tracings.	During this test, the patient can expect the following: —The patient will lie on his back with his neck slightly hyperextended. For an arterial pulse wave tracing, he will turn his head away from the carotid artery being tested. The transducer will then be applied to the skin. —If the transducer is secured with a pediatric pressure cuff, the cuff will not be uncomfortable or restrict his breathing or blood flow. —Although the procedure will be entirely painless, the patient may hear a harsh sound when the sensor is placed over his carotid artery. —The procedure will be performed by a technician. It will take about a half hour, unless other tests are performed at the same time or the tracing is continuous. —The transducer will be removed after the test, and the patient will be able to resume his usual activities immediately.
4 Discuss patient guidelines for pulse wave tracings.	The patient must lie quietly, without talking. The technician may ask him to hold his breath occasionally, so that breathing sounds do not interfere with recording.

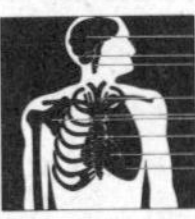

Explaining disorders

HYPERTENSION

Patient objectives	*Teaching plan content*
1 Define blood pressure.	Blood pressure is the pressure exerted by blood against the inside walls of the blood vessels as the heart rhythmically contracts and relaxes. There are two components to blood pressure: —Systolic blood pressure is the amount of pressure pushing against the walls of blood vessels (arteries) when the heart contracts and forces the blood through them; normally it is 100 to 140 mm Hg. —Diastolic blood pressure is the amount of pressure present in the blood vessels (arteries) when the heart is resting between contractions; normally it is below 90 mm Hg.

2 Define hypertension.

Hypertension is blood pressure that is too high. A blood pressure greater than 140 systolic and 90 diastolic is said to be high, or above normal. The patient should know what his blood pressure is and compare it with these standards. If it is normal, the treatment regimen is effective.

3 Identify at least three risk factors associated with hypertension.

Risk factors for hypertension include family history, age, race, smoking, and stress.
—Patients with a family history of high blood pressure are more likely to develop it than others.
—Blood pressure normally increases as one gets older.
—High blood pressure is found more often in blacks than in people of other races.
—Smoking may cause blood vessel constriction, thereby increasing blood pressure.
—Stress may increase blood pressure.

4 Explain what causes hypertension.

Two major factors that determine blood pressure are the amount of blood forced out of the left ventricle with each contraction (cardiac output) and the amount of resistance to this blood volume given by the blood vessels (peripheral vascular resistance). An increase in cardiac output or peripheral vascular resistance can, therefore, increase blood pressure.
—An increase in cardiac output can occur from increased blood volume (retaining too much sodium and water) or an increase in heart rate that increases the amount of blood forced into the blood vessels every minute.
—An increase in peripheral vascular resistance occurs when the blood vessels become narrowed. This can happen because of a disease process (atherosclerosis—buildup of fatty deposits in the blood vessel) or by constriction of the blood vessel through nervous system stimulation. Smoking is one factor that has been identified as causing vasoconstriction via the nervous system.
—The organic cause of hypertension is often unknown. In this case, it is called primary or essential hypertension, which requires lifelong treatment.
—A second type of sustained hypertension (secondary hypertension) results from another abnormality in the body, notably kidney, heart, hormone, or neurologic disorders.

5 Explain the importance of hypertensive therapy.

Reasons for treating hypertension, even in asymptomatic individuals, include the following:
—People with hypertension die younger than people

with normal blood pressure.
—Hypertension is a risk factor for cardiovascular disease. (In the United States cardiovascular disease is the leading cause of death.)
—Hypertension can damage the kidneys, eyes, blood vessels, and heart, increasing the risk of kidney failure, blindness, stroke, or heart attack.

6 Discuss the goals of hypertensive therapy.

Goals of hypertensive therapy include the following:
—Lowering blood pressure to a safe level (below 140/90)
—Keeping blood pressure under control
—Decreasing or preventing complications, such as damage to the kidneys, eyes, blood vessels, and heart.

7 Identify the components of the treatment regimen for hypertension.

Components of a hypertension treatment regimen requiring lifelong compliance include the following:
—Dietary modifications
—Medications
—Stress management
—Regular exercise
—Blood pressure self-measurement
—Regular medical follow-up.

8 Discuss the dietary measures to control hypertension.

Dietary measures include the following:
—Salt intake should be reduced. Too much salt (Na) makes the body retain fluid, increasing the pressure within blood vessels. Instructions for a reduced salt (low-sodium) diet are as follows:

- Do not add salt to food at the table or while cooking.
- Avoid foods with a high sodium content. (The nutritionist can provide a list.)
- Do not use salt substitutes unless the physician approves.
- Read food labels and avoid foods preserved with sodium.

—Weight should be reduced, if ordered by the physician. Obesity may increase blood pressure. Steps to follow in adhering to a weight-control diet include the following:

- Modify food choices and quantities as necessary to maintain a reduced calorie intake.
- Modify eating behavior to help stick to the diet.

9 Describe the medication regimen.

Some drugs commonly used for this disorder are atenolol, captopril, clonidine hydrochloride, furosemide, hydralazine, hydrochlorothiazide, metoprolol tartrate, methyldopa, minoxidil, nadolol, prazosin hydrochloride, propranolol hydrochloride, timolol, and verapamil. See Chapter 9, Drug Therapy, for specific medication instructions.

10 Describe at least two ways to reduce stress using deep relaxation.

Five deep relaxation techniques that may be used to reduce stress are taped relaxation exercises, relaxation cues, deep breathing, imagery, and progressive muscle relaxation.

—In using a tape recording of a programmed relaxation exercise, the patient should listen to it twice daily, preferably not at bedtime. (If he associates the exercise with sleep, he may fall asleep during practice sessions during the day.) He must follow all the instructions on the tape; this encourages him to concentrate on relaxing. With practice, he may be able to relax without the tape.

—The use of relaxation cues is similar to the previous technique, but it does not require a tape recording or any other special equipment. The patient can use it anywhere, anytime. He must select a cue that he associates with deep relaxation. The cue can be anything easily noticed—his watchband, for instance, or a sign on a door near his workplace. Then he concentrates on the cue as he relaxes. In time, simply looking at the cue may help him relax within minutes.

—In deep breathing, the patient breathes rhythmically while staring at a cue object. As he breathes, the nurse helps him establish a rhythm by slowly counting; for example, "in, 2, 3, 4; out, 2, 3, 4." When he has established a comfortable, relaxing rhythm, the patient concentrates on feeling a little more relaxed with each exhalation. He focuses on how he feels as he relaxes: weightless, pulsating, tingling, warm, or heavy.

—In using imagery, the patient thinks of a place where he usually feels relaxed and carefree—the beach or some other vacation spot, for example. He mentally transports himself to that place and concentrates on the details of every sound, sight, smell, and touch he associates with that location.

—Progressive muscle relaxation depends on the patient's ability to systematically tense and relax muscle groups throughout his body. This technique is performed as follows:

- Focus on a particular muscle group (start with the muscles in the hands).
- Tense these muscles.
- After 5 to 7 seconds, relax the muscles. Concentrate on the difference between the relaxed and tense states.
- Then concentrate on another group of muscles;

tense and then relax them. Continue the procedure until all the muscle groups throughout the body have been tensed and relaxed.

—Another muscle relaxation technique (sometimes called the Benson response) involves progressively relaxing the muscles from feet to head—without tensing them first. When relaxed, the patient performs deep breathing for about 20 minutes.

11 Describe a regular exercise program to control hypertension.

Systolic blood pressure can be 25% lower after aerobic exercise (exercise that increases oxygen use). Over a period of time, a regular program of aerobic exercise can permanently lower at-rest (diastolic) blood pressure.

—The physician must provide exercise guidelines before the patient begins any exercise program.

—The patient should avoid isometric exercises, such as weight lifting, push-ups, waterskiing, pulling a heavy golf cart, shoveling, carrying heavy bundles, moving furniture, mopping floors, pushing a vacuum cleaner, sawing hardwood, opening stuck windows or jar lids, judo, and karate, because they dramatically increase blood pressure.

—He should choose one aerobic activity (for example, walking briskly, jogging, running, swimming, bicycling, cross-country skiing, aerobic dancing, climbing stairs, handball, racquetball, or soccer) and stay with it. By sticking to one activity he will condition his cardiovascular system more efficiently. Obviously, it should be one he enjoys so it becomes part of his life. It should not be expensive, and it should be something he can do year-round in some form.

—No matter what activity he chooses, he should plan to exercise:

- frequently, at least three times a week
- for a sustained period—gradually building up to 20 or 30 minutes each time
- vigorously, so his heart works at 70% to 80% of its maximum rate.

—If the patient is not athletic or if he has health problems in addition to his hypertension, walking is a good choice. He can plan walks where he will see new sights every day; a walk around town, for example, is more interesting than six laps around the same block. In bad weather, he can walk in a shopping mall during off-peak hours (he can walk faster without crowds around). He should take the stairs between floors. Brisk, uninterrupted walking is essential to exercise the heart.

—He should exercise at least every other day. After

more than 2 days without exercise, he will start to lose condition. If he exercises moderately (by brisk walking, for example), he may comfortably maintain a daily schedule. If he exercises vigorously, however, he needs a day of recovery between sessions.
—If the physician has approved routine exercise, the patient must be able to find his target heart rate and check whether he is maintaining that rate during exercise. His target heart rate should be maintained for 20 to 30 minutes, with 5 minutes or more of easier work to warm up and 5 minutes to cool down.
—As the patient's conditioning improves, his heart will work more efficiently. As a result, it will not have to beat as quickly during exertion, and its at-rest rate will gradually drop. When it beats at less than the target rate during exercise, the patient is ready for more vigorous exercise.

12 Obtain an accurate blood pressure self-measurement.

To perform blood pressure self-measurement, the patient should proceed as follows:
—For accurate results, he should rest for 15 minutes before taking a measurement.
—He should practice with the same type of equipment he will use at home. (If possible, the nurse should use a double stethoscope to check his ability to recognize Korotkoff's sounds.)
—To apply the cuff more easily, the patient should make it into a sleeve and then slide it onto his arm. If it has a D-ring, he should make a sleeve by slipping the cuff through the ring before putting it on. If it does not have a D-ring, he can make a sleeve by fastening the Velcro strips together before applying the cuff.
—No matter what method is used, he should center the cuff correctly over the brachial artery and tighten it properly. Using a piece of tape or a pen, he should mark the spot on the cuff where he should fasten it.
—To help hold the stethoscope against his brachial artery, he should make two bands out of stretch fabric (such as stretch terry cloth) to apply around his forearm. This will hold the stethoscope securely in place during readings.
—The patient must inflate the cuff to 20 to 30 mm Hg above his palpatory systolic pressure each time he takes a reading. (The pressure should be determined and written down as a reference for him.)
—If the patient cannot manage regular home monitoring, there may be community blood pressure screening clinics in his area. Even infrequent measurements are better than none at all. Or better yet, a willing family member can be taught to take the patient's blood pres-

sure readings at home. (See *Monitoring Blood Pressure at Home,* pp. 66-67.)
—The patient should maintain a written record of his blood pressure readings to show his physician on routine visits.

13 Explain the importance of routine medical follow-up.	Routine medical follow-up ensures that early treatment is effective and that long-term treatment continues to keep the patient's blood pressure down. In addition, the physician will be able to monitor the effects of the patient's blood pressure on vital organs, such as the heart, kidneys, eyes, and blood vessels. Complications can be detected earlier, and the treatment regimen can be supplemented to prevent serious consequences.

CONGESTIVE HEART FAILURE (C.H.F.)

Patient objectives	*Teaching plan content*
1 Define CHF.	CHF is the inability of the heart to pump blood effectively, causing blood to pool in the lungs, the body, or both.
2 State the cause of CHF.	The cause of CHF is weakening of the heart muscle.
3 Identify at least two health problems that can weaken the heart muscle.	Conditions that can weaken the heart muscle include the following: —Heart attacks —Ischemic heart disease —Hypertension —Disorders of heart valves —Infections of the heart layers, such as bacterial endocarditis —Cardiomyopathy.
4 Name at least five symptoms of CHF.	Symptoms of CHF include the following: —Shortness of breath —Cough —Swelling of the legs and feet —Fatigue —Weakness —Weight gain —Loss of appetite.
5 Identify the components of the treatment regimen for CHF.	Components of the treatment regimen for CHF include the following: —Low-sodium diet

—Medications
- Digitalis preparations
- Diuretics

—Monitoring pulse
—Following certain guidelines for daily living.

6 Discuss the low-sodium diet.

A low-sodium diet includes the following:
—Avoiding salt at the table and in cooking
—Avoiding foods with a high sodium content. A list of such foods can be obtained from a nutritionist.
—Avoiding over-the-counter medications that contain sodium, such as Alka-Seltzer, Rolaids, Milk of Magnesia, Maalox, Mylanta, and Di-Gel
—Avoiding water softeners, as they increase sodium content.

7 Describe the medication regimen.

Some drugs commonly used for this disorder are captopril, digoxin, furosemide, hydralazine, and isosorbide dinitrate. See Chapter 9, Drug Therapy, for specific medication instructions.

8 Obtain an accurate pulse rate for 1 minute.

To determine his pulse rate, the patient does the following:
—He should place a watch so that he can easily see the second hand.
—He should then place the index and middle finger of one hand on the underside of the opposite wrist, just below the thumb. (He should not use the thumb to feel for a pulse, because it has a strong pulse of its own and may cause confusion.)
—If he has difficulty feeling the wrist pulse, he should place his thumb on his collarbone and lay his fingers along the side of his throat. Here he should feel a strong pulse.
—Once he feels the pulse, he should count the pulsations for 1 minute.
—If the pulse is less than 60 or more than 120 beats/minute, he should call his physician immediately.
—To obtain an accurate resting pulse, the patient should relax for 15 minutes before taking his pulse, and he should take it at the same time every day.

9 State at least four guidelines for daily living with CHF.

Guidelines for daily living in managing CHF include the following:
—Avoid smoking, since it increases the work load of the heart. Because the heart muscle is already weakened, smoking can then make CHF worse.
—Get plenty of rest, to help decrease the work load of the heart. If possible, shorten the work day and set

aside time for rest periods.
—Avoid emotional stress, since it increases the work load of the heart. (If this is a problem, perform deep relaxation exercises. See the "Hypertension" teaching plan in this chapter.)
—Weigh yourself daily before breakfast, since weight gain can be a sign of worsening CHF. A weight gain of 2 or 3 lb within a day's time is a warning signal and should be reported to the physician.
—Avoid temperature extremes. When possible, stay in a cool, comfortable environment. In hot weather, perform activities in the cooler part of the day. In cold weather, dress warmly but avoid restrictive clothing, which interferes with circulation. Wrap a scarf over the nose and mouth to warm the air and make breathing easier.
—Watch for and report signs and symptoms of recurring CHF. These include weight gain, loss of appetite, shortness of breath during activity, persistent cough, frequent urination at night, and swelling of the ankles, feet, or abdomen.
—Keep regular physician's appointments.

ANGINA PECTORIS

Patient objectives	*Teaching plan content*
1 Identify the anatomic structures of the heart.	On an illustration of the heart, the patient should point out the following: —Position of the heart in the body —Chambers of the heart (right and left atria, right and left ventricles) —Heart valves (tricuspid, pulmonic, mitral, and aortic) —Location of the coronary arteries: • Right coronary artery, which supplies blood to the right atrium and ventricle and to the inferior and diaphragmatic walls of the left ventricle • Left coronary artery, which supplies blood to the anterior and lateral walls of the left ventricle and is divided into two branches—the anterior descending and the circumflex arteries —Superior and inferior vena cava and the aorta.
2 Describe the basic function of the heart.	The basic function of the heart is to pump blood throughout the body. —The right side of the heart delivers unoxygenated blood from the body to the lungs. —The left side of the heart delivers oxygenated blood from the lungs to the body.

3 Define angina pectoris.

"Angina" means pain and "pectoris" means chest, and the term means a pain in the chest.

4 Name the three types of angina pectoris.

Angina pectoris may be classified as stable, unstable, or atypical.
—Stable angina refers to episodes of chest pain related to physical activity or emotional stress.
—Unstable angina refers to episodes of chest pain that occur with either activity or rest.
—Atypical angina refers to episodes of chest pain that occur mostly at rest.

5 Explain the development of angina pectoris with atherosclerosis.

Atherosclerosis is involved in the development of angina pectoris in the following manner:
—Atherosclerosis is the buildup of fatty materials, such as cholesterol, triglycerides, and phospholipids, on the inside walls of the blood vessels.
—This buildup is thought to begin early in life and to progress slowly over the years.
—As the buildup of fatty materials occurs, the channels through which blood flows in the arteries become narrow and/or blocked.
—Chest pain occurs when the heart needs more oxygen than the restricted blood flow through the coronary arteries can supply.
—Physical exertion is a common precipitator of chest pain when atherosclerosis is present, because the heart increases its requirement for oxygen during exercise. When the activity is stopped, the chest pain subsides.

6 Describe the chest pain of angina pectoris.

The type and location of angina pain may vary from individual to individual.
—Words typically used to describe the chest pain include *heaviness, a feeling of indigestion, tightness, burning,* or *squeezing.*
—The pain may be felt over the heart; between the shoulders or upper back; in the neck, shoulder, or arm; or even in the jaw or teeth.
—The pain generally lasts from 2 to 20 minutes. If it lasts longer than 20 minutes, medical attention should be sought immediately.

7 Identify at least three circumstances in which angina pectoris may occur.

These circumstances are known to trigger angina pectoris because they increase the heart's need for oxygen:
—Large meals
—Cold weather
—High altitudes
—Hot, humid weather
—Strenuous exercise

—Walking uphill
—Strong emotional responses
—Sexual activity.

8 Identify the components of the treatment regimen for angina pectoris.

Components of the treatment regimen include the following:
—Dietary modifications
—Medications
—No smoking
—Control of high blood pressure and diabetes, if present
—Planned exercise program
—Control of stress.

9 Discuss the dietary modifications used in the management of angina pectoris.

Dietary modifications may include limiting cholesterol and fat, limiting salt intake if hypertension is present, limiting calorie intake if the patient is overweight, and altering eating habits.

—Guidelines to control fat and cholesterol include the following:

- Eat more poultry (with the skin removed) and fish. If beef and pork are eaten, use only lean cuts.
- Use polyunsaturated fats (vegetable fats) that are usually liquid at room temperature instead of saturated fats (animal fats) that are solid at room temperature.
- Limit the intake of eggs, shellfish, and organ meats. (The nutritionist should provide specific limitations.)

—Guidelines for reducing salt intake include the following:

- Avoid using salt at the table and while cooking.
- Avoid foods with a high salt content. (The nutritionist should provide a list of these.)
- Do not use salt substitutes unless approved by the physician.

—Guidelines for weight reduction include the following:

- Understand the basic concept of weight loss (less intake, more expenditure).
- Understand the calorie-restricted diet. (The nutritionist should be consulted, as needed.)
- Avoid foods high in calories (fatty fried foods and sweets).
- Count calories and measure intake.
- Learn behavior modification techniques and select a strategy for sticking to the diet.

—Family members, particularly the person responsible for preparing the meals, should also be aware of these dietary guidelines.

—The patient should know how to maintain his diet

while eating out. (The nutritionist should be consulted.)
—The patient should avoid large, heavy meals because the process of digesting food increases the heart's need for oxygen. He should eat several small meals throughout the day and rest after eating.

10 Describe his medication regimen.

Some drugs commonly used for this disorder are atenolol, diltiazem, erythrityl tetranitrate, isosorbide dinitrate, metoprolol tartrate, nadolol, nifedipine, nitroglycerin, prazosin hydrochloride, propranolol hydrochloride, timolol, and verapamil. See Chapter 9, Drug Therapy, for specific medication instructions.

11 Explain the importance of not smoking.

Smoking causes the heart to beat faster and constricts blood vessels. In the presence of atherosclerosis, smoking will further decrease the amount of oxygen delivered to the heart, increasing the likelihood of chest pain. A person with angina pectoris runs a greater risk of having a heart attack if he smokes. (Programs are usually available in the community to help patients stop smoking.)

12 Explain the importance of controlling high blood pressure and diabetes.

Hypertension and/or diabetes mellitus must be kept well controlled because of their effect on the heart. (See the "Hypertension" teaching plan in this chapter and the "Diabetes Mellitus" teaching plan in Chapter 5, Endocrine Disorders.)
—Hypertension increases the work load of the heart, thereby increasing the amount of oxygen needed by the heart.
—Diabetes mellitus is associated with an acceleration of atherosclerosis, especially if it is uncontrolled.

13 State the rationale for a planned exercise program.

A planned exercise program can help the heart by improving its blood supply.
—The program must avoid putting too much strain on the heart if the patient has atherosclerosis.
—The physician should determine the kind and amount of exercise that would be beneficial for the patient.
—The patient should receive explicit instructions on the exercise program specified by the physician.

14 Identify two ways to control stress.

Two ways to help control stress are practicing deep relaxation techniques (see the "Hypertension" teaching plan in this chapter) and discussing stressful feelings with another person. If these measures are not effective, the patient should seek counseling for stress management. Stress needs to be controlled because it causes the heart to beat faster, thereby increasing the oxygen needs of the heart.

MYOCARDIAL INFARCTION (M.I.)

Patient objectives	*Teaching plan content*
1 Identify the anatomic structures of the heart.	See the "Angina Pectoris" teaching plan in this chapter for the anatomic structures of the heart.
2 Describe the basic function of the heart.	See the "Angina Pectoris" teaching plan in this chapter for the basic function of the heart.
3 Define MI.	MI is the death of tissues in the heart muscle (myocardium), which results from oxygen deprivation due to the narrowing or blockage of an artery that supplies oxygenated blood to those tissues. The area of dead tissue, called an infarct, will gradually be replaced by scar tissue.
4 Explain the relationship between atherosclerosis and MI.	See the "Arterial Occlusive Disease" teaching plan in this chapter for the relationship between atherosclerosis and myocardial infarction.
5 Identify at least three risk factors for MI.	Risk factors for MI include family history, hypertension, smoking, high levels of fats (lipids) and cholesterol in the blood, diabetes mellitus, obesity, a sedentary or stressful life-style, and age. —Patients with a family history of MI are more likely to develop it than others. —Hypertension raises the oxygen requirement of the heart muscle, which must work harder to pump blood against high pressure. —Smoking may cause constriction of the blood vessels and increase the blood pressure. —Elevated serum lipid and cholesterol levels are thought to speed the process of atherosclerosis. —Diabetes mellitus is associated with accelerated atherosclerosis. —Obesity predisposes the patient to hypertension, diabetes, and elevated cholesterol levels. —With a sedentary life-style the heart muscle is less efficient than when the patient gets regular exercise. —A stressful life-style may diminish blood flow to the heart muscle by causing constriction of the blood vessels. It may also raise the oxygen requirements of the heart by increasing the blood pressure. —With increasing age, there is a greater chance of de-

veloping atherosclerosis, which makes the heart less efficient and increases the risk of MI.

6 List at least three symptoms associated with MI.

Symptoms of MI include the following:
—Chest pain, which is described as persistent, crushing substernal pain that may radiate to the left arm, the jaw, the neck, or the shoulder blades. (Other descriptions include heaviness in the chest or a squeezing sensation. Some people, particularly patients with diabetes and elderly individuals, may not feel pain at all; in others, the pain is mild and often mistaken for indigestion.)
—Shortness of breath
—Perspiration
—Nausea/vomiting
—Dizziness
—Weakness
—A feeling of impending doom
—Cold, clammy skin
—Anxiety
—Restlessness.

7 Identify the components of the treatment regimen for MI.

A post-MI treatment regimen consists of the following:
—Dietary modifications
—Medications
—Activity changes
—Monitoring pulse rate and rhythm
—Guidelines for daily living.

8 Discuss the dietary modifications used in the management of MI.

Dietary modifications include reducing cholesterol, fat, and salt as well as calories, if the patient is overweight. (For specific instructions, see the "Angina Pectoris" teaching plan in this chapter.) The rationales for these modifications are as follows:
—Cholesterol and fats may increase the risk of atherosclerosis, a known risk factor for MI.
—Salt causes fluid retention in the body, which in turn increases the work load of the heart.
—Obesity puts an additional work load on the heart, thereby increasing the risk of myocardial infarction.

9 Describe the medication regimen.

Some drugs commonly used for this disorder are aspirin, atropine sulfate, heparin, nitroglycerin, procainamide hydrochloride, propranolol hydrochloride, quinidine sulfate, and warfarin sodium. See Chapter 9, Drug Therapy, for specific medication instructions.

10 Obtain an accurate pulse rate for 1 minute.

See the "Congestive Heart Failure" teaching plan in this chapter for instructions on how to take the pulse.

11 Describe relevant exercise limitations.

Exercise limitations may vary from patient to patient. General guidelines include the following:
—The patient should exercise at home as much as he did while still hospitalized.
—Unless restricted by his physician, the patient should gradually increase his walking until he is up to 1 to 2 miles a day. He should be cautious, however, to walk only in good weather and on level ground.
—His physician will inform him when he will be able to return to work and resume his normal activities.
—He should avoid or modify activity after meals, stress, or exposure to temperature extremes.
—The patient and his sexual partner should understand that sexual activity increases the heart's need for oxygen. They can expect to resume their previous sexual activity about 4 or 5 weeks after the MI, based on approval from the physician. If chest pain occurs during sexual intercourse, the activity must be stopped.
—The patient should avoid isometric exercises, as they increase the strain on the heart. Types of isometric activities include straining during a bowel movement (ask for a laxative instead), lifting anything heavy (children, groceries, or suitcases), pushing or pulling anything heavy, or trying to open a stuck window or unscrew a stuck jar lid.
—If a cardiac rehabilitation program will be part of his discharge plans, the patient should understand the nature of the program and what to expect. (A conference with the nurse at the rehabilitation center can help to prepare him.)

12 Discuss patient guidelines for daily living.

For guidelines the patient will need to follow when he is discharged, see *Some Heart-Saving Advice after Discharge*, pp. 70-71.

ARTERIAL OCCLUSIVE DISEASE

Patient objectives	*Teaching plan content*
1 Define arterial occlusive disease.	Arterial occlusive disease is the obstruction or narrowing of the channels of the aorta and/or its major branches, causing an interruption of blood flow, usually to the legs and feet.
2 State the function of arterial blood flow.	The function of arterial blood flow is to deliver oxygen and nutrients to the tissues so that the cells making up the tissues can perform their functions and stay alive.

3 Trace blood flow through the major arteries commonly affected by arterial occlusive disease.

On an illustration, the patient should be able to locate the aorta, the major arteries that branch off it, and the areas of the body affected by the blood flow from these arteries.
—The ascending aorta supplies blood to the coronary arteries.
—The aortic arch supplies blood to the structures in the head, the neck, and the upper extremities through branches called the innominate artery, the left common carotid artery, and the left subclavian artery. The innominate artery further branches into the right common carotid artery and the right subclavian arteries.
—The thoracic aorta supplies blood to the chest cavity.
—The abdominal aorta, a continuation of the thoracic aorta through the abdominal cavity, supplies blood to the structures of the upper abdomen.
—Through terminal branches called the internal and external iliac arteries, the abdominal aorta supplies blood to structures in the lower abdomen and the lower extremities. The external iliac arteries then further subdivide into the right and left femoral arteries, which in turn become the popliteal arteries.

4 Explain the relationship between atherosclerosis and arterial occlusive disease.

The relationship between atherosclerosis and arterial occlusive disease may be explained as follows:
—Atherosclerosis is the buildup of fatty materials, such as cholesterol, triglycerides, and phospholipids, on the inside walls of blood vessels (arteries).
—As the buildup slowly progresses, the arteries become narrowed or blocked, making it difficult or impossible for oxygenated blood to get to the tissues.
—As the blood flow decreases, blood clots may form abruptly, stopping the flow of blood to sites beyond the clots.
—In either case, if the tissues are not given oxygenated blood, they will die, and the function of that area of the body is lost.

5 Identify at least three risk factors associated with arterial occlusive disease.

Risk factors for arterial occlusive disease include the following:
—Smoking
—Hypertension
—Diabetes mellitus
—Obesity
—Hyperlipidemia.
Smoking can cause constriction of the blood vessels; the other factors can accelerate the atherosclerotic process.

6 Name at least three symptoms associated with arterial occlusive disease.

The symptoms of arterial occlusive disease, which are most common in the legs and feet, include the following:
—Pain (the major symptom) may occur in one or both legs during exercise. If the disease is advanced, pain may occur even during rest. The pain is usually described as sharp—like a stabbing knife or a vise squeezing the leg. Sometimes a feeling of unusual tiredness is experienced in one leg when walking. The pain should quickly subside when the patient stops walking. If the pain occurs at rest, he may feel the pain first in his toes, head, and the dorsum of his foot. He may experience the pain as a severe throbbing or ache that wakes him up at night.
—Temperature changes may be apparent. The patient may experience a burning sensation or the skin may feel cool to the touch.
—Ulcers may appear because of tissue breakdown.
—Skin color may change from normal to pallor (the degree of occlusion will determine the degree of pallor).

7 Identify the components of the treatment regimen for arterial occlusive disease.

Components of the treatment regimen include the following:
—Modification of risk factors
—Regular exercise
—Medications
—Special care of the lower extremities
—Surgery to improve blood flow—reserved for severe cases. (See the "Vascular Bypass Grafting" teaching plan in this chapter if surgery is to be performed.)

8 Discuss how risk factors may be modified.

Modifying risk factors identified in the patient may slow the atherosclerotic process and improve arterial blood flow.
—Giving up smoking is of primary importance because it constricts blood vessels, resulting in reduced blood flow. Community programs are usually available to help a person stop smoking.
—Hypertension and diabetes mellitus can reduce arterial blood flow if left uncontrolled. (See the "Hypertension" teaching plan in this chapter and the "Diabetes Mellitus" teaching plan in Chapter 5, Endocrine Disorders.)
—Obesity and hyperlipidemia must be controlled, as they can speed up the atherosclerotic process, thereby diminishing arterial blood flow to the tissues. (See the "Angina Pectoris" teaching plan in this chapter for dietary modifications.)

9 Describe the exercise program for arterial occlusive disease.

Walking is the best way to increase collateral circulation (new blood vessel formation), thereby increasing the ability to walk further before pain occurs.
—The patient should walk at least 30 minutes two or three times daily.
—He can rest during the walk, but not at the instant he begins to feel discomfort. He should walk until pain forces him to stop. When the pain goes away, he should resume walking.
—The patient may become discouraged at first if the distance he is able to walk without pain decreases instead of increases. This is common. However, if he persists, he will soon be walking twice as far without needing a rest.

10 Describe the medication regimen.

Some drugs commonly used for this disorder are cyclandelate, isoxsuprine hydrochloride, and pentoxifylline. See Chapter 9, Drug Therapy, for specific medication instructions.

11 Explain patient guidelines for caring for the lower extremities.

Guidelines for caring for the lower extremities include the following:
—Wash feet daily and wear clean, well-fitting socks.
—Trim nails straight across, but not too closely.
—Clean small cuts carefully with mild soap and water, and protect them from further injury.
—Call the physician to report any persistent leg problem.
—Do not go barefoot.
—Do not let the legs become extremely cold.
—Do not wear clothes that constrict the legs or feet.
—Do not let the legs get sunburned.
—Do not cut or file corns or calluses. Do not use chemical corn and callus remedies.
—Do not put a hot water bottle, heat lamp, or heating pad directly on the affected area. Instead, put the heat source on the lower back or abdomen. This will warm the legs in about 15 minutes.

VARICOSE VEINS

Patient objectives	*Teaching plan content*
1 Define varicose veins.	Varicose veins are enlarged subcutaneous blood vessels that may have a bulging or twisted appearance. They are usually most obvious in the legs.

2 Explain the function of veins in the body.

The function of veins is to return unoxygenated blood from tissues to the right side of the heart. Much of the blood must flow against gravity, and valves are located inside the veins to keep the blood flowing toward the heart.

3 Explain how varicose veins develop.

Varicose veins develop when the valves inside the veins become damaged and are unable to function properly. The blood flow through the veins then becomes slower. Where blood accumulates, or pools, in the veins, they become swollen and twisted in appearance.

4 Identify at least two causes of varicose veins.

The causes of varicose veins include the following:
—The valves may be congenitally weak. Varicose veins seem to occur more frequently in certain families.
—Diseases of the venous system, such as an infection (thrombophlebitis), may weaken the valves or damage the venous wall.
—Sustained pressure increases within the veins can damage the valves. Elevated pressure may occur with excessive abdominal weight in obesity or pregnancy and with prolonged standing in certain occupations.

5 Identify at least three symptoms associated with varicose veins.

Some patients are asymptomatic, and symptoms may vary. They include the following:
—A feeling of heaviness, itching, or burning in the general area of the vein
—A diffuse, dull aching sensation after prolonged standing or walking
—Leg cramps at night
—Fatigue
—Swelling
—Palpable nodules.

6 Name the two methods used to manage varicose veins.

Medical and surgical methods are used to manage varicose veins.
—Medical management includes supportive measures and exercise programs.
—Surgical management is reserved for severe varicose veins.

- One procedure, stripping and ligation, involves tying off the saphenous vein at its juncture to the femoral vein and removing the saphenous vein by a stripping procedure.
- In another procedure, injection of a hardening agent into small affected vein segments closes them off.

7 Discuss patient guidelines for the medical management of varicose veins.	The following patient guidelines are part of the medical management of varicose veins: —During the day, the patient should wear the antiembolism stockings prescribed by his physician, or support hose to support the veins and improve circulation. He should put them on immediately after getting out of bed. —He should elevate his legs (higher than the level of the heart) throughout the day whenever possible and should avoid prolonged standing or sitting. If he must sit for a prolonged period of time, he should move both feet in circles about 20 times every 15 to 30 minutes. This will help the blood flow back to the heart. He should also avoid crossing his legs at the knee when sitting. —If the patient is overweight, he should reduce his weight to help reduce pressure within the veins. —If the patient is a female, she should avoid garters, knee-high stockings, and knotted elastic hose or stockings around the knee, which will impede circulation. —The patient should develop a regular exercise program, such as walking, because muscular contraction during exercise forces blood through the veins, thereby minimizing venous pooling. —He should notify his physician if swelling, pain, or discomfort continues despite the above measures.

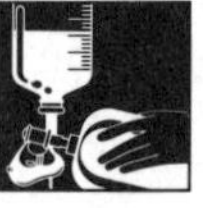

Explaining treatments

PACEMAKER INSERTION

Patient objectives	*Teaching plan content*
1 State the purpose of a pacemaker.	The purpose of a pacemaker is to produce the electrical impulses necessary to keep the heart working properly.
2 Describe the procedure used to insert the pacemaker.	The insertion procedure is simple, requires only a local anesthetic, and takes less than 1 hour. The incision site is usually the right deltopectoral groove and, while it may feel sore initially, it should not be painful. Once the bandage over the incision is removed—usually after 1 day—a bulge may be visible, depending on the size of the pulse generator and the amount of fatty tissue at the insertion site. Later, this bulge can be easily obscured by wearing loose clothing or a scarf.

3 Explain patient guidelines for pacemaker incision care.	To care for his incision, the patient should do the following: —Keep the incision clean and dry until it heals (usually 7 to 10 days). After that, he may wash as usual. —Wear loose clothing, to avoid putting pressure on the pacemaker. (For example, a woman with a pacemaker should not wear a tight bra.) —Check the implantation site. It usually bulges slightly. If it reddens, swells, drains, or becomes warm or painful, he should notify the physician immediately.
4 Obtain an accurate pulse rate for 1 full minute.	The patient should check his pacemaker by counting his pulse for 1 full minute once a day. —To check his pulse, he should place his index and middle fingers on his wrist just below the thumb. (He should not use the thumb to feel for a pulse, because it has a strong pulse of its own and may cause confusion.) If he has difficulty feeling the wrist pulse, he should place his thumb on his collarbone and lay his fingers along the side of his throat. When he feels the pulse, he should count the pulsations for 1 full minute. —He should record the pulse rate, noting the number of beats, the date, and the time. —The patient should know the pulse rate set by his pacemaker. If his pulse rate is below that, he should call his physician immediately.
5 Discuss long-term care of the pacemaker.	See *How to Care for Your Pacemaker,* pp. 72-73. In addition, the patient should be told if the manufacturer of his pacemaker provides a take-home transmitter kit, which can be leased to the patient to allow checkups over the phone. If the kit is available, the patient should understand the manufacturer's specific instructions.

CORONARY ARTERY BYPASS GRAFTING (C.A.B.G.)

Patient objectives	*Teaching plan content*
1 State the purpose of CABG.	The purpose of CABG is to increase blood flow and, thus, the supply of oxygen and nutrients to heart tissue affected by ischemia (lack of an adequate blood supply).
2 Describe the procedure used in CABG.	After the patient is anesthetized, the surgeon will make an incision in at least one arm or leg to remove a vein segment and a second incision in the chest to allow this vein segment, or graft, to be connected to the

aorta and then to the coronary arteries at a point beyond the occluded areas. (An illustration can be used to demonstrate the anatomy of the heart, if necessary.) Once the graft is sutured into place, oxygenated blood will flow from the aorta through the grafted blood vessel to the heart tissue.

3 Discuss the routine preoperative procedures for CABG.

Routine preoperative procedures include the following:
—An anesthetist will visit the patient the day before surgery to determine which anesthetic is best for him. CABG is always done under general anesthesia, and the patient will not awaken during surgery.
—The surgeon will also visit to explain the CABG procedure and the risks involved. The patient should write down any questions he would like to ask the surgeon. He will be asked to sign the operative permit giving his consent for CABG at that time. He should not sign it until all his questions have been answered and he understands the purpose and the risks involved.
—The patient will be shaved from his chin to his toes, because hair harbors bacteria that may cause an infection at the incision sites.
—He will receive a sleeping pill the night before surgery to help him relax and sleep. On the day of surgery he will receive sedation by intramuscular injection just before going to the operating room. This will make him feel drowsy and relaxed.
—The patient should not drink or eat anything after midnight the night before the procedure. (This is to prevent him from vomiting during surgery.)
—He will be transported to the operating room by stretcher.

4 Describe postoperative procedures in the intensive care unit (ICU) following CABG.

The patient should know the following facts about the ICU:
—He will see unfamiliar equipment and hear unusual noises in the recovery room and the ICU. However, specially trained nurses will interpret these strange surroundings for him. They will check him frequently to reassure him. (If time permits, the patient and his family should tour the ICU before surgery.)
—He will be attached to a ventilator and a cardiac monitor following surgery and will have in place an indwelling (Foley) catheter, chest tubes, and a pulmonary artery catheter.
—The patient will have to do deep-breathing and coughing procedures during recovery. He will be taught to use an incentive spirometer.
—The physical therapist will implement the postoperative exercise program.

	—The patient will receive medication for postoperative pain.
5 Discuss patient guidelines for postoperative care.	Once the special equipment has been removed, the patient will be transferred from the ICU to a regular unit in the hospital for further recuperation. During this time, he should prepare for discharge by reviewing the following guidelines: —He should continue to follow a low-salt, low-fat (and, if ordered, calorie-restricted) diet. (See the "Angina Pectoris" teaching plan in this chapter if further instructions are needed.) —Specific activity guidelines will be provided by his physician. Generally, all activity should be gradually increased, and an exercise program, such as walking, should be included in his daily activities. —He should understand the medication regimen. (See Chapter 9, Drug Therapy, for specific medication instructions.) —The incision sites must be kept clean and dry while healing occurs. He can expect itching and discomfort, but any increase in discomfort, redness, swelling, or drainage around the incision sites should be reported to the physician. —The patient may feel he is cured following CABG, but he must be aware that the underlying problem, atherosclerosis, is a lifelong condition requiring close medical follow-up.

PERCUTANEOUS TRANSLUMINAL CORONARY ANGIOPLASTY (P.T.C.A.)

Patient objectives	*Teaching plan content*
1 State the purpose of PTCA.	The purpose of PTCA is to increase blood flow to heart tissue affected by ischemia (lack of an adequate blood supply).
2 Define PTCA.	PTCA is a radiologic technique used to dilate an obstructed coronary artery without performing open-heart surgery. (The procedure is limited to use in small obstructed areas. Larger obstructions require coronary artery bypass grafting.)
3 Describe the procedure used in PTCA.	The procedure is performed in a special room in the hospital. —The physician begins by injecting an anesthetic at a spot where the blood vessels are close to the surface (for example, behind the knee). After the skin is numb, he makes a small incision into an artery.

—Then, he inserts a tiny balloon-tip catheter through a guiding catheter and into the artery, threading it to the narrowed section of the coronary artery.
—Once there, the balloon tip of the catheter is inflated with a solution containing a dye, and the physician looks at its position on a TV screen. The inflated balloon compresses the obstruction against the arterial walls, dilating the coronary artery and allowing more blood to pass through the artery.
—The physician then removes the balloon catheter. He leaves the introducer catheter in place for several hours after the procedure in case dilation of the artery needs to be repeated or special medications need to be given.

4 Discuss patient guidelines for PTCA.

The patient will usually require 2 days of medical evaluation before PTCA, bed rest in the coronary or telemetry unit afterward, and 1 to 2 days of evaluation after the procedure.
—He will be awake during PTCA, which usually lasts 1 to 4 hours, and will be asked to hold deep breaths periodically to allow visualization of the balloon catheter on the TV screen.
—He may experience angina, especially during inflation of the balloon catheter. He should report this to the physician.
—He will receive anticoagulant therapy (see Chapter 9, Drug Therapy, for further medication instructions) for 6 to 9 months after PTCA.
—A stress thallium imaging test to check the blood flow of the coronary arteries will be performed 1 to 2 days after PTCA and will be repeated at 3- to 6-month intervals, and cardiac catheterization will be performed 6 to 9 months after PTCA.

VASCULAR BYPASS GRAFTING

Patient objectives	*Teaching plan content*
1 State the purpose of vascular bypass grafting.	The purpose of vascular bypass grafting is to restore adequate blood flow to an ischemic area of the body (usually a lower extremity).
2 Describe the procedure used in vascular bypass grafting.	The surgeon will divert the blood flow around the obstructed arterial segment by attaching a graft to the artery with sutures above and below the obstruction. The graft will be either a segment of one of the patient's veins (usually the saphenous vein) or a Dacron graft. (An illustration can be used to demonstrate the procedure.)

3 Discuss the routine preoperative procedures for vascular bypass grafting.

The preoperative procedures used are the same as those for coronary artery bypass grafting (see the "Coronary Artery Bypass Grafting" teaching plan in this chapter), except for the area shaved. The extent of the shaved area required for vascular bypass grafting varies, depending on the location of the obstruction and the type of graft planned (for example, femoropopliteal or aortofemoral).

4 Describe postoperative procedures for vascular bypass grafting.

The patient probably will be in the ICU for the first 24 hours after surgery.
—Specially trained nurses there will explain the unfamiliar equipment and the unusual noises in the recovery room and the ICU. A nurse will check him frequently to reassure him. (If time permits, the patient and his family should tour the ICU before surgery.)
—The patient will have to do deep-breathing and coughing procedures during recovery.
—When he is transferred from the ICU to a regular unit in the hospital, he will be asked to get out of bed and walk frequently.
—Pain medication will be available; he should ask for it when needed.

5 Discuss patient guidelines for postoperative care.

After discharge, the patient should adhere to the following guidelines:
—He should report immediately any recurrence of symptoms, since the graft may fail.
—If antiembolism stockings are ordered, they should be put on immediately after getting out of bed. The patient should not wear constrictive apparel, such as garters or tight hose, around the knee.
—If he is receiving anticoagulants, he should take measures to prevent bleeding, such as using an electric razor. He should also avoid trauma, tobacco, and aspirin.
—He should immediately report any signs of bleeding (bleeding gums, tarry stools, easy bruising).
—The patient must continue to follow the prescribed medical regimen for his underlying arterial occlusive disease. (See the "Arterial Occlusive Disease" teaching plan in this chapter.)
—He should see his physician for follow-up studies to monitor anticoagulant therapy.

EXTRAANATOMIC BYPASS (E.A.B.)

Patient objectives	*Teaching plan content*
1 Define EAB.	EAB is an artificial vascular graft threaded under the skin (subcutaneously) to carry oxygenated blood from a body area with a good supply of blood to an area with a poor supply of blood.
2 State the purpose of EAB.	The purpose of EAB is to restore adequate blood flow to a deprived area (usually a lower extremity).
3 Describe the procedure used in EAB.	The two most common forms of EAB are the axillofemoral and femorofemoral bypasses. (An illustration can be used to demonstrate the procedures.) —To perform an axillofemoral bypass, the surgeon will make an incision below the clavicle to expose the axillary artery and will suture the graft to this artery. • He will then make an incision in the midaxillary line between the axillary and femoral sites to begin the tunnel. • Then a groin incision will be made, allowing the second segment of the tunnel to be completed, and the graft will be pulled through the tunnel and sutured to the recipient femoral artery. —To perform a femorofemoral bypass, an incision will be made at each groin to expose the femoral arteries. • A subcutaneous suprapubic tunnel will be made. • The graft will then be sutured to the donor femoral artery that had been passed through the tunnel and sutured to the recipient femoral artery.
4 Discuss the routine preoperative procedures for EAB.	The preoperative procedures used are the same as those for coronary artery bypass grafting (see the "Coronary Artery Bypass Grafting" teaching plan in this chapter), except for the area shaved. The area to be shaved varies depending on the type of EAB to be done.
5 Describe postoperative procedures for EAB.	Hospital policy determines whether a patient with EAB routinely goes to the ICU or back to his preoperative unit. If he is going to the ICU, see the "Coronary Artery Bypass Grafting" teaching plan in this chapter. (If time permits, the patient and his family should tour the ICU before surgery.) —If an axillofemoral bypass is done, he should not let anyone take his blood pressure on the side of the graft. Also blood should not be taken from the side of the graft or from the groin area of the incision site(s).

	—He should avoid lying on the side of the graft and should avoid excessive flexion of the axilla side of the graft (if an axillofemoral bypass was performed) and both groins. —He will have to do deep-breathing and coughing procedures during recovery. —Pain medication will be available; he should ask for it when needed. —He will probably be expected to get out of bed the day after surgery.
6 Discuss patient guidelines for postoperative care.	After discharge, the patient should adhere to the following guidelines: —The patient should check the graft pulse by placing his index and middle fingers on the graft, which is easily visible through the skin at the tunnel site. If at any time he cannot detect the graft pulse or if he experiences any symptom of arterial insufficiency (such as pain, temperature changes, or skin color changes), he should call his physician at once. —He should clean the incision(s) with soap and water and report any drainage to the physician. —The patient must continue his medication regimen for the underlying arterial occlusive disease. (See the "Arterial Occlusive Disease" teaching plan in this chapter.)

STREPTOKINASE INFUSION

Patient objectives	*Teaching plan content*
1 Define streptokinase infusion.	Streptokinase infusion is the administration of a medication to dissolve a clot occluding an artery (a blood vessel carrying oxygenated blood).
2 State the purpose of streptokinase infusion.	The purpose of streptokinase infusion is to restore blood flow to the area supplied by the artery. If it is being used to treat a myocardial infarction, it may limit the amount of heart tissue damaged.
3 Describe the procedure used in streptokinase infusion.	There are two methods of streptokinase infusion. The procedure to be used is determined by the patient's physician. —For an intracoronary artery infusion, the patient will be taken to the cardiac catheterization laboratory. There, the physician will inject an anesthetic at a spot where the blood vessels are closest to the surface (indicate the site, usually the antecubital or inguinal area). • After the skin is numb, he will insert a hollow needle into the area and then will pass a narrow

tube (catheter) through the needle and into an artery that leads to the heart.
• A fluoroscope, which looks like a TV screen, will show the catheter as it is inched toward the heart. Once the catheter is safely in place, the physician will inject a dye to visualize the coronary artery blood vessels and to locate the clot.
• Once it is located, a medication called nitroglycerin will be injected through the catheter to reduce any narrowing of the blood vessels caused by spasms that may have occurred as a result of the catheter's introduction.
• Then, the physician will inject streptokinase into the catheter, and X-ray–like pictures will be taken every 15 to 20 minutes to identify any remaining clots.
• When the clot has dissolved, or 60 to 90 minutes have elapsed since the medication was started, the catheter will be removed and the patient will be transferred to the coronary care unit for observation for several days.

—For an intravenous infusion, an intravenous line will be started and streptokinase will be administered on a continuous basis for a predetermined period of time, as ordered by the physician. Once the streptokinase infusion is completed, the intravenous line will be left in place for a period of time.

4 Discuss what to expect after streptokinase infusion.

The nurse will check the patient frequently after streptokinase infusion, as standard protocol. Frequent checks do not mean something has gone wrong or his condition is worse.
—The patient should keep the involved extremity straight, to prevent bleeding from the infusion site.
—He can expect to have blood drawn frequently to monitor his bleeding and clotting times.
—In addition, anticoagulant therapy will be administered to prevent further clots from forming. (See Chapter 9, Drug Therapy, for further medication instructions.)
—He should know what to expect regarding his disorder. (For example, see the "Myocardial Infarction" teaching plan in this chapter or the "Pulmonary Embolism" teaching plan in Chapter 3.)

Patient-Teaching Aid

MONITORING YOUR HEART RATE

Dear Patient:
Your physician has given you exercise guidelines. Follow these special instructions: ______________________________
____
____
____
____
____
____
____
____
____

During exercise, monitor your heart rate, as the nurse taught you. Use this patient-teaching aid as a reminder of what you have learned.

You target heart rate is ________ beats/minute. Try to maintain this rate when you exercise.

How can you check your heart rate? First, get a watch with a second hand. Then, as soon as you stop exercising, take your pulse.

Place your index and middle fingers on your wrist just below the thumb or into the groove between your windpipe and the large muscle in your neck, just below the angle of the jaw, as shown below. (Do not use your thumb to feel for a pulse—it has a strong pulse of its own, which may confuse you.)

Count the pulse beats for 15 seconds; then, multiply by 4. This gives you a reliable estimate of your working heart rate for 1 minute. (Do not count your pulse for a whole minute. Because your heart rate drops quickly when you rest, that figure will not be reliable.)

If your working heart rate is 10 beats or more above your target heart rate, do not work so hard next time. But if your working heart rate is lower than your target rate, work a little harder next time. For instance, if you walk, walk faster—or even jog, if your physician approves.

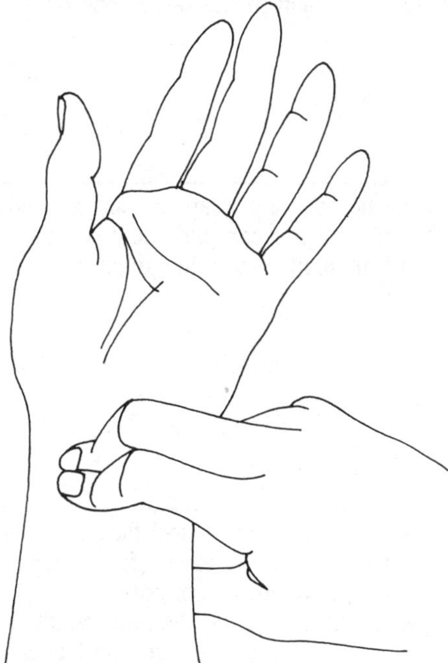

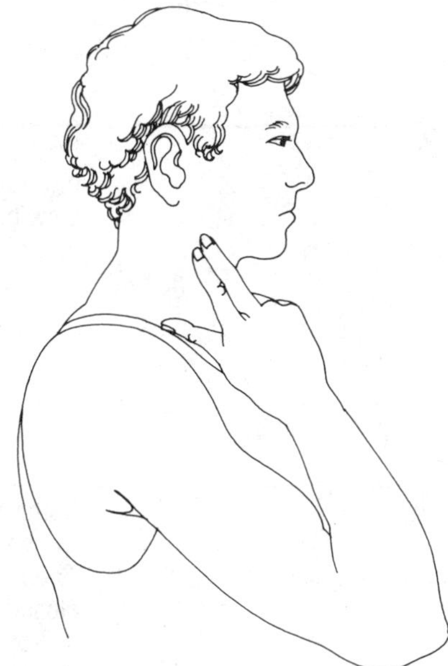

Patient-Teaching Aid

MONITORING BLOOD PRESSURE AT HOME

Dear Patient:
The nurse has taught you how to take blood pressure readings for a family member. Use these instructions at home, as a reminder.

Measure the patient's blood pressure at these times:

____

Notify the physician if: ______________________

____

____

____

____

1

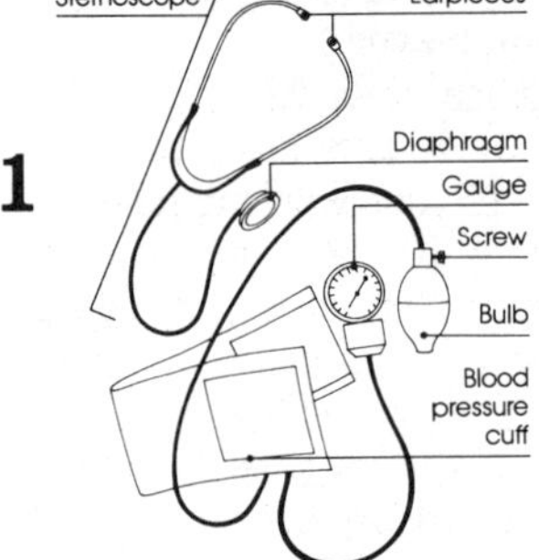

To begin, gather this equipment: a stethoscope and a blood pressure cuff with a gauge.

2

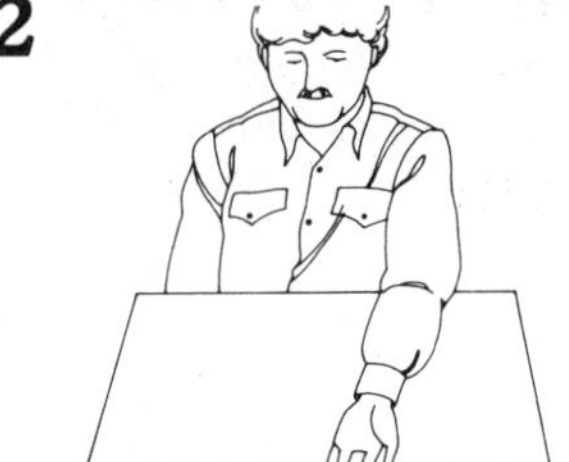

Ask the patient to sit down in a comfortable position and rest his arm on a table, so his arm is level with his heart. (Use the same arm in the same position each time.)

3

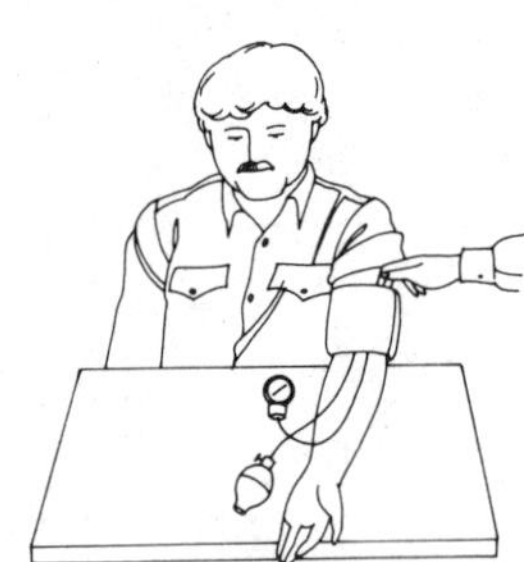

Push up his sleeve and securely wrap the cuff around his upper arm. Wrap it so you can slide only two fingers between it and his arm. Place the gauge where you can easily see it.

4

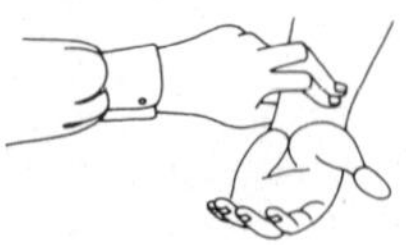

Using your middle and index fingers, feel for a pulse in his wrist. (Do not use your thumb to feel for a pulse.) Then, turn the bulb's screw clockwise, until it is closed. Inflate the cuff by squeezing the bulb rapidly.

Note the reading on the gauge when you no longer feel the pulse. Continue to inflate the cuff until the pressure is 20 points higher than this reading.

MONITORING BLOOD PRESURE AT HOME—*continued*

5

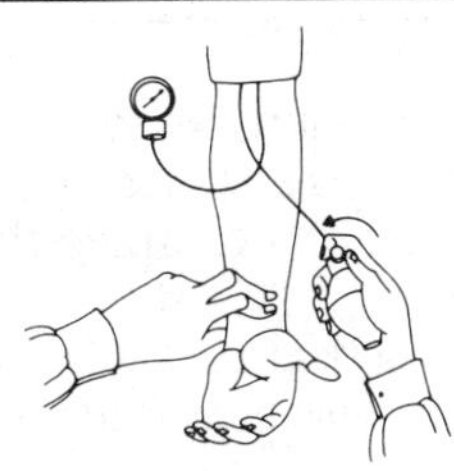

Keeping your fingers at the same spot on his wrist, slowly release the air in the cuff by loosening the screw. Now, make a mental note of the reading on the gauge when the pulse returns. This reading is called palpatory pressure.

6

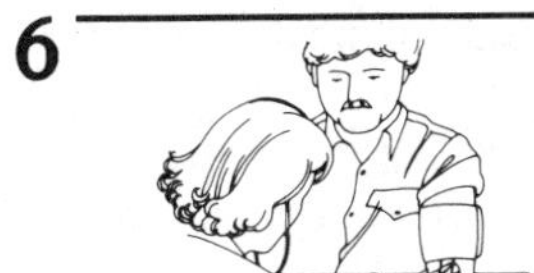

Wait 30 seconds before taking another reading. Then, place the stethoscope's earpieces in your ears. Be sure they are angled forward. Then, place the stethoscope's diaphragm over his brachial pulse (the pulse in the crook of his arm).

7

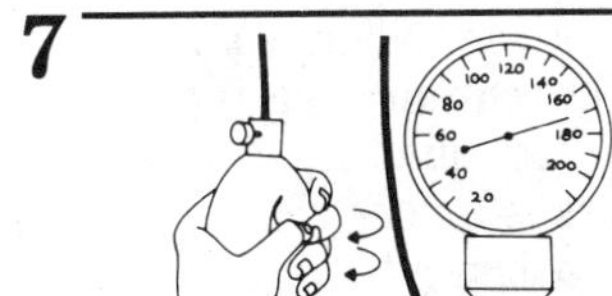

Again tighten the screw and quickly inflate the cuff, until the gauge shows a pressure 20 points higher than the palpatory pressure.

8

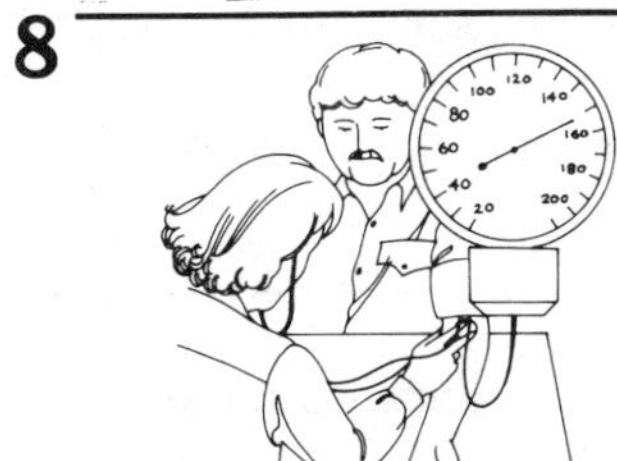

Loosen the screw to allow air to slowly escape from the cuff. Listen for the first beating sound you hear through the stethoscope. When you hear it, note the number on the gauge. This is the systolic pressure (the top number of a blood pressure reading).

9

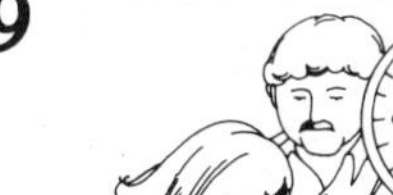

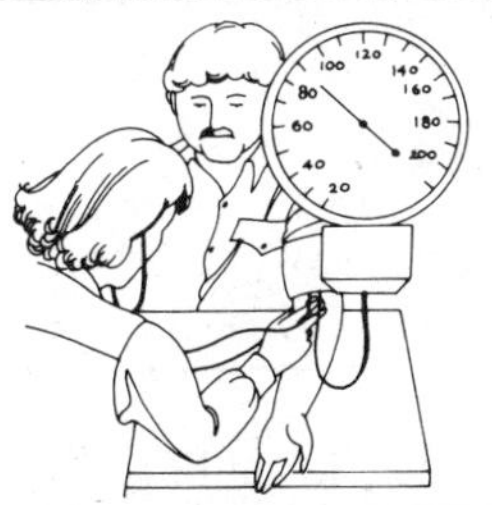

Continue to slowly deflate the cuff, and listen for the beating to stop. As soon as the beating stops, again note the number on the gauge. This is the diastolic pressure (the bottom number of a blood pressure reading).

Allow the cuff to deflate quickly and remove it.

10

DATE	TIME	BP
10/22	8 PM	150/90
10/24	8^{30} PM	156/86
10/27	7^{45} PM	150/84

Keep a written record of each blood pressure reading you take, including the date and time.

Patient-Teaching Aid

CUTTING DOWN ON SODIUM

Dear Patient:
To help control your high blood pressure, avoid as many salty foods as possible. This means including more low-sodium foods in your diet and breaking the habit of adding salt to your food.

Read what follows for some practical advice. Then, review this chart for details on low-sodium foods to enjoy and high-sodium foods to avoid.

- Season foods with herbs and spices instead of with salt.
- Use fresh tomatoes whenever possible for soups and sauces, or use unsalted canned tomatoes, tomato paste, or unsalted tomato juice.
- Season vegetables with vegetable oil, margarine, or approved seasonings, such as parsley or sweet basil.
- Rinse canned foods (including vegetables and tuna) under running water to reduce their sodium content.
- Read product labels carefully, remembering that additives are listed in order of greatest quantity. Avoid a product if one of these additives is among the first five listed: salt, sodium benzoate, sodium nitrate, or monosodium glutamate (MSG).
- At restaurants, order boiled, baked, broiled, or roasted foods. Skip gravies, juices, soups, and cheesy dressings.
- Avoid salt substitutes and light salt, unless your physician approves.

MEAT

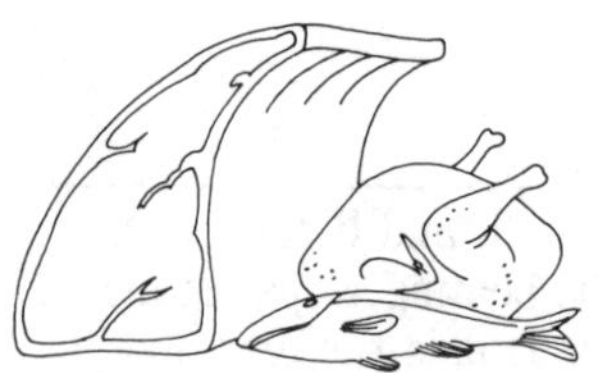

Low-sodium foods
Poultry, fresh or frozen fish, veal, lamb, pork, beef
High-sodium foods
Sausage, hot dogs, ham, bacon, luncheon meats, salt pork, smoked fish, herring, sardines, canned meat, TV dinners

DAIRY PRODUCTS

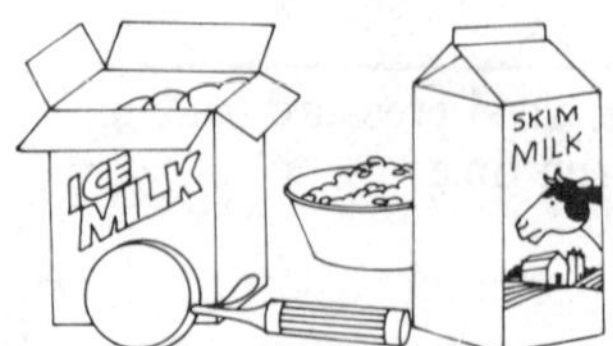

Low-sodium foods
Skim milk, low-fat cottage cheese, ice milk
High-sodium foods
Cheese (especially processed), buttermilk, ice cream

CUTTING DOWN ON SODIUM—*continued*

FRUITS AND VEGETABLES

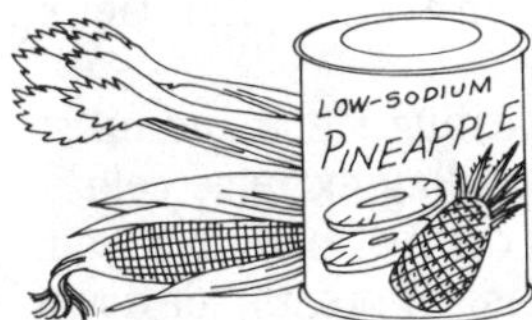

Low-sodium foods
All fresh, frozen, and low-sodium canned fruits and vegetables
High-sodium foods
Olives, pickles, sauerkraut, canned vegetables

BREADS AND CEREALS

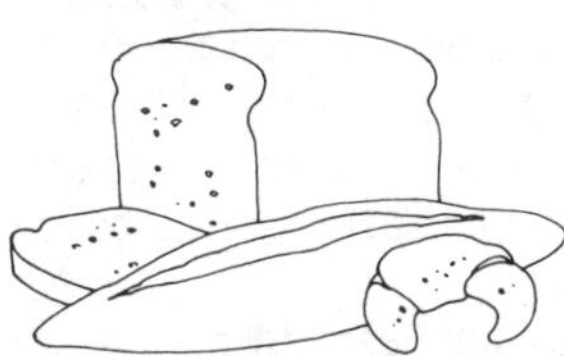

Low-sodium foods
Most commercial and homemade breads
High-sodium foods
Salted crackers, pretzels, rye rolls

SNACK FOODS

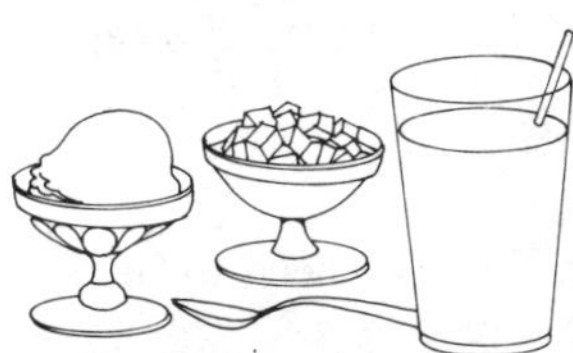

Low-sodium foods
Sherbet, fruit ice, gelatin, fruit drinks
High-sodium foods
Potato chips, pork rind, salted nuts, salted popcorn

SEASONINGS

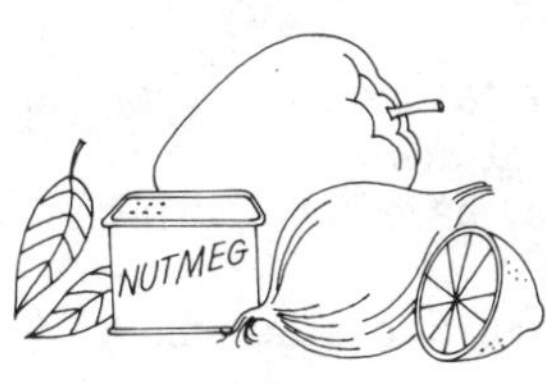

Low-sodium foods
Fresh garlic, fresh onion, bay leaf, pepper, dill, nutmeg, rosemary, green pepper, lemon juice
High-sodium foods
Salt, garlic or onion salt, bouillon, soy sauce, meat tenderizers, canned soups

Patient-Teaching Aid

SOME HEART-SAVING ADVICE AFTER DISCHARGE

Dear Patient:

During the first weeks at home, continue to be as active as you were on the last day in the hospital. Get up and get dressed every day.

- Continue with daily walks, avoiding steps and hills. Walk outside in nice weather, avoiding extreme cold, heat, or wind. Plan to walk after a rest period. If you have chest discomfort or shortness of breath, sit down on the steps or curb, take nitroglycerin if you have some, and wait until you feel better. Tell your physician about this pain when you see him.
- Eat four small meals a day; eat them slowly. Follow your fat-controlled diet. It is an important part of your physician's plan to help reduce your blood cholesterol.

After a meal, your heart is already working to digest your food. Therefore, rest for an hour after eating before doing any heavy exercise.

- Plan your activities to allow your heart to rest. Avoid overload by resting between chores. If you get tired, no matter what you are doing, stop and rest for 15 to 20 minutes. Do not push yourself. Plan a 30-minute rest period twice a day. Get 6 to 8 hours of sleep each night.

General advice

- Climb stairs only once a day. You may need to take only a few steps at a time before resting.
- Avoid working with your arms above shoulder level. For example, do not wash windows or hang clothes.
- Continue the recommended physical therapy exercises.
- Stop smoking. Smoking cigarettes increases your chance of having another heart attack.

If your physician says you may have liquor, drink in moderation.

- Avoid situations, people, and conditions that make you tense, upset, or angry.
- Avoid doing anything that tenses your body:

—Ask your physician for a laxative to avoid straining when having a bowel movement.
—Do not lift anything heavy.
—Avoid pushing or pulling anything heavy.
—Do not try to open a stuck window or unscrew a stuck jar lid.

SOME HEART-SAVING ADVICE AFTER DISCHARGE—*continued*

• Check with your physician before you take a long trip.
• If you develop pain, numbness, or shortness of breath, stop what you are doing, take your nitroglycerin, and rest for several minutes. When the discomfort disappears, continue what you were doing at a slower rate.
• As with other activities, you should not have sex if you are tired—take a 30-minute nap first; if you have just eaten a heavy meal; if you have been drinking; if you are angry with your mate; or if the temperature of the room is uncomfortably warm or cool.

If you begin to have chest discomfort, STOP. The next time, try taking nitroglycerin beforehand. Remember, it's normal for your heart to beat faster and your breathing to speed up during sexual activity. Your heartbeat and breathing should slow down and return to normal shortly afterward.
• During later weeks home, ask your physician when you may start resuming some of your regular activities, such as driving, returning to work, and going to a movie. When your physician says you may work, try to arrange to go back part-time at first and then slowly increase your working time.

You may have other questions about your activities, diet, medication, or illness. If you do, feel free to ask your physician.
• Notify your physician immediately whenever you have:
—heavy pressure or squeezing pain in the chest, which may spread to the shoulder, arm, neck, or jaw and is not relieved in 15 minutes by resting and/or nitroglycerin.
—increased shortness of breath.
—unusual fatigue.
—swelling of feet and ankles.
—fainting.
—very slow or rapid heart rate.

Patient-Teaching Aid

HOW TO CARE FOR YOUR PACEMAKER

Dear Patient:

Your physician has inserted a pacemaker in your chest to produce the electrical impulses necessary to keep your heart working properly. Now that you have a pacemaker, you must learn how to take care of it. Here are some things you should know:

- Keep the incision clean and dry until it heals (usually 7 to 10 days). After that, you may wash as usual.
- Wear loose clothing to avoid putting pressure on the pacemaker. For example, a woman with a pacemaker should not wear a tight bra.
- Normally, the implantation bulges slightly. If it reddens, swells, drains, or becomes warm or painful, notify the physician immediately.
- Depending on which type of pacemaker you have, it should give 3 to 4 years' service. See the physician regularly, usually every week during the first month or sooner if you have problems. Call the physician if you experience chest pain, dizziness, shortness of breath, prolonged hiccups, muscle twitching, nausea, vomiting, diarrhea, or a very fast or very slow heart rate. He may have you check your pacemaker periodically by transtelephonic monitoring, which enables you to transmit your EKG over the phone.
- To check your pacemaker, count your pulse at least once a day for a full minute after you have been at rest for at least 15 minutes. A good time to take a resting pulse rate is first thing in the morning. Your pulse rate reflects the number of times your heart pumps. The nurse will teach you how to count your pulse and tell you what pulse rate to expect. Report any discrepancy to the physician immediately. Also record all your pulse rates; include the number of beats, the date, and the time.
- Take your heart medication, as prescribed. This, along with your pacemaker, ensures a regular heart rate. As a reminder, note on a calendar the times when you should take your medication.
- Follow the physician's orders concerning diet and physical activity. You should exercise every day, but the physician will tell you how much exercise is right for you. You can participate in any physical activity in accordance with the physician except a contact sport, such as football. Do not overdo it. Be especially careful not to stress the muscles near the pacemaker.

HOW TO CARE FOR YOUR PACEMAKER—*continued*

• Do not get too close to gasoline engines, electric motors, or poorly shielded microwave ovens. Do not use an electric shaver directly over the pacemaker. Also stay away from high-voltage fields created by overhead electric lines. Most other electric equipment will not interfere with your pacemaker.
• If you go to the dentist or any other health care professional, tell him you are wearing a pacemaker. If you need dental work or surgery, you might require a prophylactic antibiotic to prevent infections. Consult your physician before undergoing any procedure that involves electricity, such as cautery or diathermy.
• Always carry your pacemaker emergency card. The card lists your physician, hospital, type of pacemaker (model, serial number, lead type), and date of implantation.
• You can drive a car a month after your pacemaker is implanted, but avoid long trips for at least 3 months and when the time for your battery replacement nears. Tell your physician of your travel plans in advance, and carry a list of physicians and hospitals in the area where you will be traveling.
• If you are traveling by plane, you must pass through an airport metal detector. Before doing so, be sure to alert the authorities that you have a pacemaker.
• If you have a nuclear pacemaker and plan to travel abroad, the Nuclear Regulatory Commission requires that you inform the pacemaker manufacturer of your travel itinerary, means of travel, and the name of your physician.
• Periodic short-term hospitalization is usually necessary for battery changes or pacemaker replacement.

Patient-Teaching Aid

CHECKING YOUR PACEMAKER BY TELEPHONE

Dear Patient:
Your physician has prescribed a Medtronic Teletrace Transmitter so he can check your pacemaker by telephone. The nurse has explained how the transmitter works and has shown you how to operate it. Use this patient-teaching aid as a guide after you've been discharged. If you have any questions or problems, call

____

1

Here is how the back and the front of your transmitter look. Before using your transmitter for the first time, remove the battery cover and insert the 9-volt alkaline battery supplied by the manufacturer. REMEMBER: Replace the battery every 2 or 3 months.

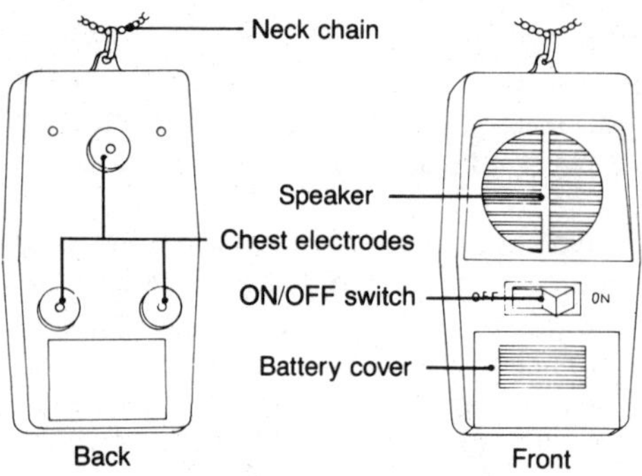

2

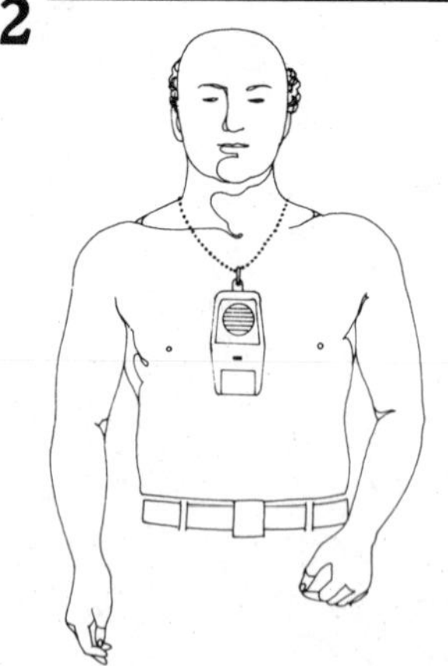

When you are ready to use the transmitter, put its chain around your neck, and adjust the chain so the transmitter hangs comfortably at the middle of your chest. Open or remove your shirt and underwear so the transmitter's chest electrodes rest against your bare skin.

CHECKING YOUR PACEMAKER BY TELEPHONE—*continued*

3

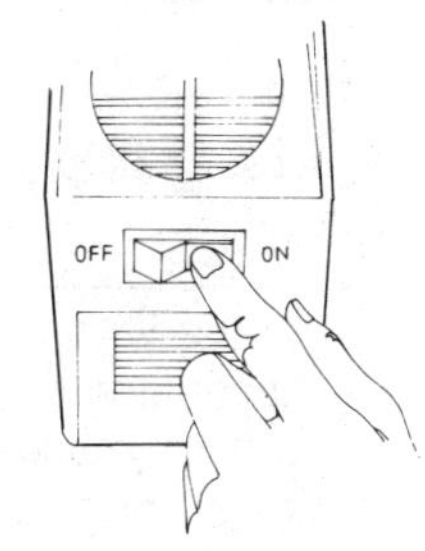

When you have contacted your physician's office by telephone, turn on the transmitter by pressing the ON/OFF switch to the *on* position. Listen for a squealing sound. If you do not hear it, change the transmitter's battery before continuing.

4

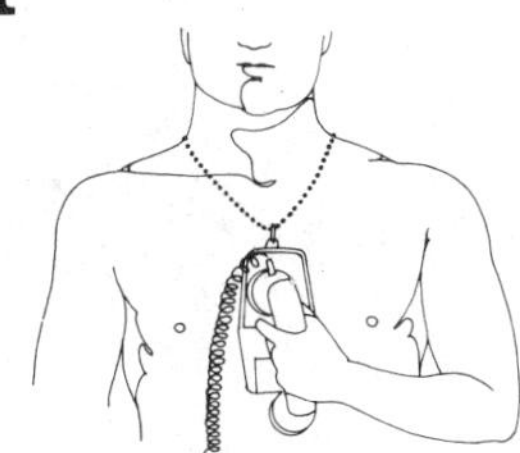

When the physician (or his assistant) is ready to receive your signal, place the telephone's mouthpiece against the transmitter's speaker. Hold the telephone as steady as you can, and try to sit still for about 30 seconds.

5

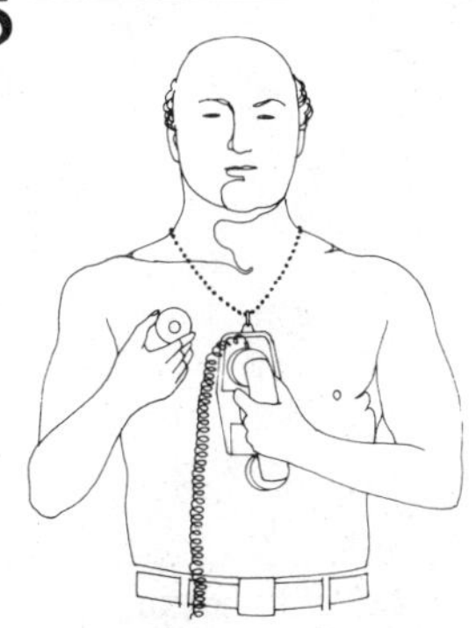

After 30 seconds, hold the telephone to your ear, and listen for further instructions. For example, the physician may want you to repeat the procedure while you hold a special magnet he has given you over the pacemaker. If so, take care to place the magnet flat against your pacemaker, and hold it as steady as possible. (If you wish, ask someone to hold it for you.) But do not use the magnet unless the physician asks you to do so.

6

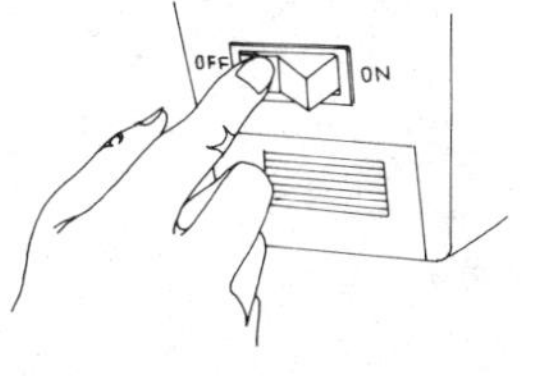

If the physician has no further directions for you, hang up the phone and remove the transmitter from around your neck. Don't forget to switch off your transmitter, and keep it switched off whenever you are not using it.

Patient-Teaching Aid

CARING FOR YOUR LEGS AND FEET

Dear Patient:
Because of poor circulation in your legs and feet, there is a danger you will develop leg ulcers. To help prevent these ulcers, follow these guidelines:

1 Keep your legs and feet clean, soft, and dry.

Wash daily and dry thoroughly by patting with a soft towel, especially between the toes. Apply lanolin or a similar mild cream to keep your skin from cracking. Wear clean, absorbent socks or stockings (preferably cotton or wool).

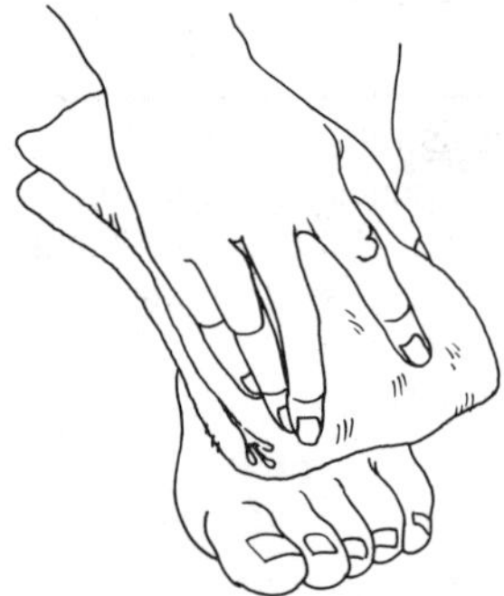

2 Inspect your legs and feet every day.

This is important because you may develop breaks in the skin that you cannot feel.

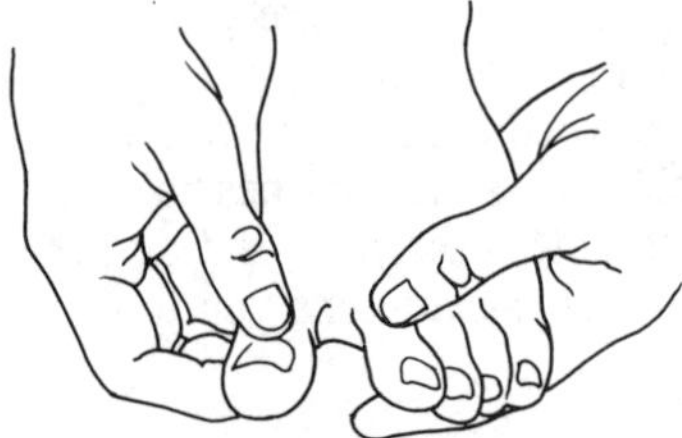

3 Avoid injury to your legs and feet.

Wear shoes that fit correctly, and avoid walking barefoot. Also put lamb's wool between your toes to prevent rubbing. Lastly, have your physician or a podiatrist cut your toenails.

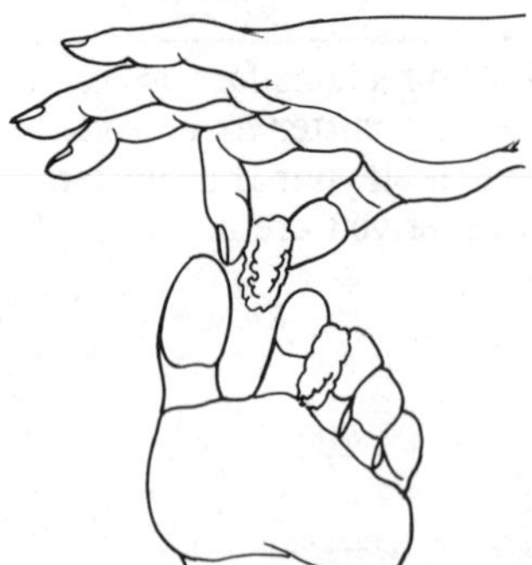

CARING FOR YOUR LEGS AND FEET—*continued*

4 Avoid foot preparations unless your physician prescribes them.

This is important because many foot plasters, corn removers, disinfectants, and ointments are strong enough to injure your feet.

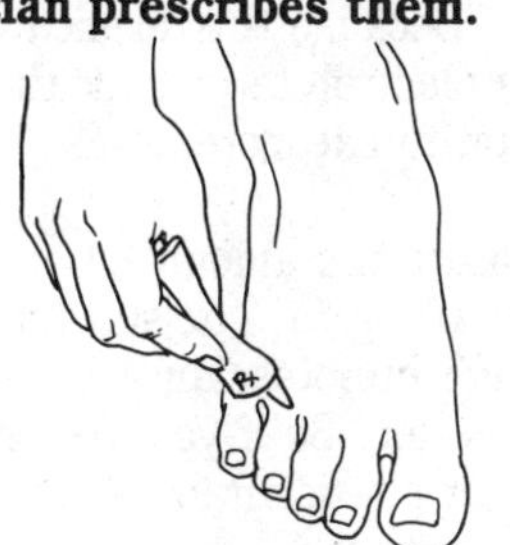

5 Avoid smoking.

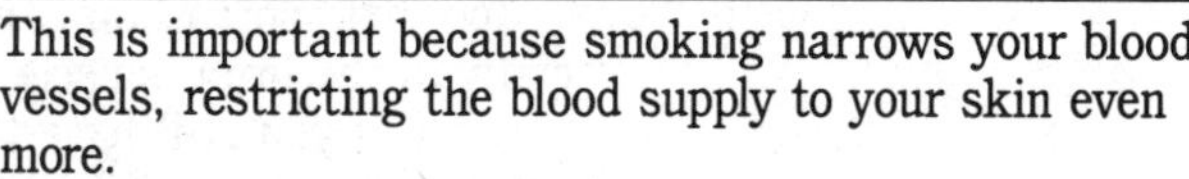

This is important because smoking narrows your blood vessels, restricting the blood supply to your skin even more.

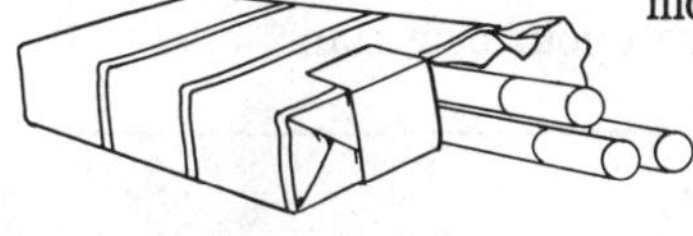

6 Avoid extremes in temperature.

Keep your feet and legs warm; wear cotton or wool socks. Never apply heat (for example, a hot water bottle) to your foot. Test bathwater with your hand (not your foot) before getting into the tub. Also avoid exposing your legs and feet to the sun, and do not swim in cold water.

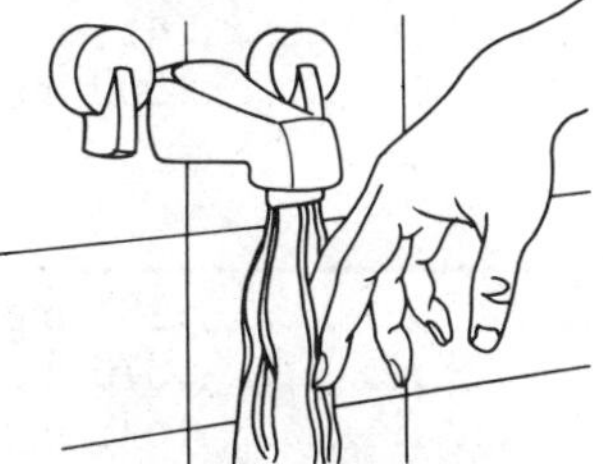

7 Avoid clothing that restricts your circulation.

Do not wear girdles, garters, or socks with tight elastic bands.

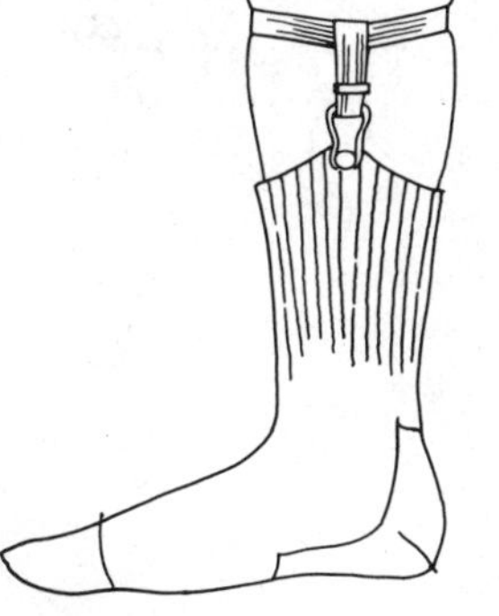

IMPORTANT: Notify your physician if you get a wound on your leg or foot. Cover the wound with a plain, sterile gauze pad. Do not put ointments (such as hydrocortisone cream) on it.

Patient-Teaching Aid

GUIDE TO POTASSIUM-RICH FOODS

Dear Patient:
Your physician has prescribed a water pill (diuretic) to help control your blood pressure. Because this medication may result in the loss of an electrolyte (chemical) called potassium, he may ask you to eat more potassium-rich foods.

The numbers listed below indicate the amount of potassium (in milligrams) found in 100 g (3½-oz serving) of food. All of these foods are high in potassium—but some of them are high in calories, too. So if you are on a low-calorie diet, check with your physician for further guidelines.

Too little potassium can cause muscle cramps (especially in the legs), muscle weakness, paralysis, and spasms. If you still have these problems after adding potassium to your diet, call your physician.

MEATS

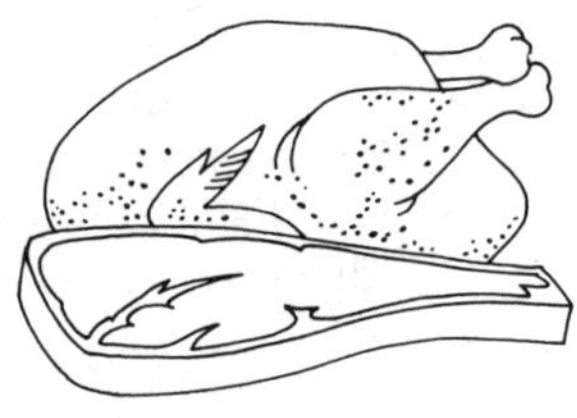

Food	Potassium
Beef	370 mg
Chicken	411 mg
Lamb	290 mg
Liver	380 mg
Pork	326 mg
Turkey	411 mg
Veal	500 mg

FRUITS

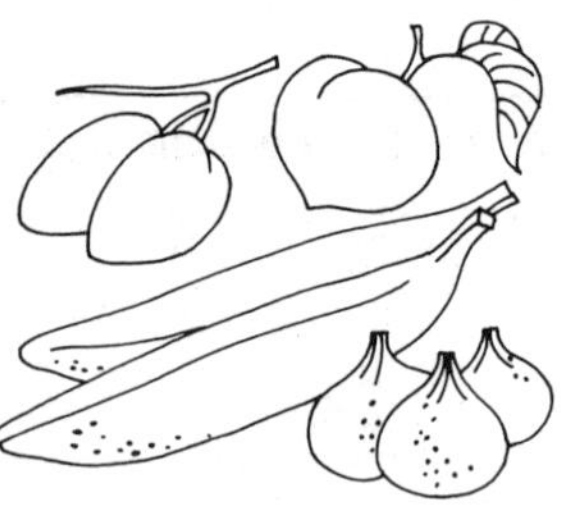

Food	Potassium
Apricots	281 mg
Bananas	370 mg
Dates	648 mg
Figs	152 mg
Nectarines	294 mg
Oranges	200 mg
Peaches	202 mg
Plums	299 mg
Prunes	262 mg
Raisins	355 mg

GUIDE TO POTASSIUM-RICH FOODS—*continued*

VEGETABLES

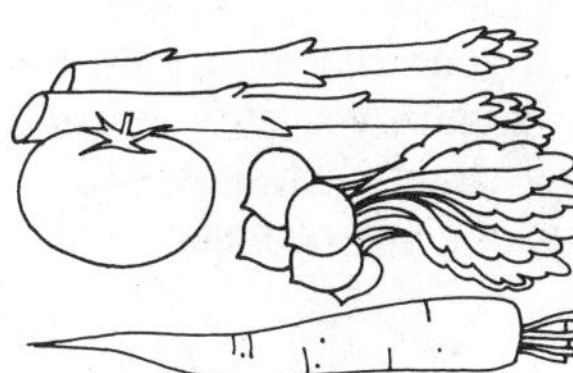

Food	Potassium
Asparagus	238 mg
Brussels sprouts	295 mg
Cabbage	233 mg
Carrots	341 mg
Endive	294 mg
Lima beans	394 mg
Peppers	213 mg
Potatoes	407 mg
Radishes	322 mg
Spinach	324 mg
Sweet potatoes	300 mg

JUICES

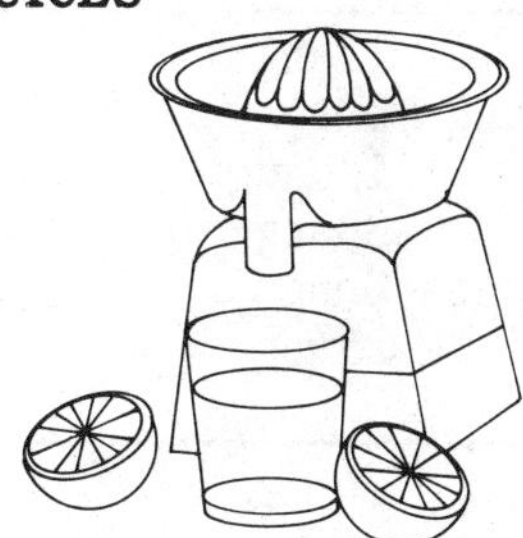

Food	Potassium
Orange, fresh or	200 mg
reconstituted	186 mg
Tomato	227 mg

FISH

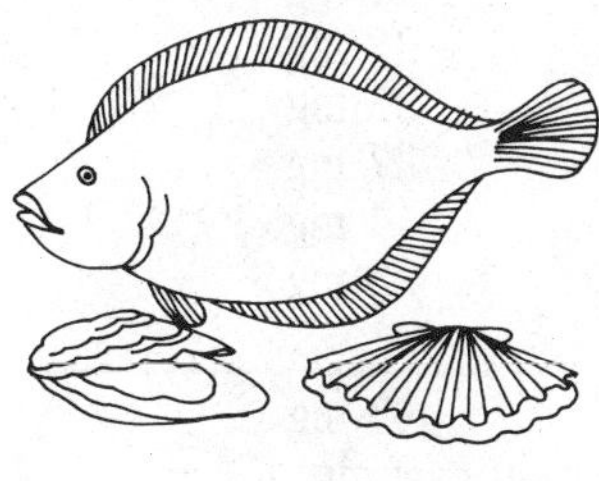

Food	Potassium
Bass	256 mg
Flounder	342 mg
Haddock	348 mg
Halibut	525 mg
Oysters	203 mg
Perch	284 mg
Salmon	421 mg
Sardines, canned	590 mg
Scallops	476 mg
Tuna	301 mg

MISCELLANEOUS

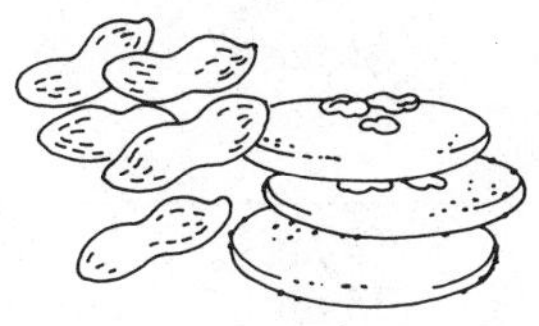

Food	Potassium
Gingersnap cookies	462 mg
Graham crackers	384 mg
Oatmeal cookies (with raisins)	370 mg
Ice milk	195 mg
Milk, dry (nonfat solids)	1,745 mg
Molasses (light)	917 mg
Peanuts	674 mg
Peanut butter	670 mg

Patient-Teaching Aid

KEEPING TRACK OF CHOLESTEROL

Dear Patient:
To help control the amount of cholesterol in your blood, the physician wants you to limit your cholesterol intake to less than 300 mg a day. Make sure you stay within this limit by using the following chart that shows the approximate cholesterol content of some common foods.

FOOD TYPE	EXAMPLE	SERVING SIZE	CHOLESTEROL CONTENT
Breads	biscuit	1	17 mg
	bread slice or roll	any amount	0 mg
	French toast	1	130 mg
	pancake	1	38 mg
	saltine crackers	any amount	0 mg
	sweet roll	1	25 mg
Cheeses	American	1 oz	30 mg
	cottage cheese		
	creamed	1 cup	45 mg
	uncreamed	1 cup	16 mg
	mozzarella	1 oz	18 mg
	Muenster	1 oz	25 mg
	Parmesan	1 oz	25 mg
	provolone	1 oz	27 mg
	ricotta	1 oz	14 mg
	Swiss	1 oz	28 mg
Cooking oils	lard	1 tbsp	12 mg
	margarine	any amount	0 mg
	vegetable oils	any amount	0 mg
Desserts	angel food cake	any amount	0 mg
	baked custard	1 cup	275 mg
	chocolate cake	1 slice	32 mg
	sherbet	any amount	0 mg
Fish	clams	1 oz	13 mg
	haddock	1 oz	23 mg
	herring	1 oz	32 mg

KEEPING TRACK OF CHOLESTEROL—*continued*

FOOD TYPE	EXAMPLE	SERVING SIZE	CHOLESTEROL CONTENT
Fish (continued)	oysters	1 oz	19 mg
	salmon	1 oz	18 mg
	scallops	1 oz	15 mg
	shrimp	1 oz	57 mg
	trout	1 oz	21 mg
	tuna	1 oz	21 mg
Meat	bacon	2 slices	15 mg
	beef (lean)	1 oz	36 mg
	beef (liver)	1 oz	123 mg
	lamb	1 oz	37 mg
	pork (ham)	1 oz	33 mg
	pork (sausages)	1 oz	27 mg
	veal	1 oz	38 mg
Milk and dairy products	butter	1 tbsp	30 mg
	egg white	any amount	0 mg
	egg yolk	1 egg	245 mg
	ice cream	½ cup	25 mg
	ice milk	½ cup	5 mg
	skim milk	1 cup	5 mg
	whole milk	1 cup	32 mg
Poultry	chicken (light meat with skin)	1 oz	22 mg
	turkey (light meat with skin)	1 oz	23 mg
Miscellaneous	chocolate sauce	any amount	0 mg
	coconut	any amount	0 mg
	gravy	¼ cup	18 mg
	low-fat cookies	any amount	0 mg
	popcorn (unbuttered)	any amount	0 mg
	potatoes	any amount	0 mg
	white sauce	¼ cup	29 mg

Patient-Teaching Aid

LIVING WITH CONGESTIVE HEART FAILURE

Dear Patient:

You have congestive heart failure, a condition that impairs your heart's ability to pump blood. Because overexertion places a tremendous strain on your heart, you will need to modify your life-style to decrease your heart's work load and minimize symptoms.

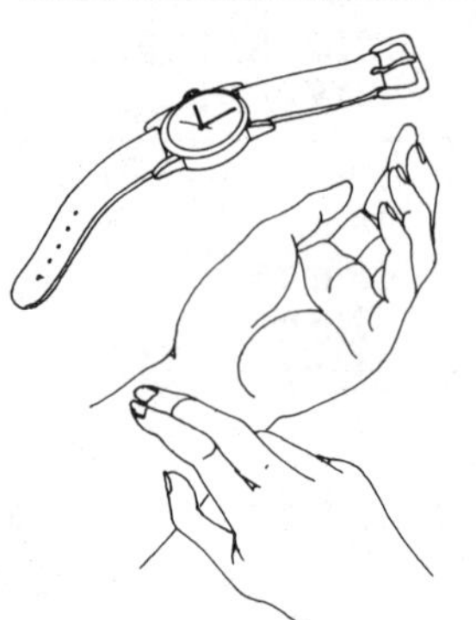

Check pulse rate before taking digitalis.

Take digitalis, as prescribed, to strengthen your heart and improve its pumping ability. Do not substitute one brand of digitalis for another without first consulting your physician. Check your pulse rate daily before taking digitalis, and call your physician immediately if it is less than 60 or more than 120 beats/minute. Also promptly report any loss of appetite, nausea and vomiting, diarrhea, fatigue, visual disturbances, headache, muscle weakness, or apathy.

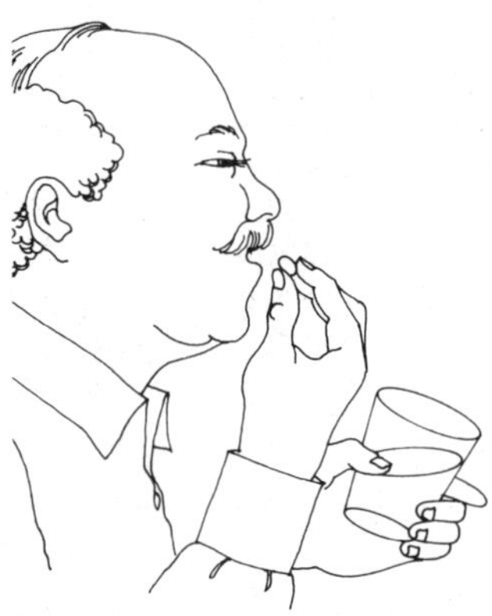

Take prescribed drugs.

Take a diuretic, if prescribed, to reduce your body's total volume of water and salt. Because a diuretic can cause loss of potassium, promptly report dizziness, nausea and vomiting, loss of appetite, abdominal distention, muscle weakness and fatigue, leg cramps, malaise, confusion, or headache. Because these symptoms may intensify if you become dehydrated, notify your physician if you cannot eat or drink normally. Do not, however, stop taking any prescribed drug without first consulting your physician.

Be sure to ask your physician before taking any over-the-counter drugs, such as cold remedies.

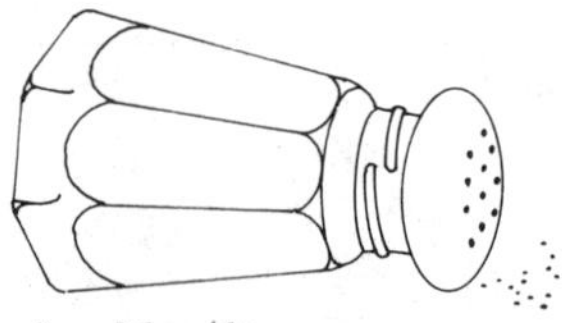

Avoid salt.

Restrict sodium intake to decrease fluid retention, thereby decreasing your heart's work load. Do not add salt to your food. Avoid salted "snack" foods, canned soups and vegetables, prepared foods (such as TV dinners), luncheon meats, cheeses, or pickles and any other food preserved in brine. Check food labels for sodium content. And finally, be sure to adhere to the diet plan provided by your physician.

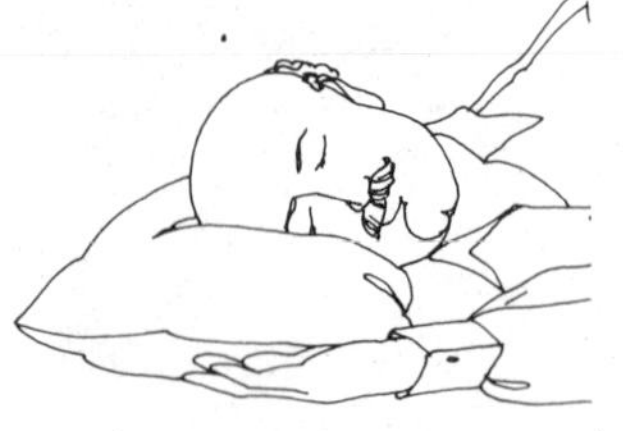

Get adequate rest.

Be sure to get adequate rest. If possible, shorten your work day and set aside a daily rest period. Also try to avoid emotional stress.

Gradually increase walking and other physical activities to your capacity. Continue at whatever activity level you can maintain without developing shortness of breath, palpitations, or severe fatigue. Also notify your physician if these symptoms increase. He may be able to adjust your medication dosage to allow increased activity.

LIVING WITH CONGESTIVE HEART FAILURE—*continued*

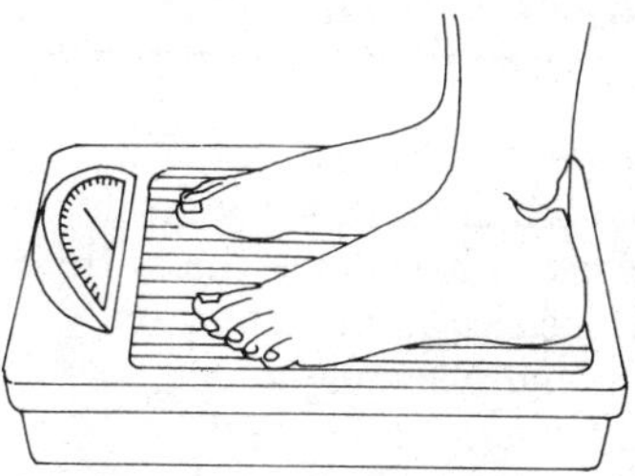

Watch for weight gain.

Try to avoid temperature extremes. When possible, stay in a cool, comfortable environment. In hot weather, perform your activities in the cooler part of the day. In cold weather, dress warmly but avoid restrictive clothing that interferes with circulation. Wrap a scarf over your nose and mouth to warm the air and make breathing easier.

Watch for and report signs and symptoms of recurring congestive heart failure. These include weight gain, loss of appetite, shortness of breath upon activity, persistent cough, frequent urination at night, and swelling of the ankles, feet, or abdomen.

Keep your regular physician appointments.

Patient-Teaching Aid

WHAT YOU SHOULD KNOW ABOUT CARDIAC CATHETERIZATION

Dear Patient:

Your physician has scheduled you for cardiac catheterization, a procedure that allows him to view the inside of your heart and examine what is happening there. He does this by making a small incision in an artery or vein near your elbow or groin and inserting a long, thin, flexible tube called a catheter.

After inserting the catheter, the physician will thread it through your blood vessels and into your heart. When the catheter is properly in place, he will perform certain tests that may include injection of a special dye. What the physician sees will help him to decide what additional treatment might improve your heart's functioning.

Before the procedure. If your catheterization is scheduled for early morning, you probably will not be allowed to eat or drink anything after midnight of the evening before the procedure.

To protect against infection, before the procedure the nurse may shave the area where your incision will be made.

Before you go to the catheterization laboratory for the procedure, she will also ask you to urinate. Then she will help you into a hospital gown. Depending on the physician's orders, she may start an intravenous (I.V.) line in your arm.

During the procedure. When you reach the catheterization laboratory, you will be placed on a padded table and probably strapped to it. During catheterization, the physician will tilt the table to view your heart from different angles. The straps will keep you from slipping out of position. Special foam pads, called leads, may be connected to a monitor and put on your chest so that your heartbeat can be monitored.

Cardiac catheterization usually takes 1 to 2 hours. You will be awake throughout the procedure, although the physician may order some medication to help you relax. (Some patients even doze off.)

When the physician's ready to begin, he will inject a local anesthetic at the insertion site. The injection may feel a little uncomfortable, but it will numb the area before he puts in the catheter. When the catheter is going in, you should feel a little pressure but no pain.

If the catheter meets a blockage—where atherosclerosis has narrowed a blood vessel, for example—the

WHAT YOU SHOULD KNOW ABOUT CARDIAC CATHETERIZATION—*continued*

physician will withdraw the catheter and start from another insertion area.

When the catheter enters your heart, you may experience a fluttering, or flip-flop, sensation. Tell the physician if you do, but do not worry, as it is a normal reaction. You are likely to feel a warm sensation, some nausea, or the urge to urinate if dye is injected, but these feelings will pass quickly. Throughout the procedure, remember to let the physician or the nurse know if you have chest pain.

During the procedure, your physician may ask you to cough or to pant like a dog. These actions help to advance the dye through your heart. The physician may also ask you to breathe deeply, which will give him a better view of your heart.

When the physician removes the catheter, he will put a special bandage on your arm or groin. Chances are the anesthetic will still be working, so you should not feel anything.

After the procedure. When you are back in your room, the nurse will probably obtain an electrocardiogram if you're not already on a cardiac monitor. She will check your bandage and your temperature, heartbeat, breathing, and blood pressure frequently, so do not be concerned. This frequent checking is standard for anyone who has had cardiac catheterization.

At this point, we will need your special cooperation. Your bandaged arm or leg must stay completely still for 6 to 24 hours, depending on your physician's orders. To help you keep from moving, the nurse may splint the arm or leg or weigh it down with a sandbag. She will check the blood flow in the affected arm or leg and will probably ask you to wiggle your toes or fingers once an hour or more.

As your anesthetic wears off, you will probably feel some discomfort at the insertion site. Let the nurse know so she can give you medication to ease the pain.

As soon as the test results are available, the physician will talk to you and your family about them. Do not hesitate to ask him or the nurse any questions you may have.

Patient-Teaching Aid

LEARNING HOW TO RELAX

Dear Patient:

The nurse has explained to you why you should relax more to help you lower your blood pressure. This patient-teaching aid will tell you how to relax—on your own, without special equipment. As with any other learning procedure, learning to relax will take practice.

First, choose a slogan that you will feel comfortable saying each time you practice, for example, "Ease up" or "Slow down." Or, if you prefer, use a short prayer. Then follow the steps shown below.

If you prefer, try this method: Breathe out slowly while concentrating on a particular muscle. Imagine a wave of relaxation starting at the muscle and spreading out to the rest of your body.

No matter which method you choose, do it twice. Then, return to whatever you were doing.

Do your relaxation exercise at least 10 times daily.

1 Stop whatever you are doing.

2

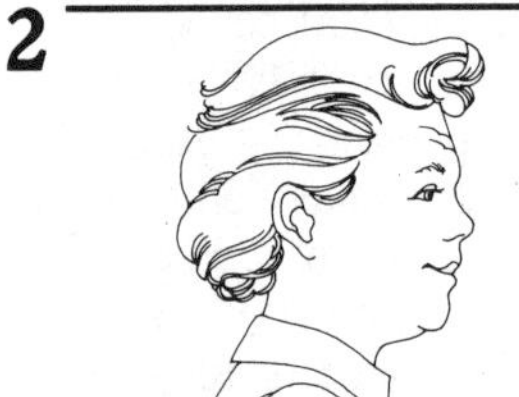

Smile—openly, if appropriate; otherwise, smile inwardly.

3

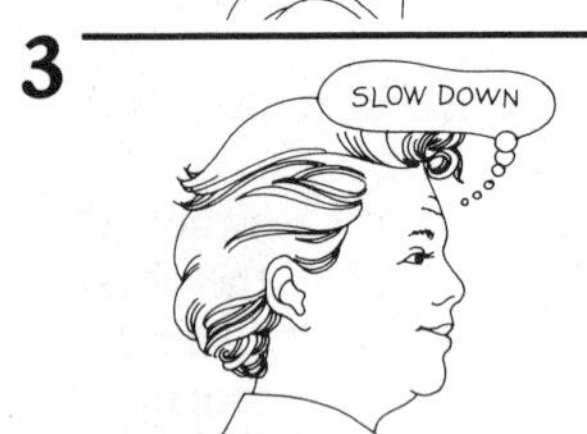

Say your relaxation slogan to yourself.

4

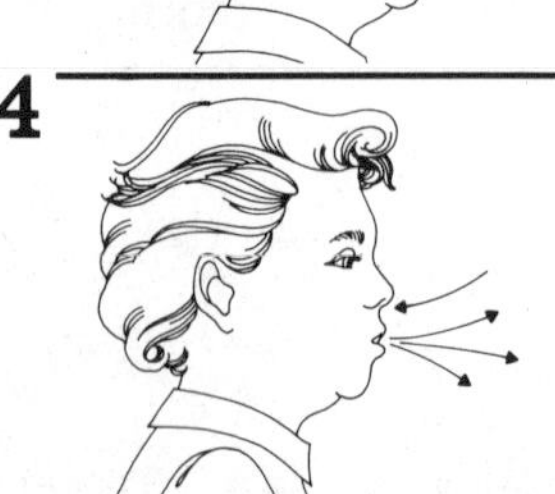

Take a long, slow, deep breath. Breathe out slowly. As you do, think about how relaxed you are feeling.

Respiratory Disorders

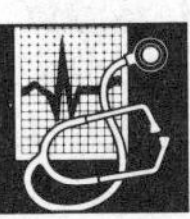

Patient-learner data base*

Areas of potential knowledge deficit

Presence of respiratory risk factors:
—Smoking
—Occupational exposure to respiratory irritants and/or pollutants
—Genetic predisposition
—Emotional/stressful life-style
—Obesity
Anatomy and physiology of the respiratory tract
Definition of respiratory disease
Causes of respiratory disease
Symptoms associated with the disease
Treatment of the respiratory disease:
—Diet
—Medications
—Exercise
—Relaxation
—Guidelines for daily living
—Additional treatments
Complications of respiratory disease

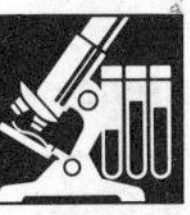

Explaining diagnostic tests

ARTERIAL BLOOD GAS (A.B.G.) ANALYSIS

Patient objectives	*Teaching plan content*
1 Define ABG analysis.	ABG analysis is a blood test that evaluates how well the lungs are delivering oxygen to the blood and eliminating carbon dioxide from the blood.

*A general assessment should be done for all patients. For general assessment guidelines, see Chapter 1, Principles of Patient Teaching.

2 State the purposes of ABG analysis.	The purposes of ABG analysis are as follows: —To evaluate the efficiency of gas exchange in the lungs —To assess the integrity of breathing (ventilatory control system) —To determine the acid-base level of the blood —To monitor respiratory therapy.
3 Describe the procedure used in ABG analysis.	A health care professional will perform the arterial puncture at the bedside. The patient should know which site will be used: the radial (wrist), brachial (arm), or femoral (groin) artery. —Just before the puncture, the technician may have the patient rest his arm on the mattress or bedside table, placing a rolled towel under his wrist (if this is the site selected) for support. —He will be asked to clench his hand into a fist, then unclench it. —He may experience a brief cramping or throbbing pain at the puncture site. —Pressure will be applied over the puncture site until bleeding has stopped (at least 5 minutes).
4 Discuss patient guidelines for ABG analysis.	Patient guidelines for ABG analysis include the following: —The patient need not restrict foods or fluids prior to the test. —He should breathe normally during the test. —He should not remove oxygen (if applicable) for 20 to 30 minutes before the test. —He should remain calm and relaxed during the procedure to alleviate possible spasm of the artery. —The patient must keep his hand, arm, or leg still.

FIBER-OPTIC BRONCHOSCOPY

Patient objectives	*Teaching plan content*
1 Define fiber-optic bronchoscopy.	Fiber-optic bronchoscopy is a test that uses a special tube to directly visualize the trachea and tracheobronchial tree.
2 State the purposes of fiber-optic bronchoscopy.	Fiber-optic bronchoscopy may be done for diagnostic or therapeutic purposes. —The diagnostic purposes are as follows: • To collect specimens for bacterial and/or cytologic analysis

• To determine the location, extent, and cause of disease
• To determine the cause of improperly functioning intubation.
—The therapeutic purposes of fiber-optic bronchoscopy are as follows:
• Removal of a foreign body or localized lesion from the tracheobronchial tree
• Removal of mucous plugs from the lower airways
• Prevention or treatment of collapsed lung tissue (atelectasis)
• Improvement of bronchial drainage.

3 Describe the procedure used in fiber-optic bronchoscopy.

The patient will be given medication before the procedure: atropine is administered to decrease secretions and a barbiturate or narcotic is usually administered I.V. to allay anxiety and provide sedation or amnesia. He will need to be relaxed and calm during this procedure.
—He will be placed in the supine position on an examination table or on his bed.
—He will be asked to hyperextend his neck and breathe through his nose.
—The room will be darkened, and the physician will spray a local anesthetic in his throat and nasal cavity.
—After being lubricated with a jellylike substance, the bronchoscope will be introduced through his nose or mouth. He will be able to breathe through and around the tube, although he may feel a fullness in his throat.
—The vocal cords will be anesthetized and the gag reflex suppressed with an anesthetic administered through the bronchoscope.
—The bronchoscope then will be advanced through the larynx into the trachea and bronchi, as the physician inspects the structure and color of the trachea and bronchi.
—The bronchoscope will be removed after the observation, biopsy, and/or specimen analysis are completed.
—The patient should know who will perform the test and where and when it will be done.

4 Discuss patient guidelines for fiber-optic bronchoscopy.

Patient guidelines for fiber-optic bronchoscopy include the following:
—The patient must fast for 6 to 12 hours before the test.
—During the test, he should remain relaxed and keep his arms at his sides.
—After the test, he can expect to have his vital signs checked frequently. Advise him that he may experience hoarseness, loss of voice, and/or a sore throat.

—He should not eat or drink anything until the gag reflex has returned (usually 2 to 8 hours after the procedure).
—Lozenges and a gargle should ease his discomfort when his gag reflex returns.

LARYNGOSCOPY

Patient objectives	*Teaching plan content*
1 Define laryngoscopy.	Laryngoscopy is a procedure that permits direct visualization of the larynx by the use of a fiber-optic endoscope or laryngoscope.
2 State the purposes of laryngoscopy.	The purposes of laryngoscopy are as follows: —To detect lesions, strictures, or foreign bodies in the larynx —To aid in the diagnosis of laryngeal cancer —To remove benign lesions or foreign bodies from the larynx.
3 Describe the procedure used in laryngoscopy.	The patient will receive a sedative and atropine about 30 to 60 minutes before the procedure. —He will be placed in the supine position. —A general anesthetic will be administered, or his mouth and throat will be sprayed with a local anesthetic. —His head will be positioned and held while the physician introduces the laryngoscope through his mouth. —During the procedure the larynx will be examined for abnormalities and secretions and/or a specimen will be obtained for analysis. —The patient should know who will perform the test and where and when it will be done.
4 Discuss patient guidelines for laryngoscopy.	Patient guidelines include the following: —He must fast for 6 to 8 hours before the procedure. —Just before the procedure, he should empty his bladder and remove dentures, jewelry, and contact lenses. —During the procedure, he should remain relaxed, breathe through his nose, and keep his arms at his sides. —After the laryngoscopy, his vital signs will be checked frequently. —An ice-collar may be applied to prevent laryngeal edema. —The patient should spit saliva into an emesis basin, rather than swallow it. —If a biopsy was performed, he should refrain from

clearing his throat or coughing, which could dislodge the clot at the biopsy site and precipitate a hemorrhage.
—He should avoid smoking until his vital signs are stable.
—Foods and fluids will be restricted until the gag reflex returns (2 to 8 hours).
—He may experience voice loss, hoarseness, and/or sore throat. These symptoms are only temporary.

LUNG SCAN (Lung perfusion scan or lung scintiscan)

Patient objectives	*Teaching plan content*
1 Define a lung scan.	A lung scan is a radiographic study in which a contrast medium is used to visualize blood flow through the lung tissue.
2 State the purpose of a lung scan.	The purpose of a lung scan is to confirm the presence of an obstruction in the lungs' vascular system. A lung scan performed with a ventilation scan assesses ventilation-perfusion (air exchange) patterns.
3 Describe the procedure used in a lung scan.	The procedure is painless and is performed with the patient sitting up or supine. —The contrast agent is injected into a vein in the patient's arm, and the amount of radioactivity is minimal. —Half the contrast agent is injected I.V. while the patient is supine, the other half while he is prone. —After the uptake of the contrast agent, the gamma camera takes a series of single stationary images of the anterior (front), posterior (back), and both lateral (side) chest views. —These images are projected onto an oscilloscope screen and show the distribution of radioactive particles. —The procedure takes 15 to 30 minutes, and the patient should know who will perform it and where and when.
4 Discuss patient guidelines for a lung scan.	Patient guidelines for a lung scan include the following: —The patient need not restrict foods or fluids before the test. —Neither the camera nor the uptake probe emits any radiation. —The patient does not have to remain perfectly still during the procedure. —He may resume his pretest activities immediately after the test.

PULMONARY ANGIOGRAPHY (Pulmonary arteriography)

Patient objectives	*Teaching plan content*
1 Define pulmonary angiography.	Pulmonary angiography is the radiographic examination of the pulmonary blood circulation, using a dye injected in a blood vessel for visualization.
2 State the purpose of pulmonary angiography.	The purpose of pulmonary angiography is to detect defects in pulmonary vascular perfusion, such as pulmonary embolism (blood clot) or aneurysm (ballooning of a blood vessel wall). It is usually performed on a patient who is symptomatic but whose lung scan shows no abnormalities.
3 Describe the procedure used in pulmonary angiography.	The patient is taken to the X-ray department, placed on the X-ray table in a supine position, and draped with sterile sheets. —EKG leads are attached to his chest to monitor his heart, and an I.V. line is inserted into his arm, if medications are needed. —After the area is cleansed, a local anesthetic (2% procaine) is injected into the catheter insertion site (the right arm or right groin). —Through a small incision, a catheter is introduced into the antecubital (arm) or femoral (groin) vein. —As the catheter is advanced through the heart (the right atrium, right ventricle, and pulmonary artery), pressures are measured and blood specimens obtained. —The contrast agent is then injected, and it circulates through the pulmonary artery and lung capillaries while X-ray films are taken and videotape recorded. —The patient's heart rate/rhythm and vital signs are continuously monitored during the procedure. —At the end of the procedure, the catheter is removed and a pressure dressing applied. —The test takes approximately 1 hour. The patient should know who will perform it and when.
4 Discuss patient guidelines for pulmonary angiography.	Patient guidelines for pulmonary angiography include the following: —The patient must fast for 8 hours before the test or as ordered. —The site where the catheter is to be inserted will be shaved and cleansed. —The patient will be asked to empty his bladder the morning of the procedure, since he will not be able to walk to the bathroom once the procedure begins. —He will be given a sedative to help him relax, but he

will remain awake throughout the procedure, as his cooperation will be needed.
—He may wear his eyeglasses and dentures; however, he should remove contact lenses to prevent discomfort and movement during the test due to eye irritation.
—He will be taken to the pulmonary laboratory via litter; how far family members may accompany him and where they will wait depends on hospital policy.
—The pulmonary laboratory should be described for the patient or, if possible, he should visit it before the procedure to meet staff members and to become familiar with the equipment and its use.
—For approximately 5 minutes after the dye is injected, the patient may experience an urge to cough, a flushed feeling, nausea, or a salty taste. He must remain still throughout the procedure.
—After the test, he will be returned to his room and may eat or drink what he chooses.
—His vital signs will be monitored closely. The dressing and the peripheral pulses of the involved extremity will be checked frequently for about 8 hours after the procedure.
—He should report any of the following side effects to the nurse immediately:

- Dyspnea
- Itching
- Palpitations
- Anxiety
- Light-headedness.

PLEURAL FLUID ANALYSIS (Thoracentesis)

Patient objectives	*Teaching plan content*
1 Define pleural fluid analysis.	Pleural fluid analysis assesses the fluid in the space around the lungs.
2 State the purpose of pleural fluid analysis.	The purpose of pleural fluid analysis is to obtain a fluid specimen and determine the cause and nature of pleural effusion (fluid collection around the lungs).
3 Describe the procedure used in pleural fluid analysis.	Pleural fluid analysis is usually done at the patient's bedside. —The patient puts on a hospital gown, and his vital signs are checked. —The area where the needle will be inserted is shaved, if necessary. —The patient is positioned in one of three ways: • Sitting on the edge of his bed with a chair or stool

supporting his feet and his head and arms resting on a padded overbed table
• Sitting up in bed with his head and arms resting on a padded overbed table
• Lying on his unaffected side with the arm on the affected side elevated above his head.

—The site is cleansed, and a local anesthetic is injected.
—The physician then inserts a needle and withdraws pleural fluid.
—After the needle is withdrawn, a small adhesive bandage is applied to the puncture site.

4 Discuss patient guidelines for pleural fluid analysis.

Patient guidelines for pleural fluid analysis include the following:
—The patient need not restrict foods or fluids before the procedure.
—He may feel a stinging sensation when the anesthetic is injected.
—He may experience some pressure during withdrawal of the fluid.
—He should not cough, breathe deeply, or move during the test.
—After the test, he will be repositioned comfortably on the affected side and should remain on that side for at least 1 hour, to seal the puncture site.
—His vital signs will be monitored frequently, and the dressing over the puncture site will be inspected.
—He should call the nurse immediately if he experiences any difficulty breathing.
—He should expect to have a chest X-ray taken to assess lung function after the fluid is removed.

PULMONARY FUNCTION TESTS

Patient objectives / ***Teaching plan content***

1 Define pulmonary function tests.

Pulmonary function tests are a series of measurements that evaluate lung function.

2 State the purposes of pulmonary function tests.

The purposes of pulmonary function tests are as follows:
—To determine the cause of dyspnea
—To assess the effectiveness of specific therapeutic regimens
—To evaluate disability for legal or insurance purposes.

3 Describe the procedure used in pulmonary function tests.

The patient is taken to the pulmonary laboratory, where the test is performed by a technician or a physician.

—The patient is asked to put on and adjust a nose clip before the test and then verify that he cannot pass any air through his nose.

—The patient is then asked to do the following breathing procedures, using various mouthpieces, as various pulmonary parameters are tested:

- For a test of tidal volume, he is told to breathe normally into the mouthpiece 10 times.
- For a test of expiratory reserve volume, he is instructed to breathe into the mouthpiece 10 times and to exhale as completely as possible at the end of each breath.
- For a test of vital capacity, he is told to inhale as deeply as possible and to exhale into the mouthpiece as completely as possible. This procedure is repeated three times; the test result showing the largest volume is used.
- For a test of inspiratory capacity, he is instructed to inhale fully, to exhale normally into the mouthpiece, and then to breathe normally 10 times, inhaling as deeply as possible after the 10th breath.
- For a test of functional residual capacity, he is told to breathe normally into a spirometer that contains a known concentration of an insoluble gas (helium or nitrogen). After a few breaths, the concentrations of gas in the spirometer and in the lungs reach equilibrium.
- For a test of force vital capacity and force expiratory volume, he is instructed to inhale as slowly and as deeply as possible and then to exhale into the mouthpiece as quickly and as fully as possible. This is repeated three times, and the largest volume is recorded.
- For a test of maximal voluntary ventilation, he is instructed to breathe into the mouthpiece as quickly and as deeply as possible for 15 seconds.

4 Discuss patient guidelines for pulmonary function tests.

Patient guidelines for pulmonary function tests include the following:

—If the patient wears dentures, he should wear them during the test to ensure a tight seal around the mouthpiece.

—He should not eat a heavy meal before the test; this can cause gastric distention, which may restrict pulmonary function.

—He should not smoke for 4 to 6 hours before the test.

—He should void immediately before the test.
—He should wear loose-fitting clothes, so his breathing is not restricted.
—The accuracy of this test depends on his cooperation, so he should listen carefully to instructions.
—The procedure is painless, and if he tires during it, he can rest.
—After the test, he should rest for a period of time; he may then resume his diet, activities, and medication as before the test.

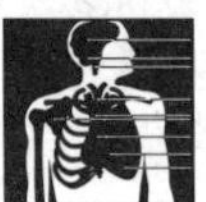

Explaining disorders

ASTHMA

Patient objectives	*Teaching plan content*
1 Define asthma.	Asthma is a chronic disease of variable severity, characterized by episodes of airway narrowing that temporarily produces breathing difficulty.
2 Identify four factors that can trigger an asthma attack.	Factors that can trigger an asthma attack include the following: —Respiratory infections —Exposure to allergens —Emotional factors —Environmental changes, such as air temperature, humidity, and dust.
3 Explain how airway obstruction occurs in asthma.	Although the exact cause of asthma is unknown, obstruction of the airway passages occurs as a result of one or more of the following: —Spasms of bronchial smooth muscles narrow the passages, possibly because of an irritant. —Inflammation may also occur, further narrowing the airways by causing swelling of the mucous membranes lining the airways. —Inflammation also produces thick mucus secretions, causing further obstruction.
4 Identify at least five symptoms associated with asthma.	Symptoms of asthma include the following: —Wheezing —Prolonged expiration —Dyspnea —Physical exhaustion

—Inability to sleep or rest
—Anxiety
—Dehydration
—Thick, tenacious mucus production
—Use of accessory muscles of respiration; retractions.

5 State the goals of treatment for asthma.

The goals of the treatment regimen for asthma are as follows:
—To help the patient maintain optimal breathing function by relieving airway obstruction and providing adequate arterial oxygenation
—To help the patient maintain an optimal activity level
—To reduce coughing and sputum production
—To treat infections
—To prevent acute asthma attacks.

6 Identify five measures for the prevention of asthma attacks.

Preventive measures include the following:
—Avoiding the following bronchopulmonary irritants:
- Cigarette smoke
- Industrial pollutants
- Animal hair
- Dust
- Powder, perfume
- Weeds, pollen, grasses
- Extreme heat or cold

—Avoiding known allergens
—Avoiding distressing situations
—Avoiding people with respiratory infections
—Practicing good oral hygiene to help prevent infection.

7 Identify the components of the treatment regimen for asthma.

Components of the treatment regimen for asthma include the following:
—Medications
—A balanced, nutritious diet with small, frequent meals
—Oxygen therapy
—Stress management
—Regular medical examinations.

8 Describe the medication regimen.

Some drugs commonly used for this disorder are aminophylline, cromolyn sodium, ephedrine sulfate, epinephrine inhalant, prednisone, terbutaline sulfate, and theophylline. See Chapter 9, Drug Therapy, for specific medication instructions.

9 Identify at least three deep-muscle relaxation techniques to reduce stress.

Deep-muscle relaxation techniques include the following:
—Taped relaxation exercises
—Relaxation cues

	—Deep breathing —Imagery —Progressive muscle relaxation. For a detailed explanation of these techniques, see the "Hypertension" teaching plan in Chapter 2, Cardiovascular Disorders.
10 Explain the importance of routine medical examinations.	Routine medical follow-up is very important even after good control has been obtained. It ensures that the treatment is maintaining optimal respiratory function. If not, damage can be detected, and the treatment regimen can be supplemented to prevent serious consequences.

BRONCHIECTASIS

Patient objectives	*Teaching plan content*
1 Define bronchiectasis.	Bronchiectasis is a chronic pulmonary condition characterized by abnormal dilation of the large air passages leading into the lungs (bronchi) and destruction of bronchial walls.
2 Explain the cause of bronchiectasis.	Bronchiectasis is caused by repeated damage to bronchial walls. The resulting destruction and bronchial dilation reduce bronchial wall movement so that secretions cannot be removed effectively from the lungs.
3 Identify at least four health problems that can cause repeated damage to bronchial walls.	Health problems that can cause repeated damage to the bronchial walls include the following: —Mucoviscidosis (cystic fibrosis of the pancreas) —Inhalation of corrosive gas —Repeated aspiration of gastric juices into the lungs —Obstruction by a foreign body/tumor, in association with recurrent infection —Immunologic disorders —Recurrent or inadequately treated bacterial respiratory tract infections, such as tuberculosis, pneumonia, or influenza.
4 Identify at least four symptoms of bronchiectasis.	Symptoms of bronchiectasis include the following: —Chronic cough —Hemoptysis (bloody sputum) —Copious, foul-smelling, mucopurulent secretions —Occasional wheezing sounds —Dyspnea

—Sinusitis
—Weight loss
—Anemia
—Malaise
—Recurrent fever
—Chills.

5 Identify the components of the treatment regimen for bronchiectasis.	Components of the treatment regimen for bronchiectasis include the following: —Medications, including antibiotics and bronchodilators —Postural drainage and chest percussion —Oxygen therapy —Bronchoscopy, which may occasionally be used to help clear secretions.
6 State the goals of treatment for bronchiectasis.	Goals of bronchiectasis treatment include the following: —Avoidance of infections —Aggressive management of existing infections —Liquefaction of sputum —Removal of secretions —Promotion of rest.
7 Describe the medication regimen.	Some drugs commonly used for this disorder are aminophylline, cromolyn sodium, ephedrine sulfate, epinephrine inhalant, penicillin G procaine, prednisone, terbutaline sulfate, and theophylline. See Chapter 9, Drug Therapy, for a discussion of bronchodilators and antibiotics.
8 State guidelines for daily living with bronchiectasis.	Guidelines for daily living with bronchiectasis include the following: —Stop smoking. —Get adequate rest. —Eat balanced, high-protein meals. —Drink fluids, to aid expectoration. —Dispose of all secretions properly. —Avoid air pollutants. —Avoid people with respiratory infections.

CHRONIC BRONCHITIS

Patient objectives	*Teaching plan content*
1 Define chronic bronchitis.	Chronic bronchitis is an inflammation of the windpipe, the large passages of the lungs, and their branches (the tracheobronchial tree) that produces hypersecretion of bronchial mucus.

2 Explain the cause of chronic bronchitis.	Chronic bronchitis is the result of tissue irritation that causes hypertrophy of mucus-producing cells in the bronchi, thus increasing mucus secretion.
3 Identify health problems that can cause hypertrophy of mucus-producing cells.	Health problems that can cause hypertrophy of mucus-producing cells include the following: —Cigarette smoke —Air pollutants —Toxic industrial gases or chemicals —Chronic respiratory infections.
4 Identify at least four symptoms of chronic bronchitis.	Symptoms of chronic bronchitis include the following: —Persistent cough with sputum production —Reduced chest expansion —Wheezing sounds —Sensation of heaviness in the chest —Fever —Dusky or cyanotic skin color —Shortness of breath (dyspnea).
5 Identify the components of the treatment regimen for chronic bronchitis.	The treatment regimen for chronic bronchitis includes the following: —Antibiotic therapy to ameliorate any respiratory infections —Bronchodilators to relieve bronchospasm and facilitate clearance of mucus —Adequate fluid intake and chest physiotherapy to mobilize secretions —Ultrasonic or mechanical nebulizer treatments to loosen secretions and aid in mobilization —Corticosteroids to alleviate the effects of inflammation —Oxygen therapy to diminish hypoxia and improve oxygenation —Breathing retraining to minimize dyspnea.
6 State the goals of treatment for chronic bronchitis.	The goals of treatment for chronic bronchitis include the following: —Minimizing bronchial irritation —Controlling chronic respiratory infections and promptly treating intercurrent acute infections —Preventing further infections —Relieving bronchospasm —Minimizing dyspnea by breathing retraining —Facilitating the raising of sputum and the clearing of air passages.
7 Describe the medication regimen.	Some drugs commonly used for this disorder are aminophylline, ampicillin, cromolyn sodium, ephedrine sul-

fate, epinephrine inhalant, prednisone, terbutaline sulfate, tetracycline, and theophylline. See Chapter 9, Drug Therapy, for specific medication instructions.

8 Discuss guidelines for daily living with chronic bronchitis.

Guidelines for daily living with chronic bronchitis include the following:

—Avoid the following bronchopulmonary irritants:
- cigarette smoke
- industrial pollutants
- dust
- powder and perfume
- known allergens.

—Use an air-conditioning unit with an effective filtering system to help minimize bronchial irritation.

—Maintain a relatively high humidity level in the home, especially during the winter.

—Prevent chronic respiratory infections by:
- avoiding people with colds, influenza, and so forth
- seeking medical care at the beginning of any respiratory infection or influenza
- notifying the physician if sputum becomes purulent or if there is any change in its color or consistency.

9 Explain the importance of routine medical examinations.

Routine medical follow-up is important even after good control is achieved. It ensures that the treatment is maintaining optimal respiratory function. If not, damage can be detected, and the treatment regimen can be supplemented to prevent serious consequences.

EMPHYSEMA

Patient objectives	*Teaching plan content*
1 Define emphysema.	Emphysema is the accumulation of air in the lungs resulting from abnormal enlargement or overinflation of air sacs in the lungs (alveoli) and destruction of lung tissue.
2 Explain the cause of emphysema.	Emphysema is primarily a defect of the alveolar walls, which may result from various disorders and from repeated exposure to environmental factors. The air spaces become overinflated, the alveolar walls rupture, and the alveolar capillary bed is destroyed.
3 Identify risk factors for emphysema.	Several disorders and environmental factors can cause irreversible enlargement of alveoli and can destroy alveolar walls, decreasing the elasticity of the lungs. These risk factors include the following:

—Deficiency of alpha-antitrypsin
—Repeated exposure to bronchopulmonary irritants, such as:
- cigarette smoke
- air pollutants
- known allergens
- toxic industrial gases or chemicals.

—Chronic respiratory infections.

---

4 Identify at least five symptoms of emphysema.

Symptoms of emphysema include the following:
—Shortness of breath
—Dyspnea on exertion
—Chronic cough
—Barrel chest
—Weight loss
—Malaise
—Use of accessory muscles of respiration
—Prolonged expiratory period, with grunting
—Wheezing sounds
—Pursed-lip breathing
—Increased respiratory rate
—Peripheral cyanosis.

---

5 Identify the components of the treatment regimen for emphysema.

The treatment regimen for emphysema includes the following:
—Bronchodilators to reverse bronchospasm and promote clearance of mucus
—Antibiotics to treat respiratory infection
—Oxygen therapy at low flow settings to treat hypoxia
—Adequate hydration
—Chest physiotherapy to mobilize secretions.

---

6 State the goals of treatment for emphysema.

The goals of treatment for emphysema include the following:
—Avoiding bronchopulmonary irritants
—Controlling chronic respiratory infections and promptly treating intercurrent acute infections
—Controlling cough
—Assisting ventilation.

---

7 State guidelines for daily living with emphysema.

Guidelines for daily living with emphysema include the following:
—Avoid bronchopulmonary irritants.
—Take vaccines to prevent influenza and pneumococcal pneumonia.
—Avoid sedatives and narcotics, which can depress respiration.
—Minimize dyspnea by breathing retraining exercises,

such as the abdominal muscle breathing pattern and pursed-lip breathing. (See *How to Avoid Tiring Easily,* p. 115.)

8 Describe the medication regimen.	Some drugs commonly used for this disorder are aminophylline, cromolyn sodium, ephedrine sulfate, epinephrine inhalant, prednisone, terbutaline sulfate, and theophylline. See Chapter 9, Drug Therapy, for specific medication instructions.
9 Explain the importance of routine medical examinations.	Routine medical follow-up is important even after good control is achieved. It ensures that the treatment is maintaining optimal respiratory function. If not, damage can be detected, and the treatment regimen can be supplemented to prevent serious consequences.

PLEURITIS (Pleurisy)

Patient objectives	*Teaching plan content*
1 Identify the anatomic structures of the pleurae.	On an illustration, the patient should identify and state the function of the anatomic structures of the pleurae. —Each pleura consists of a thin membrane that doubles back on itself at the hilum, so that one (visceral) layer encases the lungs, and the other (parietal) layer lines the inner chest wall. —The two layers are held together by negative (subatmospheric) pressure that results from the natural tendency of lung and chest wall tissue to pull in opposite directions. —A thin layer of lymphatic (pleural) fluid lubricates the pleural surfaces to prevent friction during breathing. —The airtight pleural cavity becomes a real space only in an abnormal condition.
2 Define pleuritis.	Pleuritis is an inflammation of the visceral and parietal pleurae that line the inside of the chest cavity and cover the lungs.
3 State three possible causes of pleuritis.	Pleuritis is usually a complication caused by one of the following: —Pneumonia —Tuberculosis —Viruses —Systemic lupus erythematosus —Rheumatoid arthritis —Uremia

—Dressler's syndrome
—Malignancy
—Pulmonary infarction
—Chest trauma.

4 Describe the symptoms of pleuritis.	Symptoms of pleuritis include the following: —Sharp, stabbing pain that worsens with respiration —Splinting of the afflicted area —Dyspnea.
5 Identify the components of the treatment regimen for pleuritis.	The treatment of pleuritis is aimed at relieving symptoms and may include the following: —Medications, such as anti-inflammatory agents and analgesics, for mild to moderate pain —Intercostal nerve block for severe pain —Bed rest during the acute phase —Possible thoracentesis, if pleuritis is complicated by pleural effusion —Coughing (the patient can minimize pain by applying firm pressure at the site of the pain during coughing).
6 Describe the medication regimen.	Some drugs commonly used for this disorder are aspirin and codeine. See Chapter 9, Drug Therapy, for specific medication instructions.

PULMONARY EMBOLISM

Patient objectives	*Teaching plan content*
1 Describe the anatomy of the pulmonary vasculature.	On an illustration, the patient should identify and/or discuss the anatomy of the pulmonary vasculature, including the following: —Position in the body —Location and relation to the cardiac system —Blood supply to the pulmonary system by the pulmonary and bronchial arteries —Exchange of gases between the air and blood in the terminal alveolar capillaries, which requires an intact vascular system.
2 Define pulmonary embolism.	Pulmonary embolism is an obstruction of a pulmonary or bronchial artery by a dislodged thrombus (clot) or other tissue, air, or fluid.
3 Describe thrombus/embolus formation.	A thrombus/embolus forms in the following manner: —Arterial thrombi are formed by the clumping of circulating platelets to an abnormal vessel wall. A venous

thrombus occurs in areas of stagnation and slow blood flow.
—As the thrombus becomes larger in diameter and length, it obstructs the vein.
—The newly formed venous thrombus has a tail that may become attached and develop into a pulmonary embolism.
—The embolus travels through the veins to the right side of the heart and into the pulmonary artery.

4 State the causes of pulmonary embolism.

The causes of pulmonary embolism include the following:
—Air
—Fat
—Amniotic fluid
—Neoplasms
—Thrombi.

5 Identify measures that can prevent thrombus formation.

Measures to help prevent thrombus formation include the following:
—Passive dorsiflexion of the foot and active exercises in bed for the postoperative or postpartum patient or the patient on prolonged bed rest
—Early postoperative ambulation
—Elastic support hose
—Deep-breathing exercises
—Avoidance of tight garters and girdles.

6 Identify at least four symptoms of pulmonary embolism.

Symptoms of pulmonary embolism include the following:
—Pleuritic chest pain
—Diffuse chest discomfort
—Increased respiratory rate
—Tachycardia (rapid heartbeat)
—Hemoptysis (bloody sputum)
—Anxiety, restlessness, apprehension
—Dyspnea, cough.

7 State the goals of pulmonary embolism management.

The goals of pulmonary embolism management include the following:
—Maintaining adequate heart and lung functions
—Preventing embolism recurrence.

8 Identify the components of the treatment regimen for pulmonary embolism.

The treatment regimen for pulmonary embolism includes the following:
—Oxygen therapy to maintain adequate oxygenation
—Anticoagulant therapy to prevent propagation and platelet adhesion on the surface of thrombi

	—Fibrinolytic therapy to dissolve thrombi (See the "Streptokinase Infusion" teaching plan in Chapter 2, Cardiovascular Disorders, for further instruction.) —Surgical intervention, if anticoagulant therapy is not advised or effective.
9 Describe the medication regimen.	Some drugs commonly used for this disorder are heparin and warfarin sodium. See Chapter 9, Drug Therapy, for specific medication instructions.

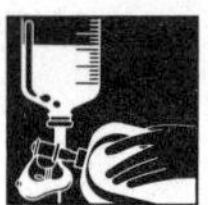

Explaining treatments

INTERMITTENT POSITIVE-PRESSURE BREATHING (I.P.P.B.)

Patient objectives	*Teaching plan content*
1 State the purposes of IPPB.	The purposes of IPPB are to expand the lung volume and promote an effective cough, to deliver aerosolized medications deeper into the air passages, and to assist in mobilizing secretions.
2 Describe the procedure used in IPPB.	The IPPB machine delivers room air or oxygen into the lungs at a pressure higher than atmospheric pressure. This delivery ceases when the pressure in the mouth or in the breathing circuit tube achieves a preset positive pressure. —The patient will sit erect in a chair, if possible, to allow for optimal lung expansion; if not, he will lie in semi-Fowler's position. —The plastic mouthpiece or mask he uses during treatment will be attached to the tubing of the IPPB machine. —He will be asked to breathe deeply and slowly through his mouth, allowing the machine to do the work. Slow, deep breathing cycles the machine which, in turn, delivers a breath to the patient. —The patient should hold each breath for a few seconds, then exhale normally. —The treatment lasts for about 15 to 20 minutes.
3 Discuss patient guidelines for the IPPB procedure.	The patient should cough and expectorate any sputum. If he wears dentures, he should leave them in place to ensure a proper seal.

INCENTIVE SPIROMETRY

Patient objectives	*Teaching plan content*
1 State the purpose of incentive spirometry.	The purpose of incentive spirometry is to establish alveolar hyperinflation for a longer time than is possible with a normal deep breath, thus preventing and/or reversing alveolar collapse.
2 Demonstrate the procedure for using an incentive spirometer.	The patient should do the following: —He should insert the end of the mouthpiece and close his lips tightly around it (a loose seal may alter flow or volume readings). —He should exhale normally and then inhale to the predetermined level. —When he inhales to the preset level, he should hold his breath for 3 seconds or until the light turns off, to achieve maximal alveolar inflation. —He should then remove the mouthpiece and exhale normally. —Next, he should relax and take a few normal breaths. —He should cough after each effort, because deep lung inflation may loosen secretions and facilitate their removal. —He should know that 10 breaths/hour while awake is adequate.

CHEST PHYSIOTHERAPY (Chest PT or CPT)

Patient objectives	*Teaching plan content*
1 State the purposes of chest physiotherapy.	The purposes of chest physiotherapy are to mobilize and eliminate secretions, to reexpand lung tissue, and to promote the efficient use of respiratory muscles.
2 Identify the components of chest physiotherapy.	Chest physiotherapy includes postural drainage, chest percussion, and coughing/deep-breathing exercises.
3 Identify at least three indications for chest physiotherapy.	Indications for chest physiotherapy include the following: —Bronchiectasis —Cystic fibrosis —Bronchitis —Emphysema —Prolonged immobility

—Postoperative decreases in chest expansion because of pain.

4 Describe the procedure used in chest physiotherapy.

Before starting chest physiotherapy, the health care provider will listen to the patient's lungs to determine a baseline respiratory status. Postural drainage encourages secretions to empty by gravity into the major bronchi or trachea and involves sequential repositioning of the patient.

—The patient will be positioned according to his physician's orders, if specific areas of the lung are affected. In generalized disease, drainage usually begins with the lower lobes and ends with the upper lobes.

—He must remain in each position for 10 to 15 minutes. During this time, the health care provider will perform percussion and vibration, as ordered.

—Three techniques are commonly used during each chest physiotherapy session: percussion, vibration, and deep-breathing exercises.

—During percussion, the patient must breathe slowly and deeply, using his diaphragm, to promote relaxation. (See *How to Breathe Easier, Using Your Diaphragm*, p. 114.) The health care provider percusses the area over each segment of the lung with cupped hands for 1 to 2 minutes, alternating hands in a rhythmic manner.

—During vibration, the patient must inhale deeply and then exhale slowly through pursed lips. During exhalation, the health care provider firmly presses his hands against the patient's chest wall. The health care provider then tenses the muscles of his arms and shoulders in an isometric contraction to send fine vibrations through the patient's chest wall. After exhaling in three short huffs, the patient must inhale and cough deeply.

—To perform deep-breathing exercises, the patient must assume a sitting position to promote optimal lung expansion. Then he proceeds as follows:

- He places one hand on his chest and the other on his abdomen just below his ribs, to feel the rise and fall of his diaphragm.
- He inhales slowly and deeply, pushing his abdomen out against his hand, to provide optimal distribution of air to the alveoli.
- He then exhales through pursed lips and contracts his abdomen.
- He must perform the exercises for 1 minute, then rest for 2 minutes.

—If chest physiotherapy is to be continued at home, he will be told who will provide the service and when. (If the patient will be responsible for postural drainage, specific home care instructions must be provided. See *How to Do Postural Drainage Exercises,* pp. 116-117.)

OXYGEN THERAPY

Patient objectives	*Teaching plan content*
1 State the purpose of oxygen therapy.	The purpose of oxygen therapy is to prevent or reverse hypoxia (decreased oxygen level) and improve tissue oxygenation.
2 Identify at least three indications for oxygen therapy.	Indications for oxygen therapy include the following: —Decreased oxygen level —Decreased cardiac output (decreased blood flow from the heart) —Dysrhythmias (rhythm changes of the heart), particularly ventricular —Myocardial infarction (heart attack) —Hypovolemia (low blood volume) —Increased vascular resistance —Atelectasis (lung collapse) —Carbon monoxide poisoning —Burns —Methemoglobinemia —Chronic obstructive pulmonary disease.
3 Describe the procedure used to initiate oxygen therapy.	One of three types of oxygen delivery equipment is commonly used to initiate oxygen therapy: cannula, catheter, or mask. —For the oxygen to be effective, the equipment must be used correctly and consistently. —The patient should keep his skin dry under the oxygen devices and tubing to prevent breakdown caused by humidity and perspiration. —Because the mask must be removed for eating, the physician may order a cannula for use during meals if the patient becomes short of breath.
4 Discuss patient guidelines for home use of oxygen therapy.	Guidelines for using oxygen therapy at home include the following: —There must be absolutely no smoking in the vicinity of oxygen. —Only properly grounded (three-pronged) electrical devices (for example, clocks and radios) should be used in the vicinity of the oxygen. —Since oxygen has no odor, color, or taste, its source must be checked regularly for patency and possible chemical contamination.

—If an oxygen cylinder is being used, a second cylinder should be kept readily available.
—Gauze squares placed behind the ears and at pressure points help to alleviate the problems of skin breakdown.
—The oxygen flow rate must be correctly set.
—For instructions on the use of oxygen at home, see *How to Care for Oxygen at Home,* p. 121.

VENA CAVA UMBRELLA

Patient objectives	*Teaching plan content*
1 State the purpose of the vena cava umbrella.	The purpose of the vena cava umbrella is to obstruct the flow of emboli into the pulmonary vasculature.
2 Describe the procedure used to insert the vena cava umbrella.	This device has been developed for use in patients who are unable to tolerate major surgery under a general anesthetic. —An umbrella-like filter is inserted under a local anesthetic, either percutaneously or transvenously (by cutdown), usually in the jugular vein, and advanced to the inferior vena cava below the renal veins. —The filter device, which is folded around the catheter tip, is then opened, much like an umbrella, to obstruct the flow of emboli while not obstructing blood flow.
3 Describe postoperative care for the vena cava umbrella procedure.	The patient will be taken to the intensive care unit (ICU) immediately after the procedure. —The patient and his family should know that he will see unfamiliar equipment and hear unusual noises in the recovery room and the ICU. If time permits, a preoperative visit to the operating room and ICU for the patient and his family would be helpful. See also Appendix B, *Preoperative and Postoperative Teaching,* in this manual. —A nurse will check him frequently and explain this strange environment. —The patient may be connected to a mechanical ventilator (breathing machine) or a cardiac monitor following surgery. —He may have an indwelling urinary drainage system (Foley catheter), possibly an arterial line, and a central venous pressure or pulmonary artery pressure line. —He must do deep-breathing and coughing exercises during his recovery. —He should ask for medication as he begins to experience any postoperative pain.

4 Discuss patient guidelines for the postoperative/recuperative phase.

Postoperative guidelines after vena cava umbrella insertion include the following:

—Once the special equipment has been removed and the patient's physical parameters are stable, he will be transferred from the ICU to a regular unit in the hospital.

—The patient should follow these guidelines at home:

- Wear elastic stockings daily.
- Do not sit with crossed legs in bed.
- Avoid sitting in a chair with the legs dependent.
- Perform active and passive leg exercises at least twice a day, or walk in accordance with the level of activity permitted.
- Notify the physician immediately if sudden shortness of breath or chest pain occurs, because reembolization is still possible.

Patient-Teaching Aid

EFFECTIVE BREATHING TECHNIQUES

Dear Patient:
To help prevent acute episodes of chronic obstructive pulmonary disease, learn to control your breathing by using either the abdominal or pursed-lip method. By practicing these methods regularly and using them during all your activities, you can keep your lungs free of stale air and gain confidence in managing your disorder.

1 Abdominal breathing

Lie comfortably on your back with your knees bent, and relax your abdomen.

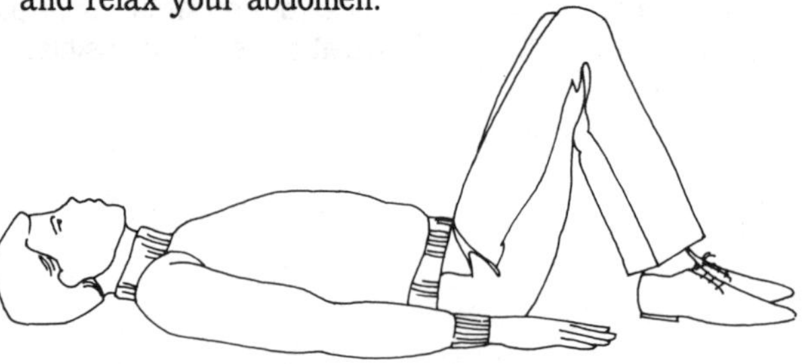

2

Next, press your hands (or place a book) lightly on your abdomen to create resistance.

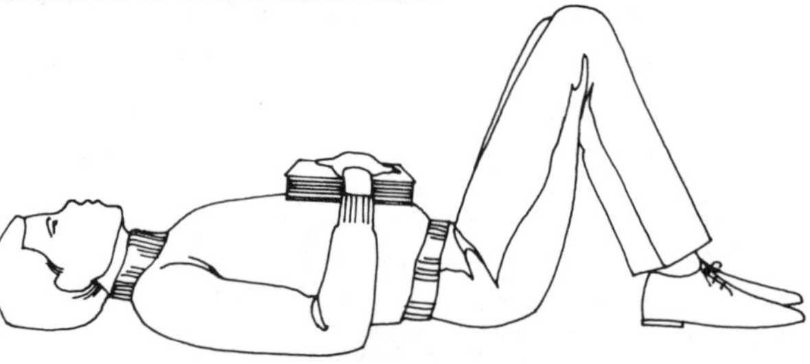

3

Keeping your chest still, begin breathing abdominally. You are performing the technique correctly if your abdomen and hands (or book) rise as you breathe in and fall as you breathe out.

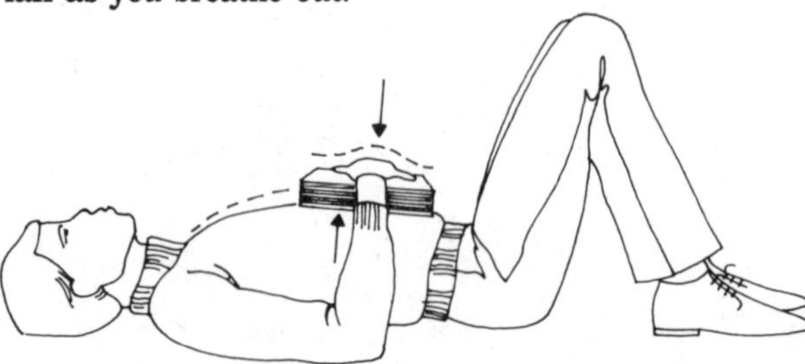

EFFECTIVE BREATHING TECHNIQUES—*continued*

1 Pursed-lip breathing

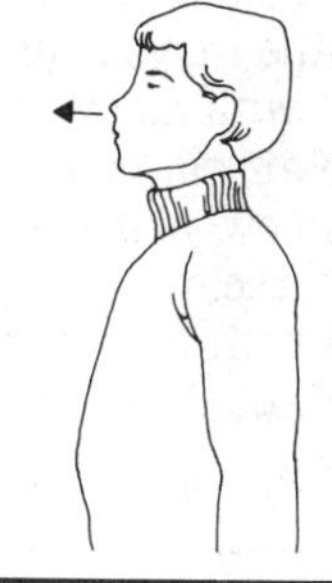

Close your mouth and breathe in through your nose, taking a normal breath. (If you take too large a breath, you will have to exhale much more air.)

2

Now, purse your lips as you would to whistle, and breathe out slowly through your mouth, without puffing your cheeks. Take at least twice the time you took to breathe in. Use your abdominal muscles to squeeze out every last bit of air you can.

3

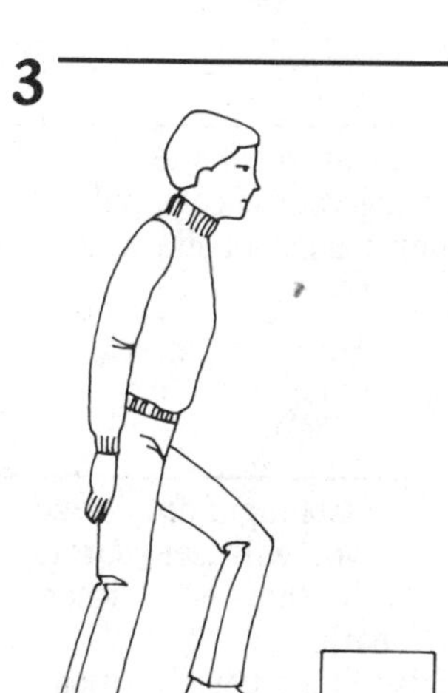

During physical activity, always inhale before exerting yourself; exhale while performing the activity. For example, when walking up stairs, inhale between steps; exhale while climbing.

Patient-Teaching Aid

HOW TO BREATHE EASIER, USING YOUR DIAPHRAGM

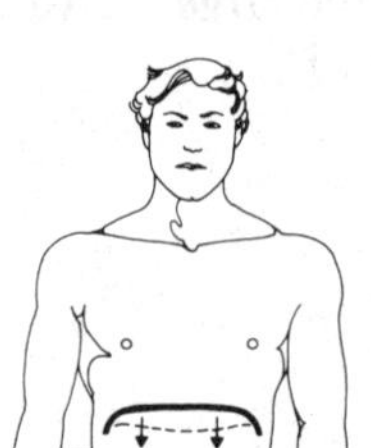

Dear Patient:
The diaphragm is a dome-shaped muscle between your lungs and abdomen. When you breathe in, your diaphragm drops so your lungs can fill with air. When you breathe out, it rises and pushes the air out of your lungs. The illustration at left shows how your diaphragm changes position as you breathe.

You can breathe more deeply and with less effort by letting your diaphragm work for you. Learn to use it effectively by following these steps:

1

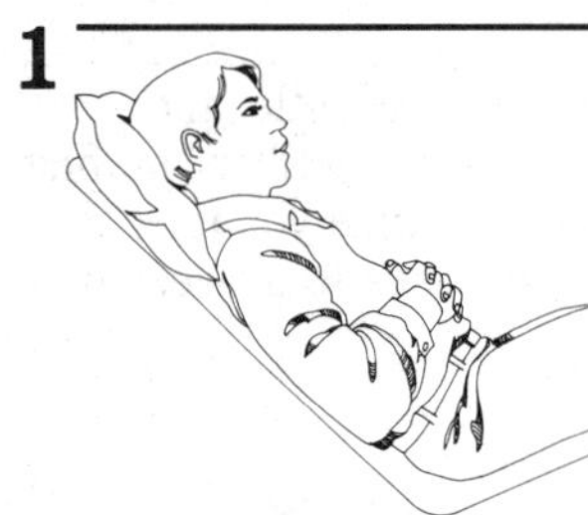

Sit in a comfortable, reclining position with your back well supported, as shown here. Support your head with a pillow. Place both hands on your abdomen just below your ribs. Relax your neck, shoulders, and arms.

2

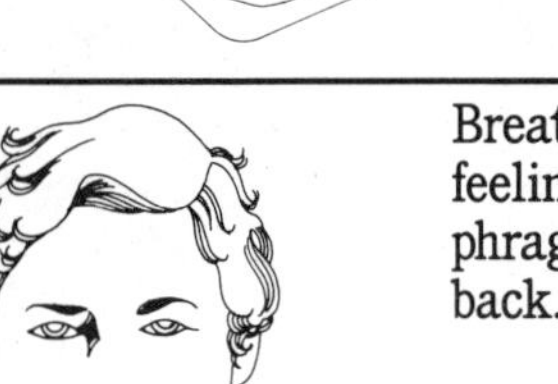

Breathe in gently through your nose. Concentrate on feeling your abdomen rise, which allows your diaphragm to drop. Stay relaxed, and do not arch your back.

3

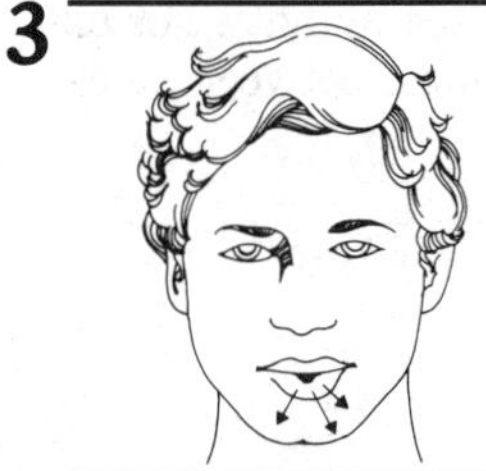

Purse your lips as if you were about to whistle. Breathe out gently without letting your cheeks puff out. Concentrate on feeling your abdomen sink, which allows your diaphragm to rise.

4

If you have trouble making your diaphragm drop, take a quick sniff through your nose—you will feel your abdomen rise. Now, try to produce the same effect when you take a longer and slower breath.

After you can do this exercise in a sitting position, practice it in other positions: lying flat on your back with a pillow under your head, sitting upright, and standing.

Use this exercise whenever you feel short of breath. With practice, you can even use it to help you breathe more easily while walking.

Patient-Teaching Aid

HOW TO AVOID TIRING EASILY

Dear Patient:

The nurse taught you various deep-breathing exercises while you were in the hospital. Now that you are going home, observe the following guidelines to help you breathe better and tire less quickly.

— Avoid rushing by planning your day carefully. For example, if you have a scheduled activity, get up a little earlier. That way, you will have time to get ready for the activity without hurrying.

—Spread your activities out over the day. For example, do not do all your chores in the morning. Save some for the afternoon or the next day.

—Rest between activities.

—Practice deep breathing regularly, at least every 2 hours while you are awake. Remember to use your abdominal muscles. Breathe out with your lips pursed. Breathing out should last twice as long as breathing in. Also use an incentive spirometer if you have one.

—Use deep breathing while performing any active movement, such as sweeping or mopping, or with any activities that require you to raise your arms, such as lifting packages or combing your hair. Coordinate your movement with breathing, as shown below.

NOTE: Whenever possible, avoid working with your arms raised, which can tire you more quickly. Work with objects at waist level instead.

1

Inhale deeply, using your abdominal muscles.

2

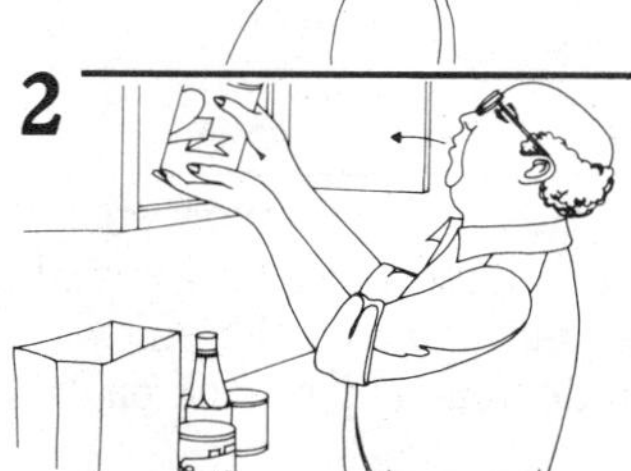

Exhale through pursed lips, lift your arms, and put a package on the shelf.

3

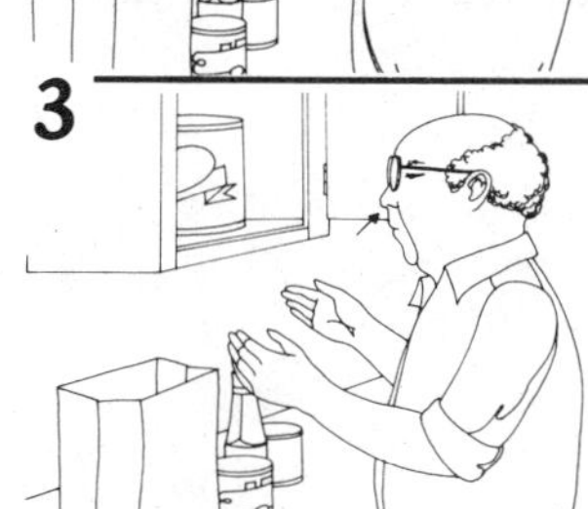

Lower your arms and inhale again.

Then raise your arms while exhaling, and put another package on the shelf.

Repeat these steps as necessary. REMEMBER: Always perform the activity while exhaling.

Patient-Teaching Aid

HOW TO DO POSTURAL DRAINAGE EXERCISES

Dear Patient:
These exercises will help you clear your lungs of mucus. You will need a helper. Do not forget to take deep breaths, fully expand your chest, and cough with each new position.

When the exercises call for clapping, have your helper cup his hands, keeping his fingers and thumb close together. The sound made by the cupped hand tapping the chest must be hollow, not slapping. Have him use both hands in a uniform rhythm, keeping his wrists flexible and elbows slightly bent. Continue for 1½ to 2 minutes. During clapping, always cover the chest with a gown or towel.

When exercises call for vibration, have your helper place his hands flat, directly on the percussed area. Take a deep breath. As you exhale, have your helper vibrate his arms. Repeat the vibration at least three times. Make sure the pressure applied is forceful but not excessive.

1

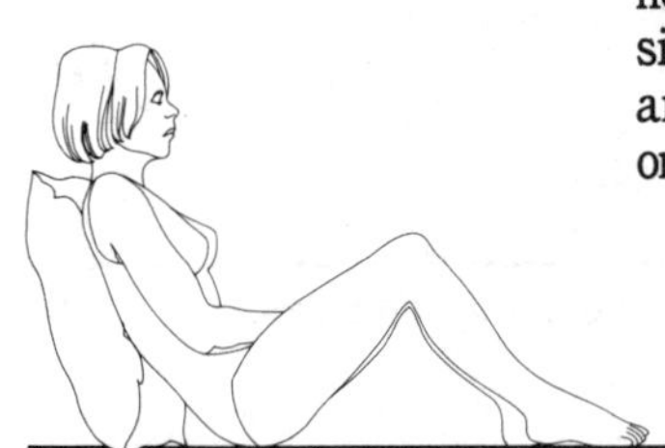

With pillows behind you, sit on a chair and lean back from your waist at a 30-degree angle. Have your partner clap your upper chest just below the collarbone, one side at a time. He should stand behind you, placing one arm around your neck so that both hands fit easily on one side of your chest.

2

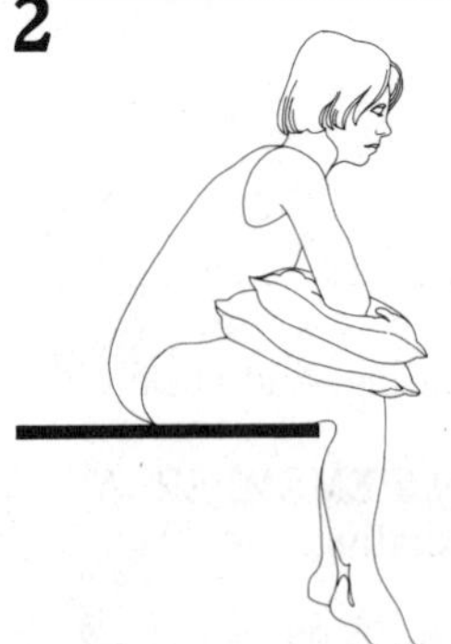

Sit on the edge of your bed. Place a folded pillow on your lap or over the back of the chair and lean forward at a 30-degree angle, resting your arms on the pillow. Have your helper clap or vibrate your upper back on the shoulder blades.

HOW TO DO POSTURAL DRAINAGE EXERCISES—*continued*

3

Lie down. Place pillows under your hips and legs to keep your legs about 16″ (41 cm) higher than your head. Lie on your left side, with a small pillow under your head and pillows behind your back. Lean back slightly on the pillows. Have your helper clap or vibrate the front of your chest over the nipple and just below it on the right side.

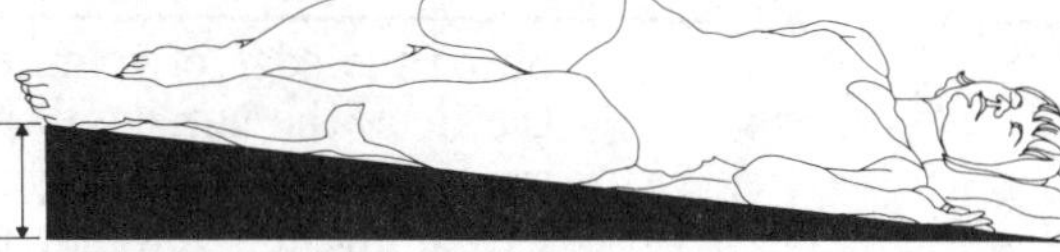

4

Position yourself as you did for Exercise 3, but this time turn to your right side. Have your helper clap the left side of your chest.

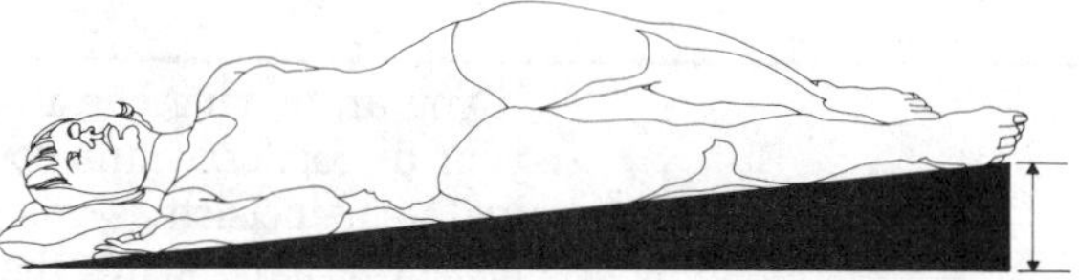

5

Include this important exercise in each set of exercises you do. Lie on your left side. Elevate your legs about 20″ (51 cm) higher than your head. Place a pillow in front of you to support your chest as you lean forward. Use another pillow under your right leg, which is flexed for support. Have your helper clap and vibrate your lower ribs beneath your right armpit, being careful not to hit your abdomen.

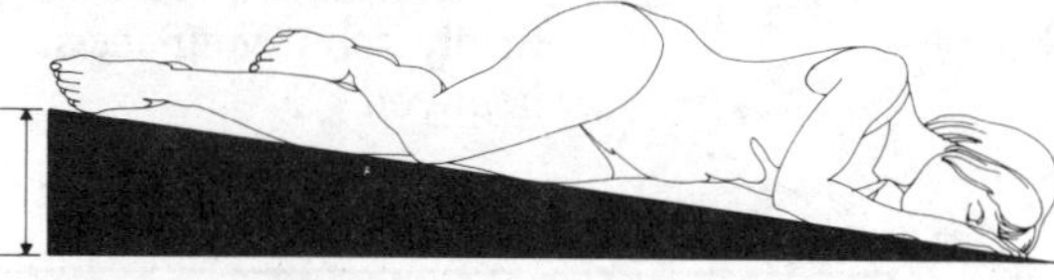

6

Position yourself as for Exercise 5, but this time lie on your right side with your left leg flexed. Have your helper clap and vibrate your lower ribs beneath your left armpit.

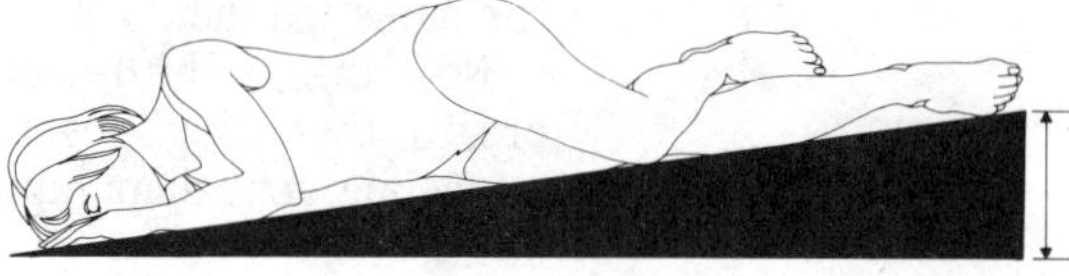

Patient-Teaching Aid

HOW TO COUGH EFFECTIVELY

Dear Patient:

After your surgery, the nurse will ask you to do coughing exercises at least every 2 hours. Coughing helps keep your lungs free of secretions. You should practice coughing before your surgery, so you can do it easily afterward. Follow these instructions:

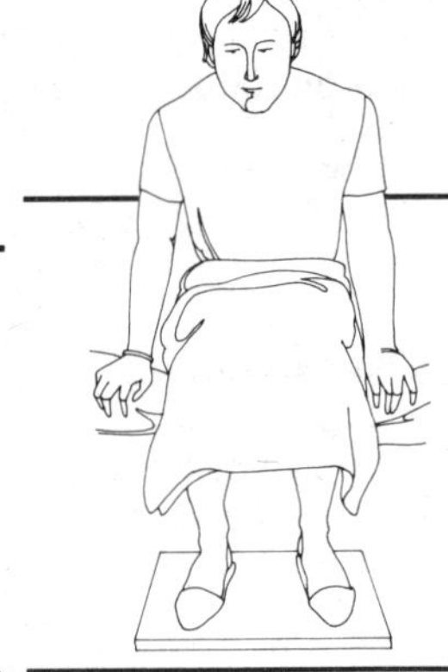

1 Sit on the edge of your bed. If your feet do not touch the floor, the nurse will give you a stool to rest them on. Bend your body slightly forward, as shown here. (After surgery, you may perform this exercise while lying in a comfortable position, instead of sitting on the edge of the bed.)

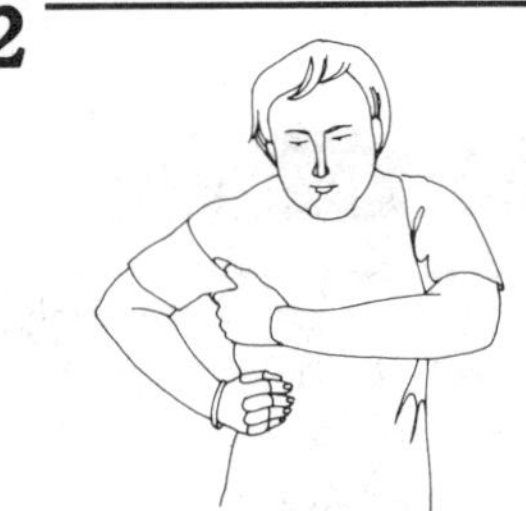

2 If you are having chest or abdominal surgery, reduce your discomfort while coughing by splinting (supporting) your incision as you cough. To splint your incision, place one hand above the incision and one hand below it, as shown here.

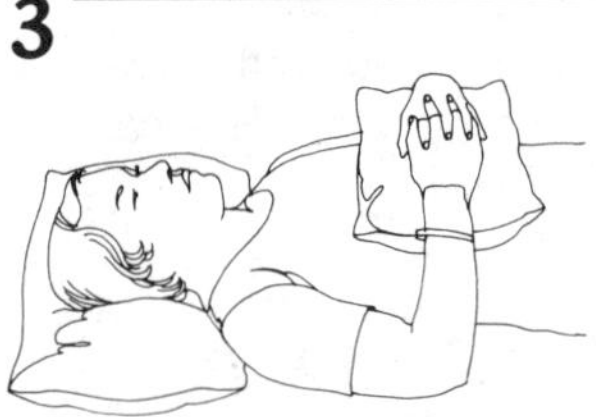

3 If you are lying down, you can splint a chest or abdominal incision by putting a pillow over it and lacing your fingers together over the pillow.

Immediately after surgery, you may feel too weak to firmly splint your incision. Do not worry; the nurse will help you.

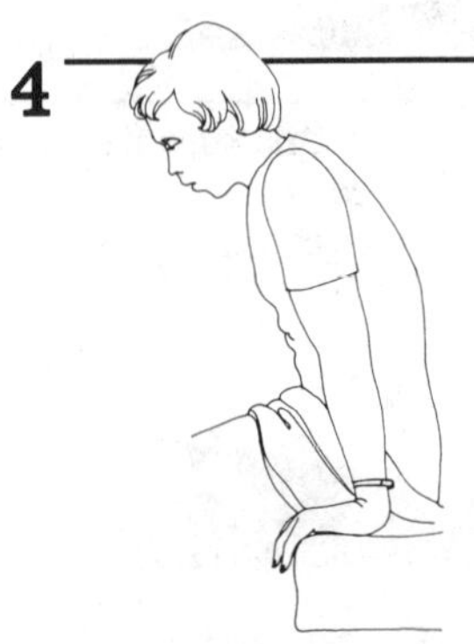

4 To help stimulate your cough reflex, take a slow, deep breath. Breathe in through your nose, and concentrate on fully expanding your chest. Breathe out through your mouth, and concentrate on feeling your chest sink downward and inward. Then take a second breath in the same manner.

Now, take a third deep breath. This time, hold your breath; then cough vigorously. As you do, concentrate on feeling your diaphragm force out all the air in your chest.

Repeat this exercise at least one more time.

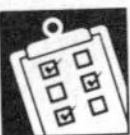

Patient-Teaching Aid

HOW TO USE AN INCENTIVE SPIROMETER

Dear Patient:
The physician wants you to use a breathing aid called an incentive spirometer. Using this aid will expand your lungs, helping you to breathe in more oxygen and avoid lung complications.

1

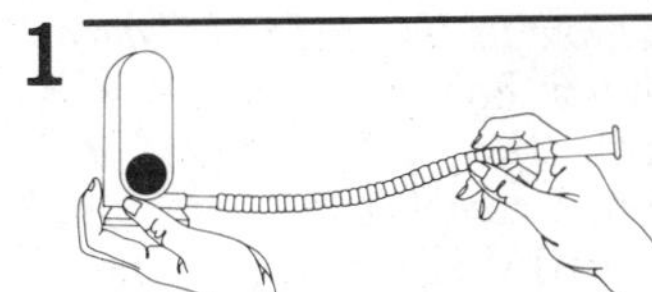

First, hold the spirometer upright in your hand. Be careful not to tilt it.

2

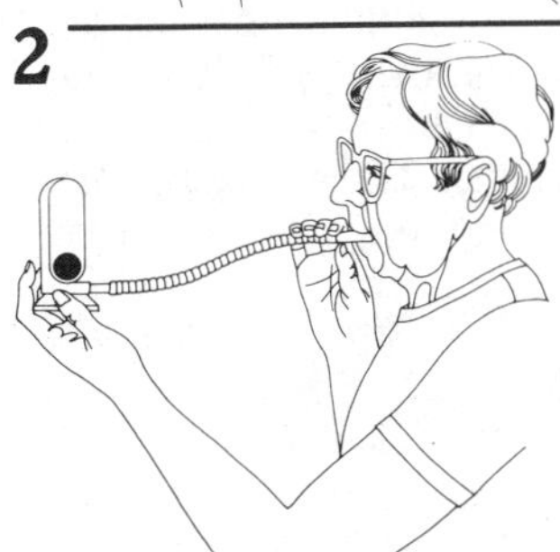

Now, exhale normally, and place your lips tightly around the spirometer's mouthpiece.

3

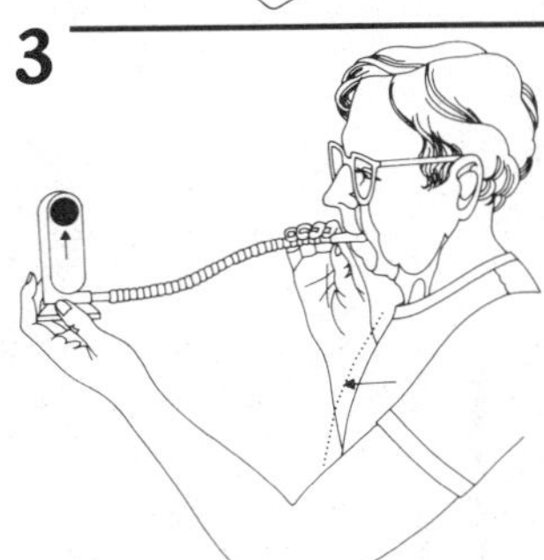

Inhale deeply, until the ball in the chamber rises to the top. Hold your breath for a count of three (even though the ball drops).

4

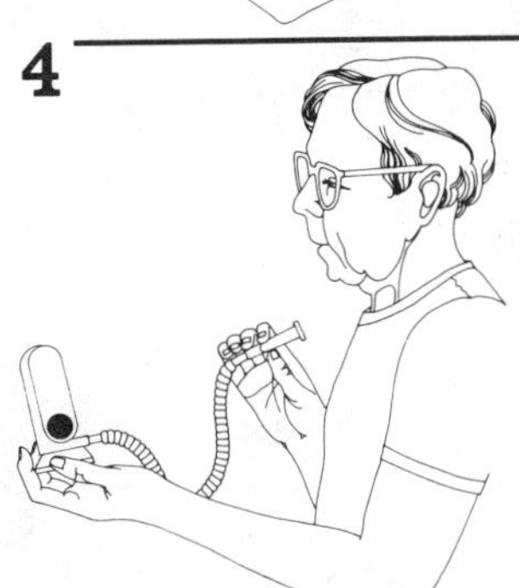

Finally, remove the mouthpiece from your mouth, and exhale normally. Rest for a moment. Repeat the exercise several times, resting after each time.

Use the spirometer to deep-breathe at least once every 2 hours while you are awake.

Patient-Teaching Aid

SETTING UP AN OXYGEN TANK FOR USE

Dear Patient:

The physician has instructed you to use oxygen at home. Follow these steps to set up your equipment:

First, obtain from your supplier an oxygen tank that is patient-ready. It will have a flow meter, a regulator, and a humidifier bottle attached to it.

Now, unscrew the humidifier bottle, fill it with distilled water, and reattach it to the flow meter. NOTE: Be sure to change the water every day. Also check the water level throughout the day. Whenever you need to refill the bottle, first pour out all the water.

Open the tank by turning the knob on top of the tank counterclockwise (as shown in the illustration), until you see the needle on the regulator gauge move, registering pressure. Now, attach the nasal cannula to the humidifier bottle. The nurse will give you another patient-teaching aid, *How to Use a Nasal Cannula,* to teach you how to do this.

Then turn the flow meter knob counterclockwise and adjust it to _____liters/minute (see inset). You should see the water bubbling in the humidifier bottle.

Continue oxygen therapy for the prescribed period. When you are finished, turn off the oxygen. Make sure the needle on the regulator drops to zero. Then turn off the flow meter.

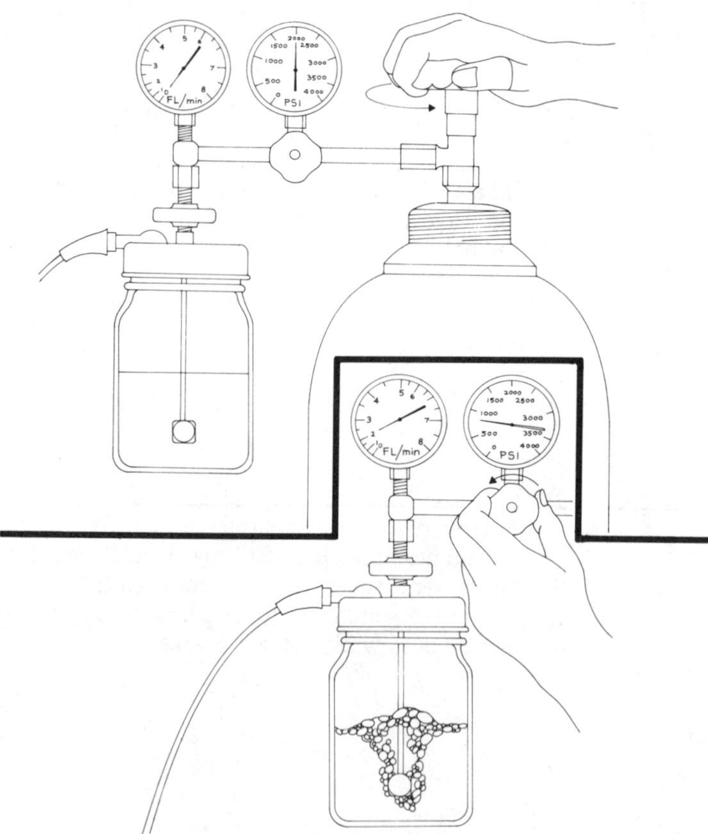

Patient-Teaching Aid

HOW TO CARE FOR OXYGEN AT HOME

Dear Patient:

To help you breathe more easily, your physician wants you to continue using oxygen at home. Follow these instructions:

—Rent or buy the oxygen therapy equipment you will need. If you are able to move around, and need oxygen all the time, you will want to obtain a portable unit in addition to your main source.

—Always keep at least a 3-day supply of oxygen on hand. Plan ahead for any long holiday weekends when your supplier will be closed. If you decide on oxygen with a continuous electrical source, talk to your supplier about getting a small emergency tank to use in case of a power failure.

—Be sure your supplier teaches you and your family how to change oxygen cylinders properly.

—Make sure a NO SMOKING sign is posted on the door of your house and your room.

—Make your family and visitors aware of oxygen's hazards and the precautions they should take.

—Use common sense when using electrical appliances, such as radios and television. Check to be sure all appliances are properly grounded and the wires are in good condition.

—To prevent the possibility of electric shock or sparks, avoid close contact with electrical appliances.

—Keep all oxygen containers away from electrical baseboard vents, gas or kerosene heaters, radiators, stoves, and grills.

—Close all valves when the oxygen is not in use, even those on an oxygen container that registers empty.

—Adjust the cylinder's flow meter so you are receiving _____liters of oxygen/minute.

—Add water to the humidifier as necessary to maintain the proper level. Change all water in the container daily.

—Clean the ends of your nasal cannula daily. Use water-soluble ointments to lubricate your nostrils. Never use oil-based products, such as mineral oil, or flammable products, such as rubbing alcohol.

—Advise a family member to call your physician immediately if you develop any of the following signs and symptoms: increased trouble breathing, irregular breathing, rapid heartbeat, blue lips or nail beds, confusion, or restlessness.

—If the family member is unable to reach your physician, have him take you to the nearest hospital emergency department.

Patient-Teaching Aid

HOW TO USE A NASAL CANNULA

Dear Patient:
Because your physician has ordered a low oxygen concentration for you, you will be using a nasal cannula to receive it. To use it, follow these steps:

1

First, check the distilled water level in the humidifier bottle attached to your oxygen source. If you need to fill it, first dispose of all water already in the humidifier. NOTE: Be sure to change the water at least once daily.

2

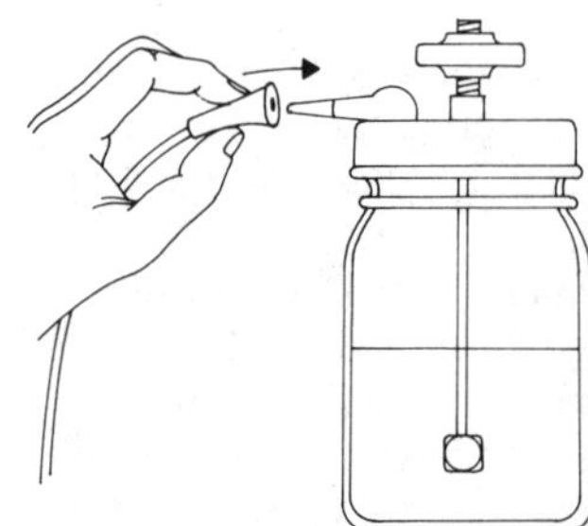

Attach the end of the oxygen tubing to the humidifier nipple, as shown here.

Next, turn on the oxygen.

3

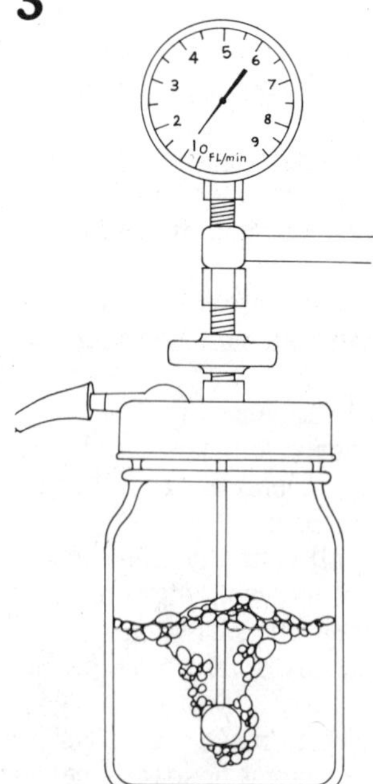

Now, set the flow rate at ______ liters/minute. IMPORTANT: Never change the oxygen flow rate without your physician's permission.

If you are receiving oxygen at 2 liters/minute or more, you should feel it flowing from the prongs. If you cannot, briefly turn up the flow rate. Then turn it back to the prescribed level. NOTE: At the same flow rate, you should see water bubbling in the humidifier. If you do not, see if the oxygen source is open.

HOW TO USE A NASAL CANNULA—*continued*

4

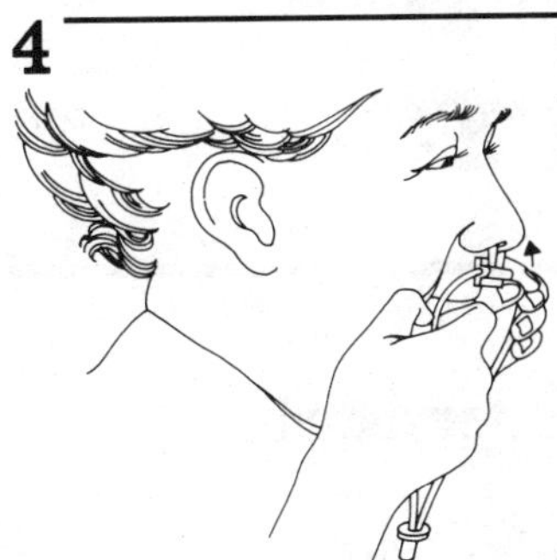

Next, insert the two prongs of the cannula in your nostrils, with the tab facing up. Make sure the prongs follow the curve of your nose.

5

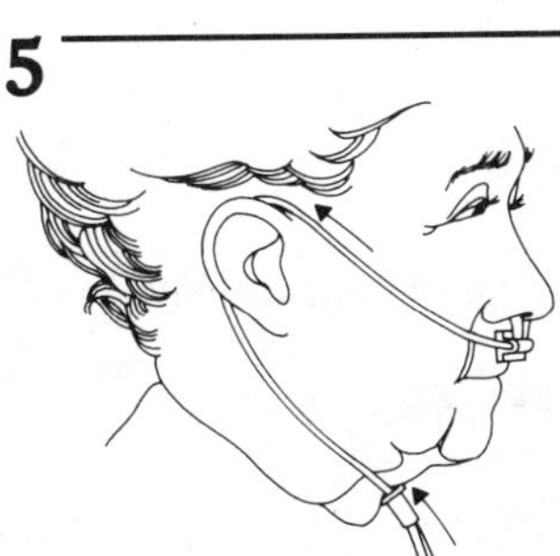

Then position the tubing over and behind each ear. Secure it by sliding the adjuster under your chin. Be careful not to adjust it too tightly.

6

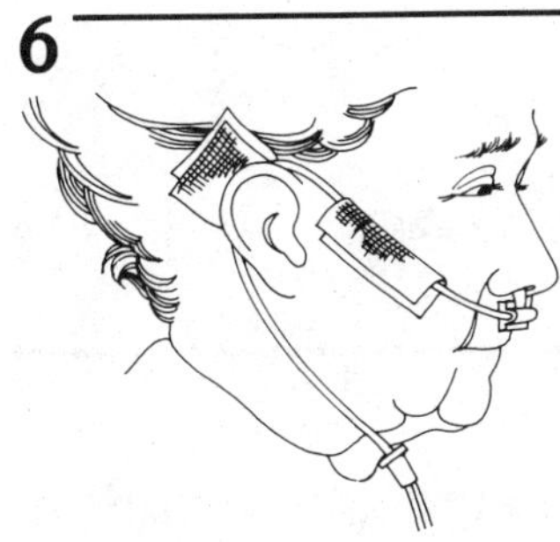

To guard against skin irritation, pad the tubing with 2″ × 2″ gauze pads, placing them against your cheeks and behind your ears. Every 2 hours, check for reddened areas under your nose and around your ears. Massage these areas if you see redness. Notify your physician if you develop any skin problems.

You may moisten your lips and nose with a water-soluble lubricating jelly (such as K-Y Lubricating Jelly), but take care not to plug the cannula.

Every 8 hours, remove the cannula and wipe it clean with a wet cloth.

IMPORTANT: Keep emergency phone numbers taped to your phone, in case you have any problems with oxygen use.

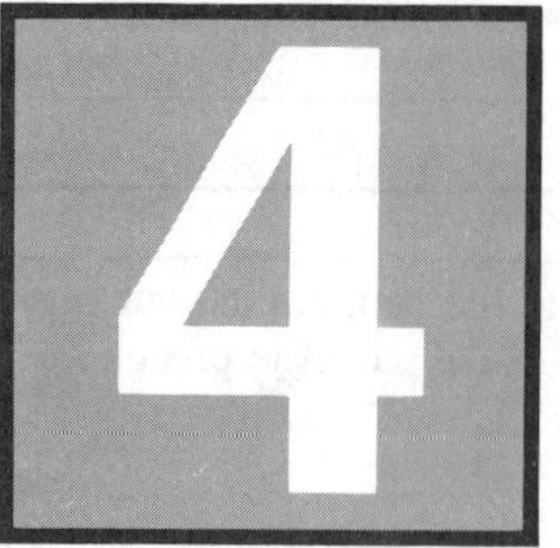

Neurologic Disorders

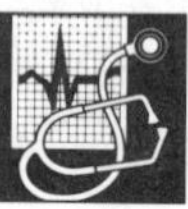

Patient-learner data base*

Areas of potential knowledge deficit

Presence of neurologic symptoms that affect learning ability
—Level of consciousness
—Expressive/receptive aphasia
—Motor ability
—Bowel/bladder dysfunction
—Sensory deficits: visual and hearing disturbances
—Sexual dysfunction
Anatomy and physiology of the nervous system
Definition of the neurologic disorder
Cause(s) of the neurologic disorder
Symptoms associated with the neurologic disorder
Treatment of the neurologic disorder
—Medications
—Rehabilitation program
—Guidelines for daily living
—Prevention of complications
—Coping strategies (for both patient and family)

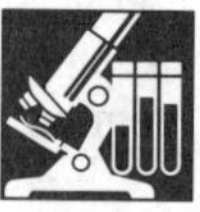

Explaining diagnostic tests

SKULL AND SPINE RADIOGRAPHY

Patient objectives	*Teaching plan content*
1 Define skull and spine radiography.	Skull and spine radiography is a procedure in which X-ray pictures are taken of the skull and/or spine.

*A general assessment should be done for all patients. For general assessment guidelines, see Chapter 1, Principles of Patient Teaching.

2 State the purpose of skull and spine radiography.	The purpose of skull and spine radiography is to identify injured bone and tissue and surrounding structures. This information helps the physician establish a diagnosis or rule out conditions that are not causing the patient's symptoms.
3 Describe the procedure used in skull and spine radiography.	Routinely, more than one view of the skull or spine is taken to obtain a complete picture of the structures. —The patient will be placed in a supine position on the X-ray table or seated in a chair (for skull X-rays only). A head band, foam pads, or sand bags may be used to immobilize his head and/or spine during the procedure. —When the X-rays are taken, the patient may hear a noise from the machine, but he will not feel or see anything. —After each X-ray, the patient will be repositioned by the X-ray technician, who will let him know when the procedure is finished. It takes about 15 minutes. —He must wait until the films are developed and checked for quality before he can leave the X-ray department. If the films are not of good quality, he will be asked to repeat the procedure. —He should know who will perform the test and where and when it will be done.
4 Discuss patient guidelines for skull and spine radiography.	Patient guidelines for skull and spine radiography include the following: —The patient need not restrict food or fluids. —He should remove glasses, dentures, jewelry, and metal objects in the X-ray field. —He may be asked to undress and wear a gown during the procedure for spine X-rays. —The procedure is painless, but he must remain still while the X-rays are taken.

BRAIN/SPINAL COMPUTED TOMOGRAPHY (C.T.)

Patient objectives	*Teaching plan content*
1 Define brain/spinal CT.	CT is a noninvasive test that uses X-rays to provide clear, cross-sectional images of the brain and spine. It does this through computer reconstruction of radiation levels absorbed by various tissues.
2 State the purpose of brain/spinal CT.	The purpose of brain/spinal CT is to help detect intracranial or intraspinal lesions and abnormalities.

3 Describe the procedure used in brain/spinal CT.	The patient will be placed in a supine position on the X-ray table, with his head and/or body immobilized by straps. His face will be uncovered. The X-ray table will then be moved into a machine. —The procedure is painless and lasts approximately 30 minutes. During this time a series of X-ray films will be taken. —At the completion of the procedure, the table will be removed from the machine. —In some cases, the physician may wish to enhance tissue density by administering contrast dye I.V. The dye accumulates in masses or lesions (except in areas of poor blood supply) and helps the physician see an area for minutes—rather than seconds. —If contrast dye is used, the patient may feel flushed and warm and experience a transient headache, a salty taste, or nausea and vomiting. —After the dye is injected, he will be placed back into the machine, and another series of X-rays will be taken. —He should know who will perform the test and where and when it will be done.
4 Discuss patient guidelines for brain/spinal CT.	Patient guidelines for brain/spinal CT include the following: —Unless contrast enhancement is scheduled, the patient need not restrict food or fluids. If contrast enhancement is scheduled, he should fast for 4 hours before the test. —He should wear a hospital gown (if an outpatient, he may wear any comfortable clothing) and remove all metal objects and jewelry in the X-ray field. —During the procedure he should lie still. However, he may talk if he can do so without moving his head. —If the patient has difficulty lying still, the physician may prescribe sedation to help him relax.

ELECTROENCEPHALOGRAPHY (E.E.G.)

Patient objectives	*Teaching plan content*
1 Define EEG.	EEG is a noninvasive test that graphically records a portion of the brain's electrical activity.
2 State the purpose of EEG.	The purpose of EEG is to assess brain wave patterns for abnormalities.

3 Describe the procedure used in EEG.

EEG is usually performed in a room designed to eliminate electrical interference and minimize distractions. The patient will be positioned comfortably on a bed or a reclining chair.
—A technician will attach 17 to 21 contact electrodes to his unshaven scalp. If needle electrodes are used, he will feel pricking sensations when they are inserted.
—The EEG machine merely records brain activity; it does not discharge electricity, nor can it read minds or indicate mental or emotional stability.
—During the test, the patient will be asked to close his eyes, relax, and remain still. However, if he becomes tired or uncomfortable, he should reposition himself, because restlessness and fatigue can alter brain wave patterns. The technician will note the movement so that it will not interfere with the recording.
—The patient will be alone in the room during the recording to eliminate any distractions. He will be observed, however, through a window.
—The recording of his brain waves begins when he is lying or sitting still with his eyes closed and his muscles relaxed.
—After the EEG is performed in a resting state, more recordings may be taken while he performs certain activities (for example, breathing deeply and rapidly for 3 minutes, observing a flashing light or a black and white checkerboard pattern, or listening to sounds through earphones), in order to detect any abnormal patterns not obvious in the resting state.
—The electrodes will be removed at the completion of the test.

4 Discuss patient guidelines for EEG.

Patient guidelines for EEG include the following:
—The patient need not restrict food or fluids before the test. (In fact, skipping the meal before the test can cause a low blood glucose level that may alter brain wave patterns.)
—He should voice any questions, concerns, or fears he might have about the test, as mental tension can affect brain wave patterns.
—If ordered, he must not take anticonvulsants, tranquilizers, barbiturates, and other sedatives for 24 to 48 hours before the test. He should also avoid stimulants, such as coffee, tea, cola drinks, and chocolate.
—Following the test, if contact electrodes were used the patient may wash his hair immediately. However, if needle electrodes were used he must wait 48 hours. Other than that, no special care is needed.

BRAIN SCAN

Patient objectives	*Teaching plan content*
1 Define a brain scan.	A brain scan is a procedure in which a series of X-rays taken in rapid succession scan the brain for abnormalities.
2 State the purpose of a brain scan.	The purpose of a brain scan is to detect abnormalities in the brain, such as an intracranial mass or vascular lesion, or to locate areas of ischemia, cerebral infarction (necrosis of brain tissue), and intracerebral hemorrhage.
3 Describe the procedure used in a brain scan.	A brain scan is performed in a special area of the X-ray department, where the patient will be placed in a supine position on the X-ray table. —An intravenous line will be inserted and a dye containing radioisotopes will be injected. —The patient may feel a slight burning sensation as the dye is injected. The radiation poses no danger to him or his visitors and should be cleared from his body within 6 hours. —Immediately following injection of the dye, the scanning machine will move back and forth close to his head, taking pictures. This enables the physician to follow the dye as it goes through the arteries in the neck and into the brain. Although the scanning machine may make some noise, the procedure is painless. —After 1 hour, a second series of films will be taken. —The patient may need to return to the X-ray department 3 to 4 hours after the dye has been injected for another series of films, if previous pictures were unclear. Dye accumulation is observed more clearly at this time. —Each series of films takes 1 to 1½ hours.
4 Discuss patient guidelines for a brain scan.	The patient need not restrict food or fluids before or after the test. He must remove all metal or jewelry in the X-ray field. His only role during the procedure will be to remain still.

CEREBRAL ANGIOGRAPHY

Patient objectives	*Teaching plan content*
1 Define cerebral angiography.	Cerebral angiography is a procedure that allows radiographic examination of the blood vessels in the brain after injection of a contrast medium.

2 State the purpose of cerebral angiography.

The purpose of cerebral angiography is to examine cerebral circulation. It allows the physician to check for structural abnormalities (aneurysms, malformations) and vessel displacement from tumors, hematomas, edema, herniation, and hydrocephalus (a condition of abnormal fluid accumulation in the cranium). He may also use the angiogram to check for abnormal bloodflow patterns. In addition, the angiogram can reveal vessel patency, narrowing, or occlusion.

3 Describe the procedure used in cerebral angiography.

Cerebral angiography is performed in a special area of the X-ray department. The patient will be placed in a supine position on an X-ray table with his head immobilized.

—The injection site for the contrast medium will be chosen (carotid, brachial, or femoral artery), shaved and cleansed with an antiseptic solution.

- If the carotid artery is to be used, the patient's neck will be hyperextended and a rolled-up towel or sandbag will be placed under his shoulders. His head will then be immobilized with a restraint or tape.
- If the brachial artery (least common) is to be used, a blood pressure cuff will be placed far from the injection site and inflated before injection, to prevent the contrast medium from flowing into the forearm and hand.

—Then the skin of the selected injection site will be cleansed with alcohol, and a local anesthetic will be injected.

—After placement of the needle, the contrast dye will be injected. The patient will probably feel a transient burning sensation as the contrast dye is injected. He may feel flushed and warm and may experience a transient headache, a salty taste, or nausea and vomiting after the dye is injected.

—Next, a series of X-rays will be taken, developed, and reviewed. Depending on the results of this initial series, more dye may be injected and another series of X-rays taken.

—When an acceptable series of X-rays has been obtained, the needle will be withdrawn and pressure will be applied to the puncture site for 15 minutes.

—The procedure takes about 2 hours, and the patient should know who will perform it and when it will be done.

4 Discuss patient guidelines for cerebral angiography.

Patient guidelines for cerebral angiography include the following:

—The patient must fast for 8 to 10 hours before the test.

—He must wear a hospital gown and remove jewelry, dentures, hairpins, and other radiopaque objects in the X-ray field.
—During the procedure he will need to lie still, with his arms at his sides.
—After the procedure he will need to stay in bed for 12 to 24 hours.
—If he experiences any discomfort, he should ask for pain medication; an icebag applied to the injection site may also ease his discomfort.
—A nurse will check him frequently during this time; this is routine and does not imply that something is wrong.
—If the injection site was in the neck (carotid artery), the patient should alert the nurse if he experiences any difficulty swallowing or breathing and if he develops any weakness or numbness in his extremities.
—If the groin (femoral artery) or arm (brachial artery) was used as the insertion site, he must keep the affected extremity straight for at least 12 hours.
—Because it is difficult to keep the arm straight for an extended period of time, an immobilizer may be used.

LUMBAR PUNCTURE

Patient objectives	*Teaching plan content*
1 Define a lumbar puncture.	A lumbar puncture is a procedure in which a needle is inserted into a space (subarachnoid space, under the middle layer of the meninges) in the spinal canal to measure pressure and to extract cerebrospinal fluid (CSF). (An illustration can be used to identify the structures and area of the insertion site.)
2 State the purposes of a lumbar puncture.	The purposes of a lumbar puncture are as follows: —To measure CSF pressure for evidence of obstruction. —To obtain a sample of CSF for laboratory analysis, to help identify various central nervous system disorders, such as tumors, hemorrhage, or infection.
3 Describe the procedure used in a lumbar puncture.	A lumbar puncture is performed at bedside by a physician. The patient will be asked to lie on his side and bring his knees up toward his head, or to sit up and bend his chest and head toward his knees. (These positions open the spaces between the vertebrae, allowing the physician to insert the spinal needle more easily.) —Once the patient is positioned, the puncture site will be cleansed and then anesthetized. He will feel a transient burning sensation as the physician injects the local anesthetic. After he receives this drug, he will feel

only slight pressure in his lower back.
—The physician usually will insert the spinal needle between the spinous processes of the vertebrae (usually between the third and fourth lumbar vertebrae).
—The physician will then collect a sample of CSF and take a pressure reading.
—Then the needle will be removed, the puncture site cleansed with antiseptic, and a small bandage applied.
—The procedure takes approximately 15 minutes.

4 Discuss patient guidelines for a lumbar puncture procedure.

Patient guidelines for a lumbar puncture include the following:
—The patient need not restrict food or fluids before the test.
—During the procedure he must remain still and not move or twist his spine. He must not move suddenly or cough. He should breathe slowly and deeply through his mouth.
—He will be expected to lie flat for 8 to 10 hours after the procedure.
—A headache is the most common side effect of a lumbar puncture, but his cooperation during the test can help minimize the risk.
—Although he must not raise his head, he can turn it from side to side.
—He should drink plenty of fluids during this time.

MYELOGRAPHY

Patient objectives	*Teaching plan content*
1 Define myelography.	Myelography is a study in which a contrast medium (dye or air) is injected into the spinal subarachnoid space and/or the cisterna magna (a reservoir for CSF located under the cerebellum and near the medulla). On an illustration, the patient should identify the spinal cord layers, the subarachnoid space, and the cisterna magna.
2 State the purpose of myelography.	The purpose of myelography is to determine abnormalities in the spinal subarachnoid space, such as bony changes, partial or complete obstruction, congenital lesions, and spinal cord tumors.
3 Describe the procedure used in myelography.	Myelography is performed in a special area of the X-ray department by a physician. Just before the study, a nurse will check the patient's blood pressure, pulse and respiratory rates, and neurologic status. Then he will be positioned on his side at the edge of the X-ray table,

with his knees drawn up to his abdomen and his chin on his chest.
—A lumbar puncture will be performed (see the "Lumbar Puncture" teaching plan in this chapter), and a fluoroscope (a screen that looks like a TV) will be used to watch the placement of the needle. Some CSF may be removed for routine analysis.
—Then the patient will be placed on his abdomen and will be secured with straps across his upper back, under his arms, and across his ankles. His chin will be hyperextended and supported in this position with a towel or sponge.
—Next, the contrast medium will be injected, and the patient may feel a transient burning sensation. This is normal. He may also experience a flushed warm feeling, a headache, a salty taste, or nausea and vomiting. Even if he feels ill, he should remain in the position he has been placed in. A technician or nurse will help him if he vomits.
—The table will be tilted so that the contrast medium will flow through the subarachnoid space. The fluoroscope will show the flow of the contrast medium, and X-rays will be taken.
—When the required X-rays have been obtained, the contrast medium will be withdrawn, if necessary, and the needle will be removed.
—The puncture site will be cleansed, and a small adhesive bandage will be applied. The patient will then return to his room on a stretcher or in a wheelchair.
—The test takes 1 hour or more.

4 Discuss patient guidelines for myelography.

Patient guidelines for myelography include the following:
—He must restrict food and fluids for 8 hours before the test.
—He must remove any jewelry and metal objects in the X-ray field and should urinate just before the test.
—If the patient receives a sedative, he must stay in bed once he has been sedated. He should use the call bell if he needs something.
—After the test, he can expect one of two things, depending on the type of contrast medium used during the test:

- If iophendylate was used, he will return to his room on a stretcher and will be expected to lie flat for 24 hours.
- If metrizamide was used, he will return to his room in a wheelchair or on a stretcher with his head elevated at least 60 degrees. He must keep his head at this angle for 8 hours, because the contrast medium can irritate the nerve roots in his neck and the

structures in his head.
—Personnel in the X-ray department will let him know which position he should maintain.

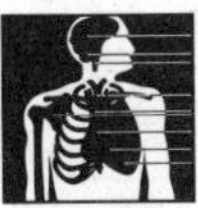

Explaining disorders

CEREBROVASCULAR ACCIDENT (C.V.A., or stroke)

Patient objectives	*Teaching plan content*
1 Define a stroke.	A stroke is a sudden interruption in the flow of blood to the brain.
2 Explain the causes of a stroke.	The following three things can interrupt the flow of blood to the brain, causing a stroke: —A blood clot traveling in the bloodstream (an embolus) lodges in an artery in the brain, thereby blocking the flow of blood. —A stationary blood clot (a thrombus) blocks an artery. —Hemorrhage from the rupture of a weakened area of an artery occurs within the brain.
3 Discuss how a stroke produces neurologic damage.	Blood carries oxygen and nutrients to the brain to nourish brain cells and tissue. When inadequate amounts of blood reach a section of the brain, the brain cells and tissue in this area develop hypoxia (oxygen deficiency) and die quickly. The symptoms the patient exhibits reflect which brain cells died. —If the patient is paralyzed on the left side, the brain cells that control movement for that side of the body have been affected. —If the patient is aphasic (unable to speak or communicate), the cells within the speech center have suffered damage. —Sometimes only the cells that carry instructions from the controlling center in the brain to the muscles are damaged. If this happens, the patient may be able to regain control of the muscles by learning to use other nerves that bypass the damaged area.
4 Identify the relevant components of the treatment regimen for a stroke.	Treatment for a stroke may include the following: —Medications to prevent further blood clots from forming —Physical therapy to teach the patient how to use his paralyzed muscles

—Speech therapy to help the patient learn to communicate
—Bowel and bladder training to help the patient regain control
—Safety precautions to help the patient compensate for sensory loss
—Guidelines for daily living to reduce the risk of another stroke.

5 Describe the medication regimen.

Some drugs commonly used for this disorder are aspirin, dipyridamole, and heparin. See Chapter 9, Drug Therapy, for specific medication instructions.

6 Demonstrate and explain the rationale for the prescribed exercises.

The physical therapist will provide instruction on specific exercises, and the patient should be able to demonstrate them. (The nurse should know what exercises are being taught, in order to reinforce the instruction; if necessary, she should demonstrate them first.) For home use, the patient should have written instructions to help him remember the exercises. (See *How to Strengthen Your Muscles and Joints*, pp. 170 to 174.)
—Exercises for the affected limbs are necessary to stretch soft tissues and prevent joint contracture (fixation).
—They also improve circulation and help prevent blood clot formation.
—With repetitive exercise, new pathways form in the nervous system and help the patient improve control and range of motion in the limbs.
—The patient can increase his muscle strength and maintain range of motion only through daily exercise.

7 Demonstrate the transfer procedure (if applicable), using the stand-pivot technique (family objective).

If the patient is confined to a wheelchair as a result of his stroke, the family should know how to transfer him to and from the wheelchair. This transfer can be performed easily at home. (The nurse should demonstrate the procedure to the family and have them repeat the demonstration.)

The following example outlines the procedure used in the bed-to-wheelchair transfer, but it may be adapted for use in transferring the patient from chair to wheelchair, car to wheelchair, and so forth.
—To begin, lower the side rail and position the wheelchair next to the bed. Always position the wheelchair on the patient's unaffected side. Lock the wheels on the chair and the bed (if a hospital bed will be used at home). If possible, detach the chair's leg rests or move them out of the way.
—Seat the patient on the edge of the bed with his legs

hanging over the side. Allow him time to regain his equilibrium. Put shoes on his feet, and be sure his feet are touching the floor. If they are not, lower the bed.
—Next, move close to the patient and place your knees against his knees. Squat slightly and slide your arms under his arms. Then lock your arms around his waist. Tell him to lock his unaffected arm around your back. Ask him to help you as much as possible. Push your knees against his to keep them stable.
—Then assist him in reaching a standing position. Again, allow him a few seconds to regain his equilibrium. Now pivot toward the wheelchair. Continue to support his knees with your knees as you turn his back toward the chair. Stop turning when his back is directly in front of the wheelchair.
—With his unaffected hand the patient should grasp the wheelchair's armrest. Then, as you squat down to lower him into the chair, he will be able to guide himself into the seat.

8 Demonstrate how to walk with a cane (if applicable).

In walking with a cane, the patient must wear properly fitted shoes, and his cane should be the right height.
—He should slide to the edge of the bed and place his feet flat on the floor 6″ (15.2 cm) apart. A family member can help him into a standing position, standing slightly to the patient's weakened side.
—The patient should hold the cane in his unaffected hand with the tip about 4″ (10.2 cm) to the side of his foot. He should distribute his weight evenly between his feet and the cane and keep the cane's rubber tip(s) on the floor at all times. As he prepares to walk, he must look ahead instead of looking at his feet.
—Next, he should shift his weight to his unaffected leg as he moves the cane forward about 4″.
—With his weight supported by his unaffected leg and the cane, he should move his affected leg forward parallel with the cane.
—Then, he should shift his weight to his affected leg and the cane, and move his unaffected leg forward ahead of the cane about 4″. (If he does this correctly, his heel will be slightly beyond the tip of the cane.)
—To complete the gait sequence, he should move his affected foot forward so that it is even with his unaffected foot.
—He should begin another sequence immediately, shifting his weight to the unaffected leg and moving his cane forward as before.
—The sequence should be repeated until the patient and the nurse feel he is ready to try it alone. (See *Going Home With a Cane,* pp. 176 and 177.)

9 State at least four guidelines to follow when communicating with an aphasic family member (family objective).

When a person's brain is damaged by a stroke, he may suffer aphasia, a loss of the ability to express or comprehend language. Many patients with aphasia can recover some of their ability to speak and comprehend during the first several months after a stroke with the help of a speech therapist. The following guidelines may help family members communicate with the aphasic patient:
—Talk to the patient as an adult; aphasia does not mean he has lost his intelligence.
—Speak slowly and use simple, short sentences along with gestures, when possible.
—Do not shout; hearing loss is not part of aphasia and shouting will not help the patient understand.
—Speak to him frequently; do not neglect him because he does not understand what you say or has trouble communicating. This approach may cause him to feel isolated, and he may withdraw into silence.
—Be honest with him; do not pretend you understand if you do not. He may be trying to tell you something important.
—Be aware that he may experience extreme frustration as he attempts and fails to perform tasks that were previously routine. Anticipate displays of emotion as he tries to cope with his incapacity, and offer him reassurance as these feelings surface.
—Avoid the tendency to talk for him or frequently supply him with words; have patience with his efforts, slow as they may be.
—Check whether he has auditory comprehension by asking him a question that requires a "no" answer; for example, "Did you have soup for breakfast this morning?" (Patients who lack comprehension are more likely to answer "yes" to all questions.)
—Use a set of cards with such words as "bedpan," "thirsty," or "hurt," to help him communicate needs and reduce frustration. Encourage him to communicate by writing, if he can. (Do not use these approaches alone, without efforts to communicate verbally.)
—Avoid tiring him; aphasia worsens with fatigue or emotional upset.

10 Discuss guidelines for bladder training (if applicable).

See Chapter 7, Genitourinary Disorders, for instructions on bladder training.

11 Discuss gudelines for bowel training (if applicable).

The patient and/or his family should follow these guidelines for bowel training:
—The goal is to establish a pattern close to the patient's normal bowel habits before his stroke.

—A high intake of fluids (if not contraindicated) and a diet adequate in roughage may help.
—The patient should attempt to have a bowel movement at the same time every day. A good time choice is immediately after breakfast, because food in the stomach after an 8- to 12-hour fast acts as a stimulus on the bowel.
—To move his bowels, the patient should take a deep breath, if he can, and push inward with his hand against his abdominal muscles at the moment he feels the urge to evacuate. This imitates the normal pushing movement that may be lacking in his weakened muscles. Drinking a hot liquid upon arising can also be helpful.
—A record should be kept of when each bowel movement occurs.
—If a bowel movement has not occurred in several days, the patient or family should discuss the need for a laxative or enema with the physician. If a bowel movement does not occur even with a laxative or enema, the patient or family should obtain further instructions from the physician; a bowel obstruction can occur if corrective action is not taken.
—The patient should not strain during a bowel movement, because this raises the pressure in the brain's blood vessels, risking rebleeding if hemorrhage caused his stroke.

12 Explain safety precautions used to compensate for sensory loss.

The patient with sensory loss must use certain safety precautions in order to avoid injury:
—He should test the temperature of bath water with his unaffected hand to avoid burns.
—He should use a footboard on his bed as a means of stimulating pressure sensations and proprioception (stimulation received within the tissues regarding spatial position).
—The patient should touch, grasp, and manipulate objects of different sizes, textures, and weights throughout the day in an effort to stimulate tactile (touch) and proprioceptive sensations.
—Hot water bottles and heating pads can be hazardous and should be avoided.
—If a visual field deficit is present, the patient should scan his surroundings to avoid obstacles and to help judge distances. He must move slowly to compensate for his altered depth perception. If double vision is present, he or a family member should learn how to patch the affected eye.
—To prevent further injury to the affected body parts, the family should remind him to wash and dress all body areas.

13 Identify four premonitory signs of stroke.

The following are premonitory signs of stroke and should be reported to a physician at once:
—Severe headache
—Drowsiness
—Confusion
—Dizziness.

14 Identify at least three measures to help prevent another stroke.

Measures to help prevent another stroke include the following:
—Control such diseases as diabetes (accelerates the rate of atherosclerosis in all blood vessels, including cerebral blood vessels) and hypertension (increases pressure in weakened cerebral blood vessels, which may cause them to rupture).
—Avoid obesity. Follow a low-salt, low-cholesterol diet. (See Chapter 2, Cardiovascular Disorders, for further instructions, if needed.)
—Avoid sudden increases in activity and stress, which can increase blood pressure.
—Be as active as possible. Prolonged bed rest favors clot formation.
—Avoid smoking, which constricts the cerebral blood vessels, thereby decreasing the amount of blood available to vital brain tissue. (Smoking cessation programs are available in many areas.)
—See the physician regularly.

SPINAL CORD INJURY

Patient objectives	*Teaching plan content*

1 Identify the anatomic structures of the spinal cord and surrounding tissues.

The anatomic structures of the spinal cord and surrounding tissues include the vertebral column, the membranes enclosing the cord, the cord itself, and the spinal nerves. (An illustration can be used to demonstrate these structures in as much detail as necessary for the patient to understand his injury.)
—The vertebral column consists of five segments: cervical, thoracic, lumbar, sacral, and coccygeal. (The patient should be able to point to the area where his lesion occurred.)
—The membranes enclosing the spinal cord are the dura mater, the arachnoid, and the pia mater.
—The spinal cord consists of gray matter (an H-shaped mass revealed in cross-sectional illustrations), which contains nerve fibers that relay sensations and control reflexes; and white matter (surrounding the gray matter), which is made up of nerve fibers that carry messages to and from the brain.

—The spinal nerves, attached to the spinal cord by the anterior and posterior roots, transmit sensory and motor messages between the body and the spinal cord: 8 cervical (C1 to C8), 12 thoracic (T1 to T12), 5 lumbar (L1 to L5), 5 sacral (S1 to S5), and 1 coccygeal.

The anterior root (on the front of the cord) relays motor impulses from the spinal cord via the spinal nerves to glands and muscles. The posterior root (on the back of the cord) relays sensory information from the outlying regions of the body via the spinal nerves to the spinal cord.

A dermatome map, which is an illustration showing the body surface areas supplied by the spinal nerves, demonstrates the relationship between these nerves and particular segments of the body. (The patient should be able to point to the surface area affected by his injury.)

2 Describe the two major functions of the spinal cord.

The two major functions of the spinal cord are to serve as a relay center and to serve as reflex center.

—As a relay center, it functions as follows:

- The spinal cord picks up sensory messages from the body and transmits them to the brain for interpretation. Primary sensory messages include pain, touch, vibration, and position.
- It picks up motor messages from the brain and transmits them to the body. Motor messages travel down the spinal cord along two major pathways: the pyramidal pathway (nerve fibers in the white matter of the spinal cord) controls fine, voluntary movement; the extrapyramidal pathway (nerve fibers in the spinal cord outside of the pyramidal pathway) controls gross motor movements.

—In functioning as a reflex center, the spinal cord depends on:

- a mechanism called "the reflex arc." This is a primitive system that combines both sensory and motor functions by sensing the presence of a harmful stimulus and initiating a motor response for quick removal of the endangered body part without having to send or receive input from the brain.

3 Discuss the relationship between spinal cord injury and neurologic dysfunction.

The spinal cord may be completely or partially transected (severed) when a foreign object or a displaced vertebral bone penetrates it. This causes neurologic dysfunction by interrupting motor/sensory pathways in the cord below the lesion site. Normal function will remain above the lesion site.

—Complete transection of the cord results in loss of function below the lesion site. Loss of voluntary motor and sensory function is permanent; loss of reflex, auto-

nomic, bladder, bowel, and sexual function is called spinal shock and is temporary, lasting from weeks to months.
—The symptoms of spinal shock may include a drop in blood pressure from loss of vasomotor tone (muscle tone within blood vessels, affecting the size of the blood vessels), temperature changes from loss of thermoregulation, bladder sphincter contraction, some muscle atony (weakness), bowel distention, and reflex erection of the penis.
—As spinal shock resolves, the patient may slowly regain muscle excitability, changing his flaccid paralysis into spastic paralysis. Spasticity results because motor coordination messages are unable to get through from the brain.
—The term "paraplegic" denotes a person who has lost motor function and sensation in his legs and lower body parts; the term "quadriplegic" denotes a person who has lost motor function and sensation in all four of his limbs.
—Partial transection of the cord may result in loss of some sensory and/or motor function below the lesion, depending on the damage done to ascending pathways (which control sensory function) and/or descending pathways (which control motor function).

4 Identify at least four components of the home care program for spinal cord injury.

The components of the home care program are as follows:
—Range-of-motion exercises to prevent deformities
—Transfer technique (if paraplegic)
—Bowel training (if applicable)
—Bladder training (if applicable)
—Self-catheterization (if applicable)
—Care of an indwelling (Foley) catheter (if applicable)
—Measures to prevent skin breakdown
—Sexual options
—Safety precautions (if sensory loss is present).

5 Demonstrate passive range-of-motion (ROM) exercises.

Passive ROM exercises are needed to prevent contractures and deformities. Their purpose is to stimulate the normal muscle contraction and relaxation that is absent in the paralyzed extremities. To achieve this, the exercises should be done slowly and gently several times a day. A joint should never be forced to move beyond resistance or to continue movement beyond the point of pain. If muscle spasm is present, the joint should be moved slowly and only to the point of resistance. Then, a gentle steady pressure is exerted until the muscle relaxes. The bed should be raised to a working height that is comfortable for the person performing the exercises. After a nurse or physical therapist demonstrates how to perform these exercises, the patient or family member will repeat the demonstration to help identify and remedy any difficulties. Each exercise should be done three times. (See *Performing Passive ROM Exercises,* pp. 178 to 180.)

—For the neck, exercises are performed as follows:

- Extension-flexion: Place the patient in a supine position on the bed, without a pillow. Support the back of his head with one hand and his chin with the other. To perform extension, bend the neck backward, so the patient looks at the ceiling; to perform flexion, bend the head forward at the neck, bringing the chin toward the chest. Ideally, the patient should be able to rest his chin on his chest.
- Lateral flexion: Place one hand on each side of the patient's face. Tilt the head laterally, bringing the right ear toward the right shoulder; then slowly tilt the head back toward the left shoulder.
- Rotation: With your hands in the same position as for lateral flexion, turn the patient's head from right to left, as if he were looking over his shoulder.

—For the shoulders, exercises are performed as follows:

- Extension-flexion: If possible, place the patient in a prone, side-lying, or sitting position, or remove the headboard and slide the patient down in bed. (These exercises are most effective, however, when the patient is in the prone, side-lying, or sitting position.) With the patient's arm in the natural extended position (at his side, palm facing his body), place one hand under his elbow and grasp his wrist with the other. Keeping the patient's elbow straight, bring the arm straight up until it reaches the ear (flexion). If necessary, bend the elbow so the forearm reaches above the head.
- Vertical abduction-adduction: Assume the same starting position as for extension-flexion. Then swing the patient's arm outward from the side, staying in the plane of the body (abduction). Return the arm to his side, then direct it across the midline toward the other arm (adduction). To achieve full range of motion, externally rotate the arm at the shoulder, bring the arm up to the ear, and then return it to the starting position.
- Horizontal abduction-adduction: Place the patient's arm in vertical abduction, then bend the elbow (horizontal abduction). Grasp the elbow with one hand and the wrist with the other. Carry the patient's arm across the body so the hand touches the opposite shoulder (horizontal adduction).

• Internal-external rotation: Place the patient's arm in horizontal abduction. Grasp the wrist with one hand and the elbow, bent at a 90-degree angle, with the other. Keeping the shoulder at a 90-degree angle to the mattress, gently lower the forearm until the palm touches the bed (internal rotation). Return to the starting position, then gently push the dorsal forearm toward the mattress so the back of the hand touches the bed (external rotation).

—For the elbow, exercises are performed as follows:

• Extension-flexion: Place the patient's arm at his side, with the palm facing upward (extension). Grasp the wrist so the hand will not droop. Keeping the upper arm on the bed, bring the hand up toward the shoulder (flexion).

—For the forearm, the supination-pronation exercise is performed as follows: With the patient's arm in the natural extended position, lift the hand into the air, keeping the elbow on the bed. Grasp his wrist with one hand and his hand with your other hand. Twist the hand to bring the palm up (supination); then, twist it back again to bring the palm down (pronation).

—For the wrist, exercises are performed as follows:

• Extension-flexion: With the patient's arm in the same position as for forearm exercises, bend the hand back toward the dorsal forearm (extension); then bend it forward (flexion).

• Lateral flexion: In the same position as for extension-flexion, rock the hand sideways.

• Circumduction: In the same position as for extension-flexion, rotate the hand in a circular motion.

—For the fingers and thumb, exercises are performed as follows:

• Extension-flexion: Keep the arm in the same position as for the forearm exercises. Grasp the palm and wrist with one hand, and gently straighten the fingers with the other (extension). Then place your hand on the back of the patient's fingers, and gently bend his hand into a fist (flexion). Repeat these two motions with each finger, individually flexing each joint.

• Abduction-adduction: In the same position as for extension-flexion, spread two adjoining fingers apart (abduction) and then bring them together (adduction). Repeat this exercise for all fingers and the thumb.

• Opposition: In the same position as for extension-flexion, pinch the thumb and each fingertip together, one at a time.

• Circumduction: In the same position as for extension-flexion, rotate the thumb in a circle.

—For the hip and knee, exercises are performed as follows:

- Extension-flexion: With the patient's leg flat on the bed in the natural extended position, place one hand under the ankle and the other hand under the knee. Bend the hip and knee toward the chest, sliding your hand out from under the knee to allow full joint flexion.
- Abduction-adduction: Place your hands under the ankle and knee. Move the leg sideways, out and away from the other leg (abduction), and then back, over, and across it (adduction).
- Internal-external rotation: With the patient's leg flat on the bed, grasp its dorsal side above the ankle and at the knee. Roll the leg toward the midline (internal rotation) and then away from the midline (external rotation).

—For the ankle, exercises are performed as follows:

- Dorsiflexion–plantar flexion: Place one hand under the heel and the other on the ball of the foot. Push the foot toward the head and pull the heel back (dorsiflexion). Then move your hand from the ball to the dorsal surface. Pull the foot down toward the bed and push the heel back (plantar flexion).
- Circumduction: Place one hand under the ankle, and grasp the foot with the other hand. Then rotate the ankle in a circular motion.

—For the foot, the inversion-eversion exercise is performed as follows: Maintaining the starting position as for ankle circumduction, hold the ankle securely. Twist the foot with the sole toward the midline (inversion) and then away from the midline (eversion).

—For the toes, exercises are performed as follows:

- Extension-flexion: Hold the ankle securely with one hand, and curl the toes toward the sole with the other hand (flexion). Then straighten and stretch the toes back toward the dorsal surface of the foot (extension).
- Abduction-adduction: Spread two adjoining toes apart (abduction) and then bring them together (adduction). Repeat for all toes.

---

6 Demonstrate transfer technique using a transfer board (if paraplegic).

The transfer procedure is performed as follows:

—Make sure the wheelchair has removable armrests and leg rests. Position the wheelchair next to the bed so the right side of the chair is next to the left side of the bed. Lock the chair's wheels in place.

—Remove the wheelchair's leg rests. Then adjust the bed so it is level with the wheelchair seat. Remove the wheelchair's right armrest and hang it from the wheelchair handles.

—The patient should shift his weight onto the right buttock. Slide the transfer board under the buttocks and upper thighs. Extend the other end of the board onto the wheelchair. Before transfer begins, make sure the board is resting securely on the wheelchair seat and the bed.
—The patient should raise the buttocks and begin to inch across the board toward the wheelchair. Grasp the chair's left armrest with his left hand.
—Upon reaching the chair, guide the legs over the board and onto the chair.
—Place the right hand on the transfer board. Grasping the transfer board with the right hand, shift the weight to the left buttock. Then pull the board from underneath the buttocks.
—Replace the armrest and leg rests and put socks and shoes on the patient.

7 Discuss guidelines for bowel training (if applicable).

The goal of bowel training is for the patient to have a bowel movement approximately every 1 to 3 days without using an enema. Bowel training works in most patients with spinal cord injuries, because large-bowel innervation is independent of the spinal cord lesion.
—The patient's diet should be high in fluids and fiber. Refined foods, such as pastries and white bread, which can promote constipation, should be avoided.
—Gravity and a change of body position can help move the stool out of the body. Activity increases peristalsis; therefore, the patient's position should be changed frequently. The patient should sit in a chair to aid gravity.
—Timing is important; the bowel routine should be performed at the same time each day.
—If needed, bowel stimulation should be performed, as ordered by the physician. The equipment needed includes two or three bed-saver pads, a paper bag, a water-soluble lubricant, soap, a basin, a washcloth and towel, and a glove.

- The person performing bowel stimulation should insert a suppository about 30 to 40 minutes before bowel stimulation.
- The person performing the procedure should place the bed-saver pads on the bed and wash his hands.
- Then he should position the patient in left Sims' position (lying on his left side with his left leg extended and right knee and thigh drawn up) or place him on a bowel stimulation chair.
- Then he should put on a glove and lubricate his gloved finger. He should insert the gloved finger ½″ to 1″ (1.27 to 2.54 cm) into the patient's rectum. After moving his finger in a rotating manner, he should gently pull the rectum to one side.

• He should allow 15 minutes for the bowel to empty. If any bleeding occurs, he should stop immediately and notify the physician. If, after 15 minutes, the patient's bowel has not emptied, he should wait 24 hours before repeating the procedure.
• When the procedure is completed, he should remove and dispose of the glove, cleanse the patient's perineal area with soap and water, dry it thoroughly, and remove and dispose of the soiled bed-saver pads. Then he should make the patient comfortable.

8 Discuss guidelines for bladder training (if applicable).

See Chapter 7, Genitourinary Disorders, for instructions on bladder training.

9 Demonstrate self-catheterization (if applicable).

See Chapter 7, Genitourinary Disorders, for instructions on self-catheterization.

10 Demonstrate care of an indwelling (Foley) catheter (if applicable).

See Chapter 7, Genitourinary Disorders, for instructions on care of an indwelling (Foley) catheter.

11 Explain skin care measures used to prevent skin breakdown.

To prevent skin breakdown, the following skin care measures should be used:
—The patient should change position regularly. If he cannot do this himself, the family will need to help. If the patient is a paraplegic, he should shift position at least every 15 minutes while sitting in a wheelchair.
—Special equipment, such as an egg-crate, air, or water mattress; flotation pads; and heel and elbow protectors, is available to minimize pressure on the patient's body. The patient should know how to obtain and use these positioning aids, if needed.
—A high-protein, low-calcium, high-fluid diet helps maintain healthy skin, which is less prone to skin breakdown. All skin surfaces, especially bony prominences, should be inspected regularly for pressure signs, such as blanched or reddened areas. (The paraplegic can do this himself with a hand-held mirror.) Reddened areas should be gently massaged (especially over bony prominences) to stimulate circulation. The skin must be kept clean and dry. If breakdown occurs, the physician should be consulted for treatment measures.

12 Discuss options for sexual gratification.

The patient with a neurologic disorder may enhance sexual experiences in the following ways:
—The patient should let his sexual partner know what his needs are, what he likes, and what he does not like. For example, the patient should let his partner

know which body parts he can move, areas where he has no feeling, and areas where he is sensitive to touch.

—Regardless of his disorder, he may still be able to use his hands, eyes, and tongue, as well as conversation, imagination, and mechanical aids, to increase sexual enjoyment. These sexual options will permit participation and help provide intimacy and personal satisfaction.

—If the patient has functional use of his hands, he can use them to sexually stimulate or even satisfy his partner. He can try body massage to identify areas that are most sexually stimulating to his partner.

—If the patient does not have functional use of his hands, he can use oral sex, involving sucking, nibbling, and tongue stimulation of his partner's body. Oral stimulation can be sexually satisfying.

—Because of the patient's physical limitations, he may want to experiment with sexual positions; for example, man on top of woman; woman on top of man; woman sitting on partner's lap facing him and both moving in a rocking motion; anal intercourse; woman in crawling position with partner entering her from the back; and man and woman lying sideways, face to face.

—If the patient has a catheter, it is not always necessary to remove it before intercourse. After the penis is erect, the catheter may be bent and folded along the penile shaft. If the patient is female, the catheter can be pushed aside and positioned out of the way.

—If the patient has an ostomy, he should empty the pouch before sexual intercourse. He may also want to use a pouch cover.

—If the patient is female and has vaginal lubrication difficulties, she can use a water-soluble lubricant, such as K-Y Lubricating Jelly.

—To achieve better motion during sexual activity, the patient and his partner may want to consider a water bed. Another way to achieve better movement is to take advantage of muscle spasms.

—If the patient is a paraplegic or quadriplegic, or is not always capable of maintaining an erection, he may want to consider using some of the mechanical aids available:

- The penis stiffener is a formed piece of hard rubber that fits over the patient's penis and holds it erect for penetration.
- The dildo is an artificial penis, usually made of semihard rubber, that is strapped on or above the penis. A dildo can also be hand-held.
- The vibrator is an artificial penis made of hard plastic. It is battery-operated and hand-held.

• The flexible rubber sheath can be placed over the vibrator for greater vaginal or anal stimulation.
• The diaphragm inserter straps around the patient's wrist and aids in diaphragm insertion and removal.

13 Explain safety precautions to use in sensory loss.	See the "Cerebrovascular Accident" teaching plan in this chapter for safety precautions used to compensate for sensory loss.

EPILEPSY

Patient objectives	*Teaching plan content*
1 Define epilepsy.	Epilepsy is a chronic condition of the brain characterized by a susceptibility to recurrent seizures.
2 Define a seizure.	A seizure is a sudden discharge of abnormal electrical activity in the brain that produces erratic physical movements.
3 Describe the two types of epilepsy.	Epilepsy is categorized according to cause. —In idiopathic epilepsy, the cause of the seizures is unknown. (It is currently thought that a brain chemistry abnormality may cause electrical instability of brain cells.) This type of epilepsy tends to run in families. —In acquired epilepsy, the seizures are a symptom of conditions affecting the electrical activity of the brain. These conditions include the following: • anoxia (lack of oxygen) or hypoxia (diminished oxygen), which can result from heart or lung problems that prevent sufficient oxygen from reaching the brain, or from birth trauma that diminishes the flow of blood to the brain • infectious diseases, such as meningitis • fever • exposure to toxic substances • head injury • metabolic disorders, such as low blood sugar • nutritional disorders, such as vitamin B_6 deficiencies.
4 Discuss how seizures occur.	Seizures result from brain cell irritation. —When brain cells become irritated, they become excited. The excitation sets off rapid discharges of electrical activity (as many as 1,000 per second) from the brain. —The body responds to the rapid discharges by producing erratic sensory manifestations or physical move-

ment, depending upon which area of the brain is being irritated. The patient should be familiar with the anatomy of the brain (an illustration or model can be used to demonstrate), including the following structures:

- frontal lobe (motor cortex, sensory cortex)
- parietal lobe (sensory discrimination and body image)
- temporal lobe (hearing, smell, sensation, speech, short-term memory)
- occipital lobe (vision).

5 Describe the symptoms of the relevant types of seizures.

Epileptic seizures are classified according to the symptoms produced. The patient should know the symptoms of the types of epileptic seizures (based on the international classification), he experiences:

—If the patient has simple partial seizures (focal and jacksonian), the irritable focus is located in the portion of the brain responsible for motor activity (motor cortex of the frontal lobe). Since a large portion of the motor cortex controls face and hand movements, most motor seizures affect these areas. A focal motor seizure affects a focal area, such as the hand. A jacksonian seizure is a focal motor seizure with a "marching" spread of activity to adjacent areas. It may start in the fingers, then expand to the hand, arm, face, or an entire side of the body. The activity appears to march along the body part as the focus involves adjacent areas of the cortex.

—In motor seizures, convulsive activity is usually clonic, beginning with slow, repetitive jerking that may increase in intensity. It may last from 5 seconds to several minutes. During the postictal phase (the period immediately after a seizure), the affected body part may experience temporary paralysis, which may last from a few minutes up to 24 hours.

—Complex partial seizures are most often associated with alterations in consciousness. One of the most common types is the psychomotor (temporal lobe) seizure. Here, the irritable focus occurs in the temporal lobe. Manifestations include automatisms (lip smacking, chewing, swallowing, grimacing, or patting or picking movements of the hands) and sometimes outbursts of rage and violence. Sensory experiences, including olfactory, visual, and auditory hallucinations, often precede the automatisms. The patient may appear wild-eyed and speak in jumbled, repetitive phrases. Psychomotor seizures may last from 30 seconds to several minutes. Afterward, the patient usually will be confused; he will not remember any of the events, including the rage attacks.

—Generalized absence (petit mal) seizures affect 6% to

12% of children with seizures, but they also occur in adults. Usually, the onset occurs between ages 4 and 12. Manifestations include briefly altered levels of consciousness (absences) lasting 5 to 30 seconds. The patient stares and may occasionally blink his eyelids. Usually, absence seizures produce no premonitory symptoms, aura (a motor or sensory phenomenon signaling the onset of a seizure), or postictal state. The patient can resume normal activity after it passes.
—Generalized tonic-clonic (grand mal) seizures occur commonly and at all ages. Typically, they are associated with a prodromal symptom and/or an aura. These seizures begin suddenly and are marked by an abrupt loss of consciousness with tonic muscle spasms and an epileptic cry. The patient falls at the onset of the tonic phase, which lasts about 1 minute and is characterized by apnea and cyanosis. The clonic phase then follows, as the patient shows rapid, synchronous muscle jerking and hyperventilation. He may also show simultaneous tongue and lip biting, bladder and bowel incontinence, hypertension, pupillary dilation, tachycardia, sweating, and heavy salivation that looks like foaming at the mouth. Most tonic-clonic seizures last 2 to 5 minutes. Immediately after the clonic phase, the patient experiences postictal fatigue, confusion, memory loss, muscle weakness, and irritability. Full recovery may take a few minutes or several hours.

6 Identify at least five common factors that can trigger epileptic seizures.

Common precipitating factors include the following:
—Nontherapeutic drug levels:
- drug withdrawal
- noncompliance
- alteration of drug regimen.

—Physiologic stress:
- fatigue
- lack of sleep
- hypoglycemia
- alcohol intake
- water intoxication
- febrile states
- constipation
- certain odors
- certain musical rhythms (steady, pounding beat)
- loud noises
- being startled or frightened
- menstruation/pregnancy
- flashing lights (TV, video games, strobe lights).

—Emotional stress.

7 Describe the medication regimen.

Some drugs commonly used for this disorder are carbamazepine, diazepam, phenobarbital, phenytoin, and primidone. See Chapter 9, Drug Therapy, for specific medication instructions.

8 Discuss guidelines for prevention of seizures.

Guidelines for the patient and his family include the following:

—Good nutrition is essential.
- Take vitamin supplements, as ordered.
- Avoid water and sodium retention (for women who have premenstrual seizures).
- Consult with a dietitian or nutritionist for help in meal planning.

—Activities of daily living may have to be modified.
- Take tub baths instead of showers to avoid falling.
- Avoid stress, exhaustion, and contact sports. (Moderate physical exercise is permitted.)

9 Describe the care required during and after seizures (family objective).

The patient's family can deal with a seizure, using the following guidelines:

—Remain calm. Reassure the patient if he has not lost consciousness.

—Stay with the patient until the seizure has passed. The convulsions may last only 2 to 5 minutes. If he is left unattended, he may injure himself or choke to death.

—If he is out of bed, help him to the floor to prevent falling. (If he has grand mal seizures, the side rails of his bed should be padded and kept raised; the bed should always be in the low position.)

—If his jaws are not yet clenched, place something soft, like a folded handkerchief, between his teeth to keep him from biting his tongue. If he has dentures or an orthodontic appliance, try to remove it quickly, but take care not to be bitten. To avoid injury, never force anything between his clenched teeth. However, if he moves his jaws in a chewing motion, try to put something between his teeth when his mouth is open.

—Remove or loosen tight clothing, such as a scarf, tie, or belt.

—Turn the patient on his side with his face slightly downward and his head back (hyperextended). This lets secretions and vomitus drain from his airway and lets the tongue fall forward.

—Place a small pillow, folded jacket, or other padding under his head, but take care not to flex his neck and obstruct his airway.

—Do not move him unless he is near something that might cause injury, such as a radiator. Instead, try to move dangerous objects away from him. If he is in bed, remove extra pillows and bedclothes that could block his airway. (Avoid using pillows to pad side rails.)

—Do not attempt to restrain him during a seizure.

This will usually only worsen his convulsions and may cause injury. His hands can be gently held to prevent them from banging. (A patient wandering around during a temporal lobe seizure should not be restrained unless he is in danger.)
—If possible, protect him from curious onlookers. In a public setting, simply ask bystanders to leave.
—Reassure and reorient him if the seizure has left him frightened or disoriented.
—If another seizure starts before he regains consciousness, this may signal the onset of status epilepticus, a medical emergency. The first priority is to support respiration. Have someone call a physician, the police, or an ambulance immediately. Stay with the patient, maintain a patent airway, and observe the above precautions until help arrives.

PARKINSON'S DISEASE

Patient objectives	*Teaching plan content*
1 Define Parkinson's disease.	Parkinson's disease is a chronic degenerative disease of the nervous system characterized by progressive degeneration of the brain structures that coordinate motor functions (the basal ganglia) and gradual loss of the chemical dopamine. The cause of these changes is unknown.
2 Identify the area of the brain affected by Parkinson's disease.	The general area of the brain involved in Parkinson's disease is the basal ganglia. (An illustration can be used to demonstrate the location of these structures in the brain.)
3 Explain the function of dopamine.	Dopamine is a chemical used by the brain cells within the basal ganglia to control posture, support, and voluntary motion used in fine motor skills.
4 Identify the four major symptoms of Parkinson's disease.	Progressive degeneration of the basal ganglia and gradual loss of dopamine cause the following four major symptoms: —Slowness in starting and carrying out voluntary movement (bradykinesia) —Loss of postural reflexes, which prevents the patient from making fine adjustments necessary to maintain a stable center of balance and causes a propulsive gait —Tremor at rest, which often involves the hands in a characteristic "pill-rolling" tremor, with the thumb and index finger rubbing against each other in a circular motion as though the person were forming a pill —Rigidity (the arms, legs, and neck). Characteristi-

cally, the rigidity in Parkinson's disease gives way with little jerks when the affected muscle is stretched, giving rise to the term "cog-wheel" rigidity. Occasionally, the rigidity is smooth ("lead-pipe" rigidity).

5 Identify the components of the treatment regimen for Parkinson's disease.

While there is no cure for Parkinson's disease, treatments help control the symptoms. These include the following:
—Medications
—Strengthening exercises
—Measures to improve motor independence
—Guidelines for daily living.

6 Describe the medication regimen.

Some drugs commonly used for this disorder are amantadine hydrochloride, levodopa, levodopa-carbidopa, and trihexyphenidyl hydrochloride. See Chapter 9, Drug Therapy, for specific medication instructions.

7 Demonstrate range-of-motion (ROM) exercises.

ROM exercises are prescribed to strengthen the muscles, thereby keeping the patient as functional as possible. Prescribed active (performed by the patient) and passive (performed on him by a family member) ROM exercises must be done regularly. (See the "Spinal Cord Injury" teaching plan in this chapter for complete instructions on passive ROM exercises and *How to Strengthen Your Muscles and Joints,* pp. 170 to 174, for active ROM exercises.)

8 Identify at least five measures to promote motor independence.

Measures the patient can use to promote motor independence include the following:
—Bring the toes up with every step. In Parkinson's disease, never begin to walk without lifting the toes.
—Spread the legs (10" [25 cm] apart) when walking or turning, to provide a wide base and a better stance and to prevent falling.
—For greater safety in turning, use small steps with the feet widely separated. Never cross one leg over the other when turning. Practice walking a few yards and then turning. Walk in the opposite direction and turn. Do this 15 minutes a day.
—Practice walking into tight corners of a room to overcome fear of close places.
—To ensure good body balance, practice rapid excursions of the body, backward, forward, and to the right and left, for 5 minutes several times a day. Do not look for a wall when you start to fall; it may not be there. Practice body balance daily.
—When the legs feel frozen or "glued" to the floor, lift the toes to eliminate muscle spasm and the fear of falling. (It sometimes helps to raise the arms in a sudden,

short motion.) Then begin to walk again.
—Swing the arms freely when walking. This helps to take body weight off the legs, lessens fatigue, and loosens the arms and shoulders.
—If getting out of a chair is difficult, rise quickly to overcome the pull of gravity. Sitting down, however, should be done slowly, with the body bent sharply forward, until the buttocks touch the seat. Practice this at least 12 times a day.
—If the body lists to one side, carry a shopping bag loaded with books or other weights in the opposite hand to decrease the bend.
—Keep the fingers busy with repetitive actions performed many times a day—tear paper, jingle coins, play the piano, and so on.
—For speech, facial, or chewing difficulties, practice making faces in a mirror; massage the face vigorously when washing and bathing.
—Practice any task that is difficult, such as buttoning a shirt or getting out of bed. (If practiced 20 times a day, it becomes easier the 21st time.)
—Take a warm bath every morning and night to relax the muscles.

9 Explain at least four guidelines for daily living with Parkinson's disease.

Guidelines for daily living with Parkinson's disease focus on diet and eating behavior, elimination, position changes, dressing, speech, and medical follow-up.
—Dietary guidelines: Because of his slowness and untidiness in eating, the patient may not eat properly, putting himself at risk for a nutritional deficiency. He needs protein (if not contraindicated) to maintain his strength and fiber and plenty of liquids (at least 3,000 ml/day) to prevent constipation. Semisolids are the easiest foods to manage if a tremor and difficulty in swallowing are present. Also, it is easier to drink liquids if a straw is used. If the patient is below his ideal body weight, he should drink nutritional supplements, such as Sustacal, eggnog, and milk shakes, between meals. The patient and his family should allow plenty of time for meals. If necessary, the patient should use feeding devices. (See *Learning About Special Feeding Devices,* pp. 182 and 183.) Such devices include the following:

- Plate guards, which block food from spilling off the plate, can help patients who have difficulty feeding themselves. Attach the guard to the side of the plate opposite the hand the patient uses to feed himself. Guiding the patient's hand, show him how to push food against the guard to secure it on the utensil. Then have him try again with food of a different consistency. When the patient tires, feed him the rest of the meal. At subsequent meals, encourage him to feed himself for progressively longer periods until he can feed himself an entire meal.

- Universal cuffs help the patient with flailing hands or diminished grasp. The cuff contains a slot that holds a fork or spoon. Attach it to the hand the patient uses to feed himself, then place a fork or spoon in the slot. If necessary, bend the utensil to facilitate feedings.
- Utensils with built-up handles can help the patient with diminished grasp. They are commercially available, but can easily be made by wrapping tape around the handle of a fork or spoon.
- Long-handled utensils can help the patient with a limited range of elbow and shoulder motion.
- Swivel spoons can help the patient with a limited range of forearm motion. They can be used with universal cuffs.

—Elimination guidelines: Because of decreased intestinal mobility in Parkinson's disease, constipation can occur. To avoid this problem and subsequent dependence on enemas, a high-fiber diet, high fluid intake, and exercise are important. Urinary hesitation, frequency, and incontinence may also occur. If any of these symptoms do occur, the physician should be notified. Use of a condom (for the male patient) and sanitary pads (for the female patient) will control odor from incontinence.

—Position-change guidelines: To increase the patient's independence in getting out of bed, tie a strong rope to the foot of his bed and put the other end on top of the covers, with a knot at the end. This will allow the patient to grab the knot and pull himself up without help. To help him get up from a sitting position, he should plant his feet farther apart than normal (to provide balance), then push against the arms of his chair to stand up. The family should put sturdy armchairs in his favorite rooms. If the patient has severe bradykinesia (slowness of movement and speech), blocks should be placed under the back legs of the chair to tip it forward.

—Dressing guidelines: Finger bradykinesia can pose a problem in dressing. If this occurs, a family member can sew Velcro strips close to the front of his shirt and sew the buttons on top of the buttonholes for a natural look. Zippered sport shirts and neckties that clip under the collar facilitate dressing. Loafers are a practical alternative to shoes with laces.

—Speech guidelines: The patient can improve his speech by consciously slowing it down and exaggerating his enunciation and inflection. He can practice at home by reading aloud or singing in the shower.

—Medical follow-up: Because of the progressive nature of Parkinson's disease, close medical follow-up is essential.

ALZHEIMER'S DISEASE

Patient objectives	*Teaching plan content*
1 Define Alzheimer's disease.	Alzheimer's disease is the premature loss of brain cells, resulting in progressive loss of intellectual and physical functions. The cause of Alzheimer's disease is unknown, and there is no effective treatment available to stop its progression.
2 Explain the disease process in Alzheimer's disease.	The area of the brain involved in Alzheimer's disease is the cerebral cortex, especially the frontal lobe. The cerebrum performs motor, sensory, associative, and mental functions in specialized areas. One of these specific areas, the frontal lobe, controls voluntary muscle movements and contains motor areas (including the motor area of speech). It is the center for personality and behavioral and intellectual functions, such as judgment, memory, and problem solving. It is also the center for emotional responses. As brain cells die, the brain shrinks and neurologic dysfunction appears.
3 Identify five early symptoms of Alzheimer's disease.	Symptoms of Alzheimer's disease in its early stage vary, depending upon how rapidly cells die and which cells are the first to die. However, common symptoms include the following: —Gradual development of forgetfulness —Anomia (inability to name objects) or aphasia (inability to communicate or comprehend speech) as memory loss progresses —Spatial disorientation (for example, confusing left and right or feeling lost in familiar surroundings) —Poor judgment —Behavioral changes —Myoclonic jerks —Restlessness —Muscle rigidity.
4 Identify the symptoms of advanced Alzheimer's disease (family objective).	Symptoms of advanced Alzheimer's disease include the following: —Severe dementia (complete senility) —Incontinence —Bizarre behavior and paranoia.

5 Discuss coping strategies for the early stages of Alzheimer's disease (family objective).

Coping strategies for the early stages of the disease include the following:
—The major goal, since there is no effective treatment, is to keep the patient functioning as long as possible. The patient will feel more secure and less frustrated in an orderly and rather ritualistic environment. Consistency in his daily routine is crucial. Memory aids, such as labeling doors, drawers, and cabinets, can be very helpful.
—Family members should not endorse senile behavior. They should not agree with confused statements in order to placate the patient and should avoid letting the patient ramble; instead, they should direct him back to the present.
—When the patient is restless and agitated, family members can use warm baths, warm milk, and back massage to help decrease his restlessness. These periods can be very trying, but family members should always remember that the patient does not know what he is doing. Showing understanding and compassion can enhance the patient's sense of security.
—The family should give the patient gentle but constant reassurance when he is disturbed. They will probably need to repeat the same statements over and over, because the patient simply may not be able to remember what was said from one moment to the next.
—The patient must receive sufficient sensory input. He should be reminded of the time, date, and place so he can remain oriented for as long as possible. (This will be impossible in advanced stages of the disease.) Clocks and calendars with large, easy-to-read numbers should be placed throughout the house. The family should discuss familiar things with the patient to help promote a sense of security. Rooms should be kept well lighted, as shadows and darkness can enhance confusion and fear. "Sundowning" (a worsening of the patient's mental abilities at night) may occur. Night-lights can be helpful.
—The family should respect the patient's territorial rights, even though his behavior may appear to indicate that he does not care about his personal space. Family members should not rearrange his personal belongings or change his room. For the patient's sense of security, he should be able to see and use his personal belongings. The patient should be encouraged to dress daily, rather than stay in his nightclothes and slippers; the familiarity of his nightclothes may confuse day and night for him.
—Communicating with the patient can be frustrating. The family should speak to him in short, simple sentences when he is confused (early in the disease, he

will have lucid periods). They should maintain eye contact with him throughout the conversation and should attempt to convey a comforting attitude at all times by listening, smiling, and touching. His questions should always be answered, no matter how irrelevant they seem.
—During the patient's confused periods, which may appear abruptly, he should not be left alone. His lucid periods will become shorter and less frequent as the disease progresses.

6 Describe management strategies for advanced Alzheimer's disease (family objective).

Management strategies the family can use in the advanced stage of the disease include the following:
—A care giver must be in attendance at all times to prevent injury to the patient. The family should explore ways to provide this type of care. (They may need information about long-term facilities.)
—The family may be interested in joining a local support group for families of patients with Alzheimer's disease. (They may need the name and phone number of a contact person.)
—Family members can use relaxation techniques to help reduce their own stress. (See the "Hypertension" teaching plan in Chapter 2 for specific instructions.) They should be aware of the need to maintain their health and should seek referrals for care, as appropriate.

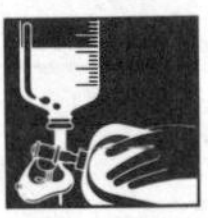

Explaining treatments

INTRACRANIAL PRESSURE (I.C.P.) MONITORING

Patient objectives	*Teaching plan content*
1 Define ICP monitoring.	ICP monitoring measures the pressure exerted by brain tissue, blood, and cerebrospinal fluid against the skull.
2 State the purpose of ICP monitoring.	The purpose of ICP monitoring is to detect an elevation in ICP before physical danger signs develop. Prompt intervention can help avert or diminish nerve damage caused by cerebral hypoxia (oxygen deprivation) and shifts of brain mass.
3 Describe the procedure used in ICP monitoring.	The device used to monitor ICP may be inserted at the bedside if the patient is in the emergency department or intensive care unit, or in the operating room if the

patient is undergoing surgery to open the skull (a craniotomy).
—If the device will be inserted during a craniotomy, see the "Craniotomy" teaching plan in this chapter.
—If the monitoring device will be inserted at bedside, the patient will be placed in a supine position, with the head of his bed elevated to approximately 30 degrees.
—A small area on his head will be shaved or his hair will be clipped at the selected insertion site, to decrease the risk of infection. His head and face will be lightly covered with sterile towels.
—A nurse will scrub the site with an antiseptic and will hold the patient's head between her hands throughout the procedure.
—After numbing the area, the physician will make a small hole in the patient's skull. He will then insert the monitoring device and position it in the correct spot.
—The device will then be connected to a machine that records the intracranial pressure.
—The physician will suture the device to the patient's scalp and apply a sterile dressing.
—Every 24 hours, or more often if needed, a nurse will change the dressing and cleanse the area.
—Every hour or so, she will check the patient and the machine to obtain readings.
—The device will be removed when the physician feels that the patient is no longer in danger of increased ICP. It will not affect brain tissue or function and, once removed, the puncture site will heal.

4 Explain patient guidelines for ICP monitoring.

Patient guidelines for ICP monitoring include the following:
—If the patient is awake and alert during the insertion procedure, he should be careful not to move his head.
—Once the device is in place, he will be repositioned frequently by the nurse. If he becomes uncomfortable, he should call the nurse to reposition him.
—He should avoid flexing his neck, turning onto his abdomen, or lifting his head off the pillow, as these positions can increase ICP.
—He should also avoid bearing down (Valsalva's maneuver) when he is on the bedpan and should avoid isometric muscle contractions (such as forcefully pulling or pushing the bed's side rails).

CRANIOTOMY

Patient objectives	*Teaching plan content*
1 Define a craniotomy.	A craniotomy is the surgical opening of the skull.

2 State the purpose of a craniotomy.

A craniotomy may be performed to remove a brain tumor, a hematoma, or an abscess or to repair an aneurysm (an outpouching of a blood vessel).

3 Explain the procedure used in a craniotomy.

First, the surgeon will make a large incision in the skull, forming a bone flap; next, he will make an incision in the brain to remove the tumor, hematoma, or abscess or to repair the aneurysm; finally, he will suture the brain, skull, and skin flap.

4 Describe preoperative procedures for a craniotomy.

The patient's head will be shaved before surgery. (The hair will grow back in time.) For further information, see instructions for preoperative teaching in Chapter 1, Principles of Patient Teaching. (See also Appendix B, *Preoperative and Postoperative Teaching.*)

5 Describe postoperative care for a craniotomy.

The patient will be taken to the intensive care unit (ICU) immediately after the procedure.

—He will awaken with a large bandage on his head, temporary swelling, discoloration around his eye on the affected side, and, possibly, a headache. He will receive pain medication.

—He will spend his first few postoperative days (or longer, as ordered by his physician) in the ICU. (If time permits, the patient and his family should visit the ICU ahead of time.) He should know that he will see unfamiliar equipment and hear unusual noises in the recovery room and the ICU.

—The patient should be familiar with any special equipment he will have in place after surgery, such as an indwelling (Foley) catheter, a heart monitor, or an intracranial pressure monitor. (See the "Intracranial Pressure Monitoring" teaching plan in this chapter, if applicable.)

—A nurse will check him frequently and will answer any questions he may have.

—The patient should avoid straining during bowel movements or coughing, as these activities increase ICP. When his physician feels he is ready, the patient will be transferred to a regular unit in the hospital to recuperate.

Patient-Teaching Aid

HOW TO PERFORM A FORWARD-BACKWARD SITTING TRANSFER

Dear Patient:
Before you leave the hospital, your physician wants you to learn how to get from your bed to your wheelchair. To learn how to do this transfer, follow these guidelines:

1

First, remove the wheelchair's leg rests. If they are not removable, swing them aside. Then, position the front of the wheelchair as close as possible to the side of your bed. Lock its wheels. If you cannot position the wheelchair yourself, ask someone to do it for you. The seat of the wheelchair should be facing the side of the bed.

Make sure you are sitting in bed with your legs extended.

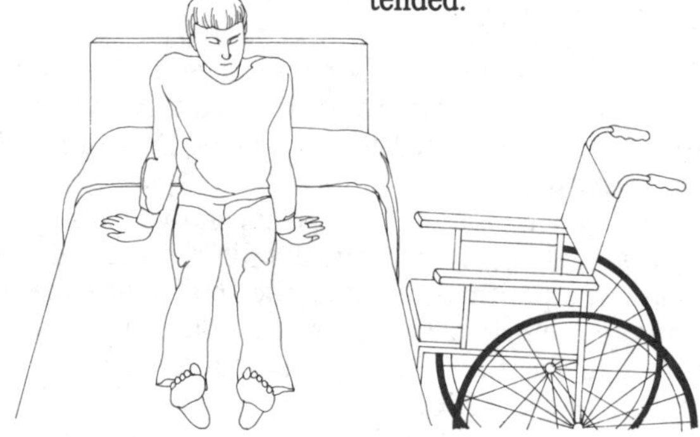

2

Next, lean slightly forward. Pushing your hands against the mattress, lift your buttocks slightly off the bed. Keeping your legs extended across the bed, inch backward to the side of the bed—close to the wheelchair. Stop when your back is directly in front of the wheelchair.

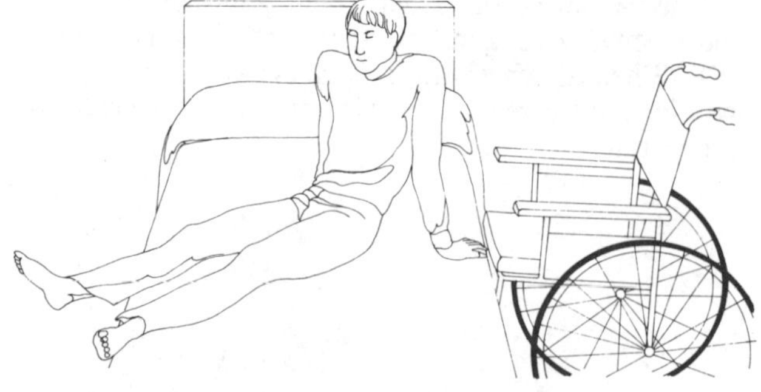

HOW TO PERFORM A FORWARD-BACKWARD SITTING TRANSFER—*continued*

3

Now, firmly grasp the armrests of the wheelchair, and gradually lift your buttocks onto the seat. Unlock the wheels. Then, push yourself away from the bed, and position yourself properly in the wheelchair.

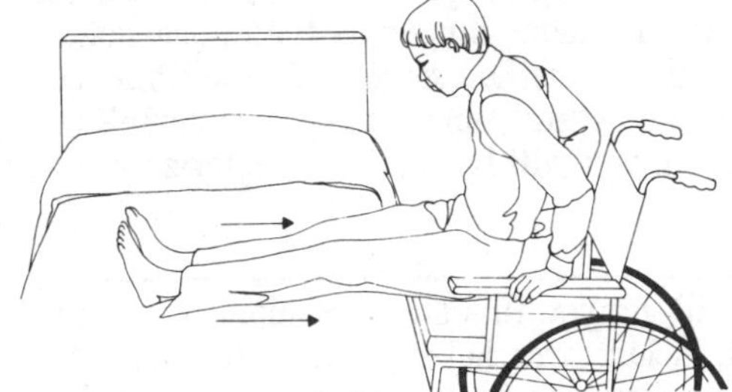

4

To get back into bed, position the wheelchair seat so it faces the bed. Remove your legs from the leg rests. Then, swing the leg rests out of the way. Now, raise your legs onto the bed as you position the chair as close as possible to the bed. Lock the chair's wheels.

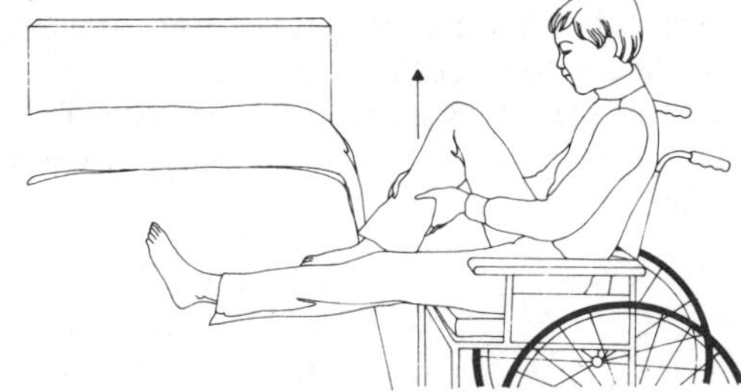

5

Next, grasp the armrests of the wheelchair, and lift your buttocks slightly off the seat. Keeping your legs extended across the bed, inch forward to the middle of the bed.

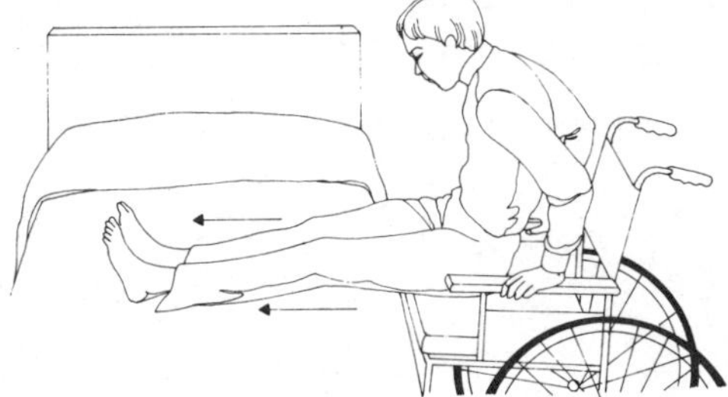

Patient-Teaching Aid

HOW TO CATHETERIZE YOURSELF USING STERILE TECHNIQUE (For the female patient)

Dear Patient:
This aid will help you learn how to catheterize yourself. During your hospital stay, you must catheterize yourself using the cleanest possible methods, because hospital germs are more dangerous than household germs. We call this method *sterile technique.* Practice sterile technique several times under your nurse's supervision. Soon, you will be able to catheterize yourself easily.

1

The nurse will get you this sterile equipment: a catheter care kit, including catheter, three cotton balls, forceps, sterile waterproof drape, povidone-iodine packet, water-soluble lubricant, container for draining urine, and two sterile gauze pads. She will give you sterile gloves if your kit does not include them. She will also give you a paper bag for discarding used equipment.

Use a mirror the first few times you catheterize yourself to help you locate your meatus, but do not become dependent on the mirror. After a few catheterizations, you should no longer need it.

Before catheterizing yourself, try to urinate. To make this easier, press on your abdomen or stroke your inner thighs.

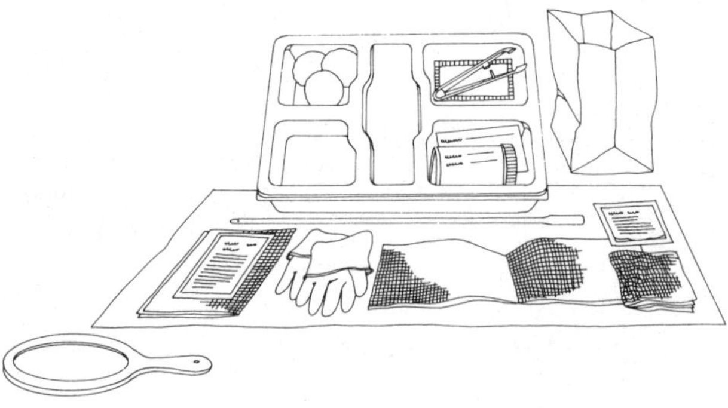

HOW TO CATHETERIZE YOURSELF USING STERILE TECHNIQUE (For the female patient)—*continued*

2

Wash your hands thoroughly. Now, position yourself correctly. For your first few catheterizations, you may find it convenient to sit on a bed, with your legs bent and your knees apart. After you become more skilled, you may sit on a toilet. Arrange your clothing so it is out of your way.

The nurse will get a small table for your equipment. Then, open the kit, making sure you do not touch its insides.

3

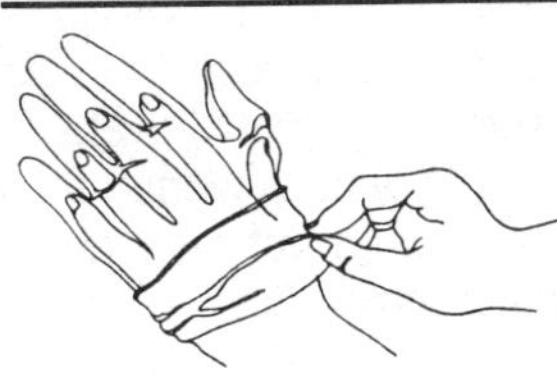

Now, put on the sterile glove, by grasping the folded edge of the cuff.

4

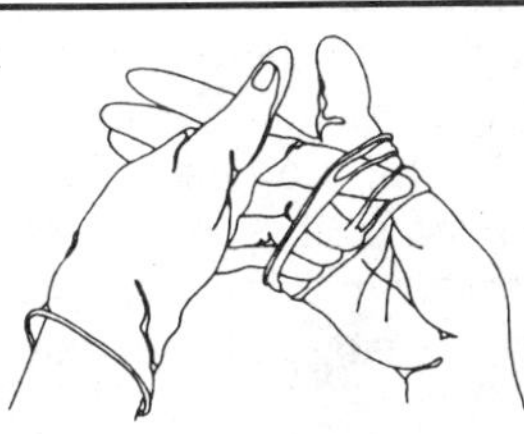

Then, place the fingers of your gloved hand in the cuff of the second glove and pull on the second glove, too.

5

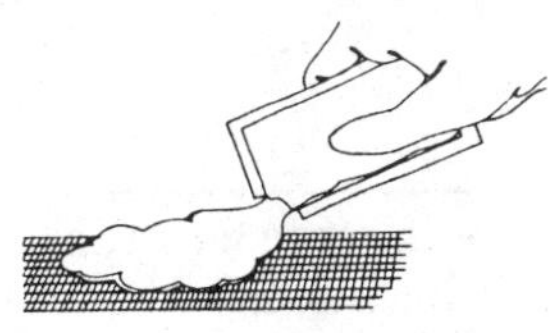

Now, lay down the sterile drape with the shiny, coated side down. Squirt sterile lubricant onto the drape. Then, open the povidone-iodine solution packet. Pour the povidone-iodine solution on the cotton balls.

6

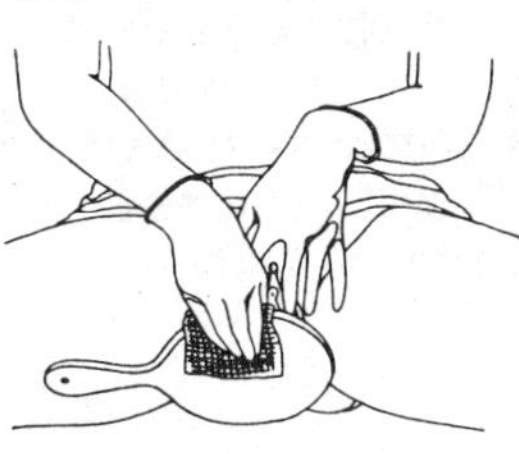

Now, use the gauze pads in your dominant hand to pick up the mirror. Be careful to touch only the gauze pads and not the mirror. Using the mirror, find your vaginal folds and urethral meatus. Hold the folds apart with your index and second finger. Identify the meatus. Remember, the hand you use to hold apart your vaginal folds is now contaminated. Do not touch anything sterile with it.

HOW TO CATHETERIZE YOURSELF USING STERILE TECHNIQUE (For the female patient)—*continued*

7

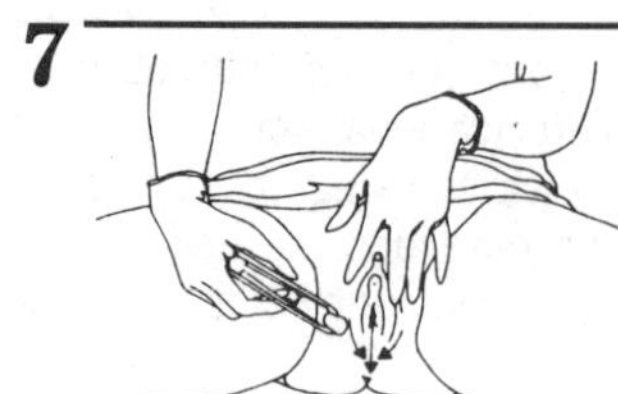

Now, clean your vaginal area. To do this, pick up the soaked cotton balls with the forceps. Clean the area between the folds with three downward strokes, using one cotton ball on the right downstroke, one on the left downstroke, and one down the center. Throw the cotton balls into the trash bag.

8

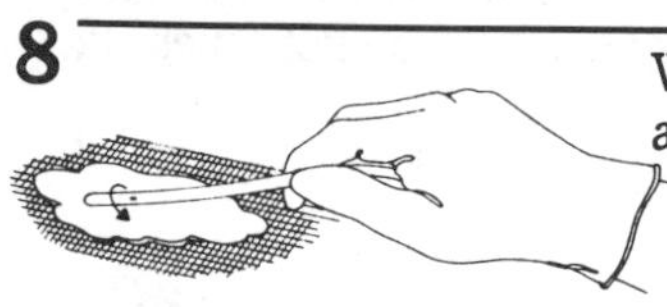

With your uncontaminated hand, pick up the catheter and roll the first 3″ of it in the lubricant.

9

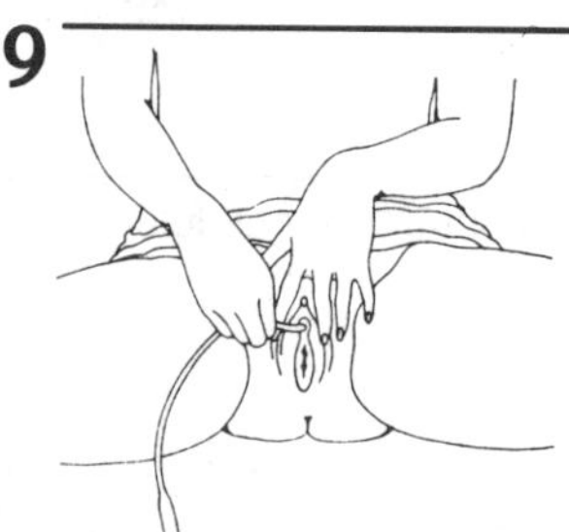

Holding your vaginal folds apart with your contaminated hand, use your other hand to grasp the catheter like a pencil or a dart. Insert it upward into the urethra. When urine begins to flow, gently push the catheter about 1″ farther. Then, allow all urine to drain from the bladder. Press down with your abdominal muscles and move the catheter in and out once or twice to help drain your bladder completely.

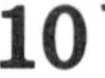

10

When the urine stops draining, pinch the catheter near its tip, to prevent urine from leaking into the urethra. Remove the catheter slowly. Tilt the tip upward as it comes out of the meatus, to avoid spilling urine on yourself. Then, throw the catheter into the trash bag. Dress yourself and dispose of the bag and used equipment.

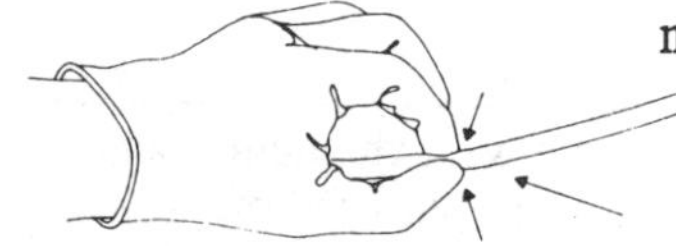

11

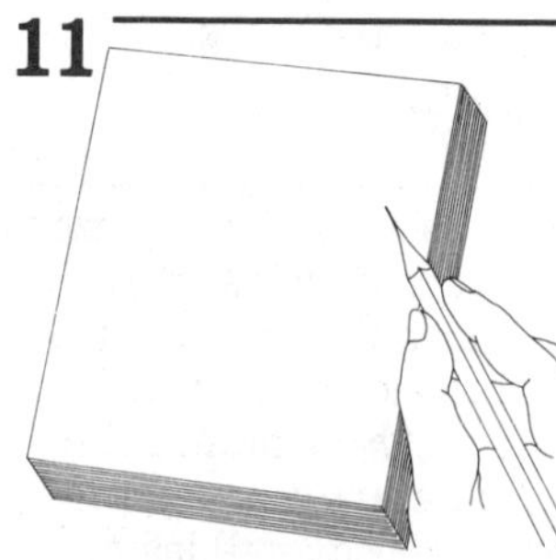

Finally, if your physician requires it, write down the amount, color, and odor of the urine. Also, write down whether the urine is clear or cloudy. Note any particles or blood in the urine and tell your physician about them at once. Let your physician know immediately if the amount of urine increases or decreases; if you have difficulty catheterizing yourself; or if you experience pain or burning during catheterization.

Patient-Teaching Aid

HOW TO CATHETERIZE YOURSELF USING STERILE TECHNIQUE (For the male patient)

Dear Patient:
This aid will help you learn how to catheterize yourself. During your hospital stay, you must catheterize yourself using the cleanest possible method, because hospital germs are more dangerous than household germs. We call this method *sterile technique.* Practice sterile technique several times under your nurse's supervision. Soon, you will be able to catheterize yourself easily.

1

The nurse will get you this sterile equipment: a catheter care kit, including catheter, three cotton balls, forceps, sterile waterproof drape, povidone-iodine packet, container for draining urine, and water-soluble lubricant. She will give you the sterile gloves if your kit does not include them. She will also give you a paper bag for discarding used equipment.

Before catheterizing yourself, try to urinate. To make this easier, press on your abdomen or stroke your inner thighs.

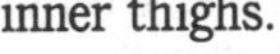

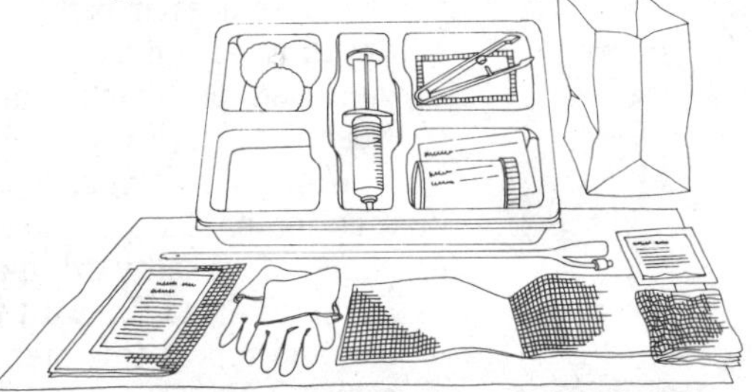

2

Wash your hands thoroughly. Sit on the toilet or on a chair for your first few catheterizations. Later, when you are more skilled, you can stand over the toilet. Arrange your clothing so it is out of your way.

The nurse will get a small table for your equipment. Or, if you are standing over the toilet, use the toilet-tank top.

Open the kit, without touching its insides.

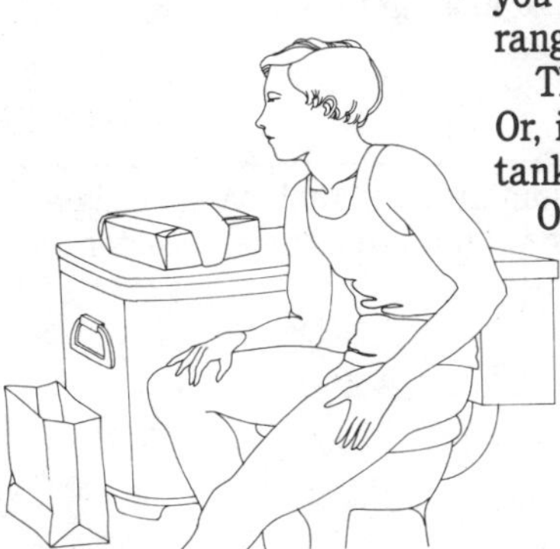

HOW TO CATHETERIZE YOURSELF USING STERILE TECHNIQUE (For the male patient)—*continued*

3

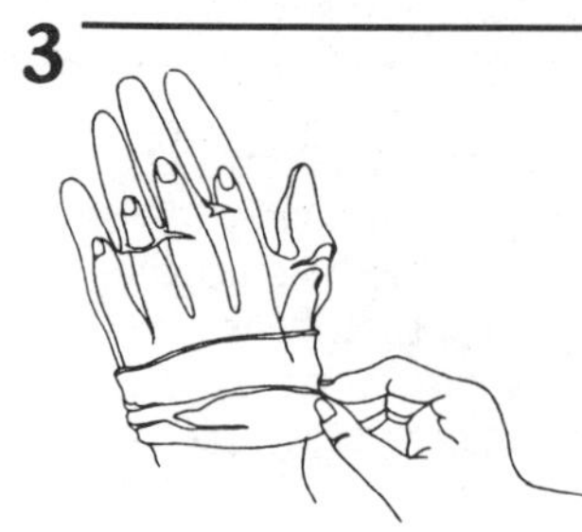

Now, put on one glove by grasping the folded edge of the cuff. Then, place the fingers of your gloved hand in the cuff of the second glove and pull on the second glove, too. Then, position the drape shiny, coated side down and lay out your equipment.

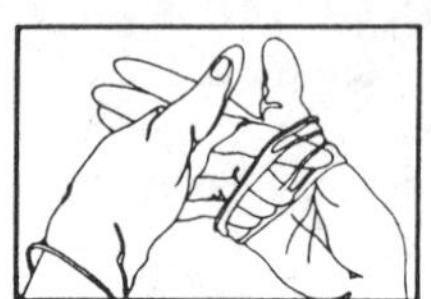

4

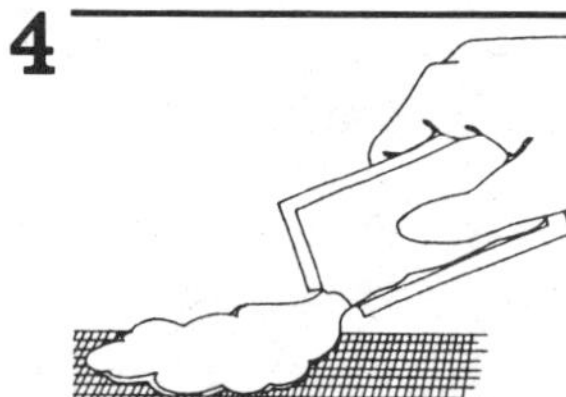

Next, squirt out the sterile lubricant onto the drape. Then, open the povidone-iodine solution packet. Pour the povidone-iodine on the cotton balls.

5

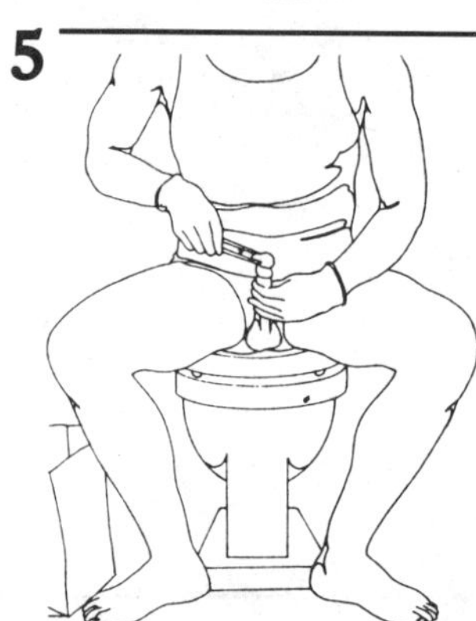

Now, you are ready to clean your penis with the saturated cotton balls. With your nondominant hand, grasp the sides of your penis. NOTE: Do not use this hand for anything else during the procedure. If you are uncircumcised, pull back your foreskin with the same hand. Keep the foreskin pulled back for insertion.

With your dominant hand, use the forceps to pick up a cotton ball. Begin cleaning at the opening of your penis. Move outward in a spiral motion to the edge of the penis head. Discard the cotton ball into the paper bag and repeat this step until you have used all three cotton balls.

6

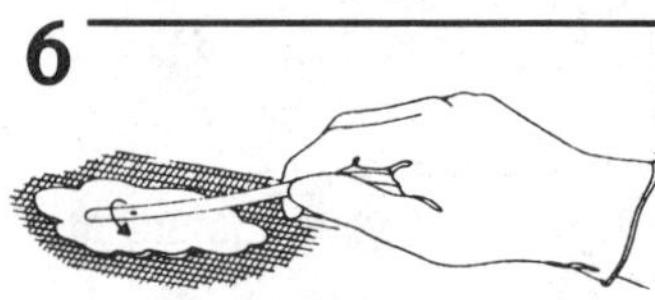

With the same hand, pick up the catheter and roll the first 7″ to 10″ of it in the lubricant.

7

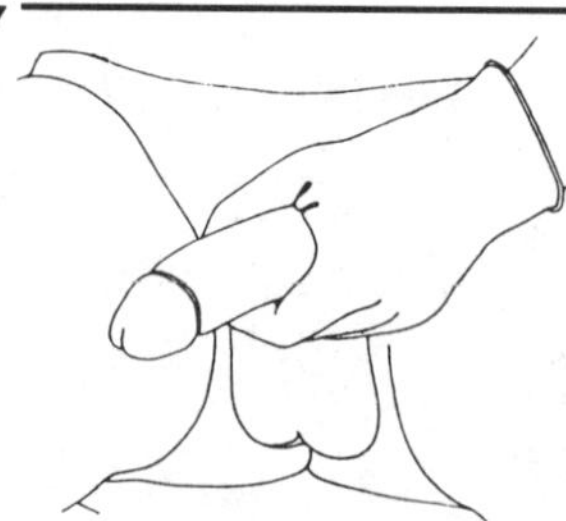

Now, using your nondominant hand, hold your penis at a right angle to your body, and prepare for catheter insertion.

HOW TO CATHETERIZE YOURSELF USING STERILE TECHNIQUE (For the male patient)—*continued*

8

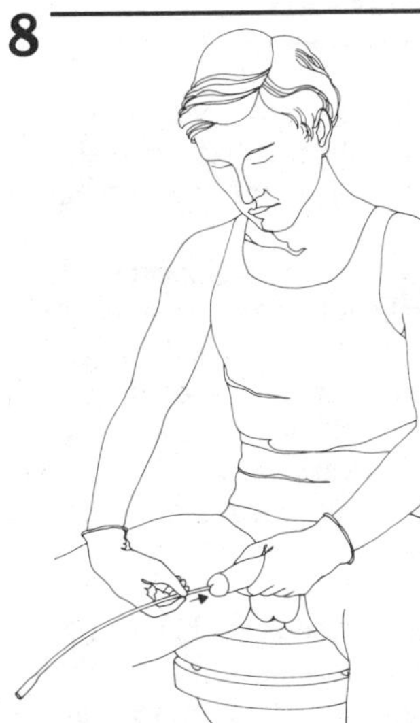

Holding the catheter like a pencil or a dart, gently advance the catheter 7″ to 10″ into your urethra.

Never force the catheter. However, when the catheter is about halfway inserted, you may feel resistance. Applying firm but gentle pressure to the catheter will help relax tight muscles and permit the catheter to pass.

NOTE: If you are inserting a coudé-tipped Tiemann catheter, keep the tip pointed up at all times.

When the urine begins to flow, gently push the catheter 1″ farther. Allow all urine to drain into the toilet or container; press down with your abdominal muscles to completely empty the bladder.

9

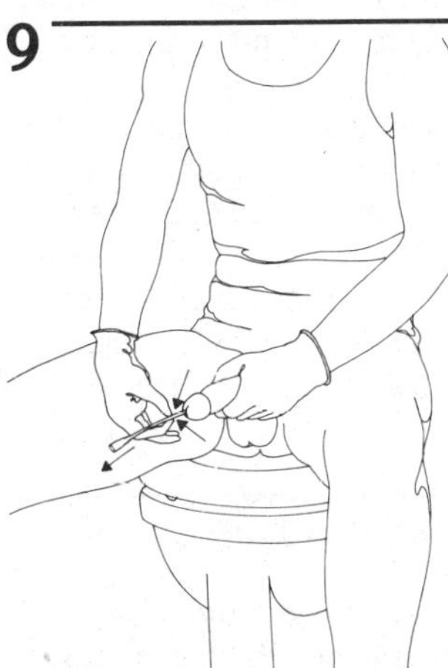

When the urine stops draining, pinch the catheter near its tip and remove it slowly. Tilt the tip upward as it comes out of the meatus, to avoid spilling urine on yourself. Discard the catheter in the paper bag. If you are uncircumcised, pull the foreskin forward again. Dress yourself and discard the paper bag and used equipment in the trash can.

10

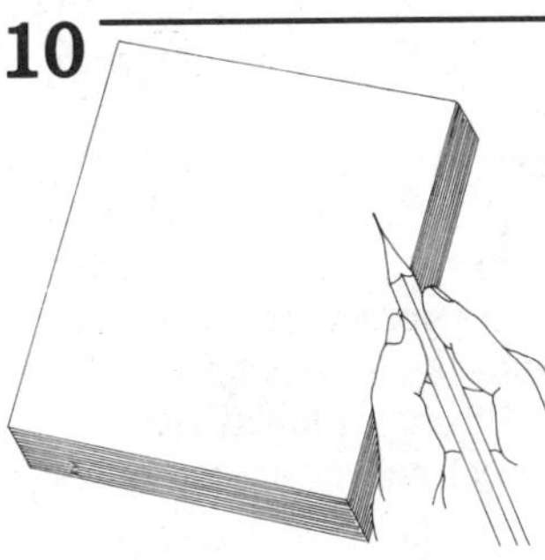

Finally, if your physician requires it, write down the amount, color, and odor of the urine. Also write down whether the urine is clear or cloudy. Note any particles or blood and tell your physician about them at once. Also, let your physician know immediately if the amount of urine increases or decreases, if you have difficulty catheterizing yourself, or if you experience pain or burning during catheterization.

Patient-Teaching Aid

HOW TO CATHETERIZE YOURSELF USING CLEAN TECHNIQUE (Male and female)

Dear Patient:

When you return home from the hospital, you will not have to use sterile technique to catheterize yourself. Just remember to take the few simple precautions outlined here.

In home self-catheterization, it is very important to follow your catheterization schedule strictly. Otherwise, you will retain urine, which can lead to infection, a stretched bladder, or urine leakage. Never postpone catheterization for any reason, such as not having soap and water handy. Cleanliness is very important, but on the rare occasions when you cannot wash, you must perform the procedure anyway to avoid the greater medical risks.

Remember that intermittent catheterization is only one component of controlling incontinence. By carefully regulating your fluid intake, you can help prevent incontinence and still maintain a good level of hydration. Also, you must remember to take your prescribed bladder medications regularly.

To catheterize yourself using clean technique, you will need a rubber catheter, a clean washcloth, soap and water, a small package of water-soluble lubricant, and a plastic bag for used catheters. Also, obtain a container for draining urine if a toilet is not available or if you need to measure your urine. Make sure you have good lighting. Before catheterization, try to urinate, then wash your hands.

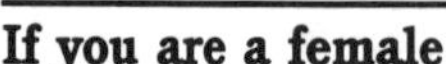

If you are a female

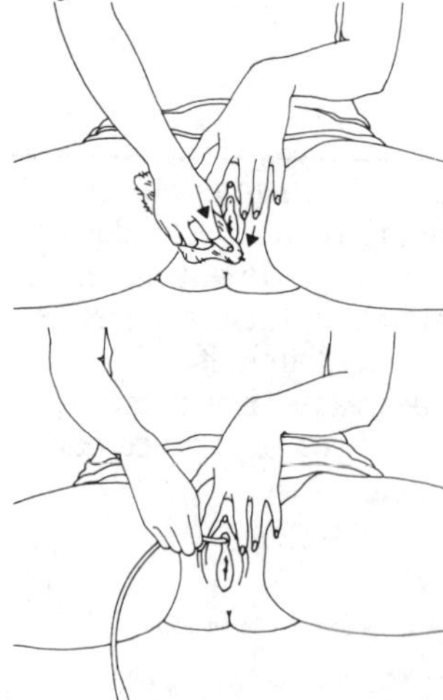

Position yourself on a bed or toilet. Arrange your clothing so it is out of your way.

Separate your vaginal folds with one hand. Use downward strokes with the washcloth to wash the area thoroughly.

Lubricate the first 3″ (7.6 cm) of the catheter with water-soluble jelly.

Now you are ready for insertion. Hold the catheter as if it were a pencil, about ½″ (1.3 cm) from its tip. Keeping the vaginal folds separated, slowly insert the lubricated catheter about 3″ into your urethra. Press down with your abdominal muscles to empty your bladder. Allow all urine to drain through the catheter. When the urine stops draining, remove the catheter slowly.

HOW TO CATHETERIZE YOURSELF USING CLEAN TECHNIQUE (Male and female)—*continued*

Wash the catheter in warm, soapy water. Then rinse it inside and out, and dry it with a clean towel. Place it in the plastic storage bag for used catheters.

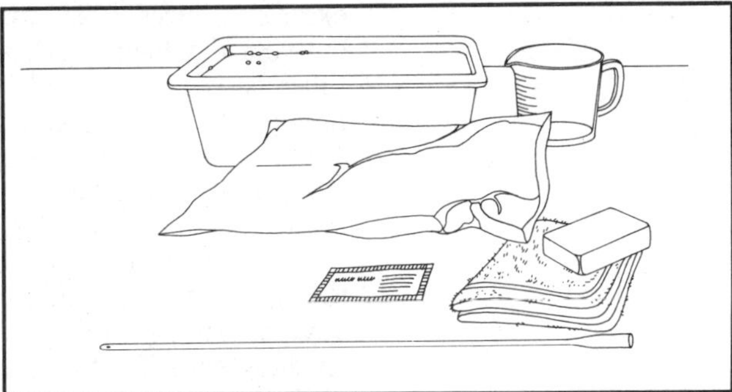

If you are a male

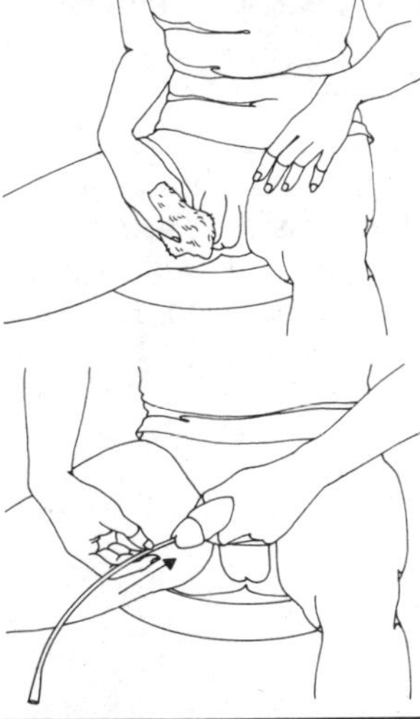

Position yourself on a bed or toilet. If you are uncircumcised, pull back the foreskin of your penis and hold it back throughout the catheterization. Then, wash the end of your penis thoroughly with soap and water.

Lubricate the first 7″ to 10″ (17.8 to 25.4 cm) of the catheter with water-soluble jelly.

Then, hold your penis at a right angle to your body. Grasp the catheter as you would a pencil, and slowly insert it 7″ to 10″ until urine begins to flow. Then gently push the catheter 1″ farther. Allow all urine to drain.

When urine stops draining, slowly remove the catheter. If you are uncircumcised, pull your foreskin forward again. Wash the catheter in warm, soapy water. Then rinse it inside and out, and dry it with a clean towel. Place the catheter in the used-catheter storage bag.

Remember

Buy a new catheter supply each month or when catheters become brittle. Use each catheter only once. When you have used all but the last one, boil the catheters for 20 minutes. Drain the water and store the catheters in a clean towel. Each time you use a catheter, be sure to put it in the plastic storage bag for used catheters, not back with the clean catheters.

Patient-Teaching Aid

HOW TO STRENGTHEN YOUR MUSCLES AND JOINTS

Dear Patient:
Now that you are ready to return home, you will need to continue strengthening and toning your muscles. By exercising twice a day, you will find it easier to carry out your day-to-day activities. Repeat each exercise five times on the muscle or joint being strengthened.
IMPORTANT: If you feel severe pain when performing any of these exercises, stop immediately. If pain persists, notify your physician. Never force or overstretch a muscle, as you may cause further damage.

And remember, to get the maximum benefit out of this program, perform each exercise slowly and gently. Try performing all the exercises the nurse has circled on these sheets in the morning and again before dinner. Work the exercises into your daily routine; for example, exercise as you bathe or while watching TV.

NOTE: If you are performing the exercises in a bed or chair with wheels, make sure they are locked before you begin.

Use these instructions as a guide:

1 Neck exercises

Keeping your shoulders level, touch your chin to your right shoulder or as close to it as possible. Then, touch your chin to your left shoulder or as close to it as possible. Do not raise your shoulder to your chin. Return to the starting position.

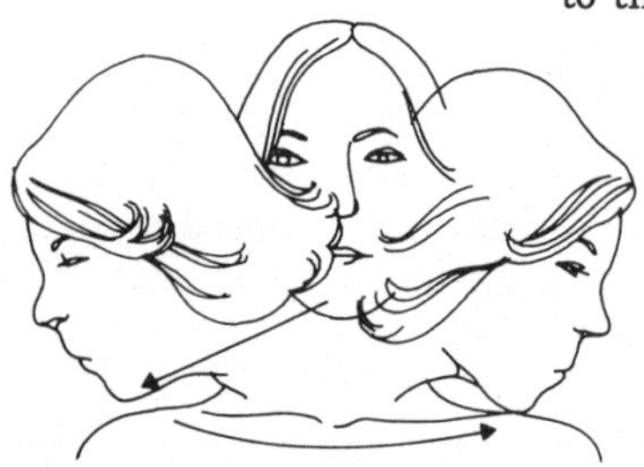

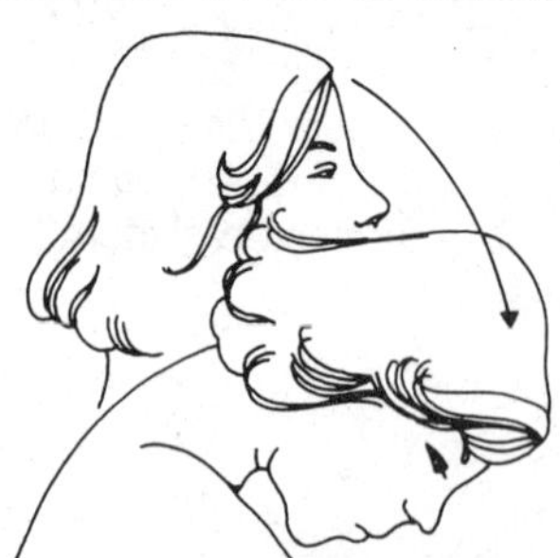

Now, touch your chin to your chest or as close to it as possible. Raise your chin to starting position.

HOW TO STRENGTHEN YOUR MUSCLES AND JOINTS—*continued*

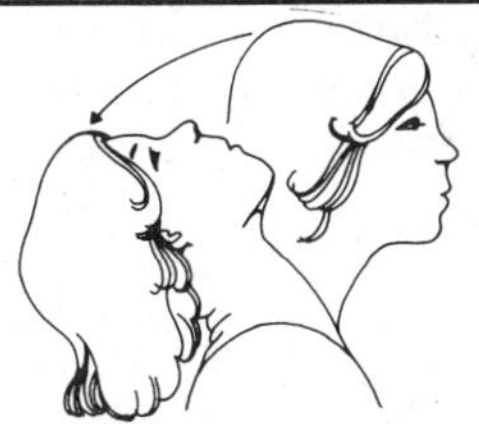

Next, bend your head and neck backward as far as possible. Return your head to starting position.

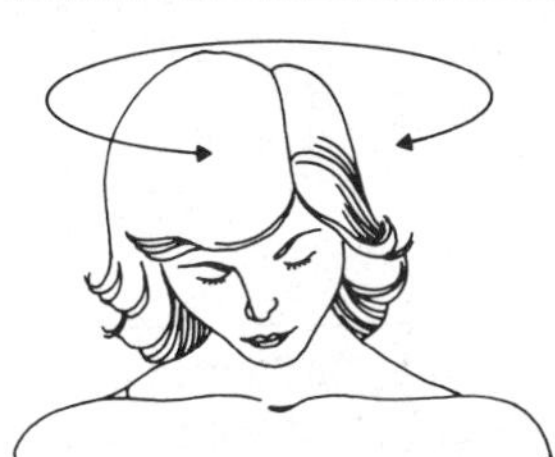

Rotate your head and neck clockwise. Then, rotate your head and neck counterclockwise.

2 Trunk exercises

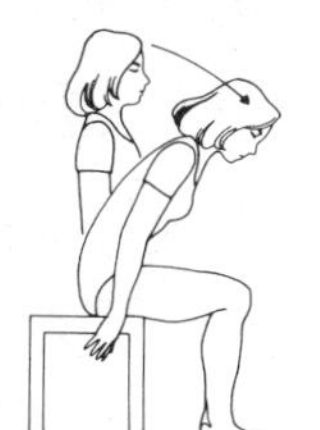

Sit on a chair so your legs are straight and your arms hang loosely at your side. Bend forward as far as possible. Return to starting position.

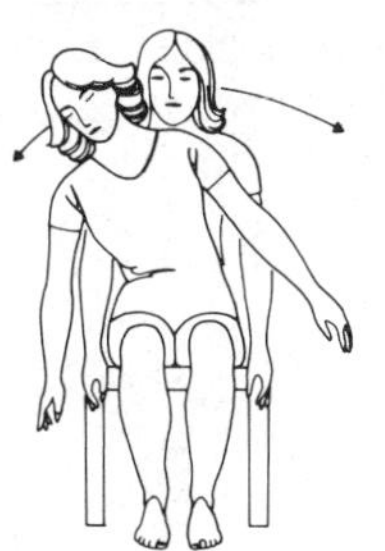

Now, maintaining the same position, bend to the right side, making sure you bend from the waist. Then, bend to the left. Return to starting position.

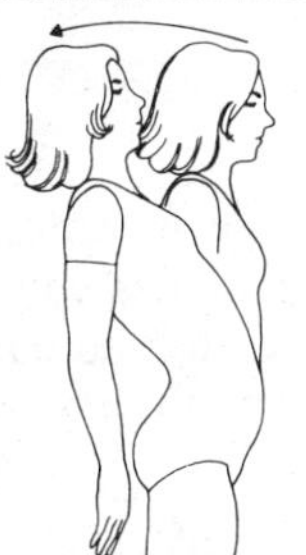

Next, stand with your feet 2″ (5 cm) apart. Let your arms hang loosely at your sides and—without bending your knees—bend backward, as far as possible. Return to starting position.

HOW TO STRENGTHEN YOUR MUSCLES AND JOINTS—*continued*

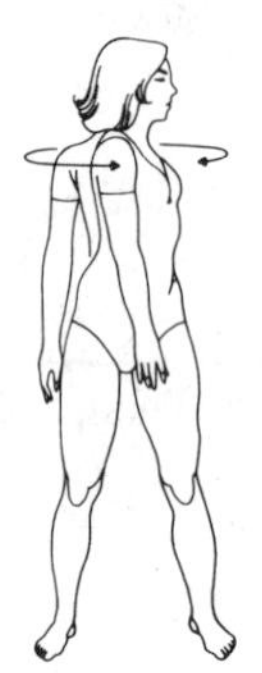

Keeping your hips facing straight ahead, twist your upper body to the right as far as possible. Then, twist your body to the left as far as possible. Return to starting position.

3 Shoulder exercises

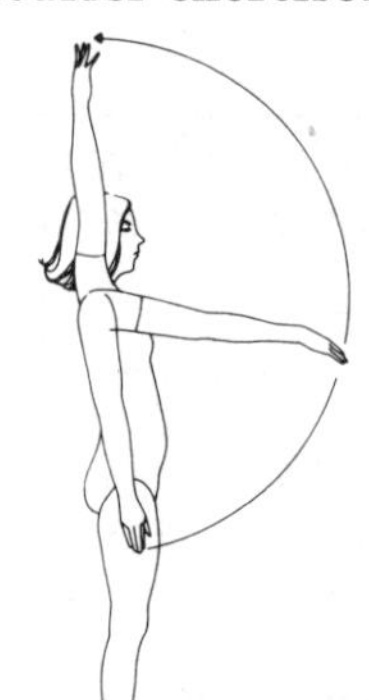

Standing straight with your arms at your sides, raise your right arm forward and upward (over your head) as far as possible. Return to starting position, and repeat the exercise with your left arm.

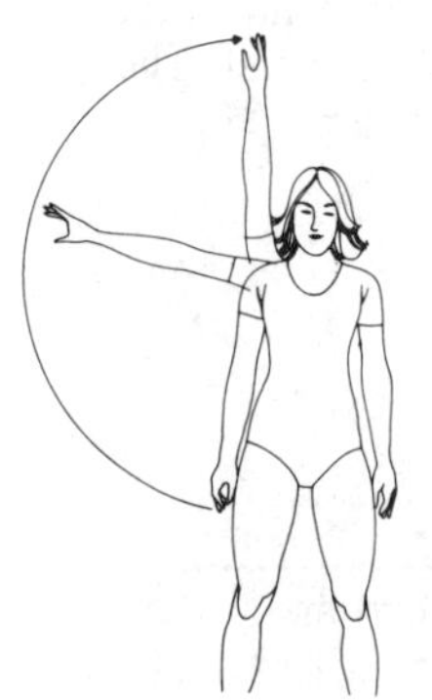

Now, standing with your arms at your sides, raise your right arm sideways and upward, over your head, or as far as possible. Return your right arm to starting position, and repeat the exercise with your left arm.

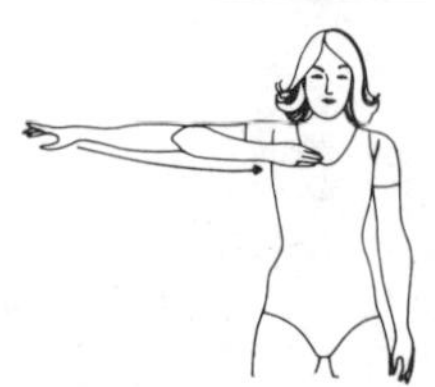

Maintaining the same position, raise your right arm to shoulder level. Then bring your arm across your body toward your left shoulder or as close to it as possible. Return your arm to starting position, and repeat the exercise with your left arm.

HOW TO STRENGTHEN YOUR MUSCLES AND JOINTS—*continued*

4 Wrist exercises

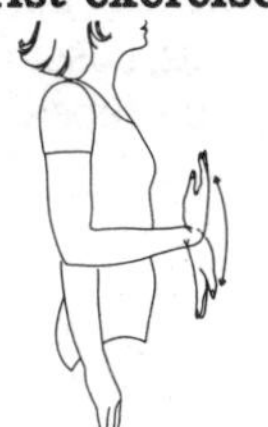

Keeping your upper right arm at your side, bend your elbow so your forearm is at a 90-degree angle to your upper arm. Turn your palm up so it is facing the ceiling. Now, without bending your elbow, raise your hand as far as possible. Then, lower your hand as far as possible. Return your hand to starting position, and repeat the exercise with your left hand.

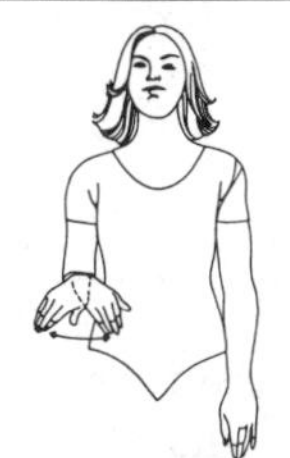

Next, maintaining the same position, move your hand toward your body as close to it as possible. Then move your hand away from your body as far as possible. Return to starting position and repeat the exercise with your left hand.

5 Elbow exercises

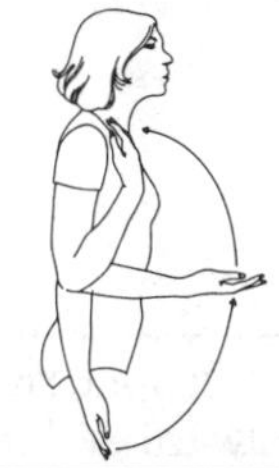

For this exercise, you can sit or stand, whichever is most comfortable. Let your arms hang loosely at your side. Then, bending your right elbow, bring your fingertips to your right shoulder or as close to it as possible. Return your right arm to starting position, and repeat the exercise with your left arm.

6 Forearm exercises

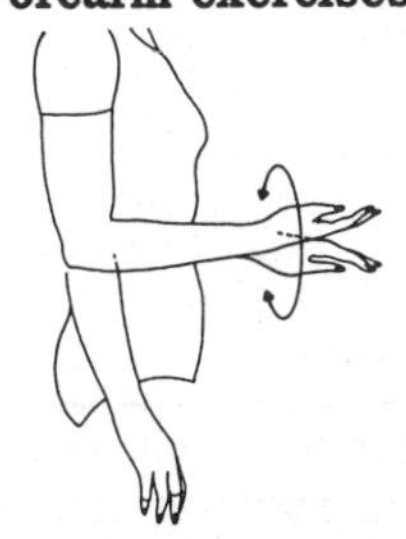

Keeping your upper right arm at your side, bend your elbow so your forearm is at a 90-degree angle to your upper arm and your palm is facing the ceiling. Turn your palm down, then up. Repeat the exercise with your left hand.

7 Knee exercises

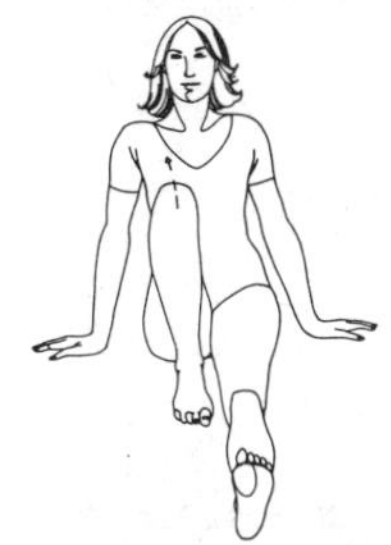

For this exercise, you can sit on the bed with your legs straight ahead of you or lie on your abdomen with your legs extended. Bend your right knee as much as possible. Return to starting position, and repeat the exercise with your left knee.

HOW TO STRENGTHEN YOUR MUSCLES AND JOINTS—*continued*

8 Hip exercises

Lie on your back and bend your right knee. Bring your knee toward your chest or as close to it as possible. Return your knee to starting position, and repeat the exercise with your left knee.

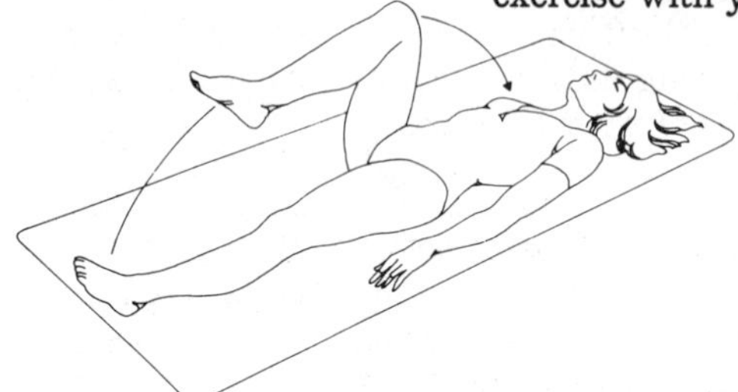

Next, keeping your knee and hip straight and toes pointed upward, move your right leg to the right as far as possible. Return to starting position, and repeat the exercise with your left leg.

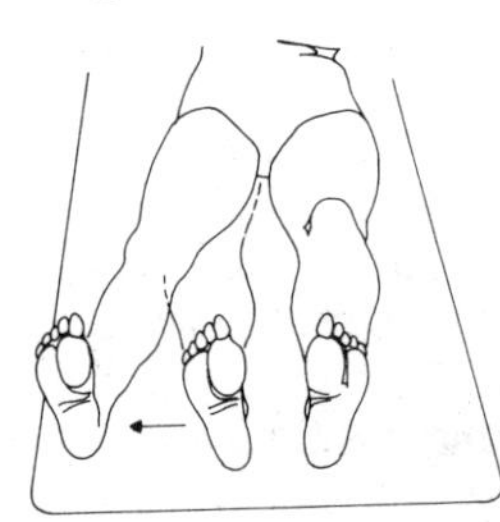

Bend your hip and knee so the bottom of your right foot is flat on the bed. Roll your leg inward as far as possible. Return to starting position, and repeat the exercise with the left leg.

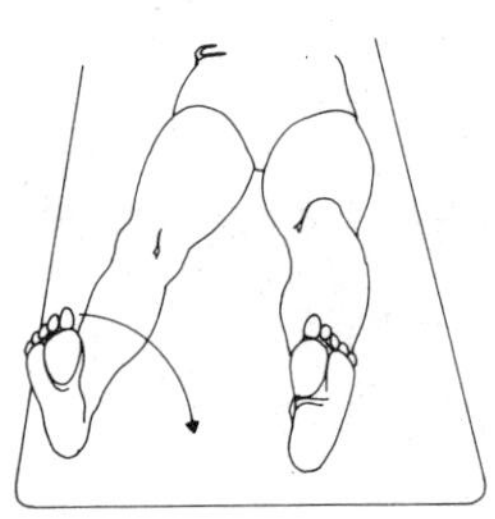

Now, maintaining the same position with your back and hips flat on the bed, raise your right leg upward as far as possible. Return your right leg to starting position, and repeat the exercise with your left leg.

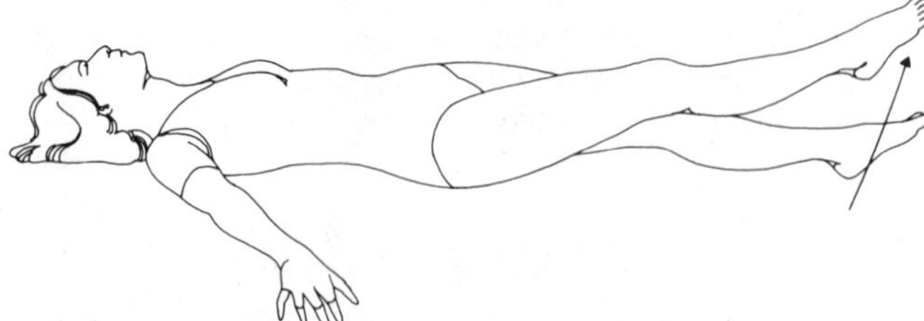

Patient-Teaching Aid

DISCHARGE INSTRUCTIONS FOR HEAD-INJURED PATIENTS

Dear Patient:

Although you have had a head injury, your physician has found no evidence of serious injury. You will not be hospitalized at this time.

However, for the next few days, you must watch your condition closely. If you develop any of the following symptoms, call the physician at once or come to the emergency department:

- Increasing drowsiness
- Difficulty waking up (NOTE TO FAMILY: Wake the patient every 2 hours during the first night.)
- Vomiting
- Slowing of pulse
- Continued headache
- Neck stiffness
- Bleeding or clear fluid dripping from the ears or nose
- Weakness of either leg or arm
- Convulsions (fits).

Patient-Teaching Aid

GOING HOME WITH A CANE

Dear Patient:
Your doctor says you are ready to return home. But he wants you to use a cane, to help you put full weight on your affected leg as you walk. The following are guidelines for a person with an affected *left* leg. If your *right* leg is affected, start with the cane on your left side, and adapt the instructions. You may want to draw the patterns for yourself.

1

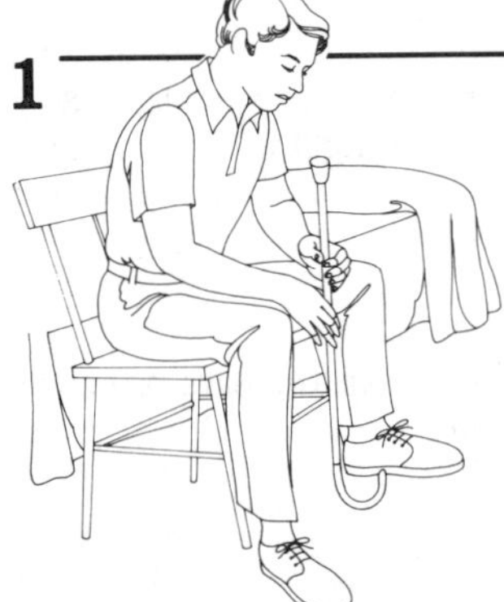

Before you begin, be sure you have on nonskid, flat-soled, supportive shoes, and check that they are buckled or tied securely. Avoid wearing slip-on shoes, such as loafers or clogs, as they do not support your weight properly. In addition, check your cane's rubber tip to be sure it has no cracks or tears and is wearing evenly. Also, make sure the tip fits securely on the cane's end.

If possible, remove throw rugs and avoid walking on slippery, wet, or waxed floors or on gravel driveways. Also, try to walk close to a wall, so you have something to lean against if you drop your cane.

2

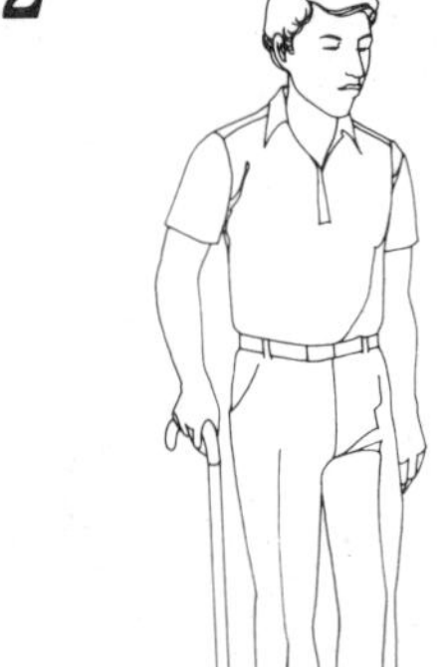

Now, position the cane about 4″ (10 cm) to the side of your unaffected leg, as shown in this illustration. Distribute your weight between your feet and your cane.

3

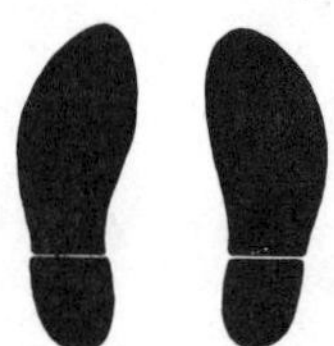

Next, shift your weight to your unaffected leg and move the cane about 4″ (10 cm) in front of you.

GOING HOME WITH A CANE—*continued*

4

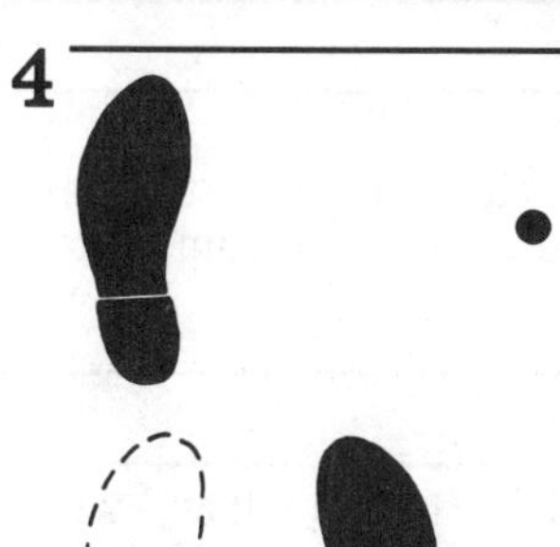

Now, you are ready to move your affected foot forward so it is parallel with the cane.

5

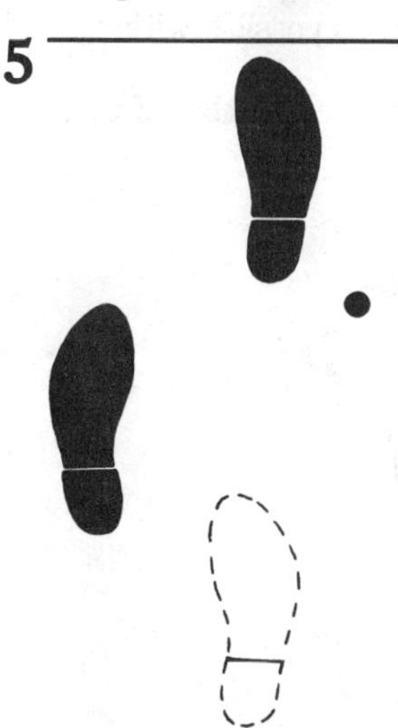

Shift your weight to your affected leg and the cane. Now, move your unaffected leg forward, ahead of the cane. If you have done this step correctly, your heel will be slightly beyond the tip of the cane.

6

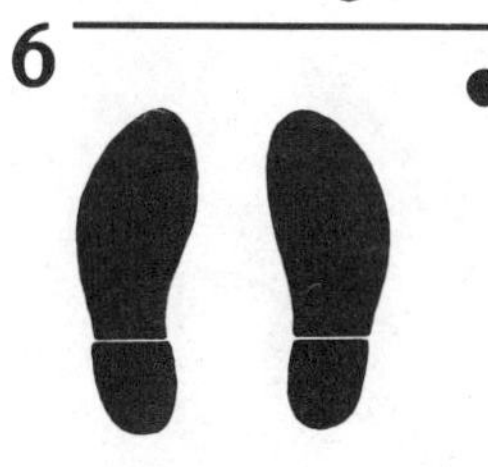

Next, move your affected foot forward, so it is even with your unaffected foot. Then, move your cane in front of you about 4″ (10 cm).

Repeat these steps. As you proceed, remember to keep your head erect, shoulders back, back straight, abdomen in, and knees slightly flexed.

Patient-Teaching Aid

PERFORMING PASSIVE R.O.M. EXERCISES

Dear Caregiver:
Remember, all these exercises should be performed slowly and gently. They should never cause pain or exceed the joints' normal ROM.

Neck exercise

Lay the patient on his back, head flat (no pillow). With one hand, support the back of his head; with the other hand, support his chin. Then, extend his neck by moving his head backward, so he looks at the ceiling, as shown here. Next, bring his head forward until his chin comes as close to his chest as possible without discomfort.

Repeat this exercise the prescribed number of times.

Move head backward

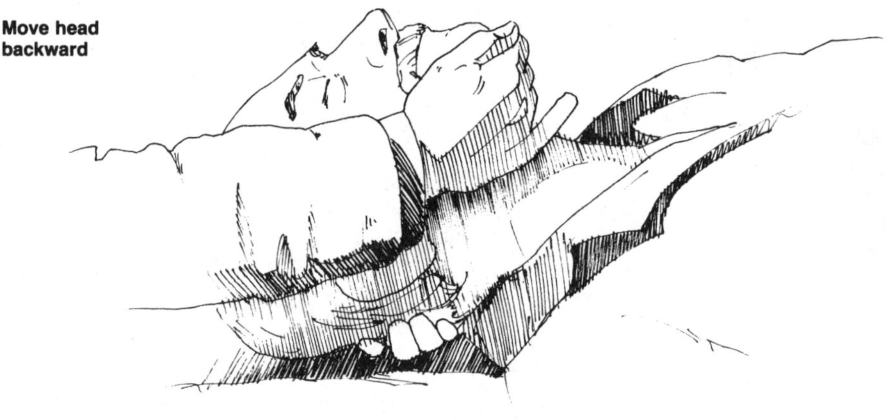

Move head forward

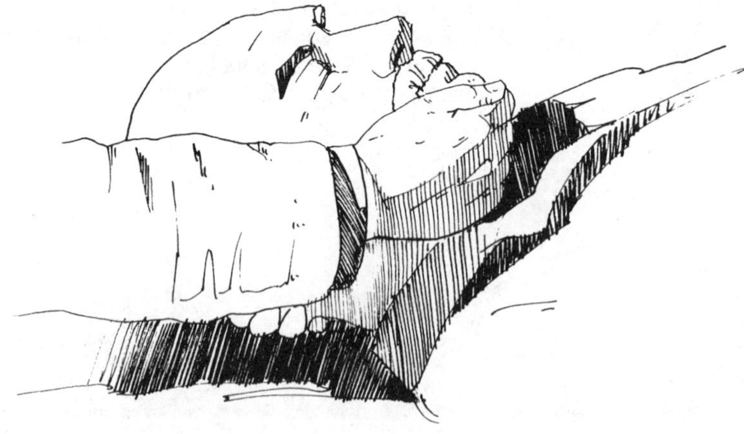

PERFORMING PASSIVE R.O.M. EXERCISES—*continued*

Shoulder exercise

With the patient sitting, standing, or lying down, extend his arm straight out to the side, with his palm facing up. Place one hand under his elbow, and use your other hand to grip his wrist. Then, keep the arm straight and bring it up until it reaches his ear. If necessary, to bring the upper arm all the way up, bend the elbow so the patient's forearm reaches over his head. Finally, return the arm to its original position.

Repeat this movement the prescribed number of times.

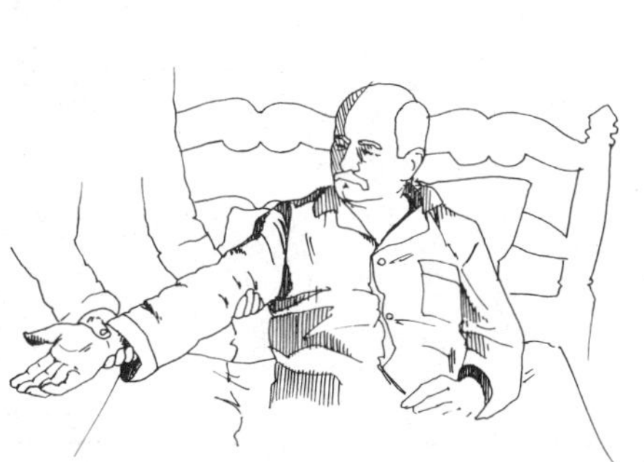

Straighten arm

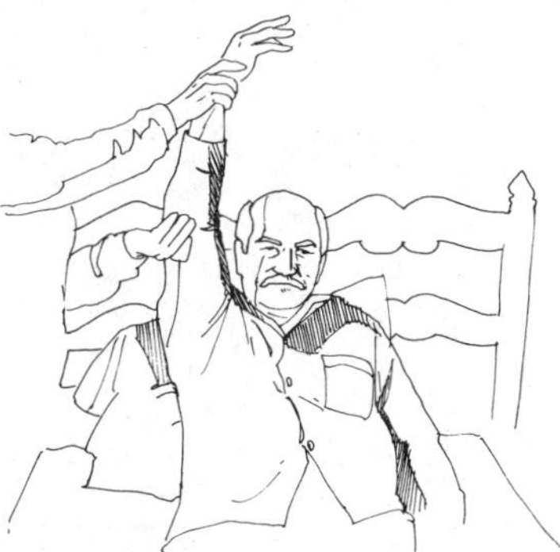

Raise arm

Elbow exercise

Extend the patient's arm straight out to the side, palm facing up. Grasp his wrist to keep his hand from drooping. Now, bend the arm at the elbow and bring it up toward his shoulder. Then, do the same thing with his other arm.

Repeat this exercise the prescribed number of times.

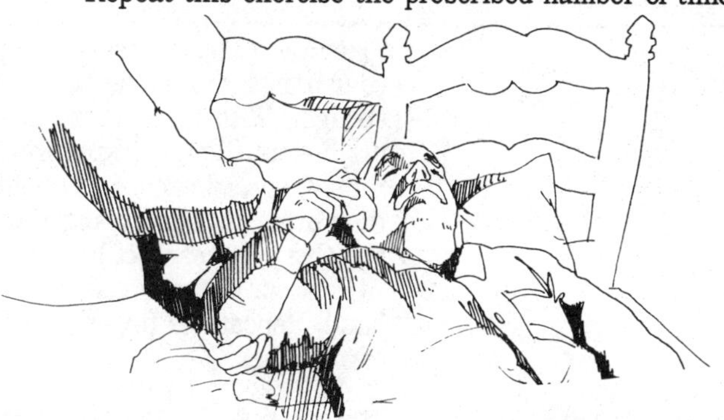

PERFORMING PASSIVE R.O.M. EXERCISES—*continued*

Forearm exercise

Place the patient's arms along his sides. Grasp the wrist and hand of one arm. Keeping the patient's elbow on the bed, raise his hand and gently twist it so his palm is up. Then twist it so his palm is down. Do the same thing with his other arm.

Repeat these movements the prescribed number of times.

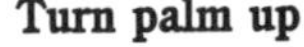

Turn palm up

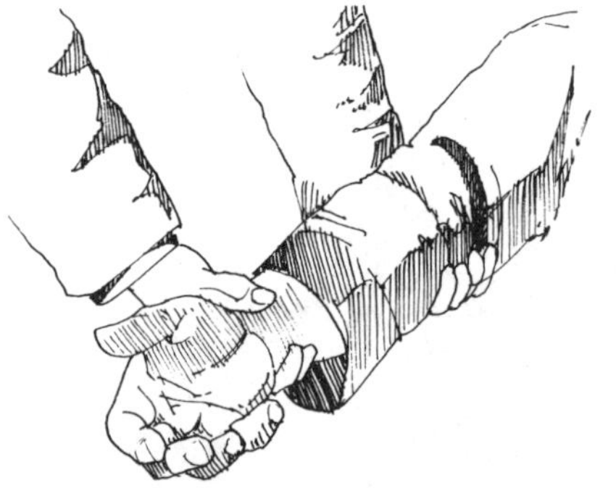

Turn palm down

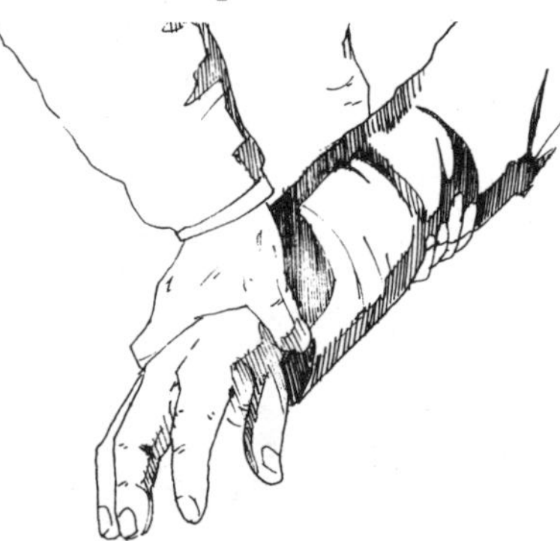

Wrist exercise

Place the patient's arms along his sides. Keeping his elbow on the bed, hold one arm slightly below the wrist and raise it. Grasp the hand, lift it, and bend it gently back, forward, and down. Then, rock the hand back and forth sideways. Gently twist the hand from side to side.

Do the same things with his other hand. Repeat the exercise the prescribed number of times.

Finger exercise

Place the patient's arms along his sides. With one of your hands, grasp one of his, keeping his wrist straight. With your other hand, gently straighten out his fingers. Now, working from his little finger to his thumb, spread each pair of adjoining fingers apart, then bring them back together. Then, pinch the thumb together with each of his fingers, one finger at a time.

Perform this exercise with the fingers of his other hand. Repeat the finger exercises the prescribed number of times.

Patient-Teaching Aid

HOW TO PERFORM CREDÉ'S MANEUVER

Dear Patient:

Credé's maneuver is a simple exercise that can help you start a stream of urine. This is how to perform it:

- While sitting on the toilet, place your hands flat on your abdomen, just below the navel. Then, firmly stroke downward about six times. This puts pressure on the bladder and stimulates your urge to void. (Women can increase pressure further by bending forward at the hips.)
- Now, place one hand on top of the other above your pubic area, as shown. Then, press firmly inward and downward. This compresses the bladder and expels urine.

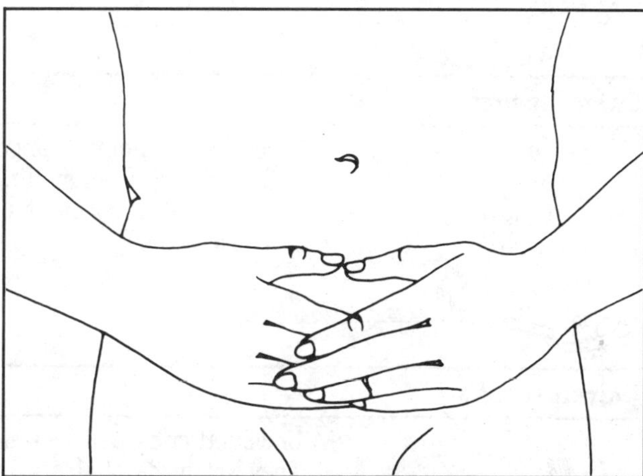

Patient-Teaching Aid

LEARNING ABOUT SPECIAL FEEDING DEVICES

Dear Patient:
You can feed yourself with some assistance.

Plate guards, scooper plates, and suction cups

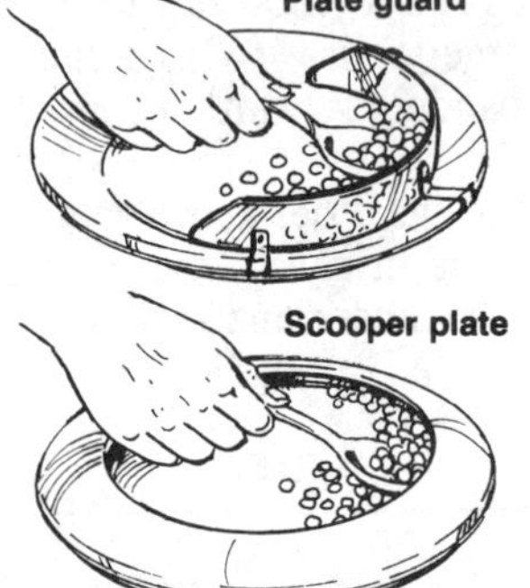

A plate guard blocks food from spilling off the plate, so you can pick it up easily with a fork or spoon. The guard should be attached to the side of the plate opposite the hand you use to feed yourself.

A scooper plate has high sides that provide a built-in surface for pushing food onto your utensil.

Suction cups attached to the bottom of a plate or bowl help prevent slipping.

Swivel spoons

If you have a limited range of motion, a swivel spoon will keep food from spilling, even if the spoon's handle is rotated. This spoon can be used with a universal cuff (see below).

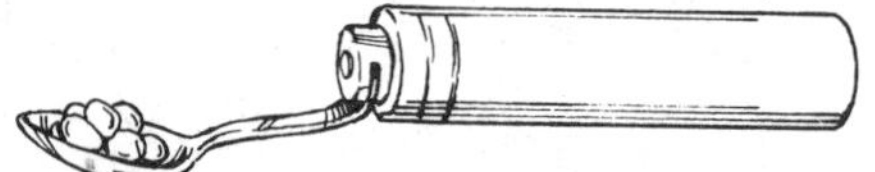

Universal cuffs

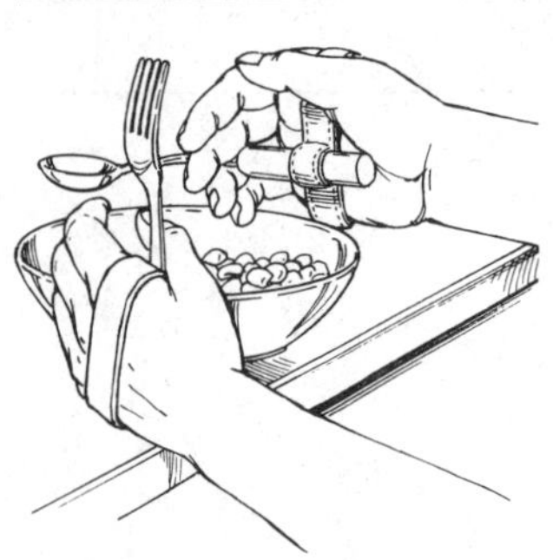

Universal cuffs will help if you have a weakened grasp. They are made of elastic or other materials. The cuff has a slot that holds a fork or spoon. It should be attached to the hand you use to feed yourself, with a fork or spoon placed in the slot. If necessary, the utensils can be bent to make feeding easier.

Long-handled utensils

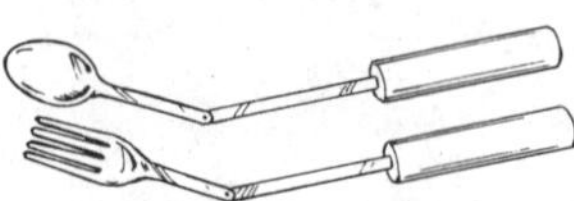

For limited range of motion in the elbow or shoulder, long-handled utensils can help you feed yourself without having to move your arm so much.

LEARNING ABOUT SPECIAL FEEDING DEVICES—*continued*

Other utensils

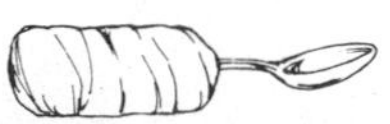

Built-up handle

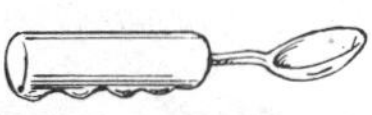

Easy-to-grasp spoon

Weighted utensil

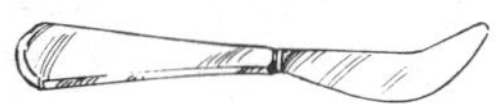

Rocker knife

Utensils with built-up handles can help if your grasp is weak. These utensils can be bought from a medical supplier, or they can be made by wrapping tape or a piece of foam rubber around the handle of a fork or spoon.

Weighted utensils can help if you have hand tremors or spasms. The extra weight will anchor and stabilize the utensil.

If you can use only one hand, you may find cutting food, buttering bread, and getting food onto a utensil difficult and frustrating. A rocker knife will allow you to cut food by rocking the curved blade over the food instead of sawing back and forth.

Special cups and mugs

A plastic mug with a weighted base and a special handle will help you if you have grasping and holding problems. A cup with a pedestal base will help you hold the cup if you have a weak finger grasp.

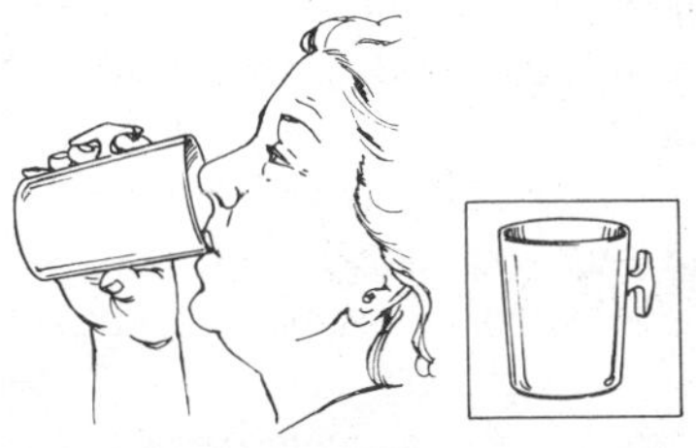

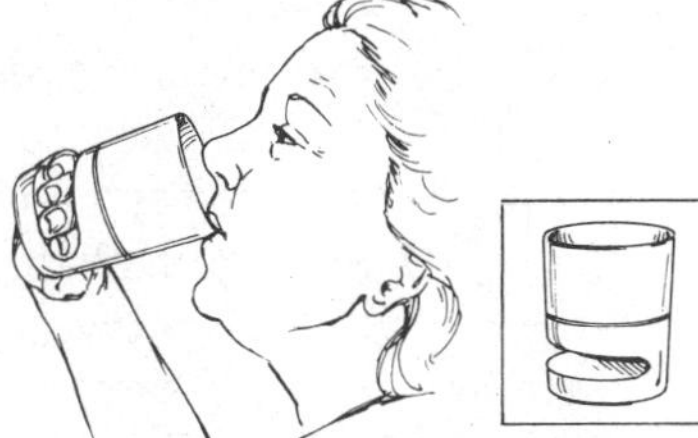

Drinking straws

Flexible or rigid drinking straws, both disposable or reusable, are available in a variety of sizes. The holes of some drinking straws are large enough in diameter for you to drink soups and thick liquids through them. To hold the straw easily, use a snap-on plastic lid with a hole for the straw.

Divided feeding tray

Special feeding trays come with deep, divided wells that hold food or dishes. Suction cups attach the tray firmly to a nonporous surface.

Endocrine Disorders

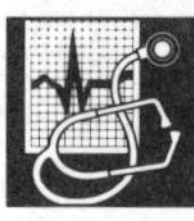

Patient-learner data base*

Areas of potential knowledge deficit

Presence of endocrine risk factors
- —Family history of endocrine disease
- —Presence of other endocrine disease
- —Recent stress
- —Overweight
- —Age
- —Presence of other immune disorders

History of complications (determine type, if applicable; frequency; treatment; and underlying causes, if known)
- —Diabetes mellitus: hypoglycemia, hyperglycemia, ketoacidosis, retinopathy, nephropathy, neuropathy, cardiovascular disease
- —Hyperthyroidism (Graves' disease): thyroid storm, exophthalmos, malnutrition, emotional state
- —Hypothyroidism: myxedema coma, cardiovascular disease, anorexia
- —Addison's disease: adrenal crisis, hypoglycemia, hypotension, dehydration, cardiac disorders

Specific level of knowledge about the endocrine disorder
- —Anatomy and physiology of specific gland(s) involved in the endocrine disorder
- —Definition of the endocrine disorder
- —Causes of the endocrine disorder
- —Symptoms associated with the endocrine disorder
- —Treatment of the endocrine disorder: diet; medications; exercise program, if applicable; guidelines used for daily living; recognition and treatment of acute complications; daily testing procedures

*A general assessment should be done for all patients. For general assessment guidelines, see Chapter 1, Principles of Patient Teaching.

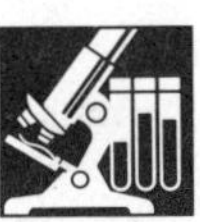

Explaining diagnostic tests

ORAL GLUCOSE TOLERANCE TEST

Patient objectives	*Teaching plan content*
1 Define oral glucose tolerance test.	The oral glucose tolerance test measures carbohydrate metabolism after ingestion of a challenge dose of glucose.
2 State the purpose of the oral glucose tolerance test.	The purpose of the oral glucose tolerance test is to confirm diabetes mellitus and/or to aid in the diagnosis of hypoglycemia and malabsorption syndrome.
3 Explain the procedure used in the oral glucose tolerance test.	The oral glucose tolerance test involves the following procedure: —A venipuncture will be performed between 7 a.m. and 9 a.m. to obtain a blood sample for a fasting blood sugar level. —The patient will then be asked to drink an overly sweet glucose solution and should know the importance of drinking it within 5 minutes. Normally, the body absorbs this solution rapidly, causing the blood glucose (sugar) levels to rise and peak within 30 minutes to 1 hour. The pancreas responds by secreting more insulin, causing glucose levels to return to normal after 2 to 3 hours. —Blood samples will be drawn at 30 minutes and at 1, 2, and 3 hours after ingestion of the glucose solution, to assess insulin secretion and the body's ability to metabolize glucose. The patient may experience transient discomfort from the needle punctures and the pressure of the tourniquet. —A urine specimen may be collected with each blood sample, depending on institutional policy.
4 Discuss the patient guidelines for the oral glucose tolerance test.	Patient guidelines for the oral glucose tolerance test include the following: —Eat a high-carbohydrate diet, containing at least 150 g, for 3 days before the test. (See *High-Carbohydrate Diet for Oral Glucose Tolerance Test (OGTT)*, p. 216.) —Withhold any medications that may affect test results, as ordered, for 3 days before the testing. —Restrict food and fluids for 10 to 16 hours before the test. —Restrict smoking and strenuous exercise for 8 hours before or during the test.

—Bring a book or other quiet diversion to the test, since the procedure usually takes 3 hours but can last as long as 6 hours.
—Immediately report symptoms of hypoglycemia (low blood sugar), such as weakness, restlessness, nervousness, hunger, and sweating, during the test.
—Lie down if feeling faint from the numerous venipunctures.
—Drink water if urine samples are to be collected throughout the test, to promote adequate urine excretion.

URINE GLUCOSE DETERMINATION

Patient objectives	*Teaching plan content*
1 **Define urine glucose determination.**	Urine glucose determination measures the amount of glucose in the urine. (Normally, no glucose is present in the urine.)
2 **State the purpose of urine glucose determination.**	The purpose of urine glucose determination is to determine the presence of glucose in the urine of patients with diabetes.
3 **Demonstrate the procedure in urine glucose determination using the copper reduction method, if applicable.**	Urine glucose determination using the copper reduction method is performed as follows: —The test may be performed on a single-voided specimen or a second-voided specimen, as ordered by the physician. If a second-voided specimen is to be used, the patient should void, then drink a glass of water. After 30 to 45 minutes, he should void again, collecting the urine in a specimen container or paper cup. —To perform the 5-drop Clinitest tablet test, the patient should: • Hold the medicine dropper vertically, and instill 5 drops of urine from the specimen container into the test tube. • Rinse the dropper with water, and add 10 drops of water to the test tube. • Add one Clinitest tablet, and observe the color change, especially during effervescence—the pass-through phase. • Wait 15 seconds after effervescence subsides, and gently agitate the test tube. If color develops at the 15-second interval, compare the color with the Clinitest color chart, and record the results. • Ignore any changes that develop after 15 seconds. • If rapid color changes occur in the pass-through phase of the 5-drop test, record the results as over 2%, without comparison with the color chart.

—To perform a 2-drop Clinitest tablet test, he should:
- Hold the medicine dropper vertically, and instill 2 drops of urine into the test tube.
- Flush urine residue from the dropper with water, then add 10 drops of water to the test tube.
- Add one Clinitest tablet, and observe the color change during the pass-through phase.
- Wait 15 seconds after effervescence stops, compare the color with the appropriate color reference chart, and record the results.

—Rapid color changes (bright orange to dark brown or green-brown) in the pass-through phase in a 5-drop Clinitest reaction indicate glycosuria of 2% or more; in a 2-drop Clinitest reaction, glycosuria of up to 5% can be measured.

—Perform this test every day as often as ordered by the physician, generally before meals and at bedtime.

4 Demonstrate the procedure in urine glucose determination, using the glucose oxidase test, if applicable.

The glucose oxidase test may be done on a single-voided specimen or a second-voided specimen, as ordered by the physician. The procedures used with the commercial, plastic-coated reagent strips (Clinistix, Diastix, Tes-Tape, Chemstrip uG) are as follows:

—Clinistix: Dip the test area of the reagent strip in the specimen for 2 seconds. Remove excess urine by tapping the strip against a clean surface or the side of the container, and begin timing. Hold the strip in the air, and "read" the color exactly 10 seconds after taking the strip out of the urine by comparing it with the reference color blocks on the label of the container. Record the results. Ignore color changes that develop after 10 seconds.

—Diastix: Dip the reagent strip in the specimen for 2 seconds. Remove excess urine by tapping the strip against the container, and begin timing. Hold the strip in the air, and compare the color with the color chart exactly 30 seconds after taking the strip out of the urine. Record the results. Ignore color changes that develop after 30 seconds.

—Tes-Tape: Withdraw about 1½" (3.8 cm) of the reagent tape from the dispenser; dip ¼" (0.6 cm) in the specimen for 2 seconds. Remove excess urine by tapping the strip against the side of the container, and begin timing. Hold the tape in the air, and compare the color of the darkest part of the tape with the color chart exactly 60 seconds after taking the strip out of the urine. If the tape indicates 0.5% or higher, wait an additional 60 seconds to make the final color comparison. Record the results.

—Chemstrip uG: Briefly (for no more than 1 second)

wet the reagent area of a Chemstrip uG by one of the following methods: totally immerse the reagent-strip test patch in a container of urine, and draw the edge of the strip along the rim of the container to remove excess urine; or hold the strip directly in the urine stream, and gently shake off excess urine. After 2 minutes, match the color of the reagent patch with the color scale to determine the results. Intermediate values can be estimated when the colors of the patch are between those on the vial. For accuracy, compare both color blocks simultaneously.

Do this test every day as often as ordered by the physician, generally before meals and at bedtime.

5 Name six precautions to use in obtaining accurate urine glucose determinations.

To obtain accurate results from urine glucose determination:

—Do not contaminate the urine specimen with toilet tissue or stool.

—Keep the test strip or tablet container tightly closed, to prevent deterioration of the strip/tablets by exposure to moisture, and store the container in a cool place (under 86° F. [30° C.]) to avoid heat degradation.

—Do not use discolored or darkened Clinistix, Chemstrip uG, or Diastix; dark-yellow or yellow-brown Tes-Tape; or dark blue Clinitest tablets.

—Do not use reagent strips or Clinitest tablets after the expiration date printed on the side of the container.

—Do not take any over-the-counter medication without the physician's approval, because many medications can alter test results. (If a prescribed medication affects test results, the physician should order a different method for urine glucose determination.)

—Avoid contact with eyes, mucous membranes, gastrointestinal tract, and clothing, if using Clinitest tablets, because the tablets and moisture produce caustic burns. Since the bottom portion of the test tube becomes boiling hot during effervescence, the test tube should be held near the top to avoid burning the hand.

6 Discuss the protocol to follow if urine glucose is present.

Normally, the urine test for glucose should be negative, but if glycosuria occurs, specific protocols should be obtained from the physician. General guidelines to observe include the following:

—Review events in the past 24 hours to determine the possible cause of glycosuria (for example, overeating, stress, illness). Correct the situation if possible (for example, return to the diet plan).

—Test urine four times a day for glucose when:

- the urine test shows 1% to 2% glucose
- signs of high blood glucose, such as excessive

thirst, frequent urination, or fatigue, are present
• under undue physical stress, such as a cold or influenza, or mental stress.
—Call the physician if urine tests that were negative previously show 2% for 1 to 2 days.
—Begin to test the urine for ketones when the urine test shows 1% to 2% glucose. (See the "Urine Ketone Determination" teaching plan in this chapter.)

URINE KETONE DETERMINATION

Patient objectives	*Teaching plan content*
1 Define urine ketone determination.	Urine ketone determination is a test that measures the presence of ketone bodies in the urine. Ketone bodies are by-products of fat metabolism.
2 State the purpose of urine ketone determination.	The purpose of this test is to determine the presence of ketone bodies in the urine; excess amounts of ketone bodies result from carbohydrate deprivation, such as starvation or diabetic ketoacidosis.
3 Demonstrate the procedure used in urine ketone determination.	One of the following procedures should be used after the patient collects a second-voided midstream specimen (NOTE: If the patient is taking levodopa or phenazopyridine or has recently received sulfobromophthalein, Acetest tablets must be used, since reagent strips will give inaccurate results.): —Acetest: Lay the tablet on a piece of white paper, and place one drop of urine on the tablet. After 30 seconds, compare the tablet color (white, lavender, or purple) with the color chart. —Ketostix: Dip the reagent stick into the specimen, and remove it immediately. After 15 seconds, compare the stick color (buff or purple) with the color chart. Record the results as negative, small, moderate, or large amounts of ketones. —Keto-Diastix: Dip the reagent strip into the specimen, and remove it immediately. Tap the edge of the strip against the container or a clean, dry surface to remove excess urine. Hold the strip horizontally to prevent mixing the chemicals from the two areas. Interpret each area of the strip separately. After exactly 15 seconds, compare the color of the ketone section (buff or purple) with the appropriate color chart; after 30 seconds, compare the color of the glucose section. Ignore color changes that occur after the specified waiting periods. Record the results as negative, or positive for small, moderate, or large amounts of ketone.

4 Name three precautions to use in obtaining accurate urine ketone determinations.	To obtain accurate results, the patient must: —Keep the urine specimen from being contaminated with toilet tissue or stool. —Keep the test strip or tablet container tightly closed, to prevent deterioration by exposure to light or moisture, and store it in a cool, dry place (under 86° F. [30° C.]) to avoid heat degradation. —Avoid using tablets or strips that have become darkened.
5 Discuss the protocol to follow if urine ketones are present.	The urine test should always be negative for ketone bodies. If ketonuria occurs, the patient should recheck the results using a new specimen. If ketone bodies are still present, he should notify his physician.

SELF–BLOOD GLUCOSE MONITORING

Patient objectives	*Teaching plan content*
1 Define self–blood glucose monitoring.	Self–blood glucose monitoring permits the patient to obtain a blood sample through a self-inflicted finger-prick and to determine his blood sugar level using a color chart or meter device.
2 State the purpose of self–blood glucose monitoring.	The purpose of self–blood glucose monitoring is to help the patient with diabetes learn to associate changes in daily blood glucose levels with when and what he has eaten, how much he has exercised, how much insulin or oral hypoglycemic agents he has taken, and what kinds of stress he is experiencing. Once he learns how these factors affect his blood glucose levels, he will be better able to fine-tune his diabetes control.
3 Demonstrate obtaining a drop of blood manually.	A drop of blood is obtained manually, as follows: —Choose a site on any fingertip, near the edge of the fingertip. Avoid using a site on the pad of the finger, where nerves and arteries are concentrated. —Wipe that fingertip with alcohol. (Omit this step if the hands have just been washed.) Allow the alcohol to dry, fanning the finger in the air to hasten drying. (Wet alcohol may interact with the reagent strip, producing an erroneously high reading.) —Squeeze the fingertip with the thumb of the same hand to well up blood at the puncture site. Keep the thumb pressed against the fingertip. —Place the fingertip against a firm surface, such as the edge of a table or counter. This will prevent instinctive motion away from the lancet. Also, by stabilizing

the finger, less force is needed to puncture the skin.
—Twist off the Monolet's round protective top. Grasp the lancet and quickly pierce the skin at the chosen site.
—Then quickly push the lancet's needle into the flat side of the protective top, to show that the lancet has been used and also to protect against accidental injury. Now stop squeezing the thumb and fingertip, to release pressure and permit blood flow.
—If a pinpoint of blood is not visible, "milk" the finger (squeeze and release it) toward the tip. If a drop of blood still is not visible, lower the hand below the waist to let gravity increase blood flow. Then milk the finger again, putting pressure on the soft tissues of the fingertip. (NOTE: The glucose concentration in the tissues is the same as in the blood, so milking will not affect the test's accuracy.)
—Continue to milk the finger until a hanging drop of blood appears that looks large enough to cover the reagent area of the test strip. Be patient; keep trying to milk the finger before making a second puncture. (NOTE: A drop of blood may also be obtained using a mechanical device. See *Using the Autoclix Device,* p. 217.)

4 Obtain an accurate blood glucose determination visually.

Three types of reagent strips are currently available for testing blood glucose visually: Chemstrip bG (Bio-Dynamics), Visidex II (Ames), and Dextrostix (Ames). (Visidex II essentially replaces Dextrostix for visual testing; Dextrostix is used more often when testing blood glucose with a meter.)
—To use Chemstrip bG:

- Remove a Chemstrip from its vial and tightly replace the vial's cap. Carefully lift the Chemstrip to the drop of blood. Note that the Chemstrip has a shiny, slippery surface; the blood will roll off if placed on the strip incorrectly.
- Let the blood completely cover the reagent area without rubbing or smearing it. If the blood smears, start again with a new reagent strip. Get another drop of blood from the same puncture, if possible. With practice, applying the blood correctly becomes easier.
- Time exactly 60 seconds, using a watch or clock. Be sure to keep the strip level.
- After 60 seconds, use a clean, dry cotton ball to gently wipe all the blood off the reagent area. Wipe three times, each time using a clean side of the cotton ball. Then wait another 60 seconds.
- Now, determine the blood glucose level by compar-

ing the two colors that have appeared on the reagent area with the two-colored blocks (on the 2-minute row) on the Chemstrip bG vial. For example, if both colors match the block labeled 80, the approximate blood glucose value is 80 mg/dl. If the two colors seem to fall between two blocks, take the average of the two numbers. For example, if the colors fall between the blocks labeled 180 and 240, the approximate blood glucose value is 210. If the reading is higher than 240 mg/dl, wait another 60 seconds. Then compare the reagent area with the blocks on the 3-minute row.

• Write the date, time, and initials on the reagent strip and store it in a tightly sealed, empty Chemstrip bG vial. The colors on the reagent area will remain stable for up to a week. Record the blood glucose reading in a logbook. Also note the date, time, and type of the following: food last eaten, insulin or oral hypoglycemic agents taken, physical exercise, and physical or mental stress. These factors, taken together, will help to explain the patterns of blood glucose highs and lows. REMEMBER: The blood glucose level is always changing.

—To use the Visidex II:

• Remove a Visidex strip from its bottle and tightly replace the bottle's cap. Compare the yellow Visidex chemical pads at the end of the strip with the "dry, unreacted reagent pads" block on the label's color chart. If the reagent pads on the strip do not match, discard that strip and use one from a new bottle. Discoloration means the reagent has deteriorated and will not give an accurate test result. Lift the Visidex strip to a large, hanging drop of blood. Let the blood completely cover both reagent pads without smearing. Time exactly 60 seconds, keeping the strip level.

• After 60 seconds, flush the blood from the pads for no more than 3 seconds, using a steady stream of water from a wash bottle or a faucet.

• Gently blot the reagent pads once on a lint-free paper towel. Do not wipe or rub.

• One reagent pad will have turned green. Immediately compare it to the green blocks on the Visidex II bottle label. If that pad is darker than the darkest green block (180 mg/dl), wait another 30 seconds for the lower pad to turn orange. Then compare the orange reagent pad to the orange blocks on the label. If the color on the reagent pad falls between two color blocks, take the average of those two values. Then record the blood glucose reading, along with all pertinent information.

	—Self–blood glucose monitoring may also be performed using a meter. (See the "Blood Glucose Monitoring With the Glucometer II," "Blood Glucose Monitoring With the Glucoscan 2000 and 3000," and "Blood Glucose Monitoring With the Accu-Chek II" teaching plans in this chapter.)
5 Discuss guidelines to follow if blood glucose determination is abnormal.	See the "Diabetes Mellitus" teaching plan in this chapter for further instructions.

THYROID SCAN

Patient objectives	*Teaching plan content*
1 Define thyroid scan.	A thyroid scan permits visualization of the thyroid gland by a special camera (scintillation camera) or scintiscanner after administration of a radioisotope.
2 State the purpose of a thyroid scan.	The purpose of a thyroid scan is twofold: First, it is used to assess the size, structure, and position of the thyroid gland; and second, it helps to evaluate how well the thyroid is functioning, in conjunction with other studies.
3 Explain the procedure used in a thyroid scan.	The procedure used in a thyroid scan involves the following: The patient will be given a radionuclide solution to drink 24 hours before the test or will be given an I.V. injection of a solution (technetium^{99m} pertechnetate) 30 minutes before the test. Once in the X-ray department, he will be asked to lie in a supine position. The special camera, or scanner, will then pass over his thyroid gland (neck area), projecting its image on a screen, paper scan, and X-ray film without discomfort.
4 Discuss the patient guidelines for a thyroid scan.	To ensure accurate results, the patient should fast from midnight the night before the test. He will not be exposed to dangerous radiation levels. The test takes 30 minutes. If the patient is on any of the following drugs, he should stop taking them (as ordered) 3 days before the test: iodine preparations, thyroid hormones, thyroid hormone antagonists, phenothiazines, corticosteroids, or aminosalicylic acid. Just before the scan, he should remove his dentures and all jewelry around the neck that may interfere with the visualization. He should continue to fast for another 45 minutes after administration of the radioisotope. Following the test, the patient may resume his normal diet and any medications discontinued before the test.

THYROID ULTRASONOGRAPHY

Patient objectives	*Teaching plan content*
1 Define thyroid ultrasonography.	Thyroid ultrasonography allows visualization of the thyroid gland by high-frequency sound waves that are converted to images on an oscilloscope screen.
2 State the purpose of thyroid ultrasonography.	The purpose of thyroid ultrasonography is to evaluate thyroid structure; it is especially useful for distinguishing cystic from solid thyroid nodules.
3 Explain the procedure used in thyroid ultrasonography.	The test is performed in the X-ray department. There, the patient will be placed in a supine position, with a pillow under his shoulder blades to hyperextend his neck. After his neck is coated with mineral oil, a transducer will scan the thyroid (neck area), projecting the image on a screen. The image will then be photographed for subsequent examination by the radiologist. To visualize the anterior portion of the thyroid, a water-filled bag covered with a contact solution may be placed between his neck and the transducer. The procedure is painless.
4 Describe the patient guidelines for thyroid ultrasonography.	Food or fluids need not be restricted before or after the test, which takes about 30 minutes. The patient must lie still when the transducer is scanning the thyroid gland, but he may resume his activities immediately after the test.

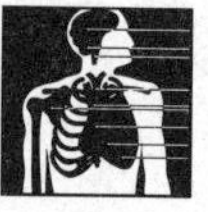

Explaining disorders

DIABETES MELLITUS

Patient objectives	*Teaching plan content*
1 Define diabetes mellitus.	Diabetes mellitus is a chronic disorder in which the pancreas does not produce enough insulin or the insulin produced is not effective. (Using an illustration, point out the proximity of the stomach to the pancreas.) The action of insulin in the body is to transport glucose (sugar) to the body cells for immediate use as energy or to be stored for future use.

2 Explain the relationship between insulin deficiency and a high blood glucose level.

Glucose comes from food in the form of three major nutrients: carbohydrates, proteins, and fats. Carbohydrates provide most of the glucose, but fat and protein can be converted into glucose by the body, if necessary. Glucose and insulin from the pancreas both enter the bloodstream. As blood flows through the body carrying glucose and insulin, insulin helps glucose leave the blood and enter a body cell that needs energy. In diabetes mellitus, because the pancreas is not producing enough insulin or the insulin produced is not effective, the glucose is unable to reach a cell that needs energy and stays in the bloodstream. As more food is eaten, more glucose enters the bloodstream; this causes the blood glucose level to rise above normal (hyperglycemia).

3 Identify a normal blood glucose level.

Normal values for blood glucose vary from one institution to another. The patient should know how his blood glucose level compares with the normal range for that laboratory, the difference between a fasting blood glucose level and a postprandial blood glucose level, and the normal range for each type.

4 Name at least three complications of diabetes mellitus.

Uncontrolled blood glucose can lead to acute and/or chronic problems:

—Acute hyperglycemia may lead to severe fluid and weight loss, loss of consciousness, and even death. These problems arise because the glucose cannot enter the cells that need its energy to function.

—Chronic hyperglycemia may affect nerves and blood vessels and may cause a variety of other chronic problems, such as heart disease, poor circulation, eye disease, kidney disease, and nerve dysfunction.

—In children, normal growth and development may be retarded.

—In pregnant women, hyperglycemia can affect the health of both mother and child.

While there is no cure for diabetes mellitus, blood glucose can be reduced with treatment.

5 Define the relevant type of diabetes.

The physician will determine whether the patient has Type I or Type II diabetes mellitus.

—Type I, also called insulin-dependent diabetes mellitus, most commonly occurs in children, although it can occur at any age. Since a person with Type I diabetes does not make enough of his own insulin, he must take insulin every day. Diet and exercise are also part of the treatment.

—Type II, also called non-insulin-dependent diabetes mellitus, is more common: more than 80% to 90% of all patients with diabetes have Type II diabetes. This type most often occurs in overweight adults over age 40. A person with Type II diabetes produces some insulin, sometimes a normal or even above-normal amount; however, the insulin produced is not very effective, and the body cells resist it. Type II diabetes may be controlled with diet and exercise, but, in some cases, medications (such as oral hypoglycemic pills or insulin) are required to control the blood glucose level.

6 Identify at least three risk factors of diabetes mellitus.

The cause of diabetes is unknown. It is known to run in families, but it is not contagious. Other factors contributing to the development of diabetes include obesity, pregnancy, physical or emotional stress (such as acute illness or accident), and aging. Diabetes is not caused by eating too much sugar. Weight gain, not sugar per se, is the contributing factor.

7 List the symptoms of the relevant type of diabetes.

Symptoms vary from person to person and between the two types of diabetes. In both types of diabetes, however, symptoms occur because blood glucose levels are high and, therefore, less energy in the form of glucose is available to the cells. (Each patient may not experience all the symptoms listed for each type of diabetes.)
—In Type I diabetes, symptoms tend to be more acute than those of Type II diabetes and come on quickly, usually within several days to a few weeks. Symptoms include increased thirst, increased hunger, increased urination, and weight loss. If the symptoms continue, the patient may develop nausea and vomiting, presence of fatty waste products called ketones in the urine, severe weight and fluid loss, rapid breathing, a fruity or sweet-smelling odor to his breath, and loss of consciousness.
—In Type II diabetes, the symptoms are usually vague and occur slowly, generally over weeks or months. The symptoms may be so mild that a person may have diabetes for a long time and not know it until a routine health examination or procedure is performed. Common symptoms include increased thirst, increased urination, visual changes, itchiness, vaginal infections in women, sores that heal slowly, fatigue, weakness, and irritability.

8 Discuss how diabetes mellitus is diagnosed.

Diabetes is diagnosed by evaluating the patient's symptoms and blood glucose level. According to the American Diabetes Association, the diagnosis of diabetes in adults is made when a random blood glucose level is 200 mg/dl or greater and the patient shows classic symptoms and signs of diabetes—increased thirst, increased hunger, increased urination, and weight loss; a fasting blood glucose level is 140 mg/dl or greater on at least two occasions; or a fasting blood glucose level is less than 140 mg/dl, but there are two abnormal glucose tolerance tests. (See the "Oral Glucose Tolerance Test" teaching plan in this chapter.) The diagnosis of diabetes in children and pregnant women varies from the adult criteria for diagnosis; obtain this information from the patient's physician, if needed.

9 Identify the components of diabetes management.

Treatment of diabetes is directed by the physician, but the responsibility for implementing the treatment rests with the patient. Therefore, to control his blood glucose, the patient will need to know how to manage the following:
—Diet
—Medications (oral hypoglycemic agents or insulin, if applicable)
—Exercise program
—Testing methods for sugar and ketone determinations
—Acute problems
- Hypoglycemia (low blood sugar)
- Hyperglycemia (high blood sugar)

—Guidelines for daily living and for skin and foot care
—Guidelines for sick days.

10 Describe the dietary measures used to manage diabetes.

Since diet has an important effect on diabetes, certain measures must be followed:
—A well-balanced diet is necessary to control the blood glucose level. An unbalanced diet, high in some nutrients and low in others, can cause wide variations in the blood glucose level. In the diabetic diet, the kinds and amounts of foods and the timing of the meals are important. The dietitian will provide the patient with his specific meal plan, and this information should be reinforced as necessary. Meals should be spread evenly throughout the day, including snacks if prescribed. The patient should eat about the same amount each day. If extra activity is anticipated, the dietitian will instruct him on the needed dietary adjustments. Include the family in these teaching sessions.
—If exchange lists are to be used, the dietitian's instructions can be reinforced by helping the patient incorporate them into his daily life. He and his family should plan meals using exchanges.
—The dietitian will provide the patient with a list of foods to avoid and will explain why these foods need to

be avoided (because they cause sudden shifts in blood glucose level).
—In addition, the dietitian will instruct the patient on how to choose a meal from a restaurant menu.
—For the overweight patient with diabetes, a reduction in calories will be part of his dietary plan. The patient should know any potential problems that may interfere with his ability to maintain the diet and must learn ways to handle the problems. A support group may be helpful.

11 Discuss the medication regimen.

Some drugs commonly used for this disorder are acetohexamide, chlorpropamide, glipizide, glucagon, glyburide, insulin, tolazamide, and tolbutamide. See Chapter 9, Drug Therapy, for specific instructions on insulin and oral hypoglycemic agents.

12 Demonstrate self-injection of insulin, if applicable.

See Appendix D, *Medication Administration,* for specific instructions.

13 Explain the role of exercise in the management of diabetes mellitus.

Exercise is as important as medication and/or diet in treating diabetes, because activity lowers blood glucose levels, increases circulation, and improves general health. To be successful, the exercise program must be consistent and part of the management routine. Because the program should be tailored to the patient's physical ability, current medical condition, and potential for developing complications, obtain exercise guidelines from his physician.

14 Discuss the different effects of aerobic and anaerobic exercise on blood sugar levels.

Not all exercise is beneficial for a person with diabetes.
—Anaerobic exercise, such as weight lifting, does not use glucose as a fuel and does not require increased oxygen. This type of exercise, while useful for building muscle mass, is likely to produce an increase in serum glucose. It may also raise the pulse and blood pressure and does nothing to improve the cardiovascular system.
—Aerobic exercise, such as walking, running, cycling, and swimming, uses glucose as a fuel and requires increased oxygen. This type of exercise is likely to produce a decrease in glucose, just what the diabetic patient needs. Aerobic exercise also offers cardiovascular benefits, making it even more valuable for people with diabetes.

15 Identify the three phases of an exercise program.

After choosing a suitable exercise, the patient will need to decide how frequently he should exercise and for how long. Ideally, he should exercise three times a

week, on alternate rather than sequential days. Each session should last between 40 and 60 minutes and should include the following phases:
—The warm-up phase usually lasts 5 to 10 minutes and involves activities designed to stretch the muscles and slowly increase the heart rate.
—The conditioning phase usually lasts 20 to 30 minutes and involves activities to reach the target heart rate, then maintain it. The target heart rate is best established by a stress electrocardiogram, but the patient can roughly determine his target heart rate by subtracting his age from 220, then multiplying the result by 0.70.
—The cool-down phase usually lasts 10 to 15 minutes and involves activities that gradually return the body systems to their normal paces.

The patient must build up gradually to 40 to 60 minutes if he is out of shape or if he must follow instructions given by his physician. Since achieving the target heart rate is the goal of the conditioning phase, the patient must know how to take his pulse (see Chapter 2, Cardiovascular Disorders, for specific instructions) and must take it regularly before, during, and after the exercise session. Initially, he should reach his target heart rate slowly and maintain it for just a short time. Over weeks, perhaps even months, he can gradually decrease the time he takes to reach his target heart rate, until finally he is maintaining it for the entire conditioning phase. He should not exceed his target heart rate. A faster heart rate provides no additional health benefits and could put too much strain on his heart.

---

16 Discuss four safety guidelines to follow when exercising.

Patient guidelines for exercising are as follows:
—He should always carry a source of carbohydrates, as well as some cash to buy food in an emergency, in case he becomes hypoglycemic.
—He should always carry identification with his name, medical condition, and medications.
—If he feels tightness or pain in his chest, severe shortness of breath, palpitations, or nausea, he should stop the activity immediately and see a physician.
—If he takes diabetic medications as part of his treatment regimen, he may develop hypoglycemia during or after the exercise session. Therefore, he should:

- not inject insulin into a part of the body that he will be exercising.
- not exercise at the peak of insulin drug activity.
- not exercise before meals, unless he wants to lower his serum glucose level.

- not drink alcoholic beverages before or during exercise.
- eat a snack before and during exercise, as appropriate.
- keep simple carbohydrates (for example, orange juice, raisins, LifeSavers) and other food available.

17 Define hypoglycemia.

Hypoglycemia means "low blood sugar."

18 Identify at least four symptoms of hypoglycemia.

Not all diabetics experience hypoglycemia in exactly the same way. Symptoms may include excessive sweating, headache, faintness, trembling, nervousness, irritability, pounding of the heart, or confusion. Hypoglycemia usually occurs abruptly. If the patient is receiving intermediate or long-acting insulins, he should know that nightmares, sleepwalking, restlessness, diaphoresis, and/or a headache upon awakening in the morning may occur.

19 Name three common causes of hypoglycemia.

The common causes of hypoglycemia are as follows:
—taking too much insulin or oral agent
—not eating enough food or delaying a meal
—participating in an unusual amount of exercise without making dietary adjustments.

20 Explain the treatment protocol for hypoglycemia.

It is important for the patient and his family to know how to treat a hypoglycemic reaction. When a hypoglycemic reaction occurs:
—The patient and his family should confirm it by taking a blood glucose reading if the patient is doing blood glucose self-determinations.
—If he is not doing blood testing and is not sure if his blood glucose level is low or high, he should treat it as if it is low.
—If he is able to swallow, he should eat or drink something with sugar in it, such as one of the following: 4 oz of orange juice or regular soda; 2 tsp of honey or sugar; or 1 tbsp of syrup. (In some patients, 1 or 2 tsp of honey or sugar may give a better response than orange juice.)
—If he does not feel better in 15 minutes, he should repeat the treatment.
—When he feels better, he should eat some supplemental, slowly absorbing carbohydrates equal to his snack, such as toast, fruit, or crackers, to prevent recurring hypoglycemia.
—If a family member finds the patient unresponsive and unable to swallow, he should administer glucagon subcutaneously (see Chapter 9, Drug Therapy, for spe-

cific medication instructions) and repeat it in 15 minutes, if necessary. If the patient does not respond to the treatment within 30 minutes, his physician should be notified; if his symptoms worsen (for example, a change in level of consciousness), he should be taken to the nearest hospital emergency department. In addition, the patient should carry some form of sugar (for example, 10 LifeSavers) with him at all times in case he experiences a hypoglycemic reaction away from home. He should not use chocolate candy to treat the reaction, because the milk fat in chocolate can delay absorption of the sugar. The patient should always wear a bracelet or necklace identifying him as diabetic.

21 Define hyperglycemia.

Hyperglycemia means "high blood sugar."

22 Identify at least four symptoms of hyperglycemia.

Not all diabetic patients experience hyperglycemia in exactly the same way. Common symptoms include increased thirst, urination, and hunger; weakness; abdominal pains; general body aches; deep, rapid breathing; loss of appetite; nausea and vomiting. Because hyperglycemia occurs slowly, daily glucose determination is important. Judging a high blood glucose level based solely on the patient's feelings is not always accurate or reliable and is not a substitute for blood or urine sugar determination.

23 Name three common causes of hyperglycemia.

Causes of hyperglycemia include lack of insulin, overeating, and stress in the form of infection, illness, or emotional upset.

24 Explain the treatment protocol for hyperglycemia.

Once hyperglycemia is confirmed by glucose determination, the patient must increase testing to every 4 hours for glucose and must begin testing his urine for ketones. (See the "Urine Ketone Determination" teaching plan in this chapter for specific instructions.) If hyperglycemia continues for more than 24 to 48 hours or if ketones are present in the urine, he should notify his physician. If hyperglycemia is a result of illness, he should do the following:

—Notify his physician when he feels too sick to eat normally or stay active.

—Continue taking his insulin, even if he cannot eat. Illness causes the body to release storage forms of sugars, which in turn cause the blood glucose level to rise, even though he is not eating. After consulting with the physician, determine how much insulin he should take during this time.

—Increase glucose determination frequency to every 4 hours.
—Begin to test his urine for ketones every 4 hours.
—Take his temperature every morning and evening, and report this, along with the glucose and ketone determination, to his physician on a daily basis during the illness.
—Stay in bed, keep warm, and drink extra fluids if his temperature is above normal (98.6° F. [37° C.]). Drink at least 12 8-oz glasses of liquid per day if he weighs more than 80 lb and if the physician approves. Check with the dietitian on dietary adjustments during illness.
—Do not stay alone. A friend or relative should stay with the patient if he lives alone and should know how to contact the patient's physician if he cannot.
—If difficulty with breathing occurs or the friend/relative notices the patient is very sleepy and cannot pay attention, seek medical attention at once.
—Return to the preillness diabetes management protocol, as instructed by the physician.

25 Demonstrate urine glucose determination using testing product of choice, if applicable.

See the "Urine Glucose Determination" teaching plan in this chapter for instructions.

26 Demonstrate urine ketone determination using testing product of choice, if applicable.

See the "Urine Ketone Determination" teaching plan in this chapter for instructions.

27 Demonstrate self–blood glucose monitoring using testing product of choice, if applicable.

See the "Self–Blood Glucose Monitoring" teaching plan in this chapter for instructions.

28 Describe skin and foot care guidelines.

Because dry skin is a common problem in diabetic patients and minor foot injuries may have serious consequences, provide the patient with guidelines for caring for his feet and skin. (See *Diabetic Foot Care,* p. 220.)

29 Discuss follow-up care for his diabetes.

Regular checkups are important because of the chronicity of diabetes and the need for periodic adjustments in the treatment regimen.
—It is important for the patient to wear a bracelet or necklace identifying him as diabetic.
—An eye examination should be performed by an ophthalmologist on a regular basis.

—Alert him to the activities of the American Diabetes Association in his area.
—Encourage him to call his physician, dietitian, and/or nurse educator with questions and problems that may arise once he is home.
—Advise him to inform his friends and employer of his diabetes and how to manage a hypoglycemic reaction.

HYPERTHYROIDISM (GRAVES' DISEASE)

Patient objectives	*Teaching plan content*
1 Define hyperthyroidism.	Hyperthyroidism is a chronic condition in which the thyroid gland produces excessive amounts of thyroid hormone.
2 Describe the basic function of the thyroid gland.	The thyroid, a butterfly-shaped gland located in the anterior portion of the lower neck, produces two substances called thyroid hormone and thyrocalcitonin. The primary function of thyroid hormone is to regulate the activity of body cells; thyrocalcitonin helps to regulate blood calcium levels.
3 Discuss the cause of Graves' disease.	Graves' disease is the most common form of hyperthyroidism, accounting for more than 85% of all cases. The cause of Graves' disease is unknown, although it is thought to result from a defect in the immune system. This defect causes production of abnormal thyroid-stimulating antibodies, which direct the thyroid gland to work harder, thereby producing more thyroid hormone than the body actually needs.
4 Explain what happens to the thyroid gland in hyperthyroidism.	The influence of the abnormal thyroid-stimulating antibodies causes both functional and structural changes in the thyroid gland when hyperthyroidism occurs. Functional changes cause excessive production of thyroid hormone. Excessive amounts of thyroid hormone stimulate cells to function more quickly, which causes hyperactivity of body functions. Structurally, the thyroid gland enlarges so it can have enough space to produce more thyroid hormone. An enlarged thyroid gland is commonly referred to as a goiter.
5 Name the classic symptoms of hyperthyroidism (Graves' disease).	Classic symptoms of Graves' disease are an enlarged thyroid (goiter), nervousness, heat intolerance, weight loss despite increased appetite, sweating, diarrhea, tremor, and palpitations. Sometimes the eyes take on a bulging appearance. Many other symptoms may also occur, as this disorder can affect virtually every body

system. This is because thyroid hormone is used by all body cells. These symptoms are a result of cellular hyperactivity.

6 State the goal of treatment for hyperthyroidism.

The goal of therapy is to reduce thyroid hyperactivity, which will provide symptomatic relief. The mode of treatment will be prescribed by the physician.

7 Discuss the medication regimen, if applicable.

Some drugs commonly used for this disorder are methimazole, potassium iodide, propranolol hydrochloride, and propylthiouracil. See Chapter 9, Drug Therapy, for instructions on antithyroid drugs used to limit the production of thyroid hormone or to limit its effectiveness. Antithyroid drugs are not a cure for hyperthyroidism and, therefore, must be taken for life if no additional treatment is prescribed.

8 Discuss radioactive iodine therapy in regard to purpose, procedure, and precautions, if applicable.

The purpose of radioactive iodine (^{131}I) therapy is to irradiate the thyroid gland (without harming other tissue), thereby decreasing its capability to produce thyroid hormone.

—The procedure is simple and painless. The patient will be asked to drink a tasteless, colorless "cocktail" containing ^{131}I. His symptoms should subside in about 3 to 4 weeks. If they do not, another dose of ^{131}I can be given after several months have elapsed.

—Treatment with ^{131}I does not carry an increased risk of leukemia or thyroid cancer, and children of parents treated with ^{131}I (but not treated during pregnancy) show no increased incidence of birth defects.

—Precautions to take with ^{131}I therapy include:

- After treatment, the patient should avoid close contact with pregnant women, infants, and children for 1 week.
- Since his urine and saliva are radioactive, the patient must carefully flush urine and use disposable plates and cutlery for the first 48 hours after treatment.
- Family contact poses no hazard, except for contact with body secretions for the first 48 hours.
- Hospitalization will be required if treatment requires a dose of ^{131}I greater than 30 mCi, in which case the hospital's radiation safety officer will advise the patient and his family concerning specific precautions.

• Signs and symptoms of hypothyroidism (see the "Hypothyroidism" teaching plan in this chapter) can be a side effect of ^{131}I therapy and can occur as late as 10 years after therapy.

9 Discuss surgical intervention for hyperthyroidism in regard to purpose, procedure, and preoperative and postoperative management, if applicable.	See the "Subtotal Thyroidectomy" teaching plan in this chapter for specific instructions.

HYPOTHYROIDISM

Patient objectives	*Teaching plan content*
1 Define hypothyroidism.	Hypothyroidism is a chronic condition in which the thyroid gland produces an inadequate amount of thyroid hormone.
2 Describe the basic function of the thyroid gland.	The thyroid, a butterfly-shaped gland in the anterior portion of the lower neck, produces two substances called thyroid hormone and thyrocalcitonin. The primary function of thyroid hormone is to regulate the activity of body cells; thyrocalcitonin helps to regulate blood calcium levels.
3 Discuss the cause of his hypothyroidism.	Hypothyroidism commonly results from Hashimoto's thyroiditis, an autoimmune disorder in which the immune system turns upon the thyroid gland and begins to destroy it. Hypothyroidism can also occur from treatment of hyperthyroidism with radioactive iodine therapy or surgery or from iodine excess or deficiency in the diet. An infrequent cause of hypothyroidism may be another endocrine dysfunction, hypopituitarism. (The pituitary gland oversees the activity of the thyroid gland.)
4 Explain what happens to the thyroid gland in hypothyroidism.	The pathophysiology of hypothyroidism relative to a specific cause is as follows: —If hypothyroidism results from Hashimoto's thyroiditis, the immune system produces antibodies against the thyroid that cause fibrosis of the thyroid gland, which interferes with thyroid hormone production. —If hypothyroidism is related to a previous treatment modality for hyperthyroidism, too much of the thyroid gland was removed (surgery) or destroyed (radioactive

iodine therapy), and the remaining thyroid tissue is unable to produce adequate amounts of thyroid hormone.
—If an iodine deficiency exists, thyroid hormone cannot be produced, because iodine is needed to synthesize thyroid hormone. In iodine excess, too much is just as harmful as too little, because iodine in large amounts blocks the ability of thyroid hormone to leave the thyroid gland.
—If hypothyroidism is caused by hypopituitarism, the pituitary gland is not functioning well and loses its ability to stimulate the thyroid gland to make thyroid hormone. As a result, hypofunction of the thyroid occurs, and, consequently, less thyroid hormone is produced.

5 Discuss the symptoms of hypothyroidism.

Symptoms of hypothyroidism reflect depressed cellular function (body cells need thyroid hormone to stimulate them to work), causing a wide variety of signs and symptoms in many body systems, such as the following:
—Neurologic effects can result in slowed speech and hoarseness, slowed mental function, apathy, poor short-term memory, and confusion in the elderly.
—Cardiovascular effects can result in slow heart rate, congestive heart failure, and high blood pressure.
—Cutaneous effects can cause vulnerability of the skin, hair, and/or nails to the effects of cellular function, resulting in cold intolerance; cool, dry, scaly skin; nonpitting edema of hands and feet; facial puffiness; coarse, broken hair; and thick, brittle nails.
—Gastrointestinal effects can result in poor appetite (anorexia) and constipation.
—Reproductive effects can result in a decreased libido in both sexes; infertility and heavy, irregular menses in females; impotence in males.
—Musculoskeletal effects can cause backache and muscles that are stiff and slow to contract and relax.

6 State the goal of therapy for hypothyroidism.

While hypothyroidism is a chronic disorder, the rate of cell function can be restored to normal by daily replacement of thyroid hormone. This replacement therapy is for life.

7 Describe the medication regimen.

Some drugs commonly used for this disorder are levothyroxine sodium, liothyronine sodium, thyroglobulin, and thyroid USP. See Chapter 9, Drug Therapy, for specific instructions on thyroid replacement therapy.

8 Discuss guidelines for daily living with hypothyroidism.	After thyroid replacement therapy begins, it is important for the patient to use the following guidelines: —Report any signs of aggravated cardiovascular disease (for example, chest pain or tachycardia) to the physician. —Force fluids (if not contraindicated); eat a high-fiber, low-calorie diet; and exercise, to combat constipation and to promote weight loss until replacement therapy can restore a normal metabolic rate in the body. —Report any signs and symptoms of recurring hypothyroidism or hyperthyroidism, such as restlessness, nervousness, sweating, or excessive weight loss, to the physician. —Because of the chronicity of hypothyroidism, see the physician on a regular basis. —Report any infection immediately, and make sure any physician who prescribes drugs knows about the underlying hypothyroidism.

ADDISON'S DISEASE

Patient objectives	*Teaching plan content*
1 Define Addison's disease.	Addison's disease is a chronic disorder of hyposecretion of the adrenocortical hormones (hormones produced in the cortex).
2 Describe the function of the adrenal cortex.	Addison's disease is a disease of the adrenal glands, which are located on top of each kidney. Each adrenal gland is divided into two parts: the inner part, called the medulla, and the outer part, called the cortex. Addison's disease affects only the cortex, which is itself divided into three zones: the zona glomerulosa, a thin outer layer making up about 15% of the cortex; the zona fasciculata, the middle layer, which constitutes about 75% of the cortex; and the zona reticularis, constituting the rest. Each zone produces certain hormones. For example, the zona glomerulosa primarily produces a hormone called aldosterone, which regulates levels of water and certain substances called electrolytes (namely sodium and potassium) in the body. The zona fasciculata produces hormones called glucocorticoids, which regulate normal use of the nutrients, carbohydrates, fats, and proteins in the body and help the body resist physical and mental stress. The adrenal glucocorticoids include the major hormone cortisol, as well as corticosterone and cortisone. The zona reticularis produces sex hormones called androgens and estrogens.

3 Identify the two major causes of Addison's disease.

The two major causes of Addison's disease are the following:
—Surgical removal of the adrenal glands
—Destruction of the adrenal cortex as a result of infections such as tuberculosis—an autoimmune process in which the immune system attacks the adrenal cortex, mistaking it for a foreign substance—or shrinkage of the adrenal gland, caused by an unknown mechanism. The major cause of destruction is thought to be the autoimmune process.

4 Explain what happens in Addison's disease.

If the adrenal glands are removed or destroyed, adrenal insufficiency results, because no other gland can reproduce the adrenocortical hormones. Adrenal insufficiency leads to a decreased utilization of the major nutrients and to loss of sodium and water in stool, urine, and perspiration; however, potassium is retained.

5 Describe the symptoms of Addison's disease related to adrenocortical hormone deficiency.

The symptoms of Addison's disease include the following:
—Glucocorticoid deficiency: A decrease in utilization of the major nutrients causes hypoglycemia (low blood sugar), which leads to weight loss, fatigue, and weakness. In addition, a variety of gastrointestinal disturbances occur, such as nausea, vomiting, anorexia, and chronic diarrhea. A deficiency of the glucocorticoid hormones also produces abnormal skin and mucous membrane coloration (the patient appears deeply suntanned), especially on the creases of the hands and over the metacarpophalangeal joints, the elbows, and the knees. A darkening of scars, areas of vitiligo (absence of pigmentation), and increased pigmentation on the mucous membranes, usually the buccal mucosa, can also occur.
—Fluid and electrolyte disturbances: The retained potassium can cause cardiac problems, such as a weak, irregular pulse and postural hypotension (drop in blood pressure when position is changed). The loss of sodium and water produces dehydration and hypotension. Other effects of adrenocortical hormone deficiency include decreased tolerance for even minor stress, poor coordination, and a craving for salty foods.

6 Identify the two components of the treatment regimen for Addison's disease.

Treatment of Addison's disease involves medication to replace the adrenocortical hormones and dietary measures to replace the lost sodium and fluid, as well as to decrease potassium consumption.

7 Discuss the medication regimen.

Some drugs commonly used for this disorder are fludrocortisone acetate, hydrocortisone, and prednisone. See Chapter 9, Drug Therapy, for specific medication instructions.

8 Discuss the dietary measures used in the treatment of Addison's disease.

Dietary measures include the following:
—Force fluids until replacement therapy is effective.
—The dietitian should provide the patient with specific instructions on a high-protein, high-carbohydrate diet, as well as instructions on how to maintain a sodium and potassium balance by dietary measures. If the patient is anorexic, he should eat six small meals a day to increase caloric intake.

9 Name two complications that can occur with Addison's disease.

Complications of Addison's disease include the following:
—Cushing's syndrome, from too much adrenocortical hormone replacement therapy.
—Adrenal crisis, from a lack of adrenocortical hormones to meet the body's immediate demands.

10 Identify four situations that can precipitate an adrenal crisis.

Four situations that increase the body's immediate demand for adrenocortical hormones include the following:
—Stress
—Infection
—Injury
—Profuse sweating in hot weather.

11 Explain how to prevent adrenal crisis.

To prevent adrenal crisis, the patient should do the following:
—Increase the dosage of steroid therapy during times of stress, infection, or injury. (Obtain specific guidelines from his physician.)
—Avoid situations that make him perspire profusely.
—Always carry a medical identification card stating that he is taking a steroid, along with the name of the drug and the dosage.
—Learn how to give himself an injection of hydrocortisone (see Appendix D, *Medication Administration,* for instructions).
—Keep an emergency kit containing hydrocortisone in a prepared syringe for use in times of stress. Any stress may require additional cortisone, to prevent a crisis.

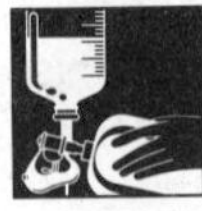

Explaining treatment and monitoring procedures

SUBTOTAL THYROIDECTOMY

Patient objectives	*Teaching plan content*
1 Define subtotal thyroidectomy.	A subtotal thyroidectomy is the surgical removal of five sixths of the thyroid gland.
2 State the purpose of a subtotal thyroidectomy.	A subtotal thyroidectomy is performed to decrease the thyroid gland's ability to produce thyroid hormone, thus preventing excessive amounts of thyroid hormone from being released in the body.
3 Discuss dietary guidelines to follow prior to subtotal thyroidectomy.	Because hyperthyroidism increases metabolic activity and causes a rapid depletion of glucogen reserves, the patient may be experiencing rapid weight loss and malnutrition. He must be well-nourished prior to surgery. If he needs to gain weight, he should increase his caloric intake, and if malnutrition is present, he should eat a well-balanced diet. If a special diet (such as a high-protein diet) has been ordered, the dietitian will provide the patient with the necessary instructions, to be reinforced as needed. The patient should avoid caffeine, commonly found in coffee, tea, sodas, and chocolate, and other stimulants, because they will aggravate his symptoms.
4 Explain his preoperative medication regimen.	The preoperative medication regimen involves the following: —Antithyroid drugs are given to suppress the secretion of thyroid hormone so that, during surgery, excessive amounts are not released into the bloodstream. —Iodine preparations are given to reduce the vascularity of the thyroid gland, thus decreasing the chance of hemorrhage. (See Chapter 9, Drug Therapy, for specific medication instructions.) Adequate preparation for surgery may take as long as 2 or 3 months, because thyroid function studies must be taken to ensure that adequate reduction has occurred.

5 Describe the preoperative events for subtotal thyroidectomy.

Preoperatively, the surgeon should explain the procedure to the patient. The incision for a subtotal thyroidectomy will be made in the lower anterior area of his neck. The disadvantages of thyroidectomy include up to a 30% risk of permanent hypothyroidism, requiring lifetime thyroid replacement therapy; a 20% risk of recurring hyperthyroidism; and a greater risk of complications if surgery is required to correct recurring hyperthyroidism. An informed consent must be signed. He should be shown the coughing and deep-breathing exercises he will be asked to do postoperatively, and he should practice until he does them correctly. (See Chapter 1, Principles of Patient Teaching, and Appendix B, *Preoperative and Postoperative Teaching.*)

6 Describe possible postoperative effects of subtotal thyroidectomy.

Events to expect after subtotal thyroidectomy include the following:

—The patient will be returned to his room from the recovery room, and the nurse will check him frequently.

—To prevent postoperative stress on his incision, the patient should raise his elbows and place his hands behind his head whenever he wants to turn.

—He should have little difficulty in swallowing, but if he experiences difficulty, he should report this at once to the nurse.

—Cold fluids and ice will help ease discomfort, and a soft diet will be given initially.

—He should talk as little as possible in the early postoperative period.

—The patient may need oxygen to facilitate breathing. He should not have any difficulty breathing, but if he does, he should report it to the nurse at once.

—He can expect to be out of bed on the first postoperative day.

—He will receive pain medication and should let the nurse know when he is in pain.

—Sutures or surgical clips are usually removed on the second postoperative day.

7 Discuss the guidelines to be followed on returning home from a subtotal thyroidectomy.

Adequate rest and nutrition are very important. The patient should have specific instructions regarding follow-up visits to his physician, who will tell him when he can return to his normal daily routine. The patient should know the signs and symptoms of hypothyroidism (see the "Hypothyroidism" teaching plan in this chapter), and he should report to his physician if he experiences any of them.

BLOOD GLUCOSE MONITORING WITH THE GLUCOMETER II

Patient objectives	*Teaching plan content*
1 List the supplies needed for testing blood glucose with the Glucometer II.	Supplies needed for testing blood glucose with the Glucometer II include: —Glucostix reagent strips —Glucometer II blood glucose meter —finger-sticking device and needle —absorbent tissue (Kleenex).
2 Describe how to calibrate the Glucometer II.	To check the calibration of the Glucometer II, the patient should do the following: —Turn the meter on by pressing the on/off button. —Check that the number shown on the meter display is the same as the one printed on the label of the Glucostix reagent strip bottle being used. —If the numbers do not match, press the program button repeatedly until they are identical.
3 Obtain an accurate blood glucose determination using the Glucometer II.	To obtain an accurate blood glucose reading, the patient should perform the following steps: —Turn the meter on and check its calibration. —Remove a Glucostix strip from the bottle and tightly replace the bottle cap. —Fold an absorbent tissue in half, then in quarters. —Obtain a large hanging drop of blood manually or by using the Autoclix device. (See the "Self–Blood Glucose Monitoring" teaching plan in this chapter and *Using the Autoclix Device,* p. 217.) —Press the start button on the meter and at the sound of the beep, apply the drop of blood to the Glucostix strip, being sure to completely cover both yellow pads. —Listen for two warning beeps that will sound at 22 and 21 seconds, shown on the display. When the beeps sound, be prepared to blot the strip, using the folded tissue. When a longer beep sounds and the number 20 appears on the display, blot the test pads by placing the reacted strip, pad side up, on the tissue. Then fold the tissue over the pads and press firmly for 1 to 2 seconds. If blood still remains on the pad, blot a second time, using a clean area on the tissue. —When blotting is completed *and* before the meter display reaches 1, open the test door and insert the strip with test pads facing the test window. Close the door.

—Read the glucose determination result that is shown in the display window and record it.
—Remove the test strip and turn the meter off.

BLOOD GLUCOSE MONITORING WITH THE GLUCOSCAN 2000 and 3000*

Patient objectives	*Teaching plan content*
1 List the supplies needed for testing blood glucose with the Glucoscan 2000 and 3000.	Supplies needed for testing blood glucose with the Glucoscan 2000 and 3000 include: —Glucoscan test strips —Glucoscan 2000 or 3000 blood glucose meter —finger-sticking device and needle —blotting paper.
2 Describe how to calibrate the Glucoscan 2000 or 3000.	To check the calibration of the Glucoscan 2000 or 3000, the patient should do the following: —Wipe the calibration test strip clean with a tissue and open the test strip door to the first position. —Insert the test strip into the test holder with the arrow pointing down and the printed side facing the display. —Close the test strip door and press the power button to turn on. The meter will show "60" on the display screen. —Press the start button until the display goes blank. (The display will begin to count down and then go blank after 2 to 3 seconds.) —After a brief delay, the calibration reading will appear and should fall within the calibration range printed on the test strip label. —Remove the calibration test strip and place it in a plastic bag or holder. —If the calibration reading falls outside the range, consult the owner's manual for further instructions.
3 Obtain an accurate blood glucose determination using the Glucoscan 2000 or 3000.	To obtain an accurate blood glucose reading, the patient should perform the following steps: —Turn the meter on and check its calibration. —Note the number "60" (representing seconds) that should appear on the display screen. Observe for a flashing "B" in the upper right hand corner. If it is present, change the batteries, following the instructions in the owner's manual. —Remove the test strip from its foil wrapper by tearing the wrapper lengthwise in the same direction as its perforations. Make sure the reagent pad is ivory—discoloration means the reagent strip has deteriorated. Be careful not to touch the reagent pad or to place it on

the blotting paper or on a wet surface.
—Obtain a large, hanging drop of blood manually or by using the Autoclix device. (See the "Self–Blood Glucose Monitoring" teaching plan in this chapter and *Using the Autoclix Device,* p. 217.)
—Press the start button on the meter to activate the countdown. Note the three "000" in the display screen. Apply a drop of blood to the test strip reagent pad, making sure the entire pad is covered, before the number "60" appears on the display screen. As the meter's counting down from "60," keep the test strip level so the blood will not roll off.
—As the countdown continues, open the test strip hatch and listen for two beeps that will sound at "23" on the display screen. When the beeps sound, be prepared to blot the strip, using blotting paper. When the beep sounds at "20" on the display screen, blot the reagent pad. Turn it upside down, and, using the other hand, gently press it on the blotting paper for 2 seconds. Reposition it on a clean area of the blotting paper and press again for 2 seconds.
—After blotting, the patient should insert the test strip into the test strip hatch with the pad down and facing him.
—When "0" appears on the display screen, immediately close the hatch door.
—Read the glucose determination result shown on the display screen and record it.
—Remove the test strip and turn the meter off.

*NOTE: Glucoscan 3000 is the same as Glucoscan 2000 but has the added feature of a memory bank data log that stores 29 test results sequentially.

BLOOD GLUCOSE MONITORING WITH THE ACCU-CHEK II

Patient objectives	*Teaching plan content*
1 List the supplies needed for testing blood glucose with the Accu-Chek II.	Supplies needed for testing blood glucose with the Accu-Chek II include: —Chemstrip bG test strips, which are specially marked for use with the Accu-Chek II (NOTE: Chemstrip bG test strips used for the Accu-Chek bG blood glucose monitor will not work in the Accu-Chek II meter.) —Accu-Chek II blood glucose meter —finger-sticking device and needle —cotton ball.
2 Describe how to calibrate the Accu-Chek II.	To check the calibration of the Accu-Chek II, the patient should do the following:

—Place the Accu-Chek II meter on a flat surface.
—Remove a calibration strip from the bottle and insert the pointed end of the test strip into the calibration compartment (left of the display) until it touches the work surface.
—Press the on/off button once.
—Pull the calibration strip through the compartment.
—The calibration is completed when a beep sounds and "ccc" appears on the display.
—If the calibration is not successful, consult the owner's manual for further instructions.

3 Obtain an accurate blood glucose determination using the Accu-Chek II.

To obtain an accurate blood glucose reading, the patient should perform the following steps:
—Turn on the meter and open its door.
—Puncture his finger and put a drop of blood on a Chemstrip, then immediately press the TIMER button. He will see the digital display count from 1 to 60. At 60 seconds, he will hear a beep. Using a clean, dry cotton ball, he should wipe the blood off the reagent strip twice, each time using a clean side of the cotton ball.
—Insert the strip under the strip guide. The timer will continue to count from 61 to 120 seconds, at which time he will hear another beep. At the beep, he should close the meter's door. His blood glucose reading will appear on the digital display. (If his reading is less than 20 (20 mg/dl), he will see "LLL" on the display; if it is more than 500 (500 mg/dl), he will see "HHH.") After recording the blood glucose reading in his logbook, the patient should remove the reagent strip from the meter, close its door, and turn it off. If he forgets to turn off the meter, it will shut off automatically after 3 minutes.

Patient-Teaching Aid

HIGH-CARBOHYDRATE DIET FOR ORAL GLUCOSE TOLERANCE TEST (O.G.T.T.)

Dear Patient:
To prepare for the OGTT and to ensure accurate results, follow a high-carbohydrate diet like the one below for at least 3 days before the test. If you find the diet too restrictive, follow your regular regimen, but eat 12 additional slices of bread each day.

BREAKFAST

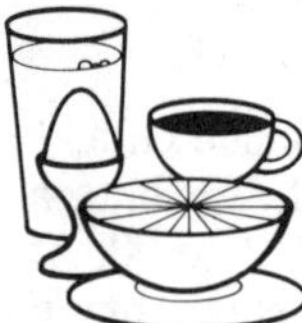

1 serving fruit
Eggs, as desired
5 bread exchanges*
1 cup milk
Butter or margarine
Coffee or tea, if desired

LUNCH AND SUPPER

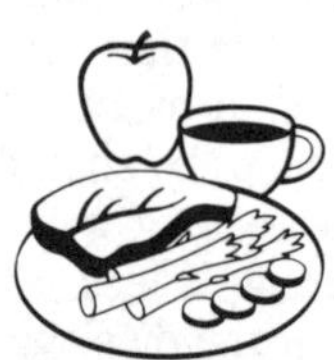

Meat, as desired
5 bread exchanges*
2 vegetables
1 serving fruit
1 cup milk
Butter or margarine
Coffee or tea, if desired

***One* of the following equals one bread exchange:**

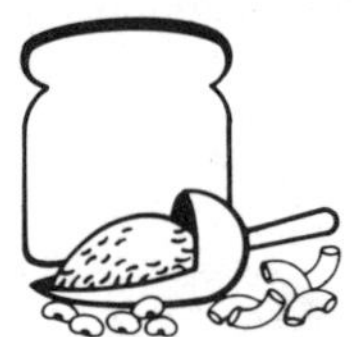

1 slice bread, white or whole wheat
1½" cube of corn bread
½ hamburger or hot dog roll
½ cup cooked cereal
¾ cup dry cereal (avoid sugar-coated varieties)
½ cup noodles, spaghetti, or macaroni
½ cup cooked dried beans or peas
⅓ cup corn or ½ small ear of corn
1 biscuit
½ corn muffin
1 roll
5 saltine crackers
2 graham crackers
½ cup grits or rice
1 small white potato
½ cup mashed potato
¼ cup sweet potato
¼ cup baked beans
¼ cup pork and beans

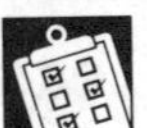

Patient-Teaching Aid

USING THE AUTOCLIX DEVICE

Dear Patient:
Your doctor has ordered self–blood glucose monitoring for you. To perform this procedure, you must first learn how to obtain a large drop of blood, which is essential for the accuracy of the test. Because many people have a natural aversion to pricking their fingers, your doctor has suggested that you use an Autoclix device. An Autoclix is a mechanical device used to prick the finger or earlobe for testing purposes.

1

Hold the Autoclix case vertically, and gently snap the platform on the tapered end of the case. Place your thumb on the plunger located at the case's base, press the plunger as close to the base as possible, and hold it there. Insert the flat end of the lancet through the hole in the platform's middle, twisting the lancet slightly as you push it into place. While keeping the plunger depressed, slowly twist off the lancet's round protective cap and put the cap aside. Release the plunger, so the lancet withdraws into the case. The case is now cocked and can be activated by pressing on the platform.

2

With an alcohol swab, thoroughly cleanse your fingertip, allowing the skin to air-dry before proceeding. Next, firmly hold the Autoclix case in your free hand, without touching the plunger, and gently press your cleansed fingertip over the platform hole. The pressure releases the lancet, which then punctures the skin.

3

Next, put the Autoclix case down and squeeze just below your fingertip, wiping away the first drop with a clean gauze pad or cotton ball. After you have collected an acceptable blood specimen and tested it, press the plunger to eject the lancet. Then, recap the lancet and discard it.

Patient-Teaching Aid

TESTING YOUR URINE FOR GLUCOSE AND KETONES

Dear Patient:
If your urine contains glucose (sugar) or ketones (waste chemicals), the glucose levels in your blood may be too high. Regularly testing your urine can help you tell whether your diabetes is under control.

Test your urine at least four times a day (before breakfast, lunch, dinner, and bedtime snack)—or as your physician or nurse directs. For convenience, use a reagent (test) strip that tests for both glucose and ketones. (Your nurse or physician can suggest reliable brands.) You will also need a watch with a second hand.

1

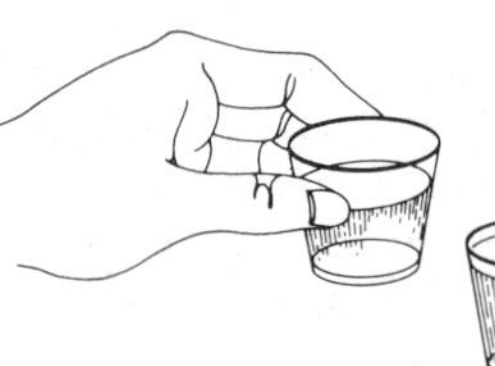

Collect a urine specimen in a clean container. Wait 30 to 60 minutes, and collect a second urine specimen in another clean container. This is the specimen you will test. (If you cannot urinate a second time within an hour, then test the first specimen you collected.)

2

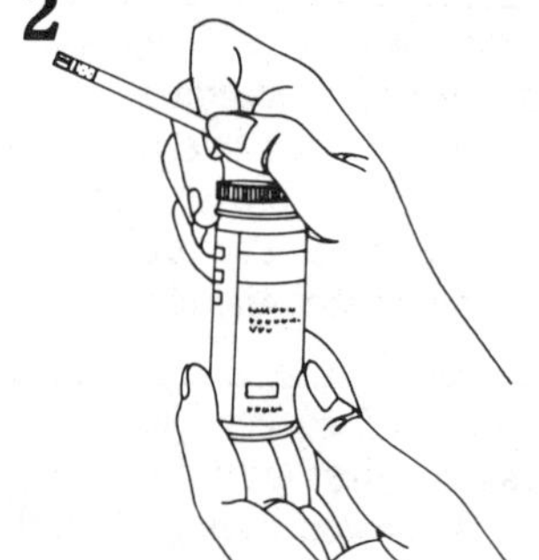

Remove one strip from the bottle and replace the cap. Hold the strip so the test blocks face up. Make sure you do not touch them.

3

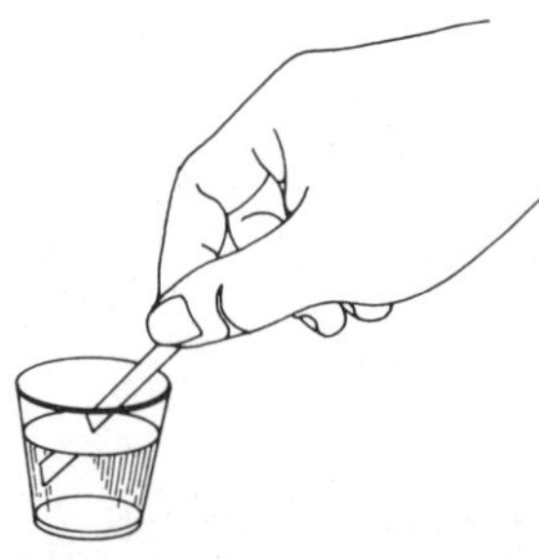

Dip the reagent strip's test blocks into the urine for about 2 seconds. Then lift the strip up and shake off excess urine. (If you prefer, you can perform the test while you urinate by simply holding the strip under the stream for about 2 seconds.)

TESTING YOUR URINE FOR GLUCOSE AND KETONES—*continued*

4

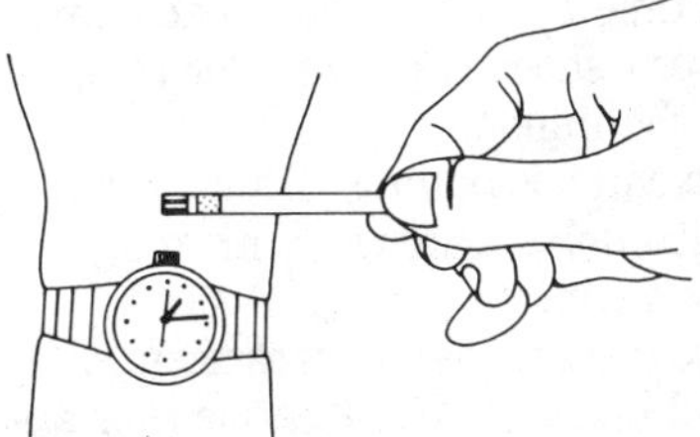

Hold the strip horizontally and immediately begin timing, following the manufacturer's directions. After waiting the recommended time, compare the ketone test block with the ketone color chart on the bottle label.

5

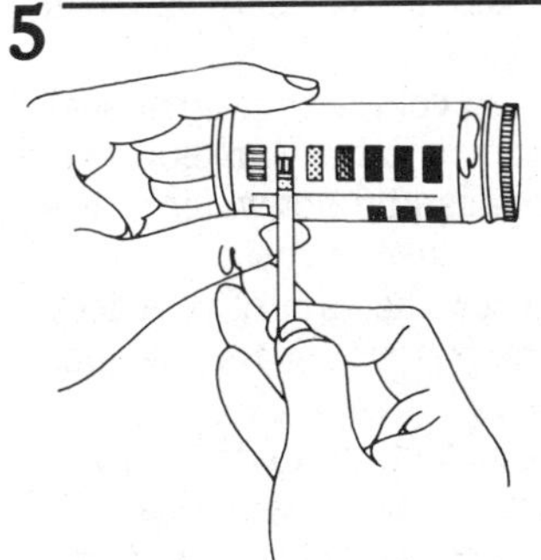

Wait the additional time that the manufacturer recommends, then compare the glucose test block with the glucose color chart. Ignore any color changes that occur after the specified time.

Keep a record of all your test results, and take it with you every time you visit your physician.

Important tips

- If your test results are positive for either glucose or ketones, test your urine again after a few hours. If the later test shows that your glucose or ketone level is still positive, call your physician or nurse.
- If you have a cold or fever, test your urine every 4 hours and notify your physician if any test results are positive. Test more frequently if you develop vomiting or diarrhea—especially if you have Type I diabetes.
- If your urine is highly colored (from a drug you are taking, for example), your urine test results may be inaccurate or unreliable. To make sure your diabetes is controlled, monitor your glucose levels with blood tests.

Patient-Teaching Aid

DIABETIC FOOT CARE

Dear Patient:

Because you have diabetes, your feet require meticulous daily care. Diabetes can reduce blood supply to your feet, so normally minor foot injuries, such as an ingrown toenail or a blister, can lead to dangerous infection. Because diabetes also reduces sensation in your feet, you can burn or chill your feet without feeling it. To prevent foot problems, follow this care routine:

- Soak your feet in warm, soapy water for 5 minutes every day. To prevent burns, check the water temperature before immersing your feet.
- Dry your feet gently and thoroughly by blotting them with a towel. Be sure to dry between the toes.
- Apply oil or lotion to your feet immediately after drying, to prevent evaporating water from drying your skin. Lotion will keep your skin soft.
- If your feet perspire heavily, use a mild foot powder. Sprinkle it lightly between your toes and in your socks and shoes.
- Do not cut your nails. Instead, file them even with the end of your toes. Do not corner nails or file them shorter than the ends of your toes. If your nails are too thick, tough, or misshapen to file, consult a podiatrist.
- Exercise your feet daily to improve circulation. Sitting on the edge of the bed, point your toes upward, then downward, 10 times. Then make a circle with each foot 10 times.
- Make sure your shoes fit properly. Break in new shoes gradually, increasing wearing time by half an hour each day. Check worn shoes frequently for rough spots in the lining.
- Wear clean socks daily. Do not wear socks with holes or darns with rough, irritating seams.
- Consult a podiatrist for treatment of corns and calluses. Self-treatment or application of caustic agents may be harmful.
- If your feet are cold, wear warm socks or slippers and use extra blankets. Avoid using heating pads and hot-water bottles, which may cause burns.
- Regularly check the skin of your feet for cuts, cracks, blisters, or red, swollen areas.
- If you cut your foot, no matter how slightly, contact the physician. Meanwhile, wash the cut thoroughly and apply a mild antiseptic. Avoid harsh antiseptics, such as iodine, which can cause tissue damage.
- Do not wear tight-fitting garments or engage in activities that can decrease circulation. Especially avoid wearing elastic garters, sitting with knees crossed, picking at sores or rough spots on your feet, walking barefoot, or applying adhesive tape to the skin of your feet.

Patient-Teaching Aid

PREVENTING NECK STRAIN AFTER THYROIDECTOMY

Dear Patient:
After your thyroidectomy, to prevent strain on your neck muscles when rising to a sitting position, support your head with a pillow and put your hands together behind your head (as shown).

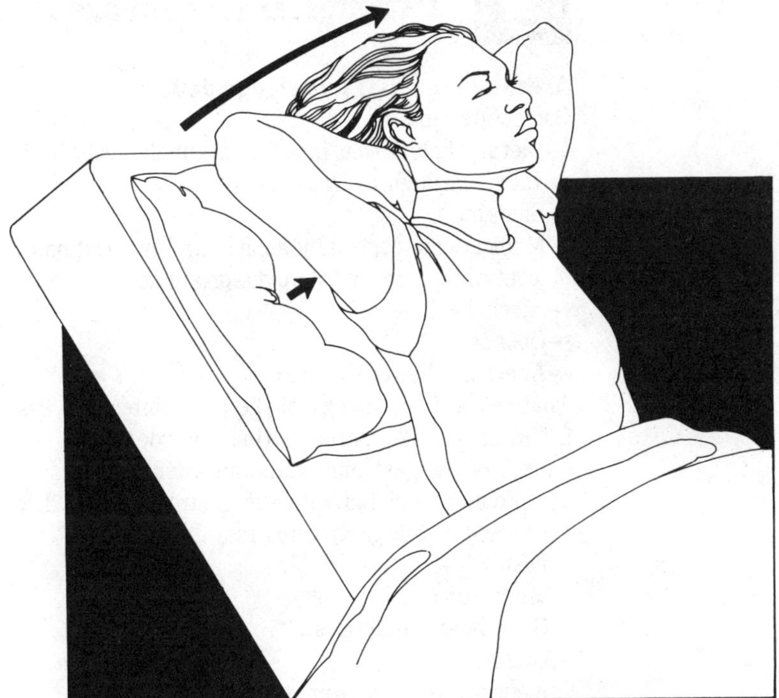

Gastrointestinal Disorders

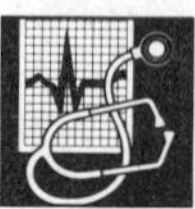

Patient-learner data base*

Areas of potential knowledge deficit

Gastrointestinal risk factors:
—Dietary habits that include an unbalanced diet low in bulk and high in irritants
—Smoking
—Medications, especially aspirin and medications containing aspirin, steroids, or anticoagulants
—Alcohol intake
—Obesity
—Abnormal bowel function

Anatomy and physiology of the gastrointestinal system
Definition of the gastrointestinal disorder
Causes of the gastrointestinal disorder
Symptoms associated with the gastrointestinal disorder
Treatment of the gastrointestinal disorder:
—Diet
—Medication
—Good health practices
—Other

Complications of gastrointestinal disease

Explaining diagnostic tests

COLLECTING STOOL SPECIMEN(S) TO DETECT OCCULT BLOOD

Patient objectives	*Teaching plan content*
1 State the purpose of collecting the stool specimen(s).	The purpose of collecting the stool specimen is to help detect abnormal gastrointestinal (GI) bleeding.

* A general assessment should be done for all patients. For general assessment guidelines, see Chapter 1, Principles of Patient Teaching.

2 Discuss patient guidelines for preparing to collect the stool specimen(s).

Patient guidelines include the following:
—The patient should maintain a high-fiber diet and refrain from eating red meats, poultry, fish, turnips, and horseradish for 48 to 72 hours before the test, as well as throughout the collection period.
—If ordered, the patient should withhold iron preparations, bromides, iodides, rauwolfia derivatives, indomethacin, colchicine, salicylates, phenylbutazone, steroids, and ascorbic acid for 48 hours before the test and also during it.
—The patient should be aware of how many specimens the physician has requested. The test usually requires collection of three stool specimens, but occasionally, only a random specimen is collected.

3 List the equipment needed to collect the stool specimen(s).

The following equipment is needed:
—A clean, dry bedpan (If the patient does not have a bedpan, he may use a large glass jar that has been cleaned and boiled.)
—A tongue depressor or small piece of cardboard
—A waterproof container with a tight-fitting lid (which the nurse or laboratory technician will give him).

4 Describe the six steps to follow when collecting the stool specimen(s).

The patient should follow these six steps:
—When he feels the urge to move his bowels, he should urinate into the toilet as he usually would; then, he should close the toilet's lid and position the bedpan or glass jar on the lid.
—Next, he should position himself on the bedpan and move his bowels. When he is finished, he should not urinate or place toilet tissue in the bedpan; doing so contaminates the stool. He should clean his perineal area with toilet tissue, using one front-to-back motion, and get dressed.
—He should now remove the lid from the container and place it flat side down, making sure he does not touch the inside of the lid or the container.
—Using the tongue depressor, he should transfer some of the bowel movement into the container, being careful not to overfill it. He should avoid touching the outside of the container with the tongue depressor. Then he should place the filled container on the sink and discard the tongue depressor.
—Then, he should put the lid on the container and wash his hands thoroughly.
—The patient should let the nurse know he has collected the specimen, so she may send the container to the laboratory immediately or refrigerate the specimen until the collection is completed. If the patient is at home, he should do the same thing.

UPPER GASTROINTESTINAL ENDOSCOPY (Esophagogastroduodenoscopy)

Patient objectives	*Teaching plan content*
1 Define esophagogastroduodenoscopy	Esophagogastroduodenoscopy is the visual examination of the esophagus, stomach, and small intestine, using a flexible tube inserted into the mouth and throat. (An illustration can be used to demonstrate the location of these structures in the body.)
2 State the purpose of esophagogastroduodenoscopy.	The purpose of esophagogastroduodenoscopy is to identify various GI abnormalities, for example, esophageal stenosis, esophagitis, inflammatory disease, tumors, Mallory-Weiss syndrome, lesions, gastritis, and polyps.
3 Discuss patient guidelines for esophagogastroduodenoscopy.	Patient guidelines include the following: —The patient should fast for at least 6 hours before the endoscopy to permit better visualization of the small intestine. —Necklaces, earrings, hairpins, or combs should be removed before the test, as should constricting undergarments such as girdles or long-line bras. If the patient wears dentures or eyeglasses, they should be removed just before the test. —Someone should accompany an outpatient home after the test. He will be groggy from the medications given before the test and will not be able to drive a car safely for about 12 hours. —The physician will speak with the patient and/or family concerning the reason for the diagnostic procedure, what the procedure entails, and possible complications.
4 Describe the procedure used in esophagogastroduodenoscopy.	Just before the procedure, the patient's blood pressure, pulse, and respirations will be taken. The blood pressure cuff will be left on his arm, and his blood pressure will be taken several times during the procedure. A heparin lock or I.V. infusion may be started in the patient's hand or arm. The line is used to administer medications (sedatives, atropine) during the procedure. —The patient will be positioned on his left side with his head bent forward, and he will be asked to open his mouth. He will then be asked to hold his breath while his mouth and throat are sprayed with a local anesthetic, which tastes somewhat bitter. This may make his mouth and throat feel swollen and may make swallowing difficult. The patient should allow saliva to drain from the side of his mouth into an emesis basin, which will be provided for him. A suction machine may

be used to remove saliva, if necessary. He will also be provided with tissues.
—A small plastic mouthpiece will be inserted so that the patient will have somewhere to rest his teeth (or gums, if he wears dentures). This will allow the physician to move the tube freely. If possible, the patient should be shown the mouthpiece and reassured that the opening in its center allows him to breathe through his mouth or nose, whichever is more comfortable.
—When the patient is groggy, the physician will ask him to open his mouth. He will lay his finger on the patient's tongue and slide the tube alongside the finger to the back of the throat. Because the patient is relaxed from the medication, he will be able to swallow the tube easily, and it will slide right down.
—During the test, the patient may feel some pressure in his stomach as the tube is moved about. He may also feel some fullness or bloating, much like that experienced after eating a large meal. This is caused by the air used to inflate the stomach. When the stomach is empty, its lining has large folds that could hide abnormalities. Inflating the stomach causes the walls to become smooth, giving the physician a better view.
—The physician will perform the test. It is usually done in the special studies laboratory and will take approximately 15 to 30 minutes. The patient should know when it will be done.

5 Discuss what to expect after esophagogastroduodenoscopy.

The patient can expect the following after the procedure:
—The nurse will check his vital signs every 15 minutes for 4 hours, every hour for the next 4 hours, then every 4 hours. This is routine.
—Food and fluids will be withheld until the gag reflex returns. The gag reflex is tested by touching the back of the throat with a tongue blade. When it returns—usually in 1 hour—fluids and a light meal will be allowed, as ordered.
—The patient may burp some insufflated air and may have a sore throat for 3 or 4 days after the procedure. Throat lozenges and warm saline solution gargles will be provided to ease his discomfort.
—If the patient experiences soreness at the I.V. site, warm soaks will be applied.
—An outpatient should watch for the following complications and notify the physician immediately if they develop: persistent difficulty in swallowing and pain, fever, black stools, or vomiting blood. He should not drive a car for 12 hours after the test because of drowsiness from the sedation.

LOWER GASTROINTESTINAL ENDOSCOPY (Colonoscopy, Sigmoidoscopy, Proctoscopy)

Patient objectives	*Teaching plan content*
1 Define lower GI endoscopy.	Lower GI endoscopy is the examination of the rectum, anal canal, or large intestine, using a flexible tube inserted into the anus. (An illustration or a model can be used to show these structures and their location in the body.)
2 State the purpose of lower GI endoscopy.	The purpose of lower GI endoscopy is to identify various problems in the lower GI tract (bowel); for example, tumors, polyps, inflammation, hemorrhoids, and bleeding.
3 Discuss patient guidelines for lower GI endoscopy.	Patient guidelines include the following: —The patient should follow applicable preparatory steps to clear his bowel of stool, since better visualization is obtained when the bowel is empty. These preparatory steps may include: • A clear liquid diet for 24 hours before the test • A laxative the evening before the test • A cleansing enema with warm tap water, given 3 to 4 hours before the test. (It may be necessary to repeat the enema to fully clear the bowel.) —The patient or a responsible family member will be asked to sign a consent form. The physician will speak with the patient and/or family concerning the reason for the diagnostic procedure, what the procedure entails, and the possible complications. —Someone should accompany an outpatient home after the test. He will be groggy from the medications given during the test and will not be able to drive a car safely.
4 Describe the procedure used in lower GI endoscopy.	Just before the procedure, a heparin lock or I.V. infusion may be started in the patient's hand or arm. The line may be used to administer medication (sedation) during the procedure. —He will receive medication that will make him sleepy (sedative), but he will remain conscious throughout the procedure. He will be adequately draped. —The patient will be asked to lie on his left side with his knees flexed while the endoscope is inserted. It is well lubricated to ease its insertion; it initially feels cool, and he may feel an urge to defecate when it is inserted and advanced. He should breathe deeply and

	slowly through his mouth to relax the abdominal muscles. —Air may be introduced into the large intestine through the endoscope to distend the intestinal wall and provide a better view of the lining and to facilitate the instrument's advance. Flatus normally escapes around the instrument due to air insufflation, and he should not attempt to control it. —A suction machine may be used to remove any blood or liquid feces that obscure vision, but this will not cause any discomfort. —The physician will perform the test. It is usually done in the special studies laboratory and will take approximately 15 to 30 minutes. The patient should know when it will be done.
5 Discuss what to expect after lower GI endoscopy.	The patient can expect the following after the procedure: —The nurse will check vital signs every half hour for 2 hours, every hour for 4 hours, then four times a day. —After the patient has recovered from sedation, he may resume his usual diet. —The patient may pass large amounts of flatus resulting from the air insufflated to distend the colon. Privacy should be provided in order to minimize embarrassment. —If a polyp has been removed, there may be some blood in his stool.

UPPER GASTROINTESTINAL SERIES (Barium swallow)

Patient objectives	*Teaching plan content*
1 Define an upper GI series.	An upper GI series is the examination of the throat, stomach, and small intestine through X-ray films. (An illustration can be used to show these structures and their position in the body.)
2 State the purpose of an upper GI series.	The purpose of an upper GI series is to identify various problems in the throat, stomach, and small intestine, for example, tumors, ulcers, hernias, and swallowing malfunctions.
3 Discuss patient guidelines for an upper GI series.	Patient guidelines include the following: —The patient should follow applicable preparatory steps to clear his GI tract of stool and decrease its activity, since the GI tract shows up clearly on X-ray only when it is empty and at rest. Preparations may include the following:

• The patient will be on a low-residue diet for 2 or 3 days before the test and will fast after midnight the night before the test.
• Smoking may not be permitted after midnight the night before the test, because nicotine alters bowel motility.
• If ordered, oral medications should not be taken after midnight the night before the test. Anticholinergics and narcotics should not be taken for 24 hours before the test, because these drugs affect GI motility. In addition, the patient may have to stop taking antacids several hours before the test if gastric reflux is suspected.
• A laxative and a saline solution or tap water enema will be given the evening before the test.

—Just before the procedure, the patient will put on a hospital gown without snap closures and remove jewelry, dentures, hair clips, or other objects that might obscure anatomic details on the X-ray film.

—The patient or a responsible family member will be asked to sign a consent form. The physician will speak with the patient and/or family concerning the reason for the diagnostic procedure, what the procedure entails, and possible complications.

4 Describe the procedure used in an upper GI series.

Just before the procedure, the patient will be asked to drink a barium milkshake. This tastes chalky, but it is important that he drink a large amount so the barium can coat his digestive tract, which then shows up clearly on X-ray.

—As the barium passes through the digestive tract, the radiologist will take X-rays from many angles at 15- to 30-second intervals. The X-ray table will be rotated and tilted in various positions to obtain proper visualization of the digestive tract. The patient will be adequately secured to the table.

—The radiologist may ask him to swallow some flavored granules. These produce air in his stomach, which improves visualization on X-rays. Or the patient may be asked to drink a carbonated drink, which has the same effect. He may feel like burping, but he should try not to do so until the procedure is finished.

—If the radiologist wants to examine the entire small intestine, he will ask the patient to drink several more cups of barium solution.

—The patient may be asked to wait in the X-ray department while the radiologist examines the film; if necessary, more X-rays will be taken before he returns to his room.

	—The radiologist will perform the test. It will be done in the X-ray department and will take between 1 and 4 hours. The patient should know when it will be done.
5 Discuss what to expect after an upper GI series.	The patient can expect the following after the procedure: —He may resume his normal diet and medications. —He should rest, since the test is very tiring. —A laxative or enema will be administered to help empty the GI tract of barium. All of the barium should be removed from the GI tract, because it can harden and cause intestinal obstruction or fecal impaction. —His stools will be light in color for 24 to 72 hours after the test.

LOWER GASTROINTESTINAL SERIES (Barium enema)

Patient objectives	*Teaching plan content*
1 Define a lower GI series.	A lower GI series is the examination of the large intestine (bowel) through X-ray films. (An illustration can be used to show the bowel and its location in the body.)
2 State the purpose of a lower GI series.	A lower GI series identifies various problems in the bowel, for example, obstructions, tumors, and inflammation.
3 Discuss patient guidelines for a lower GI series.	Patient guidelines include the following: —The patient should follow applicable preparatory steps to clear his bowel of stool, since the bowel shows up clearly on X-ray only when it is empty. Preparations may include the following: • He will be on a low-residue diet for 1 to 3 days before the test. Occasionally, intake is further restricted to clear liquids the day before the test or for the evening meal. The patient should drink water or clear liquids for 12 to 24 hours before the test to ensure adequate hydration. • He will receive a laxative the afternoon before the test. He may also receive a suppository. If ordered, other oral medications should not be taken after midnight the night before the test. • A cleansing enema of warm tap water will be given the evening before or early on the morning of the test. It may be necessary to repeat the enema to clear the bowel completely. —The patient or a responsible family member will be asked to sign a consent form. The physician will speak with the patient and/or family concerning the reason

for the diagnostic procedure, what the procedure entails, and possible complications.

4 Describe the procedure used in a lower GI series.

Just before the procedure, the radiologist will take an X-ray of the patient's bowel to make sure it is completely empty. If it is, he will position the patient on his side and prepare to insert a small tube into the rectum.

—After inserting the tube, the radiologist will allow a liquid called barium to flow gently through it. He may also introduce air through it. Both the barium and the air improve visualization of the bowel on X-ray film. The patient may experience cramping pains or the urge to defecate as the barium or air is introduced into the intestine. He should breathe deeply and slowly through his mouth to ease this discomfort.

—The patient should keep his anal sphincter tightly contracted against the rectal tube; this holds the tube in position and helps to prevent leakage of barium. If the intestinal walls are not adequately coated with barium, test results may be inaccurate. The barium enema is fairly easy to retain because of its cool temperature.

—As the radiologist takes the X-rays, he may ask the patient to change his body position. Assistance will be provided, if necessary.

—After the X-rays are taken, the patient will be permitted to empty his bowel; he will be escorted to the bathroom or given a bedpan.

—A radiologist or an X-ray technician will perform the test. It will be done in the X-ray department and will take approximately 1 hour. The patient should know when it will be done.

5 Discuss what to expect after a lower GI series.

The patient can expect the following after the procedure:

—He may resume his normal diet and medications.

—He should drink fluids to avoid dehydration and to help remove the barium.

—He should rest, since the test and the bowel preparations are tiring.

—A mild laxative or enema will be administered to empty the bowel of the barium. All of the barium should be removed from the bowel, because it can harden and cause intestinal obstruction or fecal impaction.

—His stools will be light in color for 24 to 72 hours after the test.

ORAL CHOLECYSTOGRAPHY

Patient objectives	*Teaching plan content*
1 Define oral cholecystography.	Oral cholecystography is the examination of the gallbladder through X-ray films. (An illustration can be used to demonstrate the location of the gallbladder in the body.)
2 State the purpose of oral cholecystography.	Oral cholecystography identifies various problems in the gallbladder, for example, gallstones, tumors, or inflammation.
3 Discuss patient guidelines for oral cholecystography.	Patient guidelines include the following: —The patient should follow preparatory steps that apply to him: • If ordered, he should eat a meal containing fat at noon the day before the test and a fat-free meal the evening before the test. The former stimulates the release of bile from the gallbladder, preparing it to receive the contrast-laden bile; the latter inhibits gallbladder contraction, promoting accentuation of bile. After the evening meal, the patient should restrict food and fluids, except water. • He will be given six tablets (3 g) of iopanoic acid 2 or 3 hours after the evening meal the night before the test, as ordered. Other commercial contrast agents are available (such as sodium ipodate), but iopanoic acid is most commonly used. He should swallow the tablets one at a time, at 5-minute intervals, with one or two mouthfuls of water, for a total of 8 oz (240 ml) of water. Thereafter, water should be withheld. He should tell the nurse if he vomits or moves his bowels before the test, so his vomitus and/or stool can be examined for undigested tablets. • He may receive a cleansing enema the morning of the test, if ordered. This clears the gastrointestinal tract of interfering shadows that may obscure the gallbladder. —The patient or a responsible family member will be asked to sign a consent form. The physician will speak with the patient and/or family concerning the reason for the diagnostic procedure, what the procedure entails, and possible complications.
4 Describe the procedure used in oral cholecystography.	The procedure involves making several X-rays. —X-rays will be taken while the patient is assisted to various positions.

Patient objectives	Teaching plan content
	—The patient may then be given a high-fat meal or a synthetic fat-containing agent (for example, Bilevac). Fluoroscopy is used to observe the resultant emptying of the gallbladder, and spot films are taken at 15, 30, and, if necessary, 60 minutes to visualize the common bile duct. —A radiologist or an X-ray technician will perform the test. It will be done in the X-ray department and will take approximately 45 minutes (longer if fluoroscopy is done to observe gallbladder emptying). The patient should know when the test will be done.
5 Discuss what to expect after oral cholecystography.	The patient can expect the following after the procedure: —His usual diet will be resumed if the test is normal. —A low-fat diet may be continued if test results are questionable. —If gallstones are discovered, an appropriate diet will be ordered.

LIVER-SPLEEN SCANNING

Patient objectives	*Teaching plan content*
1 Define liver-spleen scanning.	Liver-spleen scanning is the examination of these structures through radioactive scanning.
2 State the purpose of liver-spleen scanning.	Explain to the patient that this test identifies various problems in the liver and/or spleen, for example, tumors, cysts, and abscesses.
3 Describe the procedure used in liver-spleen scanning.	Just before the procedure, the patient will be injected with a radioactive substance (technetium^{99m}). The injection is not dangerous; it contains only trace amounts of radioactivity, and allergic reactions to it are rare. —After 10 to 15 minutes, the patient's abdomen will be scanned. If the gamma camera is used, the uptake probe and detector head may touch his abdomen, but this is not dangerous. If the rectilinear camera is used, it will make a soft, irregular clicking noise as it moves across his abdomen. The patient will be assisted to various positions to ensure optimal visualization of the liver and the spleen. He should lie still and breathe quietly during the procedure to ensure images of good quality. He may also be asked to hold his breath briefly. This technique helps to evaluate liver mobility and pliability. —A radiologist will perform the test. It will be done in

	the nuclear medicine laboratory and will take approximately 1 hour. The patient should know when the test will be done.
4 Discuss what to expect after liver-spleen scanning.	The nurse will take vital signs periodically to be sure that the patient has no adverse reaction to the contrast agent.

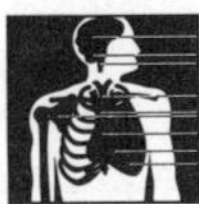

Explaining disorders

CONSTIPATION

Patient objectives	*Teaching plan content*
1 Define constipation.	Constipation occurs when the interval between the patient's bowel movements is greater than normal. (A 2- to 3-day interval between bowel movements can be normal.)
2 Describe the causes of constipation.	There are several common causes of constipation that may be applicable to the patient. —Persons with a low fiber intake, low food intake, and low fluid intake will have fewer stools. —Lack of activity or decreased activity associated with illness, age, or a change in life-style can prolong the interval between bowel movements. The usual motion of the bowel is lessened when at rest or in a recumbent position. —Travel, poor bathroom facilities, and unfamiliar surroundings can change the normal bowel routine. —During periods of emotional stress, bowel habits may change. —Ignoring the urge to pass stool and neglecting normal bowel habits disturbs the natural process of bowel elimination. —Such medications as antacids, pain medication, antihypertensives, iron, and the chronic use of laxatives may decrease the natural motion of the bowel. —Hypothyroidism, tumors, strictures, and adhesions of the GI tract affect bowel movement. —In pregnancy, pressure from the enlarged uterus against the rectum and lower portion of the colon, in addition to the relaxation of smooth muscle caused by elevated progesterone levels, contributes to a decrease in GI motility.

3 Describe the symptoms of constipation.

The symptoms of constipation include the following:
—Straining and passing of hard, dry stools
—A sensation of fullness in the rectum and a frequent urge to defecate
—Nausea, belching, regurgitation
—Abdominal pain.

4 Identify the components of the treatment regimen for constipation.

The treatment regimen for constipation may include the following:
—Diet
—Medications
- Bulk-forming laxatives
- Stool softeners

—Rest
—Exercise.

5 Discuss the dietary modifications used in the management of constipation.

The following dietary modifications may alleviate constipation:
—Drinking at least 8 to 10 glasses of liquid every day (particularly important in the older patient), since fluids help keep the intestinal contents in a semisolid state for easier passage. Before breakfast or in the evening the patient can stimulate the bowel with a drink of hot or cold water—plain or with lemon—or prune juice.
—Adding fiber to the diet with such foods as whole grain cereals (rolled oats, bran, oatmeal) to contribute bulk and induce peristalsis. However, too much bran can create an irritable bowel, so the patient should check labels on foods for fiber content (low fiber, 0.3 to 1 g; moderate fiber, 1.1 to 2 g; high fiber, 2.1 to 4.2 g). Bulk content of the diet should be increased slowly to prevent flatulence, which is sometimes a transient effect of a high-bulk diet.
—Using foods containing fat, such as bacon, butter, cream, and oil, in moderation, since they will help to soften intestinal contents; however, they sometimes cause diarrhea.
—Avoiding highly refined foods, such as white rice, cream of wheat, farina, white pastries, pie or cake, macaroni, spaghetti, noodles, and ice cream.

6 Describe the medication regimen.

Some drugs commonly used for this disorder are bisacodyl, docusate, and magnesium salts. See Chapter 9, Drug Therapy, for a discussion of any medications the physician has advised the patient to take.

7 Identify at least four good health practices to prevent and/or alleviate constipation.	Good health practices include the following: —Rest at least 6 hours every night. —Incorporate moderate exercise, such as walking, into the daily routine. —Avoid overuse of laxatives, and maintain a regular time for bowel movements (usually after breakfast). —Try such techniques as autosuggestion, relaxation, and use of a small footstool to promote thigh flexion while sitting on the toilet, to stimulate elimination. —Respond promptly to the urge to defecate. —Anticipate events that may change normal bowel habits (for example, illness or changes in work schedule). Plan diet, activity, and elimination patterns as the daily routine changes. —Establish and maintain a regular time for bowel movements.
8 Identify signs and symptoms that may warn of fecal impaction.	The patient should notify his physician immediately if he notices any of the following signs and symptoms of fecal impaction: —Malaise, anorexia —Headache, dizziness —Failure of bowel to empty in response to a laxative.

DIVERTICULAR DISEASE

Patient objectives	*Teaching plan content*
1 Define diverticulosis and diverticulitis.	Diverticulosis indicates the presence of bulging pouches, or diverticula, in the wall of the intestine. Diverticulitis is an inflammation of the diverticula, or pouches, resulting from retained fecal material in the pouch mixing with bacteria.
2 Describe the structure and function of the large intestine (colon, or bowel).	The large intestine (colon, or bowel) is divided into six parts: the cecum, ascending colon, transverse colon, descending colon, sigmoid colon, and rectum. Its major function is the elimination of the end products of digestion (stool).
3 Identify the causes of diverticular disease.	The causes of diverticular disease include the following: —Atrophy or weakening of the bowel muscle from aging —Increased pressure in the bowel that may be due to: • Chronic constipation • Straining at stool • Lack of dietary bulk • Obesity.

4 Describe the symptoms of diverticular disease.	The severity of the patient's symptoms will depend on the type of diverticular disease he has. —Diverticulosis may cause recurrent pain in the left lower quadrant of his abdomen. This pain is often accompanied by alternating constipation and diarrhea and is relieved by the passing of stool or gas. —Diverticulitis produces moderate to severe pain in the left lower quadrant of the abdomen, along with nausea, gas, and low-grade fever.
5 Identify the components of the treatment regimen for diverticular disease.	Treatment will depend on the type of diverticular disease the patient has. —In diverticulosis with abdominal pain and constipation, the goals are to reduce irritation and prevent infection by following this care routine: • Liquid or bland diet, followed by a high-fiber diet once symptoms subside • Stool softeners • Mild laxatives. —In diverticulitis, the goals are to prevent constipation and combat infection by following this care routine: • Bed rest • Liquid diet, followed by a high-fiber diet once symptoms subside • Stool softeners • Antibiotics • Medication to relieve pain. —Severe diverticulitis that does not respond to medical treatment may be treated by: • Colon resection to remove the involved portion of the bowel • Colostomy to drain abscesses and rest the bowel.
6 Discuss the dietary modifications used in the management of diverticular disease.	The patient should increase his intake of foods high in undigestible fiber, including fresh fruits and vegetables, whole grain breads, and wheat or bran cereals. (A dietary instruction sheet should be reviewed with the patient.)
7 Describe the medication regimen.	Some drugs commonly used for this disorder are ampicillin and docusate. See Chapter 9, Drug Therapy, for a discussion of the patient's discharge medications.
8 Identify the signs and symptoms of complications of diverticular disease.	The warning signs of complications of diverticular disease include the following: —Pain, abdominal rigidity, high fever, chills, hypotension, and bleeding, which may be signs and symptoms of rupture of diverticula with peritonitis —Constipation, ribbonlike stools, intermittent diarrhea,

abdominal distention, nausea, vomiting, and abdominal pain, which may be signs and symptoms of obstruction.

HIATAL HERNIA

Patient objectives	*Teaching plan content*
1 **Define hiatal hernia.**	A hiatal hernia occurs when the opening in the diaphragm through which the esophagus passes becomes weak or enlarges. This allows a part of the stomach to protrude into the chest cavity when intraabdominal pressure increases as a result of coughing, straining during bowel movement, vomiting, bending, lifting, wearing constrictive clothing, and making strenuous physical effort. There are three types of hiatal hernia. (An illustration can be used to help explain the different types of hiatal hernia.)
2 **Identify the relevant type of hiatal hernia.**	There are three types of hiatal hernia: —In a Type I sliding hernia, the stomach cardia (the area of the fundus nearest the gastroesophageal junction) "slides" upward through the opening in the diaphragm, into the chest. The lower esophageal sphincter also moves into the chest, and this impairs its ability to prevent the backflow of stomach contents into the esophagus. (This is the most common type of hernia.) —In a Type II paraesophageal, or rolling, hernia, the fundus rolls up beside the esophagus through an opening in the diaphragm. —A Type III hiatal hernia combines the features of Types I and II.
3 **Describe the normal structure and function of the esophagus, diaphragm, and stomach.**	The normal structure and function of the esophagus, diaphragm, and stomach are as follows (an illustration or model can be used to help explain): —The esophagus is a long, muscular tube that connects the mouth and the stomach. Its function is to transport food from the mouth to the stomach. A sphincter (the lower esophageal sphincter, located at the lower end of the esophagus just before it joins the stomach) prevents a backflow of stomach contents into the esophagus. (Stomach contents are very acidic and can cause heartburn and various other problems.) —The diaphragm is a large muscle that separates the chest cavity from the abdominal cavity. The diaphragm has a small opening (hiatus) through which the esophagus passes, just before it joins the stomach. —The stomach is a collapsible pouch located beneath the diaphragm and between the esophagus and the small intestine. The stomach mixes and stores food.

For descriptive purposes, it can be divided into the following three parts:
- Fundus (top portion)
- Body (middle portion)
- Antrum (bottom portion).

4 Describe the causes of hiatal hernia.

Hiatal hernias are caused by a weakening in the wall of the diaphragm. Causes of muscle weakening include the following:
—Congenital malformation (The hernia may have been present since birth, but symptoms often do not occur until mid-life.)
—Abdominal or chest injury
—Loss of muscle tone as a result of aging, pregnancy, or obesity.

5 Describe the symptoms of hiatal hernia.

Symptoms of hiatal hernia include the following:
—Heartburn, which occurs from 1 to 4 hours after eating, is caused by reflux of stomach contents into the esophagus. Aggravated by reclining, belching, and increased abdominal pressure, it may be accompanied by regurgitation or vomiting.
—Retrosternal or substernal chest pain, resulting from the reflux of stomach contents, distention of the stomach and spasm, or altered motor activity, occurs most often after meals or at bedtime and is aggravated by reclining, belching, and increased abdominal pressure. It is often confused with angina.

6 Identify the components of the treatment regimen for hiatal hernia.

The treatment regimen for hiatal hernia includes the following:
—Restriction or control of factors that increase intraabdominal pressure
—Diet
—Medications, including antacids, cholinergics, antiemetics, and cough suppressants
—Elevating the head with two or three pillows or placing 6″ to 8″ (15 to 20 cm) blocks under the legs of the head of the bed to alleviate heartburn by gravity
—Cessation of smoking, since nicotine stimulates the production of acid in the stomach
—Surgery to repair the hernia.

7 Describe factors that increase intraabdominal pressure and methods to control them.

Factors that increase intraabdominal pressure and methods to control them include the following:
—Strenuous exercise: Avoid sports, weight lifting, lifting, bending.
—Straining with bowel movement: Modify the diet to include natural laxatives, such as whole grain cereals

	and breads. Take laxatives or stool softeners, if prescribed by physician. —Coughing: Take cough suppressants, if prescribed by physician. Stop smoking. —Constrictive clothing: Avoid tight girdles, jeans, or other constrictive clothing. —Obesity: Maintain a weight-reduction diet.
8 Discuss the dietary modifications used in the management of hiatal hernia.	The following dietary modifications will reduce secretions and activity of the stomach and alleviate symptoms: —Eating small, frequent meals at least 2 hours before lying down (no bedtime snacks) —Eating slowly —Avoiding milk products; caffeine; highly seasoned, spicy foods and foods known to cause symptoms; fruit juices; and alcoholic beverages —Eating a bland diet (if ordered, a dietary instruction sheet should be reviewed with the patient).
9 Describe the medication regimen.	Some drugs commonly used in this disorder are aluminum hydroxide, bisacodyl, and docusate. See Chapter 9, Drug Therapy, for a discussion of the patient's discharge medications.
10 Identify the signs and symptoms of complications of a hiatal hernia.	The following signs and symptoms may be a warning of possible complications. The patient should notify his physician immediately if he experiences any of them. —Difficulty swallowing (dysphagia) could indicate esophagitis, esophageal ulceration, or stricture. —Bleeding may indicate esophagitis or erosion of the gastric pouch and may be mild, massive, frank, or occult. —Severe pain and shock results from incarceration, in which a large portion of the stomach is caught above the diaphragm (usually with paraesophageal hernia). It may lead to perforation of a gastric ulcer and strangulation and gangrene of the herniated portion of the stomach.

INFLAMMATORY BOWEL DISEASE (Ulcerative colitis, Crohn's disease)

Patient objectives	*Teaching plan content*
1 Define inflammatory bowel disease.	Inflammatory bowel disease is a chronic condition characterized by an inflammation of the lining of the GI tract. When the GI tract becomes inflamed, it becomes irritated and cannot perform its main functions of digestion, absorption, and elimination in the normal

manner. (An illustration or model of the GI tract can be used to help explain the disorder.)

2 Identify the relevant type of inflammatory bowel disease.

There are two types of inflammatory bowel disease.
—Ulcerative colitis is chronic inflammation of the lining of the large intestine (colon, or bowel), characterized by episodes of exacerbation and remission.
—Crohn's disease is chronic inflammation of the lining of any part of the GI tract from the mouth to the anus, characterized by a slow, progressive course.

3 Describe the causes of inflammatory bowel disease.

The causes of inflammatory bowel disease are not well understood, but they may include the following:
—Family history of the disease
—Bacterial infection
—Allergic reactions to certain foods, milk, or other substances that irritate the bowel
—Overproduction of certain enzymes that break down the lining of the bowel
—Emotional stress
—Certain autoimmune diseases, such as arthritis, hemolytic anemia, erythema nodosum, and uveitis.

4 Describe the signs and symptoms of inflammatory bowel disease.

The signs and symptoms of inflammatory bowel disease include the following:
—Rectal bleeding (more common with ulcerative colitis)
—Diarrhea (often contains blood, mucus, and pus; accompanied by cramping abdominal pain, often relieved by defecation)
—Steatorrhea (fat in stool; more common in Crohn's disease)
—Weight loss, weakness, anorexia, nausea, vomiting
—Fever.

5 Identify the components of the treatment regimen for inflammatory bowel disease.

The goals of treatment are to alleviate symptoms and to help heal the GI tract. Treatment includes the following:
—Physical rest to decrease activity of the bowel and promote healing
—Diet and/or nutritional support to allow the bowel to heal by decreasing its activity and providing the calories and nutrients necessary for cell healing to occur. During the acute phase, the patient will have nothing by mouth (I.V. feedings) or may be allowed an elemental diet (Ensure, Vivonex) with I.V. fluids. As his condition improves, his diet will be increased gradually until a bland, low-residue diet is tolerated.

—Medication to reduce inflammation, pain, and diarrhea. Drug therapy may include anti-inflammatories, antimicrobials, sulfonamides, antispasmodics (rarely), antidiarrheals (rarely), and immunosuppressives (rarely).
—Surgery, depending on the extent and the location of the problem. (See the "Ostomies" teaching plan in this chapter.)

6 Discuss the dietary modifications used in the management of inflammatory bowel disease.

The following dietary modifications will not cure the disease or prevent recurrence of an acute attack, but may alleviate symptoms or prevent them from recurring as frequently:
—Avoiding foods known to cause symptoms, including:
- Foods prepared with milk or milk products
- Spicy or high-residue foods, such as raw vegetables and fruits, whole grain cereals, spices, condiments, nuts, cellulose
- Carbonated beverages, caffeine, alcohol

—Eating small, frequent meals
—Eating slowly
—Avoiding extremely hot or cold foods or beverages
—Eating a bland diet (if ordered, a dietary instruction sheet should be reviewed with the patient).

7 Describe the medication regimen.

Some drugs commonly used for this disorder are atropine sulfate, hydrocortisone, methantheline bromide, prednisone, propantheline bromide, and sulfasalazine. See Chapter 9, Drug Therapy, for a discussion of the patient's discharge medications.

8 Identify at least three good health practices to alleviate and/or control inflammatory bowel disease.

Good health practices include the following:
—Getting adequate sleep and rest
—Avoiding excessive physical activity, which increases bowel activity. Moderate exercise may promote relaxation and relieve stress.
—Avoiding emotional stress, which increases bowel activity (If the patient anticipates problems controlling the stress in his life, he can learn to use relaxation techniques. See the "Hypertension" teaching plan in Chapter 2, Cardiovascular Disorders. If these measures are not effective, the patient may need counseling for stress management.)
—Planning carefully to avoid areas lacking adequate sanitation and preservation of food and water when traveling.

9 Demonstrate proper skin care of the rectal area.	Proper skin care helps to avoid infection and discomfort. It includes the following: —Using the softest toilet tissue possible —Cleansing the rectal area frequently with warm water —Applying a protective coating of mineral oil, karaya gel, A and D Ointment, or a similar product to prevent the next stool from direct contact with the irritated skin.

PEPTIC ULCER DISEASE

Patient objectives	*Teaching plan content*
1 Define peptic ulcer.	A peptic ulcer is a sore in the lining of the upper GI tract.
2 State the location of the ulcer.	Possible locations include the following (an illustration can be used to demonstrate): —Lower esophagus —Stomach (gastric ulcer) —Duodenum (upper portion of small bowel—duodenal ulcer).
3 Describe the causes of peptic ulcer disease.	A peptic ulcer can be caused by too much acid in the stomach or not enough mucus on the lining of the stomach or duodenum. Stomach acid digests food but can also digest living tissue. Mucus protects the lining of the stomach and duodenum from the erosive effects of stomach acid. With too much acid or too little mucus, a sore may form. Factors that may cause overproduction of stomach acid or decreased mucus include the following: —Drugs, including alcohol, aspirin, bile salts, corticosteroids, indomethacin, chemotherapeutic agents, and caffeine —Physical or emotional stress —A familial tendency for the development of ulcers (heredity).
4 Describe the symptoms of peptic ulcer disease.	Symptoms of peptic ulcer disease include the following: —Pain in the stomach between meals or during the night and/or when getting up in the morning (Pain is usually relieved by eating.) —Heartburn, which occurs approximately 2 hours after meals, whenever the stomach is empty, or after consumption of orange juice, coffee, aspirin, or alcohol —Nausea and vomiting (possibly).

5 Identify the components of the treatment regimen for peptic ulcer disease.	The goal of treatment is to neutralize the stomach acid so it is not harmful to the lining of the upper GI tract. This allows the ulcer to heal and may prevent another ulcer from developing. Treatment includes the following: —Diet —Medication —Physical and emotional rest —Surgery. (See the "Gastric Resection" teaching plan in this chapter.)
6 Discuss the dietary modifications used in the management of peptic ulcer disease.	The following dietary modifications will help to control pain and further irritation in peptic ulcer disease: —Avoiding foods that cause pain —Avoiding foods that are extremely hot or cold, as well as excessive use of caffeinic and alcoholic beverages —Initially, eating six small meals daily; then, as healing progresses, gradually returning to three reasonably sized meals a day —Eating a bland diet (if ordered, a dietary instruction sheet should be reviewed with the patient).
7 Describe the medication regimen.	Some drugs commonly used for this disorder are aluminum hydroxide, cimetidine, Maalox, Mylanta, and ranitidine. See Chapter 9, Drug Therapy, for a discussion of the patient's discharge medications.
8 Identify at least three good health practices to alleviate and/or control peptic ulcer disease.	Good health practices include the following: —Getting adequate sleep and rest —Avoiding excessive physical activity, as it increases the secretion of acid in the stomach. Moderate exercise, however, may promote relaxation and reduce stress. —Avoiding emotional stress by altering life-style to avoid stressful situations (If the patient anticipates a problem controlling the stress in his life, he can learn to use relaxation techniques. See the "Hypertension" teaching plan in Chapter 2, Cardiovascular Disorders. If these measures are not effective, the patient may need counseling for stress management.) —Avoiding medications containing aspirin —Stopping smoking, since smoking alters the body's natural ability to neutralize stomach acid.
9 Identify the signs and symptoms of complications of peptic ulcer disease.	The following signs and symptoms may warn of complications of peptic ulcer disease. The patient should notify his physician immediately if he experiences any of them.

—Black, tarry stools; blood in the stool; vomiting blood or coffee-ground material; dizziness upon standing; and paleness may indicate hemorrhage.
—Increase in pain, nausea, vomiting, anorexia, weight loss, and constipation may indicate intestinal obstruction.
—Pain over the entire abdomen, increased pulse, sweating, and dizziness may indicate gastric perforation.

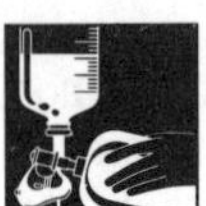

Explaining treatments

CHOLECYSTECTOMY

Patient objectives	*Teaching plan content*
1 Describe the normal structure and function of the gallbladder.	The gallbladder is located on the underside of the liver, and its main function is to store bile, which is made in the liver. Bile is used to digest the fat we eat. Digestion of fat takes place in the small intestine; bile is transported from the liver to the gallbladder and from the gallbladder to the small intestine via a system of ducts. An illustration or model of the biliary system (gallbladder and related ductal system) can be used to clarify the explanation.
2 Define cholelithiasis and cholecystitis.	Cholelithiasis and cholecystitis are medical terms that indicate a problem in the gallbladder. —Cholelithiasis is the term for gallstones. Gallstones are formed from bile and may lodge in the gallbladder or one of the ducts that lead into and out of the gallbladder. They irritate the lining of the gallbladder and make it susceptible to infection and inflammation. —Cholecystitis is inflammation of the gallbladder.
3 Describe the signs and symptoms of gallbladder disease.	The symptoms of gallbladder disease are associated with difficulty in digesting fat due to the inability of the bile to get to the small intestine, as well as to the inflammation of the gallbladder itself. Symptoms include the following: —Pain in right upper quadrant of abdomen, often following a meal rich in fat —Belching, nausea, vomiting —Chills, fever —Intolerance of fatty or fried foods.

4 Define and state the purpose of cholecystectomy.

Cholecystectomy is the surgical removal of the gallbladder. Its purpose is to relieve symptoms of gallbladder disease.

5 Describe the preoperative procedures for cholecystectomy.

In addition to routine preoperative procedures, the patient can expect skin preparation specific to cholecystectomy: His skin will be washed and shaved from nipples to mid-thigh, since hair harbors bacteria and may cause infection. (See Appendix B, *Preoperative and Postoperative Teaching.*)

6 Describe the procedure used in cholecystectomy.

After the patient is anesthetized, the physician will make an incision in the abdomen and remove the gallbladder. Once the gallbladder is removed, bile will flow directly from the liver to the small intestine to be used in the digestion of fat. The physician will also remove any gallstones from the ducts leading to and from the gallbladder so that bile will flow smoothly.

7 Describe immediate postoperative procedures for cholecystectomy.

In addition to routine postoperative procedures, the patient can expect the following:

—The patient will have a dressing over his abdomen. The nurse will check the dressing frequently for signs of drainage or bleeding. The dressing will be changed as needed.

—The patient will have one or more of the following tubes in place:

- A nasogastric tube will be placed in the stomach through the mouth or nose and kept in place to relieve gas and drainage in the GI tract. Gas and drainage may build up in the GI tract because the bowels do not function properly for 1 to 3 days after surgery. As soon as the bowels begin to function, the tube will be removed.
- A soft, plastic tube called a Penrose drain is placed in the area the gallbladder used to occupy and extends to the surface of the skin. Fluid tends to accumulate in this space for a day or two after surgery and must be drained to prevent discomfort and/or infection.
- A soft, plastic T tube may be placed in the common bile duct and brought out to the surface of the skin. Its purpose is to allow bile, which is formed by the liver, to drain into a plastic bag. This allows the ducts through which the bile would normally flow to heal. A T tube will also drain small gallstones and prevent them from blocking the common bile duct.

8 State the length of time necessary for healing of abdominal tissues.

It takes approximately 6 weeks for complete healing of the abdominal tissues, including the muscles, and it is normal to feel tired during the healing process.

9 Describe activity limitations after discharge.

Activity limitations may vary from one patient to another. The patient should follow his physician's instructions. Activity restrictions may include the following:
—Work usually is not allowed until after the first physician's checkup (usually 6 weeks after discharge).
—Driving usually is not allowed until after the first physician's checkup. The patient will receive further instructions at that time.
—Moderate ambulation around the house is encouraged. Climbing stairs should be limited to three times a day.
—Household chores should be limited. Mopping, vacuuming, and heavy lifting should be avoided until after the first physician's checkup. The patient will receive further instructions at that time.

10 Describe the dietary restrictions following discharge.

In most cases the patient will return to a normal diet. At first, fatty, rich foods may cause him some discomfort; however, his body will adjust to not having a gallbladder, and after it does, he should not have any problems. If he was on a special diet before surgery, the physician probably will advise him to resume the diet.

11 Demonstrate proper care of the T tube.

Changing the dressing, cleaning the T tube equipment, and positioning it correctly will help prevent such complications as infection and tube obstruction or dislodging. The dressing around the T tube should be changed and the wound site should be cleaned at least once every day or whenever the dressing becomes excessively wet or soiled.
—The patient should gather the necessary supplies: soap; a paper bag; five sterile 4″ × 4″ sponges; two sterile swabs soaked with povidone-iodine; one small sterile povidone-iodine ointment packet; alcohol and sterile saline and hydrogen peroxide solutions; a pair of sterile gloves; adhesive tape; a clean basin; a Velcro belt; and a sterile, disposable paper cloth. (He will be provided with enough equipment to last for a few days at home; thereafter, equipment can be purchased through his local pharmacy.)
—He should follow these steps for T tube dressing changes and wound care (written instructions should be provided):

- Wash hands thoroughly, using soap and water.

- Remove the old dressing, and discard it in the paper bag.
- Wash hands again.
- Open the package containing the sterile paper cloth. Unfold the cloth to its full length, touching only its undersurface, and spread it onto a smooth, wide worktable.
- Open the 4″ × 4″ sponges and carefully drop each one onto the sterile paper cloth surface without touching it. Also open the swab and ointment packets. Remove the tops from the bottles of alcohol, sterile saline solution, and hydrogen peroxide solution. Be careful to place the tops flat sides down on the worktable and away from the sterile cloth. Pour a little solution from each bottle into the basin; this will clean the lips of the bottles.
- Put on the sterile gloves. Decide which hand will be the "clean" hand and which one the "sterile" hand.
- Hold a 4″ × 4″ sponge in the sterile hand. Pick up the bottle of saline solution with the clean hand and thoroughly soak the sponge with solution. Wash around the wound site with the soaked sponge (still in the sterile hand). Wipe outward from the T tube wound, in a spiral fashion, to make a circle about 3″ (8 cm) wide.
- Repeat the procedure, using hydrogen peroxide solution.
- Soak a 4″ × 4″ sponge in alcohol solution. Use it to wipe about a 6″ (15-cm) length of tube, moving from the wound site toward the drainage bag. To prevent infection, never wipe the tube in the opposite direction.
- Wipe the wound site a third time with the povidone-iodine swabs. Again, remember to clean outward from the wound in a spiral fashion.
- Apply povidone-iodine ointment to the wound site by squeezing the packet with the clean hand, then letting the ointment drop onto the area. Use a sterile 4″ × 4″ sponge to spread the ointment with the sterile hand.
- Again with the sterile hand, fluff open the remaining 4″ × 4″ sponge. Completely encircle the T tube at the wound site with the fluffed sponge. Tape this dressing securely to the abdomen. Also, tape a small segment of the T tube itself to the abdomen so it will not inadvertently be pulled. Pulling could enlarge the wound, increasing drainage and the risk of infection.

—The purpose of the T tube is to form a passage so

excess bile can drain out under pressure. It should not be left in a downward position, which would create too much drainage. It can be taped anywhere on the abdomen as long as it is slightly below the T tube wound site.

12 Demonstrate proper care of the drainage bag.

The drainage bag should be emptied at about the same time each day. To do this, the patient should not disconnect the connecting tube at the end of the T tube, because it could lead to infection. Instead, he should let the bile flow from the spout at the bottom of the bag.
—He should note the amount, color, and odor of the drainage each time he empties the bag.
—When the bag is empty, he should coil up the drainage bag connecting tube and use a Velcro belt to secure the drainage bag and connecting tube to his abdomen below the wound site.
—He should not place the drainage bag higher than the level of the T tube wound site. Bile would then be able to flow back into the common bile duct.

13 Identify the signs and symptoms of complications associated with the T tube.

The following signs and symptoms may be a warning of complications. The patient should notify his physician immediately if he experiences any of them.
—Redness, swelling, warmth, firmness, pain, and, possibly, puslike drainage of the wound indicate infection. He may also have a fever, general malaise, and a faster pulse rate. If the infection spreads into the abdominal cavity, his abdomen may become rigid and tender to the touch.
—Little or no bile drainage, tenderness in the right upper abdominal quadrant, nausea, vomiting, clay-colored stools, jaundice, and malaise indicate an obstructed T tube. Use terms your patient can understand when you describe these signs and symptoms. Warn him that obstruction may also cause signs and symptoms of infection.
—Increased drainage or gradual enlargement of the wound indicate that the T tube may have moved. It may dislodge if it is pulled. Just before the patient goes home, the length of the T tube from the wound site to the end attached to the connecting tube should be measured. Using this measurement as a baseline, the patient will be able to tell later if the tube has moved.

14 Discuss removal of the T tube.

Some time after discharge, the patient's physician will schedule a cholangiogram to determine if the body passage formed by the T tube is clear; if so, the T tube will be removed. A flexible catheter will be advanced through the passage into the common bile duct, and any remaining stones will be trapped in the catheter's basket. Afterward, another cholangiogram will be performed to be sure all of the stones have been removed. The patient may have to stay overnight for observation, but he will most likely be discharged the next morning.

GASTRIC RESECTION

Patient objectives	***Teaching plan content***
1 Define and state the purpose of gastric resection.	A gastric resection is the removal of part or all of the stomach. Its purpose is to alleviate or control the following stomach disorders: —Peptic ulcer disease (See the "Peptic Ulcer Disease" teaching plan in this chapter for more information.) —Tumors (carcinoma).
2 Describe the normal structure and function of the stomach.	The stomach is a collapsible pouch located between the esophagus and the first part of the small intestine. The stomach mixes and stores food and then sends it on to the small intestine to be digested and absorbed. (An illustration or model of the stomach and related structures can be used for clarification.) For descriptive purposes, the stomach can be divided into the following three parts: —Fundus (uppermost portion) —Body (middle portion) —Antrum (bottom portion).
3 Describe the preoperative procedures for gastric resection.	In addition to routine preoperative procedures, the patient can expect the following procedures specific to gastric resection (See Appendix B, *Preoperative and Postoperative Teaching.*): —Laxatives, enemas, and antibiotics will be administered to cleanse the bowel and decrease the chance of infection after surgery. —The patient may have nothing by mouth for several days before the surgery. If this is the case, he will receive I.V. feedings (hyperalimentation) to ensure adequate nutrition. —To empty the stomach before surgery, a nasogastric tube will be placed through the patient's nose and connected to suction. —The patient's skin will be washed and shaved from nipples to thighs, since hair harbors bacteria and may cause infection.

4 Describe the procedure used in gastric resection.

After the patient is anesthetized, the physician will make an incision in his abdomen to reach the stomach. There are several types of procedures he can perform, depending upon the nature and extent of the patient's problem. (An illustration can be used to demonstrate the procedure to be used.) Possible surgical procedures include the following:

—Billroth I (gastroduodenostomy): Removal of part of the bottom portion of the stomach (antrum); connection of the remaining portion of the stomach to the first part of the small intestine (the duodenum)

—Billroth II (subtotal gastrectomy, or gastrojejunostomy): Removal of the bottom portion of the stomach (antrum) and the first part of the small intestine (duodenum); connection of the remaining portion of the stomach to the second part of the small intestine (jejunum)

—Partial gastric resection: Removal of the lower two thirds to three fourths of the stomach and the first part of the small intestine (duodenum); connection of the remaining portion of the stomach to the second part of the small intestine (jejunum)

—Total gastric resection (esophagojejunostomy): Removal of the entire stomach and first part of the small intestine (duodenum); connection of the esophagus to the second part of the small intestine (jejunum).

5 Describe immediate postoperative procedures for gastric resection.

In addition to routine postoperative procedures, the patient may expect the following:

—The patient will have a dressing over his abdomen. The nurse will check the dressing frequently for signs of drainage or bleeding. The dressing will be changed as needed.

—The patient will have one or more of the following tubes in place:

- A nasogastric tube will be placed in the stomach through the mouth or nose and kept in place to relieve gas and drainage in the GI tract. Gas and drainage may build up in the GI tract because the stomach and bowels do not function properly after surgery. As soon as the bowels begin to function, the tube will be removed.
- A soft, plastic tube called a Penrose drain is placed in the area that the removed section of the stomach used to occupy and extends to the surface of the skin. Fluid tends to accumulate in this space for a day or two after surgery and must be drained to prevent discomfort and/or infection.
- A soft, plastic gastrostomy tube is placed in the

stomach and brought out to the surface of the skin. Food can then be administered directly into the stomach through this tube. (See the "Gastrostomy Tube" teaching plan in this chapter for information.)
—The patient may not eat for 1 to 3 days after surgery until the stomach and intestines begin to function again. Once food is resumed, the patient will be started on clear liquids and will advance gradually to solid foods.
—In some cases, the patient may not be allowed to eat for more than 1 week after surgery. He will receive the nourishment he needs from special I.V. feedings, and his oral intake will be resumed gradually.

6 State the length of time necessary for healing of abdominal tissues.

It takes approximately 6 weeks for complete healing of the abdominal tissues, including the muscles, and it is normal to feel tired during the healing process.

7 Describe activity limitations after discharge.

Activity limitations may vary from one patient to another. The patient should follow his physician's instructions. Activity restrictions may include the following:
—Work usually is not allowed until after the first physician's checkup (usually 6 weeks after discharge).
—Driving usually is not allowed until after the first physician's checkup. The patient will receive further instructions at that time.
—Moderate ambulation around the house is encouraged. Climbing stairs should be limited to three times a day.
—Household chores should be limited. Mopping, vacuuming, and heavy lifting should be avoided until the first physician's checkup. The patient will receive further instructions at that time.

8 Define the term dumping syndrome.

Dumping syndrome refers to the process of food entering the small intestine at a very fast rate. The patient may develop this condition when he begins to eat solid foods again after surgery, because his stomach is no longer able to store food as well as it could prior to surgery.

9 Identify the signs and symptoms of dumping syndrome.

As the body tries to digest and absorb food at a very fast rate, the patient may experience the following signs and symptoms: abdominal cramping; diarrhea; feelings of fullness, weakness, faintness, dizziness; increased pulse rate; heart palpitations; and sweating.

10 Discuss dietary modifications to prevent and/or alleviate dumping syndrome.	Dumping syndrome can be alleviated or prevented by following these dietary guidelines: —Drink liquids 1 hour before or after meals, never during meals. Increased fluid intake during meals will worsen the signs and symptoms. —Assume a low Fowler's position, using two or three pillows, for 30 to 60 minutes after meals. This slows movement of food and fluid into the intestine. —Eat six small, high-protein, high-fat, low-carbohydrate meals. High-protein and high-fat foods stay in the stomach longer, delaying movement into the intestine. —Take anticholinergic drugs to decrease GI activity and antispasmodic drugs to slow food passage into the intestine, as ordered.

GASTROSTOMY TUBE

Patient objectives	*Teaching plan content*
1 Define and state the purpose of the gastrostomy tube.	A gastrostomy tube is a soft, plastic catheter that is placed in the stomach to administer food and medication to patients who cannot eat or drink in a normal manner because of a GI disorder. (An illustration or model of the GI tract can be used to help explain the GI disorder and the internal placement of the gastrostomy tube.) Specific GI disorders that may necessitate placement of a gastrostomy tube include the following: —Dysphagia (difficulty swallowing) —Oral or esophageal obstruction or trauma —Unconsciousness or intubation (tube in place to help breathing) —Recent GI tract surgery, for example, gastric resection.
2 Describe the procedure used in gastrostomy tube insertion.	The physician makes an opening through the abdomen and into the stomach. A soft, plastic catheter is inserted into the stomach, secured by sutures, and brought out through the skin. The abdominal wound is then closed around the tube. The gastrostomy tube may be inserted under general anesthesia during gastrointestinal surgery (for example, gastric resection), while the patient is asleep; or under local anesthesia, while the area of the abdomen through which the tube will be inserted is numbed.
3 Demonstrate proper care of the gastrostomy tube.	Changing the dressing, cleaning the gastrostomy tube equipment, and positioning the tube correctly will help prevent such complications as infection, tube obstruction, or dislodging. The dressing around the gastros-

tomy tube should be changed and the wound site should be cleaned at least once every day or whenever the dressing becomes excessively wet or soiled.
—The patient should gather the necessary supplies: mild soap and warm water, a paper bag, two precut gauze pads, sterile 4″ × 4″ sponges, adhesive tape, and petroleum zinc oxide ointment or a commercial skin protectant. (He will be provided with enough equipment to last for a few days at home; thereafter, equipment can be purchased through his local pharmacy.)
—He should follow these steps for gastrostomy dressing change and wound care (written instructions can be provided):

- Wash hands thoroughly, using soap and water.
- Remove the old dressing, and discard it in the paper bag.
- Wash hands again.
- Wash the skin around the gastrostomy site with 4″ × 4″ sponges soaked in warm water and mild soap.
- Rinse the area with 4″ × 4″ sponges soaked in warm water. Pat dry with a gauze sponge.
- Apply petroleum zinc oxide ointment or a commercial skin protectant to the skin near the opening.
- Apply precut gauze pads so the gastrostomy tube is completely encircled.
- Cover the precut gauze pads with an uncut 4″ × 4″ gauze pad.
- Secure the entire dressing with two strips of adhesive tape.
- Coil the gastrostomy tube once, lay it on top of the dressing, and tape securely.

---

4 Demonstrate the correct procedure for administering food or medications through the gastrostomy tube.

The patient should follow this procedure for administration of food or medication through the gastrostomy tube:
—For his comfort, he should make sure any fluids entering the stomach are warmed to room temperature.
—To feed or medicate himself, he should sit down and attach a clean funnel or syringe (with the plunger or bulb removed) to the tube and then unclamp the tube.
—To make sure the tube is not clogged, he should pour about 2 tablespoons (30 ml) of water into the funnel. (If the water does not flow into his stomach, the tube is probably clogged. He should stop the procedure and call his physician immediately.)
—When he is certain that the tube is open, he should pour the food or medication into the funnel. He should let it drip slowly into his stomach. Tell him not to try

to rush the procedure by forcing it.
—After all the food or medication is in his stomach, he should clear the tube by pouring 2 more tablespoons (30 ml) of water into the funnel.
—Then, he should replace the clamp on the tube and remove the funnel. (If he loses the clamp, he can fold the tube on top of itself and fasten it with a rubber band.)
—Next, he should cover the end of the tube with a gauze pad to keep it clean. Then, he should wrap a rubber band around the pad to hold it in place.
—He should stay seated upright for at least 30 minutes after his meal.
—Using warm water, he should wash the funnel thoroughly after each use.

5 Identify the signs and symptoms of possible complications associated with the gastrostomy tube.

The following signs and symptoms may be a warning of complications. The patient should notify his physician immediately if he experiences any of these signs or symptoms.
—Redness, warmth, firmness, pain, and, possibly, pus-like drainage of the wound indicate infection. He may also have a fever, general malaise, and a faster pulse rate. If the infection spreads into the abdominal cavity, his abdomen may become rigid and tender to the touch.
—If water does not flow into the gastrostomy tube from the funnel when the patient is preparing to administer food or medication, the tube is probably blocked.
—Gradual enlargement of the wound may indicate that the tube has moved. The tube also may become dislodged if it is pulled or if the wound gradually enlarges. Just before the patient goes home, the length of the gastrostomy tube from the wound site to the end should be measured. Using this as a guide, he will be able to tell later if the tube has moved. If the tube becomes dislodged, he should cover the site with a clean gauze bandage taped tightly to the abdomen.

OSTOMIES

Patient objectives	*Teaching plan content*
1 Define ostomy and stoma.	An ostomy is a surgical procedure that creates a new outside opening—a stoma—for elimination of body wastes when the colon or some part of it can no longer serve this purpose. Unlike the colon, however, the stoma cannot be controlled to permit voluntary passage of stool, nor will the patient experience the urge to defecate before the stool is passed. A stoma can be

temporary or permanent, depending on the disease and the problems involved.

2 Describe the normal structure and function of the small and large intestines.

The small intestine is divided into three parts: the duodenum, jejunum, and ileum. Its major function is to absorb the nutrition in food for use by the body for energy and cell building. The large intestine (colon or bowel) is divided into six parts: the cecum, ascending colon, transverse colon, descending colon, sigmoid colon, and rectum. Its major function is the elimination of the end products of digestion (stool).

3 State the purpose of an ostomy.

The purpose of an ostomy is to provide a route for the elimination of stool. Indications for this surgical procedure include tumor, fistula, diverticulitis, Hirschsprung's disease, ulcerative colitis, and Crohn's disease.

4 Describe the type of ostomy the patient will have.

There are two types of ostomy (an illustration or model can be used to show which one will be used):
—A colostomy is a stoma formed from the colon; it is named for the section of colon cut into—ascending, transverse, descending, or sigmoid.
—An ileostomy is a stoma made from the last part of the small intestine, the ileum; it usually accompanies the total removal of the large intestine, including the rectum.

5 Describe the preoperative procedures for an ostomy.

In addition to routine preoperative procedures, the patient can expect the following procedures related to the ostomy (See Appendix B, *Preoperative and Postoperative Teaching.*):
—Laxatives, enemas, and antibiotics will be administered to cleanse the bowel in order to decrease the chance of infection after surgery.
—Selection of the stoma site will be based on many factors, including the location of his problem, his body build, potential patient convenience, and the type of clothing he wears. The site will be marked with ink, and he should not wash it off.
—A nurse will show the patient the type of pouch that will be applied over the stoma after surgery. He may be asked to wear the pouch for 1 to 2 days before surgery, to ensure a proper fit. If he is to receive an ileostomy, the pouch will go to surgery with him and be applied immediately after surgery, as there will be continual drainage from the ileostomy stoma.
—The patient's skin will be scrubbed and shaved from nipples to thighs, since hair harbors bacteria and may cause infection.

—A visit from a representative of the local chapter of the United Ostomy Association may be arranged preoperatively or postoperatively.

6 Describe the immediate postoperative procedures for an ostomy.

In addition to routine postoperative procedures, the patient can expect the following procedures related to the surgical ostomy:
—The nurse will show the patient how to care for the stoma as soon as possible after surgery.
—If the patient has had an ileostomy, a pouch will be placed over the stoma immediately after surgery. If a colostomy has been performed, a pouch will be placed over the stoma when colostomy function begins (2 to 4 days after surgery). The patient will be encouraged to participate in his care as much as possible.
—After surgery, a nasogastric tube is placed in the patient's stomach through the mouth or nose and kept in place to relieve gas or drainage in the GI tract. Gas or drainage may accumulate in the GI tract because the intestines do not adjust to the surgery for 1 to 3 days. As soon as the ostomy is functioning normally, the tube will be removed.
—Because the intestines need to rest and recover after surgery, the patient will not be allowed to eat for approximately 1 to 3 weeks. He will receive the nourishment he needs from special I.V. feedings, and his oral intake will be resumed gradually.

7 Demonstrate the correct procedure for emptying the ostomy pouch.

The patient should demonstrate the procedure according to the instructions for emptying an ostomy pouch. (See *How to Empty Your Ostomy Pouch,* pp. 266 and 267.) The patient should have written instructions upon discharge.

8 Demonstrate the correct procedure for cleaning a reusable pouch.

To increase the life of his reusable pouch and help prevent odor, the patient should clean his pouch thoroughly every time he changes it. Having at least two pouches is advisable so that he can clean one while he is wearing the other. The patient should demonstrate the procedure according to the instructions for cleaning the pouch. (See *How to Clean a Reusable Pouch,* p. 263.) The patient should have written instructions upon discharge.

9 State the purpose and principles of stoma care.

The purpose of stoma care is to prevent infection, and correct procedures for stoma care should be practiced each time the pouch is changed.
—The patient should know the types of skin products available. A skin barrier product is used to protect the

skin from irritation, and a powder or paste is used to adhere the pouch to the barrier.
—Correct measurement of the stoma with a measuring guide is important to ensure proper fit of the pouch. The stoma will decrease in size the first few weeks after surgery, so frequent measuring is important.
—The following signs and symptoms indicate skin breakdown or infection: redness, rash, itching, warmth, swelling, pain, and drainage.

10 Demonstrate the correct procedure for skin care around the stoma site.

The patient should follow these procedures for skin care around the stoma site:
—Clean the skin around the stoma after removing the pouch by washing with mild soap and water, rinsing well with clear water, and drying. Coat the skin with a silicone skin protector and cover with a collection pouch.
—Avoid irritating the skin around the stoma. If irritation and breakdown do occur, apply a layer of antacid precipitate to the clean and dry skin, dust with karaya gum powder, allow to dry, and coat with a silicone skin protector.
—Measure the stoma, and prepare the faceplate of the pouch to clear the stoma with a ⅛″ (.32 cm) margin.
—Protect the skin from the effluent and the abrasiveness of the adhesive.
—Check the pouch frequently to make sure the skin seal is still intact.
—Control odor within the pouch by using any of the commercial products available for that purpose.

11 State the purpose and principles of colostomy irrigation.

Irrigation may allow the patient to gain control of his colostomy drainage so that eventually he may be able to replace his pouch with a gauze pad.
—Frequency varies from patient to patient; irrigation may be daily, every other day, or twice a week.
—Complications of irrigation include the following:
- Cramping caused by too much water or water that is too cold
- Ineffective evacuation caused by dehydration, drug-induced constipation, or an insufficient amount of water instilled.

12 Demonstrate the correct procedure for colostomy irrigation.

The patient should follow this procedure for colostomy irrigation:
—Hang the irrigation bag from a bent coat hanger, and then hang the coat hanger from a towel bar or plastic hook in the bathroom. (The bottom of the bag should be at shoulder level when the patient is sitting.)

—Insert the tube safely.
—Instill 1 quart (1 liter) of warm tap water slowly.

13 Discuss dietary modifications used in management of an ostomy.

The patient should follow these guidelines:
—Progress to a normal, varied diet of fats, carbohydrates, and proteins.
—Eat in moderation.
—Try foods in small servings to discover if they pose a problem.
—Take meals at fairly regular times.
—Chew food carefully and thoroughly. (Close the lips while chewing to avoid swallowing air; swallowed air causes gas to enter the colon.)
—Maintain an adequate fluid intake.
—Do not "wash down" unchewed food.
—Do not chew gum or smoke, both of which cause the swallowing of air.
—Follow these diet tips:

- Constipation may be caused by high-fiber foods, such as seeds, corn, celery, popcorn, nuts, coleslaw, grapefruit, raisins, and dried fruit, and by fried foods.
- Diarrhea may be caused by green beans, broccoli, spinach, highly spiced foods, raw fruits, or beer.
- Gas may be caused by foods from the cabbage family, onions, beans, cucumbers, radishes, or beer.
- Odor may be controlled by cranberry juice, buttermilk, or yogurt.

14 Discuss activity limitations of the ostomy patient.

The ostomy patient should understand the following activity limitations:
—Usually, a patient with an ostomy can participate in most sports.

- His physician may want him to avoid rough contact sports, such as wrestling, ice hockey, and football.
- He may also restrict participation in some individual sports (for example, weight lifting and shot putting) because they strain abdominal wall muscles and may cause a hernia in the stoma area.
- Swimming is a sport the patient will probably be able to participate in. If he plans to swim, he should eat lightly, empty his pouch, and seal it securely before entering the water. In addition, he should wear a pouch support, such as a wide-belted athletic supporter, under his swimsuit. Female patients may want to wear the type of girdle sold for swimwear.

—If the patient has an occupation that requires heavy physical labor, such as construction work or meat packing, he may not be able to resume it exactly as before. Under most circumstances, however, he can return to his job as soon as he regains his strength and the physician says it is OK.

—With advance preparation, the patient will be able to travel wherever and whenever he wants. However, he should always keep his ostomy equipment with him, because luggage checked through to his destination may get lost.

- He should take along enough ostomy supplies for the entire trip, if possible. If the patient wears a reusable pouch, he may want to pack some disposable pouches as a precaution.
- He should find out in advance where he can buy supplies he may need as he travels.
- Before any long trip, he should check with his physician. The physician may want to prescribe medication for diarrhea or constipation in case either develops.
- If the patient plans a trip to a foreign country, he should buy or borrow an up-to-date directory of English-speaking physicians. If he needs additional help planning the medical considerations of his trip, he should contact his local ostomy chapter.
- In addition, he should use only potable water for irrigations.

—If the patient had a satisfying sex life before surgery, it will usually remain so after surgery. The stoma cannot be injured by close physical contact, and the ostomy pouch, if applied correctly, will cause no problems.

- The patient should empty the pouch before sexual intercourse. He or she may also want to use a pouch cover.
- If a female patient has had surgery in the perineal area, she may experience some discomfort during intercourse until the wound heals.
- Rarely will a female patient have a physical sexual dysfunction from the ostomy, but a male patient may experience temporary impotence. Others (those who have had an ostomy because of bladder or rectal cancer) may have permanent nerve damage.
- A woman with an ostomy can become pregnant and have a normal pregnancy; however, she should discuss the subject with her physician, if possible, before she becomes pregnant. In some cases, the physician may recommend that a patient wait a year or so after ostomy surgery before becoming pregnant; this allows her body to recover completely.

—Wearing the pouch while taking a shower is a matter of preference. Soap and water will not hurt a patient's stoma as long as the shower stream is not

hitting it full force. If the patient feels uncomfortable about stoma drainage leaking in to the bath or shower, he may want to wear his pouch. If he does, he should make sure that the adhesive seal is watertight. He can ensure this by applying extra tape around the edge of the pouch opening.
—The patient will be able to wear his regular clothes as long as belts do not lie directly over his stoma. Ostomy pouches are virtually undetectable, even under swimsuits, because they are made to lie flat against the body. If a female patient wants to wear a girdle, she should wear a lightweight stretch type. A heavy, tight girdle may injure her stoma or may cause drainage to pool around it and loosen the adhesive seal.

SITZ BATH AT HOME

Patient objectives	*Teaching plan content*
1 Define sitz bath.	A sitz bath is the immersion of the pelvic area in tepid or hot water.
2 State the purpose and principles of a sitz bath.	A sitz bath is used to relieve discomfort after GI surgery or childbirth, promote wound healing by cleansing the perineum and anus, increase circulation and reduce inflammation, and relax local muscles. —The patient should perform the sitz bath as frequently as ordered by his physician. —He should know the name, purpose, correct dose, special considerations, and side effects of any medication additive(s) ordered by his physician. —Signs and symptoms of cardiovascular stress are possible complications of a sitz bath. These include fainting, dizziness, nausea, weakness, and chest pain. Tell him to discontinue the bath and lie down for 30 minutes to allow his circulation to return to normal if he experiences any of these complications. If signs and symptoms persist, he should notify his physician.
3 Demonstrate the correct procedure for performing a sitz bath.	The patient should follow this procedure for performing a sitz bath: —He should gather the necessary equipment: sitz bath kit (plastic pan and a plastic bag with attached tubing), bath thermometer, and medication (if ordered). (He may be provided with the necessary equipment. If he is to purchase the equipment, it can be bought at his local pharmacy.) —He should raise the toilet seat and fit the plastic pan onto the toilet bowl, positioning the pan so that the

drainage holes are along the back of the bowl. If he has placed the pan correctly, he will see a single slot in the front.

—Then, he should close the clamp on the bag's tubing, fill the bag with warm water, and add medication (if ordered).

—Next, using the bath thermometer, he should determine the water temperature. The water temperature should range between 110° to 115° F. (43.3° to 46.1° C.) for heat application and between 94° to 98° F. (34.4° to 36.7° C.) for relaxation or wound cleansing and healing.

—He should snap the free end of the tubing into the slot at the front of the pan, then hang the bag on the doorknob or towel bar, making sure that the bag is higher than the toilet.

—He should then sit in the pan and open the clamp on the tubing, letting the warm water flow from the bag and fill the pan. (He should not worry about it overflowing, because excess water will flow out of the drainage holes.) He should continue to sit in the pan until the water begins to cool. After his sitz bath, he should dry himself completely. If ordered by the physician, he should now apply an ointment or dressing.

Patient-Teaching Aid

HOW TO CARE FOR YOUR GASTROSTOMY

Dear Patient:
Your physician has placed a tube in the opening to your stomach. The nurse has shown you how to use it. Here are some guidelines to help you when you return home.

- For your comfort, make sure any fluids entering your stomach are warmed to room temperature.
- To feed or medicate yourself, sit down and attach a clean funnel or syringe (with the plunger or bulb removed) to the tube. Then, unclamp the tube.
- Make sure the tube is not clogged by pouring about 2 tablespoons (30 ml) of water into the funnel. (If the water does not flow into your stomach, the tube is probably clogged. Stop the procedure, and call your physician immediately.)
- When you are certain the tube is open, pour the food or medication into the funnel. Let it drip slowly into your stomach. Do not try to rush the procedure by forcing it.
- After the food or medication is completely in your stomach, clear the tube by pouring 2 more tablespoons (30 ml) of water into the funnel.
- Replace the clamp on the tube, and remove the funnel. (If you lose the clamp, fold the tube on top of itself and fasten it with a rubber band.)
- Cover the end of the tube with a gauze pad to keep it clean. Then, wrap a rubber band around the pad to hold it in place.
- Stay seated upright for at least 30 minutes after your meal.
- Using warm water, wash the funnel thoroughly after every use.
- Keep the skin around your stomach opening clean and dry. If it becomes irritated, dust it with karaya gum powder, as you were instructed in the hospital.
- Change your dressing once a day or whenever it becomes wet or soiled.
- Examine the skin around the opening. Call your physician if the skin feels sore, looks red, or seems puffy. Also call your physician if you find food or medication seeping from the insertion site or if you feel any discomfort in your stomach.

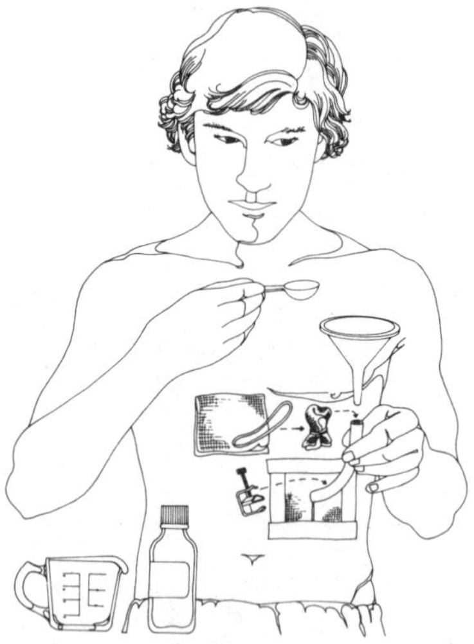

Patient-Teaching Aid

HOW TO CLEAN A REUSABLE POUCH

Dear Patient:

To increase the life of your reusable pouch and help prevent odor, clean your pouch thoroughly every time you change it. Having at least two pouches is advisable. This way you can clean one while you are wearing the other.

Here is how to clean your pouch:

1

First, remove the double-adhesive disk from the faceplate. If you cannot remove all of the adhesive, try rolling the rest of it off with your fingertips.

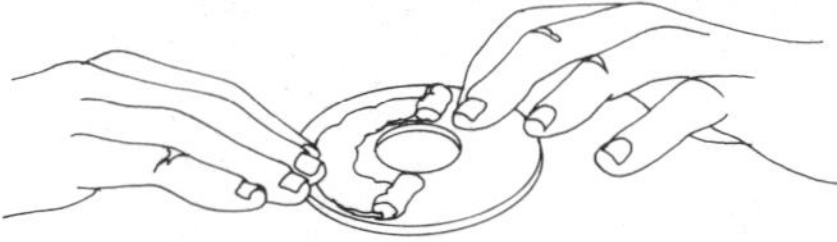

2

Or try loosening the adhesive with a gauze pad moistened in adhesive solvent. But, remember, always use solvent sparingly. Too much solvent may erode the faceplate.

3

After the adhesive is removed, rinse the pouch with cool tap water. Then, using a long-handled brush, scrub the inside with water and a mild soap or detergent (as recommended by the pouch manufacturer).

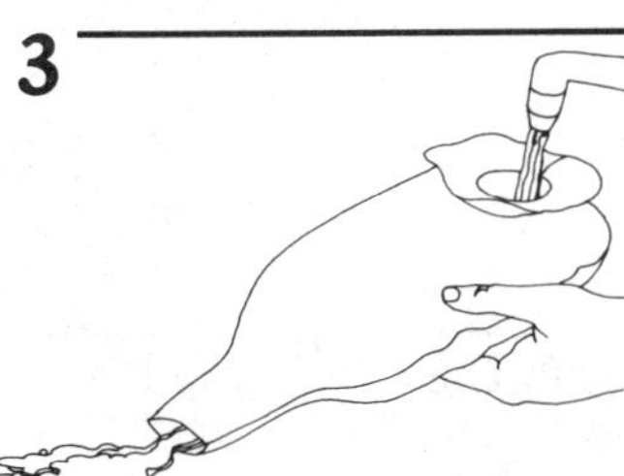

4

Rinse the bag thoroughly with cool water. Then, fill the pouch with wadded paper towels and place it on a flat surface to dry.

Or use a pouch hook to hang it over your sink.

IMPORTANT: Never dry a pouch in direct sunlight or heat.

When the pouch is completely dry, remove the paper towels, if you have used any. Store the pouch in a cool, dry place.

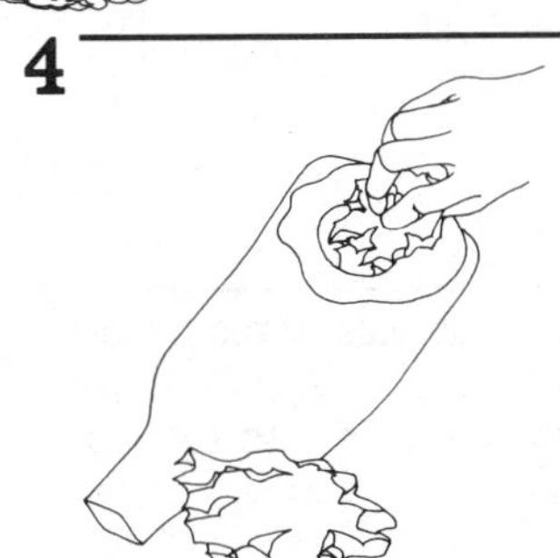

Patient-Teaching Aid

APPLYING A REUSABLE POUCH

Dear Patient:
The nurse has taught you how to apply a reusable ostomy pouch. This patient-teaching aid is designed to remind you of each step.

1

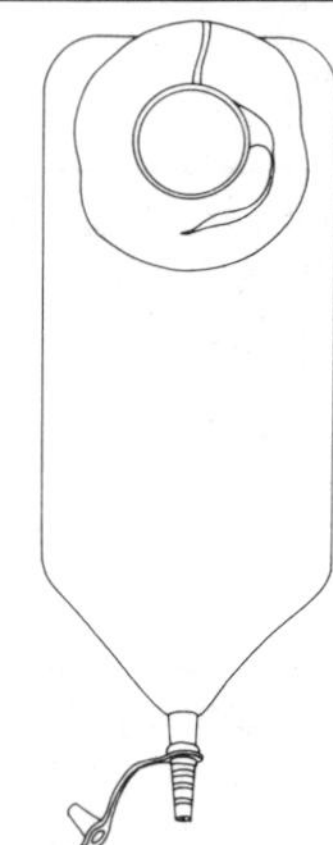

Begin by gathering this equipment: a reusable pouch, faceplate and O-ring, a double-sided adhesive foam pad, gauze pads, and a skin barrier. (You will also need scissors, if you are using a skin barrier that must be cut to size.)

Drain the urine or stool from your pouch. Wash your hands.

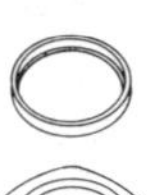

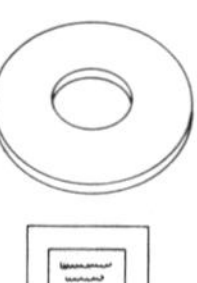

2

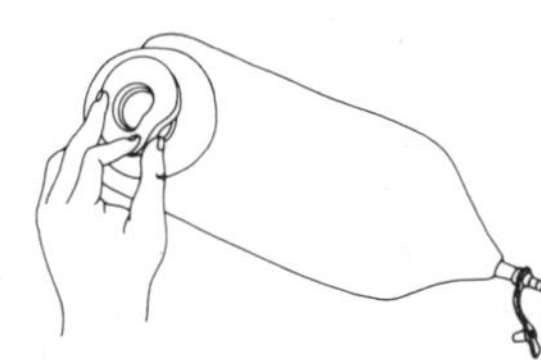

Lay the clean pouch on a flat surface, with the cup facing up. Slip the O-ring around the cup, with the O-ring's protruding edge against the pouch. Then, fold the cup down over the ring.

3

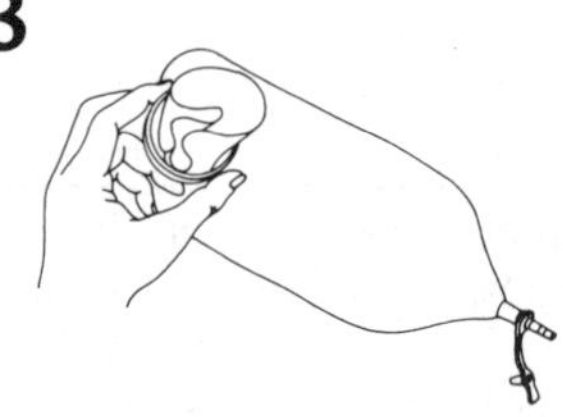

Firmly press the faceplate against the ring. Snap them together to provide a tight seal.

4

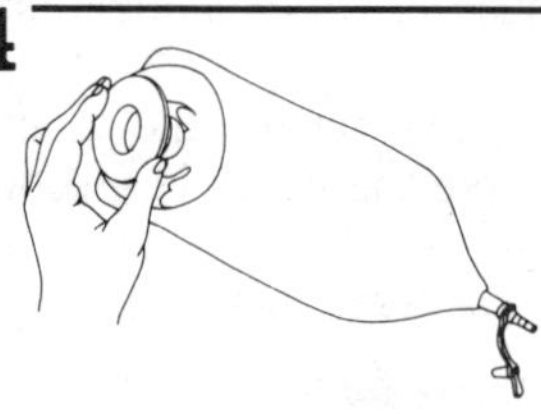

Peel off the paper backing from one side of the double-sided adhesive disk. Center the disk, sticky side down, over the faceplate. Firmly press the disk onto the faceplate.

APPLYING A REUSABLE POUCH—*continued*

5

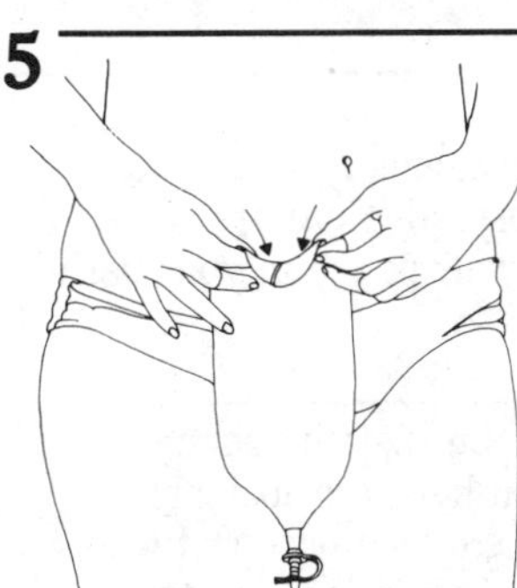

Remove the old pouch. If necessary, use warm water to loosen the adhesive. Then, set the pouch aside for later cleaning.

6

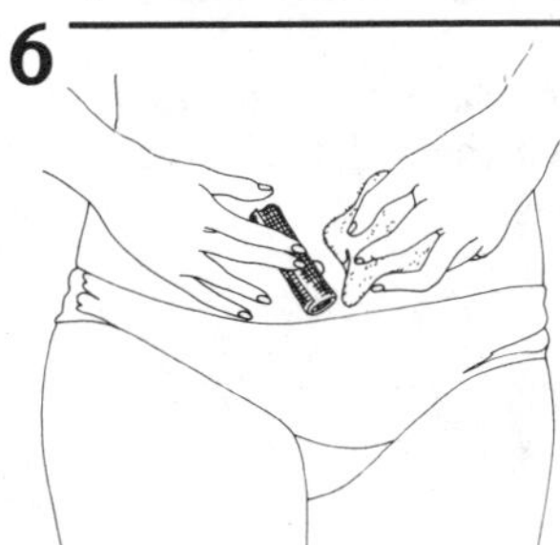

Cover the stoma with a rolled gauze pad to absorb any leaking urine. Gently wash your stoma and peristomal area with warm water, and pat the area dry. Do not rub the area dry or you will irritate the skin.

7

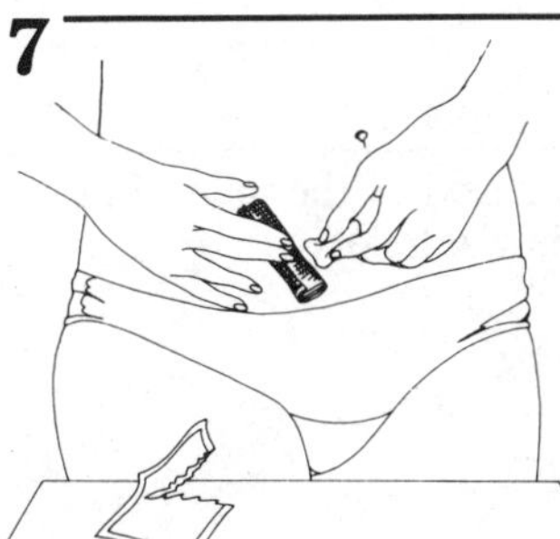

Now, still holding the rolled gauze pad over the stoma, apply the skin barrier of choice.

8

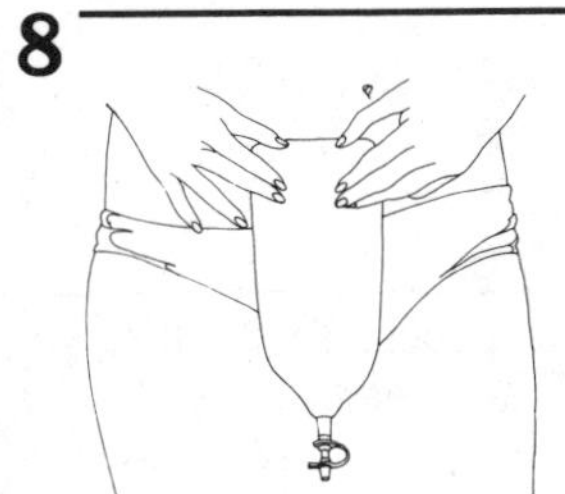

Now, remove the paper backing from the foam pad on the faceplate.

Center the faceplate over the stoma and gently press down on it. Make sure you do not wrinkle the seal. By carefully avoiding wrinkles, you will prevent urine or stool leakage.

Patient-Teaching Aid

HOW TO EMPTY YOUR OSTOMY POUCH

Dear Patient:
The nurse has shown you how to empty your ostomy pouch while you are in the hospital. Here are some guidelines to help you empty your pouch in your bathroom at home.

1

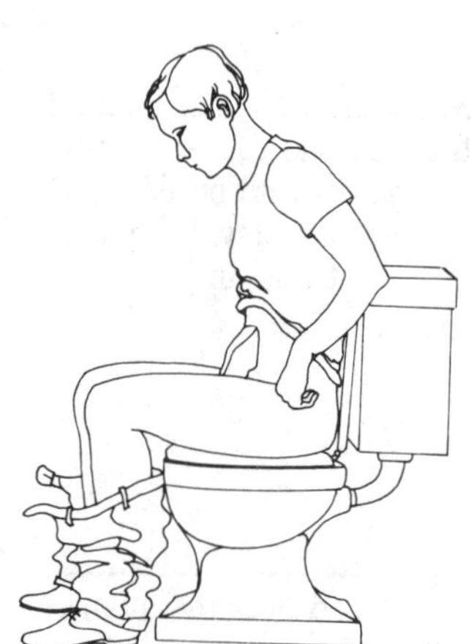

As you know, you will empty your ostomy pouch when it is about one-third full. If you have a colostomy, the pouch will usually need to be emptied once or twice daily. You will probably have to empty an ileostomy pouch five or six times daily.

To prepare for the procedure, place a cup of warm water within reach. Then, sit on the toilet with the pouch hanging between your legs.

2

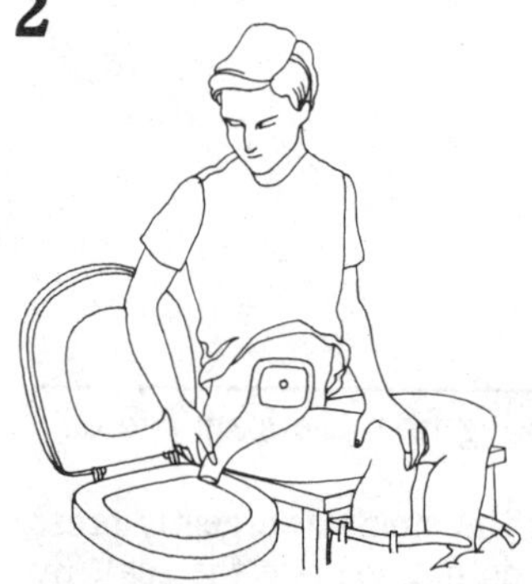

Or, if you prefer, sit on a chair next to the toilet. But be sure the pouch's opening is in the toilet.

3

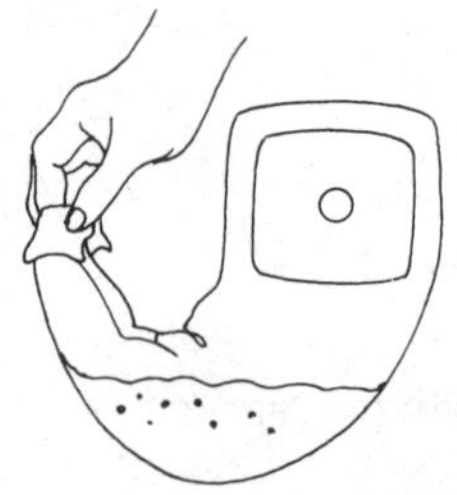

Now you are ready to empty your pouch. To do this, turn up the bottom of the pouch and remove the closure clamp.

To prevent splashing, place some toilet paper on the surface of the water, or flush the toilet as you point the pouch's unclamped opening into the bowl.

HOW TO EMPTY YOUR OSTOMY POUCH—*continued*

4

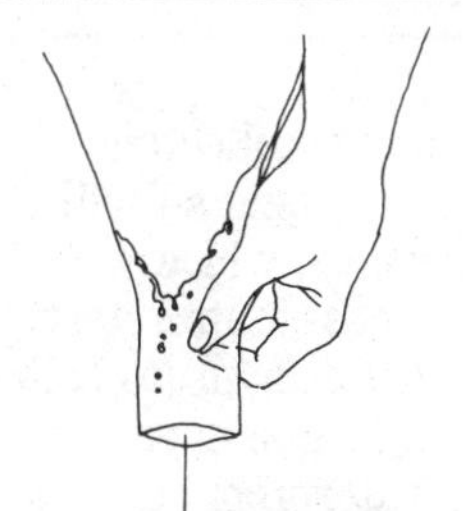

Slide your thumb and index finger down the outside of the pouch, squeezing all the contents into the toilet.

5

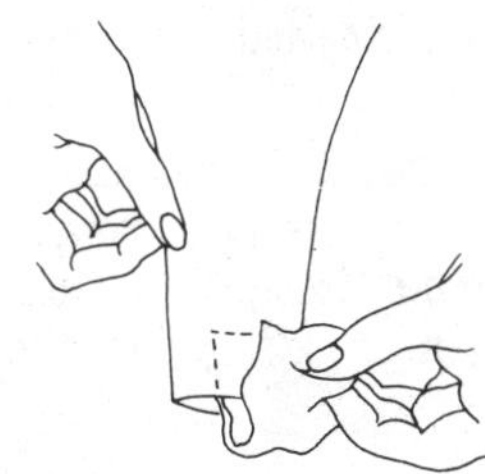

Next, use tissue or a disposable wipe to clean any remaining drainage from outside and inside the pouch opening.

6

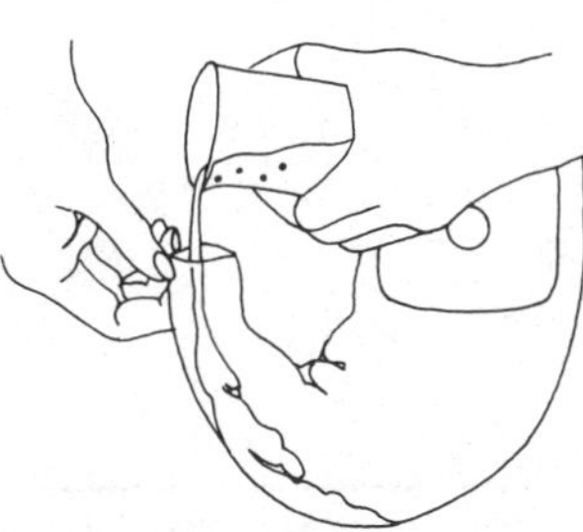

Hold the pouch opening upright and pour the cup of water into the pouch, as shown here. Swish the water around to remove any remaining drainage. As you work, avoid wetting your stoma or the pouch adhesive. Doing so could break the seal.

7

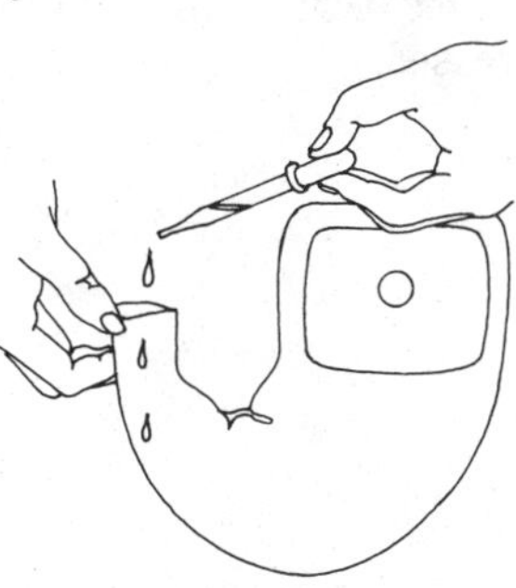

Now, direct the pouch opening into the toilet. Let the pouch drain thoroughly.

If you use a pouch deodorant, place it in the pouch, following the manufacturer's directions. Then, using a clean disposable wipe or toilet tissue, clean and dry the outside of the pouch. Finally, close the pouch with a clamp or rubber band.

Patient-Teaching Aid

COLLECTING A BOWEL MOVEMENT SPECIMEN

Dear Patient:
Carefully follow these instructions for collecting a bowel movement specimen at home. Doing so will help you avoid contaminating the specimen, which would interfere with the test results and necessitate retesting.

Make sure you have a clean, dry bedpan (to collect the bowel movement specimen), a tongue depressor or small piece of cardboard, and a waterproof container with a tight-fitting lid (which the nurse or laboratory technician will give you). If you do not have a bedpan, use a large glass jar that you have cleaned and boiled.

1

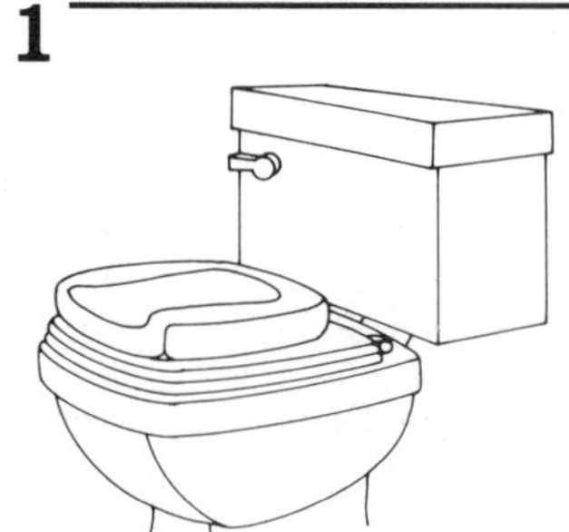

When you feel the urge to move your bowels, urinate into the toilet as you usually would. Then, close the toilet's lid and position the bedpan or glass jar on the lid, as shown.

2

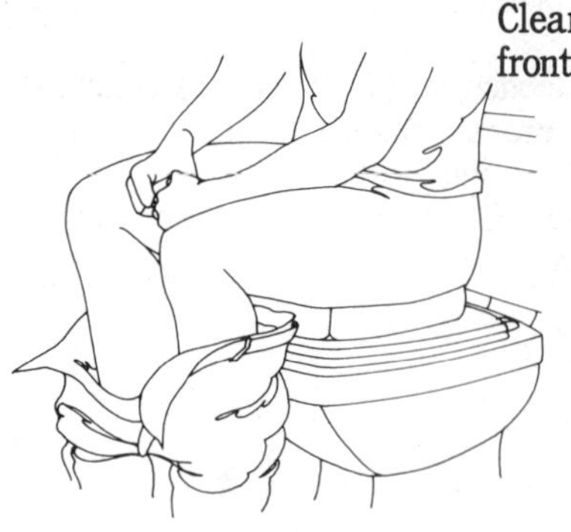

Position yourself on the bedpan and move your bowels. When you are finished, do not urinate or place toilet tissue in the bedpan. Doing so contaminates the stool. Clean your perineal area with toilet tissue, using one front-to-back motion, and get dressed.

COLLECTING A BOWEL MOVEMENT SPECIMEN—*continued*

3

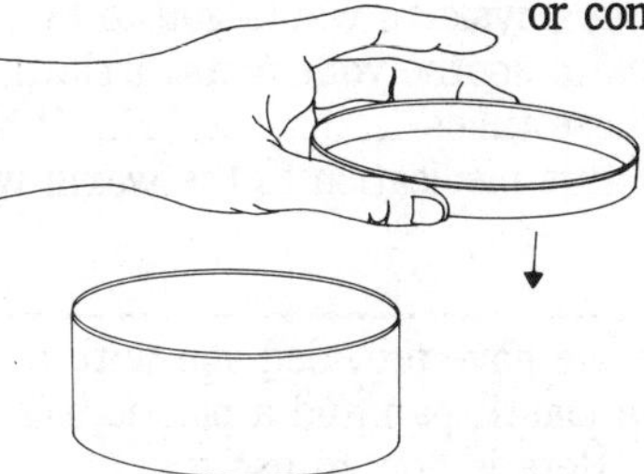

Remove the lid from the container and place it flat side down. Make sure you do not touch the inside of the lid or container.

4

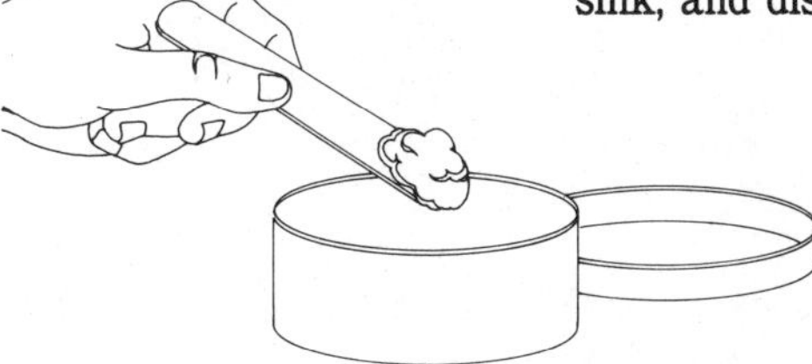

Using the tongue depressor, transfer some of the bowel movement into the container, being careful not to overfill it. Avoid touching the outside of the container with the tongue depressor. Place the filled container on the sink, and discard the tongue depressor.

5

Put the lid on the container, and wash your hands thoroughly. Then, depending on the instructions you were given, return the specimen container to the nurse, the laboratory, or the physician's office within 30 minutes. If this is impossible, place the container in a paper bag and store it in the refrigerator—away from food—until you can deliver it to the proper person or place.

Patient-Teaching Aid

GIVING YOURSELF A SITZ BATH

Dear Patient:
When you go home, the physician wants you to take warm-water sitz baths to soothe your rectal irritation. Take a sitz bath at these times: ____________. If the physician orders, add this medication to the warm water: ____________.

1

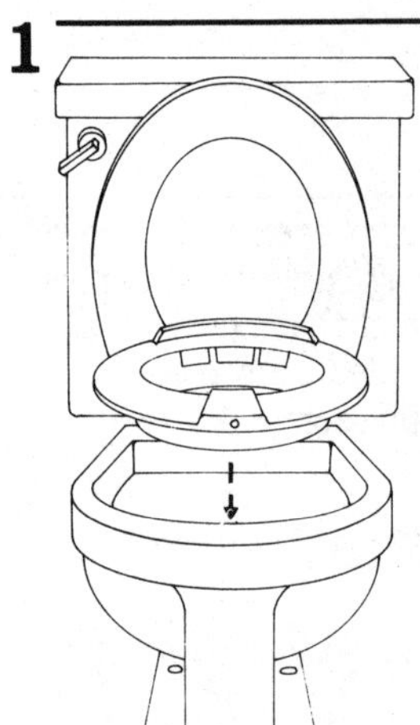

For your convenience, we have provided you with a sitz bath kit. It contains a plastic pan and a plastic bag with attached tubing. Here is how to use it:

First, raise the toilet seat, and fit the plastic pan onto the toilet bowel. Position the pan so its drainage holes are along the back of the bowl, as shown here. If you have placed the pan correctly, you will see a single slot in front.

2

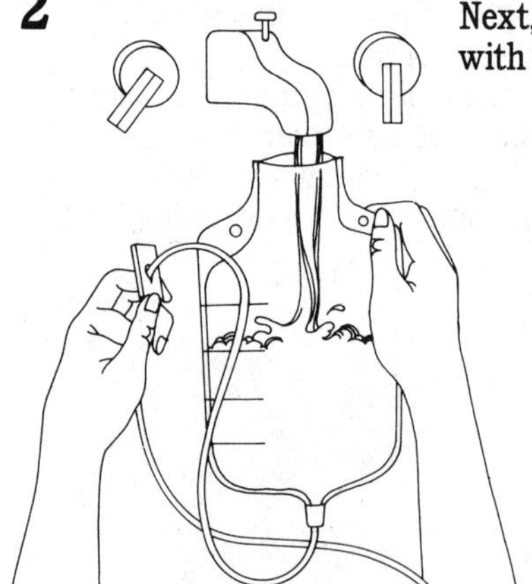

Next, close the clamp on the bag's tubing. Fill the bag with warm water and medication (if ordered).

GIVING YOURSELF A SITZ BATH—*continued*

3

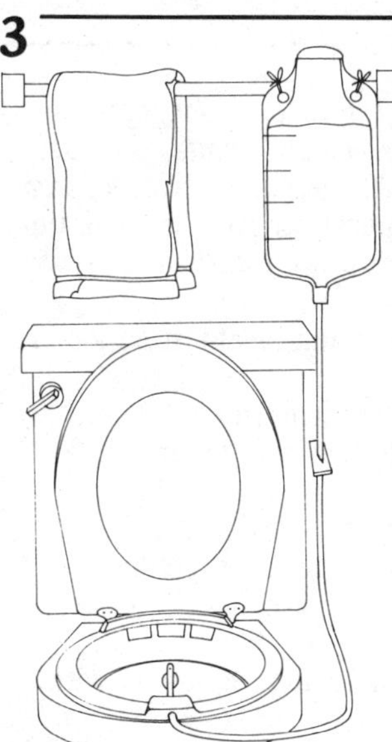

Snap the free end of the tubing into the slot at the front of the pan. Then, hang the bag on the doorknob or towel bar. Make sure the bag is higher than the toilet.

4

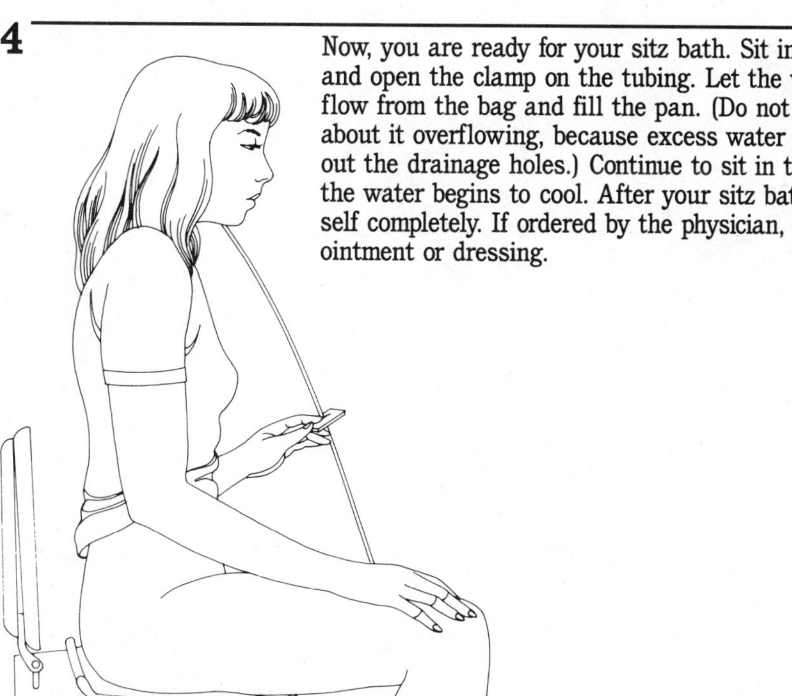

Now, you are ready for your sitz bath. Sit in the pan, and open the clamp on the tubing. Let the warm water flow from the bag and fill the pan. (Do not worry about it overflowing, because excess water will flow out the drainage holes.) Continue to sit in the pan until the water begins to cool. After your sitz bath, dry yourself completely. If ordered by the physician, apply an ointment or dressing.

Patient-Teaching Aid

ANTIFLATULENCE DIET

Dear Patient:

To help reduce gas, follow these dietary suggestions:

- Try to avoid certain vegetables and fruits, such as broccoli, brussels sprouts, cabbage, cauliflower, cucumbers, dried beans, green peppers, kohlrabi, lettuce, lima beans, melons, onions, peas, prunes, radishes, and raw apples.
- Avoid all fatty foods, such as red meats, fried foods, and pastries.
- Avoid foods or beverages that contain excess air. These include soufflés, carbonated drinks, and milk shakes.
- If you have lactose intolerance, avoid milk, cheese, ice cream, and all foods containing dairy products.
- Do not overeat, eat too rapidly, or eat while under emotional stress.
- Be sure not to drink large amounts of liquids with meals. Do not take laxatives.

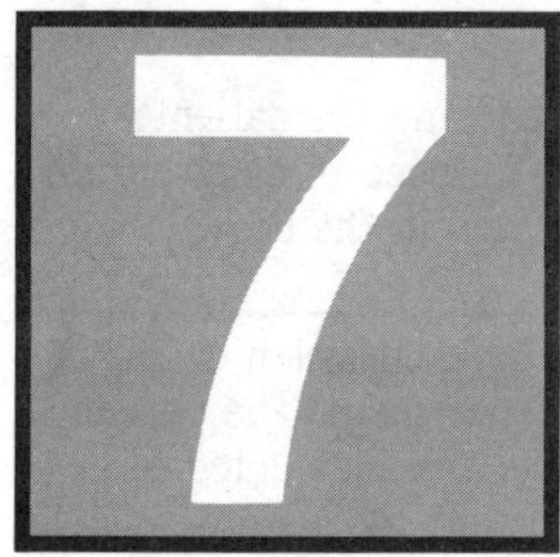

7 Genitourinary Disorders

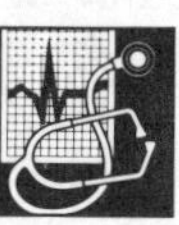

Patient-learner data base*

Areas of potential knowledge deficit
Genitourinary symptoms
—Renal/bladder disorder
—Sexual dysfunction
—Neurologic impairment
Anatomy and physiology of the genitourinary system
Definition of the genitourinary disorder
Causes of the genitourinary disorder
Symptoms associated with the genitourinary disorder
Treatment of the genitourinary disorder
—Medication
—Surgery
—Long-term therapy
—Guidelines for daily living
—Prevention of complications
—Coping strategies

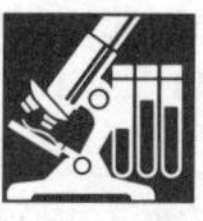

Explaining diagnostic tests

KIDNEY-URETER-BLADDER (K.U.B.) RADIOGRAPHY

Patient objectives	*Teaching plan content*
1 Define KUB radiography.	KUB radiography is an X-ray of the abdomen.
2 State the purpose of KUB radiography.	KUB radiography is often the first test performed in a urologic workup. It is done to evaluate the size, structure, and position of the kidneys, as well as to screen for any abnormalities in the region of the kidneys, ure-

*A general assessment should be done for all patients. For general assessment guidelines, see Chapter 1, Principles of Patient Teaching.

ters, and bladder that may be causing the patient's symptoms. (An illustration can be used to demonstrate where these structures are located in the body.)

3 Explain the procedure used in KUB radiography.

KUB radiography is performed by a physician or an X-ray technician in the X-ray department. The patient will be placed on the X-ray table and instructed to lie supine with his arms extended over his head. (His pelvis will be checked for symmetrical positioning.) Shielding will be provided for the male patient to prevent irradiation of the testes. (The female patient's ovaries cannot be shielded because of their proximity to the kidneys, ureters, and bladder.) A single X-ray will be taken.

4 Discuss patient guidelines for KUB radiography.

The patient need not restrict food or fluids before the test. During the procedure, he will be asked to lie very still while the X-ray is taken. (An obese patient may be asked to exhale and then hold his breath during the brief procedure.) The test causes no discomfort and takes only a few minutes, but the patient may be asked to remain in the X-ray department until the film is developed and checked for quality. He may have to go through the procedure again if the film is not of good quality.

RENAL COMPUTERIZED TOMOGRAPHY

Patient objectives	*Teaching plan content*
1 Define renal computerized tomography.	Renal computerized tomography is a test that mathematically reconstructs various X-rays to provide clear, detailed images of the inner structure of the kidneys.
2 State the purpose of renal computerized tomography.	Renal computerized tomography is performed to detect and evaluate lesions and abnormalities of the kidneys. (An illustration can be used to demonstrate where the kidneys are located in the body.)
3 Explain the procedure used in renal computerized tomography.	The patient will be placed in a supine position on the X-ray table and secured with straps. The table then will be moved into an X-ray machine called a scanner, which is operated from an adjacent room where the patient can be heard and observed. —When the scanner is turned on, it will rotate around his body, taking multiple images at different angles and making loud clacking sounds. —The physician may wish to enhance renal tissue density to help differentiate renal masses. If so, a contrast

medium will be administered intravenously after one series of X-rays has been completed.
—The patient may experience transient side effects, such as flushing, nausea, vomiting, salty taste, and headache, following injection of the contrast medium. After administration of the contrast medium and observation for allergic reactions, he will be placed back into the scanner and another series of X-rays will be taken.
—The procedure is painless and lasts approximately an hour, depending on the reason for the scan and the area to be evaluated. At the completion of the scan, the patient will be removed from the scanner.
—Information from the scan is stored on a disk or on magnetic tape, fed into a computer, and converted into images displayed on an oscilloscope screen for the physician to view.
—The patient should know who will perform the test and where and when it will be done.

4 Discuss patient guidelines for renal computerized tomography.	The patient need not restrict food or fluids before the test, unless contrast enhancement will be performed. In that case, he must fast for 4 hours before the test. He will be required to wear a hospital gown and to remove any metallic objects that could interfere with the X-rays. During the procedure, he will be asked to lie still. If he has difficulty lying still, the physician may prescribe sedation to help him relax. He or a responsible family member will be asked to sign a consent form.

NEPHROTOMOGRAPHY

Patient objectives	*Teaching plan content*
1 Define nephrotomography.	Nephrotomography is a test that uses special X-rays of the kidney to provide clear images of sections or layers of renal tissue and blood vessels.
2 State the purpose of nephrotomography.	Nephrotomography is performed to detect and evaluate renal lesions and abnormalities. (An illustration can be used to demonstrate where the kidneys are located in the body.)
3 Explain the procedure used in nephrotomography.	Nephrotomography is performed in the X-ray department by a physician or an X-ray technician. The patient will be placed in a supine position on the X-ray table. An X-ray of the kidney will be taken, followed by special X-rays after he is placed inside a machine called a scanner. Then he will be removed from the machine,

	and a contrast medium will be administered through a blood vessel in his arm: the first half in 4 to 5 minutes (the rapid phase) and the second half in the following 8 to 10 minutes (the slow phase). The patient then will be placed back inside the scanner, and a series of special X-rays will be taken at the beginning of the slow phase.
4 Discuss patient guidelines for nephrotomography.	The patient must fast for 8 hours before the test. He will be asked to lie still during the procedure, which takes less than 1 hour. He will be required to wear a hospital gown and to remove any jewelry that may interfere with the scan. He or a responsible family member will be asked to sign a consent form.

RENAL ULTRASONOGRAPHY

Patient objectives	*Teaching plan content*
1 Define renal ultrasonography.	Renal ultrasonography is a noninvasive test in which high-frequency sound waves are transmitted through the kidneys and surrounding structures, converted into electrical impulses, and displayed on a screen as images of the kidneys and surrounding structures.
2 State the purpose of renal ultrasonography.	Renal ultrasonography is performed to determine the size, shape, and position of the kidneys, their internal structures, and the surrounding tissues, and to detect any abnormalities. (An illustration can be used to demonstrate where these structures are located in the body.)
3 Explain the procedure used in renal ultrasonography.	Renal ultrasonography is performed in the X-ray department by a specially trained ultrasound technician. The patient will be placed in a prone position, and the area to be scanned will be exposed. Next the kidneys will be located, and ultrasound jelly will be applied to the area. Then a transducer will be moved over the area in many directions, and the images will be displayed on a screen.
4 Discuss patient guidelines for renal ultrasonography.	The patient need not restrict food or fluids before the test, which takes about 30 minutes. It is safe and painless; in fact, it may feel like a back rub. The patient will put on a hospital gown just before the procedure. During the test, he may be asked to breathe deeply to permit assessment of the kidneys' movement during respiration.

CYSTOURETHROSCOPY

Patient objectives	*Teaching plan content*
1 Define cystourethroscopy.	Cystourethroscopy is a test that allows direct visual examination of the bladder and urethra.
2 State the purpose of cystourethroscopy.	Cystourethroscopy is performed to detect and evaluate abnormalities of the bladder, urethra, and related structures, such as the prostate gland. It may also be done to facilitate biopsy of any suspected lesion. (An illustration can be used to demonstrate where these structures are located in the body.)
3 Explain the procedure used in cystourethroscopy.	Cystourethroscopy is usually performed in the operating room by the physician; however, when appropriate, the physician may perform it in the outpatient department, using a local anesthetic. This procedure, performed under a local or general anesthetic, involves the passage of a fiber-optic instrument through the urethra and into the bladder. —After a general anesthetic (as required) has been administered, the patient will be placed in lithotomy position on a cystoscopic table. The genitalia will be cleansed with an antiseptic solution, and he will be draped. (If a general anesthetic is not used, a local anesthetic will be instilled after the patient is positioned and draped.) —Once the anesthetic has taken effect, the physician will gently pass a well-lubricated sheath and a urethroscope through the urethra and into the bladder. While doing this, he can examine the urethra through the lighted lens of the scope. —The urethroscope then will be removed, and a cystoscope will be inserted through the sheath into the bladder. The bladder will be filled with irrigating solution, and the scope will be rotated so the physician can inspect the entire surface of the bladder wall and urethral orifices with the right-angled telescopic lens. —Then the cystoscope will be removed, the urethroscope will be reinserted, and both the urethroscope and the sheath will be slowly withdrawn, permitting examination of the bladder neck and the urethra, including the internal and external sphincters. —During cystourethroscopy, a urine specimen is routinely taken from the bladder for culture and sensitivity testing, and residual urine is measured. If a tumor is suspected, a urine specimen is sent to the laboratory for cytologic examination; if a tumor is found, a biopsy may be performed.

4 Discuss patient guidelines for cystourethroscopy.	Unless a general anesthetic has been ordered, the patient need not restrict food or fluids. If a general anesthetic will be administered, he must fast for 8 hours before the test, which takes about 20 to 30 minutes. —Just before the procedure, a sedative will be administered, as ordered, and he will be told to urinate and put on a hospital gown. —If the test is performed using a local anesthetic, he may experience a burning sensation when the instrument is passed through the urethra. He may also feel an urgent need to urinate as the bladder is filled with irrigating solution. These sensations are common and generally transient. —He may experience discomfort after the procedure, including a slight burning when he urinates. —He or a responsible family member will be asked to sign a consent form.

INTRAVENOUS PYELOGRAPHY (I.V.P. or excretory urography)

Patient objectives	*Teaching plan content*
1 Define IVP.	IVP is a procedure that permits visualization of the urinary tract by X-rays that are taken following I.V. administration of a contrast medium.
2 State the purpose of IVP.	IVP is performed to evaluate the structure and function of the kidneys, ureters, and bladder and to detect any abnormalities. (An illustration can be used to demonstrate where these structures are located in the body.)
3 Explain the procedure used in IVP.	IVP is performed in the X-ray department by a physician or an X-ray technician. The patient will be placed in a supine position on an X-ray table. A kidney-ureter-bladder radiograph will be taken, and a contrast medium will be injected. —An X-ray of the renal tissue will be obtained about 1 minute after the injection, possibly supplemented by other X-rays. Then films will be taken at regular intervals—usually 5, 10, and 15 or 20 minutes after the injection. —Ureteral compression will be performed after the 5-minute film has been exposed. This can be accomplished by inflating two small rubber bladders placed on the abdomen on either side of the midline, secured by a flannel fastener wrapped around the patient's torso. The inflated bladders occlude the ureters without

causing discomfort and facilitate retention of the contrast medium by the upper urinary tract.
—After the 10-minute film has been exposed, ureteral compression will be released.
—As the contrast medium flows into the lower urinary tract, another film will be taken of the lower halves of both ureters and then, finally, one will be taken of the bladder.
—At the end of the procedure, the patient will void and another film will be taken immediately to visualize residual bladder content or mucosal abnormalities of the bladder or urethra.
—The X-ray equipment will make loud clacking sounds during the test.

4 Discuss patient guidelines for IVP.	The patient should be well hydrated and then should fast for 8 hours before the test. He will be given a laxative the night before the test to minimize poor resolution of the X-ray films due to feces and gas in the GI tract. He may experience a transient burning sensation and a metallic taste when the contrast medium is injected. He should report any other sensations to the technician performing the test. He or a responsible family member will be asked to sign a consent form.

RADIONUCLIDE RENAL IMAGING (Renal scan)

Patient objectives	*Teaching plan content*
1 Define renal scan.	A renal scan is a procedure in which a series of special X-rays of the kidneys are taken in rapid succession after I.V. injection of a contrast medium.
2 State the purpose of a renal scan.	A renal scan is performed to evaluate the structure, blood flow, and function of the kidneys. It may also be used to assess renal transplantation or renal injury due to trauma and obstruction of the urinary tract. (An illustration can be used to demonstrate where these structures are located in the body.)
3 Explain the procedure used in a renal scan.	A renal scan is performed in the X-ray department by an X-ray technician. The patient will be placed in a prone position on the X-ray table. (If the test is being performed to evaluate transplantation, the patient will be supine.) An I.V. line will be inserted, a contrast medium containing a radioisotope will be injected, and rapid-sequence photographs (one per second) will be taken for 1 minute to assess blood flow to the kidneys. Then another radioisotope will be administered intrave-

	nously, and images will be obtained at a rate of one per minute for about 20 minutes to assess the function of the kidneys. The patient may be asked to return to the X-ray department 4 hours later for another series of X-rays (without additional contrast medium) to assess the structure of the kidneys.
4 Discuss patient guidelines for a renal scan.	The test takes about 1½ hours, but there may be a delay of several hours before the final phase is completed. The patient will receive an injection of a radionuclide containing a minimal amount of radiation, and he may experience transient flushing and nausea. Only a small amount of radionuclide will be administered, and it is usually excreted within 24 hours. The patient must remove any metallic objects in the X-ray field and remain still during the procedure. He or a responsible family member will be asked to sign a consent form. For 24 hours after the test, he should flush the toilet immediately after each voiding as a radiation precaution.

RENAL ANGIOGRAPHY

Patient objectives	*Teaching plan content*
1 Define renal angiography.	Renal angiography is an X-ray examination of the blood vessels and tissues of the kidneys after injection of a contrast medium into an artery.
2 State the purpose of renal angiography.	Renal angiography is performed to visualize the blood vessels and tissues of the kidneys and to investigate renal disease or masses. (An illustration can be used to demonstrate where these structures are located in the body.)
3 Explain the procedure used in renal angiography.	Renal angiography is performed in the X-ray department by a physician. After receiving sedation, the patient will be taken to the X-ray department and placed in a supine position on the X-ray table. —An I.V. line will be started. The skin over the arterial puncture site (usually the groin) will be shaved and cleansed with antiseptic solution, and a local anesthetic will be injected. —A catheter will be inserted into the artery, and the contrast medium will be injected. X-rays will be taken in rapid succession as the medium passes through the renal blood vessels. —If the X-rays are satisfactory in quality, the catheter will be removed and pressure will be firmly applied to the injection site for 15 minutes to prevent bleeding. —Before the patient returns to his room, the I.V. line

	will be removed and a sterile pressure dressing will be applied to the injection site.
4 Discuss patient guidelines for renal angiography.	The patient must fast for 8 hours before the test, void just before leaving his room, and wear a hospital gown during the procedure, which takes approximately 1 hour. He must lie still during the procedure. —He may experience transient discomfort (flushing, burning sensations, and nausea) during passage of the catheter and injection of the contrast medium. He should report these sensations to the physician. —After the procedure, he must remain flat in bed for 8 to 12 hours and must not get out of bed for 24 hours, depending on his physician's orders and the injection site used. —His vital signs and dressing will be checked frequently; this is routine. —He or a responsible family member will be asked to sign a consent form.

RETROGRADE CYSTOGRAPHY

Patient objectives	*Teaching plan content*
1 Define retrograde cystography.	Retrograde cystography is an X-ray examination of the bladder after instillation of a contrast medium.
2 State the purpose of retrograde cystography.	Retrograde cystography is performed to evaluate the structure and integrity of the bladder. (An illustration can be used to demonstrate the location of the bladder in the body.)
3 Explain the procedure used in retrograde cystography.	Retrograde cystography is performed in the X-ray department by a physician and a specially trained X-ray technician. After the patient is placed in a supine position, a preliminary kidney-ureter-bladder radiograph will be taken, developed immediately, and scrutinized for any abnormalities. A catheter then will be inserted into the bladder, and the contrast medium will be instilled by gravity or gentle syringe injection. Then the catheter will be clamped and, with the patient supine, an X-ray film will be taken. The patient then will be tilted to one side, then the other, and two additional views will be taken. If the patient's condition permits, he will be placed in the jackknife position, and another film will be taken. Rarely, to enhance visualization, 100 to 300 ml of air may be insufflated into the bladder by syringe after removal of the contrast medium (double contrast technique). Then the catheter will be

	unclamped, the bladder fluid allowed to drain, and another X-ray will be taken. He will hear loud clacking sounds as the X-ray films are taken.
4 Discuss patient guidelines for retrograde cystography.	The patient need not restrict food or fluids before the test, which takes about 30 to 60 minutes. He must wear a hospital gown and remove any jewelry. He may experience some discomfort when the catheter is inserted and when the contrast medium is instilled. He or a responsible family member will be asked to sign a consent form. After the test, his vital signs will be checked frequently; this is routine.

RETROGRADE URETEROPYELOGRAPHY

Patient objectives	*Teaching plan content*
1 Define retrograde ureteropyelography.	Retrograde ureteropyelography is a radiographic examination of the renal collecting system after injection of a contrast medium.
2 State the purpose of retrograde ureteropyelography.	Retrograde ureteropyelography is performed to assess the structure and integrity of the renal collecting system. (An illustration can be used to demonstrate the location of these structures in the body.)
3 Explain the procedure used in retrograde ureteropyelography.	Retrograde ureteropyelography is usually performed in the operating room by a physician. The patient will be positioned on the X-ray table with his legs in stirrups. He will then be given either a local or a general anesthetic (usually general). —After administration of the anesthetic, the physician will insert a thin, tubelike instrument called a cystoscope into the bladder, examine the bladder, and then thread a ureteral catheter up through the ureter into the kidney. —Then a small amount of the contrast medium will be instilled through the ureteral catheter, and X-rays will be taken from several angles. —After the X-rays of the kidney have been examined, a few more milliliters of the contrast medium will be injected to outline the ureters as the catheter is slowly withdrawn. Delayed films (10 to 15 minutes after complete catheter removal) will be taken to check for retention of the contrast medium, indicating urinary stasis. —If ureteral obstruction is present, the ureteral catheter may be kept in place and, together with an indwelling (Foley) catheter, connected to a gravity drainage

system until post-test urinary flow has been corrected or returns to normal.

4 Discuss patient guidelines for retrograde ureteropyelography.	If a general anesthetic is ordered, the patient should fast for 8 hours before the test. He will be given a laxative prior to the test. Generally, he should be well hydrated to ensure adequate urine flow. He may be sedated just before the procedure. He must wear a hospital gown and remove all jewelry. —He will be positioned on an examination table with his legs in stirrups. The procedure takes about 1 hour, and the position may be tiring. —If he will be awake throughout the procedure, he may feel pressure as the instrument is passed and in the kidney area when the contrast medium is introduced. He may also feel an urge to void. —He or a responsible family member will be asked to sign a consent form. —Once he is fully awake, after the procedure, he should ingest fluids liberally to maintain urine output and to help reduce the usual post-test voiding discomfort. His vital signs will be checked frequently; this is routine. —He should request pain medication, as ordered, and report any severe pain in the kidney area.

CYSTOMETRY

Patient objectives	*Teaching plan content*
1 Define cystometry.	Cystometry is a test to evaluate bladder function after instillation of normal saline solution, sterile water, or a gas.
2 State the purpose of cystometry.	Cystometry is performed to evaluate bladder muscle function and tone and to help determine the cause of bladder dysfunction. (An illustration can be used to demonstrate the location of the bladder in the body.)
3 Explain the procedure used in cystometry.	Cystometry is usually performed in a special department or in a urologist's office by a physician. The patient will urinate into a funnel attached to a machine that plots on a graph the amount, flow, and time of voiding; time and effort needed to initiate the stream, strength and continuity of the stream, and terminal dribbling are also noted. —The patient will be placed in a supine position on an examining table. A catheter will be passed into the bladder, and residual urine will be measured. —Next his response to thermal sensation will be evalu-

ated by instilling a small amount of room-temperature saline solution or sterile water, followed by an equal amount of warmed fluid. He will be asked to report his sensations (need to void, nausea, flushing, discomfort, temperature).

—Then the fluid will be drained from the bladder, the catheter will be connected to the cystometer, and normal saline solution, sterile water, or gas (usually carbon dioxide) will be slowly introduced into the bladder. He will be asked to indicate when he first feels an urge to void, then when he feels he must urinate. The related pressure and volume are automatically plotted on the graph.

—When the bladder reaches its full capacity, he will be requested to urinate to permit the recording of the maximal intravesical voiding pressure. Then his bladder will be drained and, if no additional tests are required, the catheter will be removed.

4 Discuss patient guidelines for cystometry.	The patient need not restrict food or fluids before the test, which takes about 40 minutes. He will feel a strong urge to void during the test and should describe his sensations to the physician when asked. He should not strain to void, because this can cause ambiguous cystometric readings. He or a responsible family member will be asked to sign a consent form.

VOIDING CYSTOURETHROGRAPHY

Patient objectives	*Teaching plan content*
1 Define voiding cystourethrography.	Voiding cystourethrography is a radiographic examination of the bladder and urethra after the instillation of a contrast medium through a catheter.
2 State the purpose of voiding cystourethrography.	Voiding cystourethrography is performed to detect abnormalities of the bladder and/or urethra. (An illustration can be used to demonstrate the location of these structures in the body.)
3 Explain the procedure used in voiding cystourethrography.	Voiding cystourethrography is performed in the X-ray department by a specially trained X-ray technician and a physician. The patient will be placed in a supine position on the X-ray table, and a catheter will be inserted into his bladder. The contrast medium will be instilled through the catheter until his bladder is full. —The catheter will be clamped, and X-ray films will be taken with the patient in supine, oblique, and lateral positions.

	—Then the catheter will be removed, and he will be asked to assume the right oblique position—right leg flexed to 90 degrees, left leg extended, penis parallel to right leg—and to begin voiding. —Four high-speed exposures of the bladder and urethra are usually made on one film during the voiding. (Male patients should be shielded to prevent irradiation of the gonads; female patients, however, cannot be shielded without blocking the urinary bladder.) —If the right oblique view does not delineate both ureters, he will be asked to stop urinating and to begin again in the left oblique position. The most reliable voiding cystourethrograms are obtained with the patient recumbent, but patients who cannot void recumbent may do so standing (not sitting).
4 Discuss patient guidelines for voiding cystourethrography.	The patient need not restrict food or fluids before the test, which takes about 30 to 45 minutes. He will need to wear a hospital gown, and his cooperation is vital to the successful outcome of the test. He may experience a feeling of fullness and an urge to void when the contrast medium is instilled. He or a responsible family member will be asked to sign a consent form.

CLEAN-CATCH MIDSTREAM URINE SPECIMEN

Patient objectives	*Teaching plan content*
1 Define a clean-catch midstream urine specimen.	A clean-catch midstream urine specimen is one that is uncontaminated by any organisms present near the urinary meatus.
2 State the purpose of a clean-catch midstream urine specimen.	A clean-catch midstream urine specimen is collected to obtain a virtually uncontaminated urine specimen without inserting a catheter into the patient's bladder.
3 Explain the procedure used in collecting a clean-catch midstream urine specimen.	After thoroughly cleansing the genital area, the patient voids and discards a small amount of urine. Then the patient voids into a sterile specimen cup, producing an uncontaminated specimen for laboratory analysis.
4 Discuss patient guidelines for the procedure.	Before beginning the procedure, the patient should have a clean washcloth and towel, soap, water, and a clean-catch urine kit. Then he should wash his hands thoroughly and place a clean paper towel on a nearby dry surface. —A female patient should follow these guidelines: • Remove clothing from the waist down and, using

the washcloth, wash the genital area with soap and water. Rinse the area thoroughly and dry it with a towel.

• Next open the three disposable wipes from the clean-catch urine kit, and place them on the paper towel. Remove the lid from the specimen cup. Place both the cup and the lid (flat side down) next to the wipes. Avoid touching the inside of the lid or the cup.

• Sit as far back on the toilet as possible. Spread the legs apart. Using the fingertips, separate the labia, and keep them separated for the rest of the procedure.

• With the other hand, use a wipe to clean one side of the labia, using one top-to-bottom stroke. Discard the wipe in a covered trash receptacle, not the toilet. Repeat this procedure on the other side of the labia. Then clean the urethral opening with the last wipe, and discard the wipe.

• Urinate a small amount into the toilet, then stop the flow. Hold the specimen cup a few inches from the urethra. Urinate into the cup until it is about two-thirds full. Be careful not to let the cup overflow. Place the filled cup back on the sink and, if necessary, finish urinating into the toilet.

• Place the lid on the cup, get dressed, and wash the hands thoroughly. Return the filled cup to the nurse.

—A male patient should follow these guidelines:

• Open the three disposable wipes and place them on the paper towel. Remove the lid from the specimen cup. Place both the cup and the lid (flat side down) next to the wipes. Avoid touching the inside of the lid or the cup.

• Using a wipe, clean the head of the penis. (Uncircumcised patients should first pull back the foreskin and keep it back during the procedure.) Clean from the urethral opening toward the abdomen. Then discard the wipe in a covered trash receptacle, not the toilet. Repeat this procedure with the other wipes.

• Urinate a small amount into the toilet, then stop the flow. Hold the specimen cup a few inches from the penis. Urinate into the cup until it is two-thirds full. Be careful not to let the cup overflow. Place the filled cup back on the sink. Then, if necessary, finish urinating into the toilet.

• Put the lid on the cup. Remember to wash the hands thoroughly. Then return the cup to the nurse.

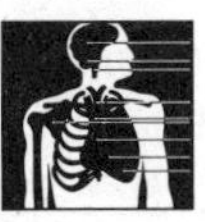

Explaining disorders

BENIGN PROSTATIC HYPERPLASIA OR BENIGN PROSTATIC HYPERTROPHY (B.P.H.)

Patient objectives	*Teaching plan content*
1 Define BPH.	BPH is a noncancerous enlargement of the prostate gland that is common in men over age 40.
2 Explain what causes BPH.	The exact cause of BPH is not clear, but recent evidence suggests a link between BPH and hormonal activity.
3 Discuss how urologic dysfunction develops in BPH.	Enlargement of the prostate affects the rest of the urinary tract. Many serious disturbances result from the effects of glandular enlargement on the urethra, bladder, kidneys, and, less frequently, the prostate itself. —As the prostate enlarges, it compresses the urethra, causing urethral obstruction. —The enlarged prostate may also obstruct the bladder neck. The flow of urine is impeded, and a gradual dilatation of the ureters (hydroureter) and kidneys (hydronephrosis) results, causing incomplete emptying of the bladder. —Hypertrophy of the bladder and urinary stasis occur, predisposing the patient to urinary tract infection and calculi formation. —Urinary flow may in time be completely obstructed, leading to urinary retention.
4 Identify the symptoms of BPH.	Symptoms the patient experiences are related to the degree of enlargement of the prostate gland and the degree of obstruction. Early symptoms may include reduced urinary stream caliber and force, difficulty starting to void (straining), hesitancy in starting the stream, feeling of incomplete voiding, and dribbling after voiding. As the obstruction increases, urination becomes more frequent, with nocturia, incontinence, and, possibly, hematuria.
5 Identify the components of the treatment regimen for BPH.	Conservative therapy may include prostatic massage, sitz baths, short-term fluid restriction (to prevent bladder distention), and antimicrobials if infection develops. However, the only truly effective treatment is surgery, particularly when urinary retention, hydronephrosis, recurrent infection, severe hematuria, and other severe

symptoms of obstruction are present. (See the "Prostatectomy" teaching plan in this chapter.)

6 Discuss discharge instructions and symptoms to be reported to the physician.

The patient should restrict his activities for a few weeks; for example, he should take only short walks and climb no more than two flights of stairs at a time.
—He should ride in a car as little as possible for the first 3 weeks, because vehicle motion may strain his bladder. He should not lift heavy objects for at least 3 weeks.
—He should drink plenty of liquids, unless the physician orders otherwise, and should not become alarmed if he sees blood in his urine during the first 2 weeks after surgery. If he does see blood, he should drink fluid and lie down. The bleeding should decrease the next time he urinates; if it does not, he should call his physician.
—If he cannot urinate at all, he should also notify his physician.
—He need not worry if he loses some control over urination, if he feels pain, or if he has a frequent need to urinate; these symptoms will disappear with time.
—The following exercise will strengthen his perineal muscles: Press the buttocks together. Hold this position for a few seconds, then relax. Repeat 10 times in succession, as ordered.
—He should not strain to have a bowel movement and should take a laxative if he is constipated. He should not give himself an enema or place anything—a suppository, for example—into his rectum for 4 weeks after surgery.
—He should avoid sexual activity for 4 weeks after surgery, because it can cause bleeding. When he does engage in sex, most of the sperm will go into his bladder instead of out his penis. This will cause his urine to become cloudy and will decrease, though not end, his fertility. He will still experience orgasm.
—He should ask his physician when he can return to work; this will vary, depending on his health, his job, and the type of surgery he has had.

URINARY TRACT INFECTION (U.T.I.)

Patient objectives	*Teaching plan content*
1 Define UTI.	A broad term, UTI refers to the presence of pathogenic microorganisms in any portion of the urinary tract. It can occur as infection of the urethra (urethritis), the urethra and bladder (cystitis), or the urethra, ureters, bladder, and kidney (pyelonephritis). It is more common in women than in men.

2 Explain the relevant causes of UTI.

Most UTIs result from ascending infection by a gram-negative enteric bacteria, such as *Escherichia coli, Klebsiella, Proteus, Enterobacter, Pseudomonas,* or *Serratia.* However, in a patient with neurogenic bladder, an indwelling (Foley) catheter, or a fistula, UTIs may result from multiple pathogens.

—UTIs may also occur after viral infections, such as mumps, measles, herpes, adenovirus, or cytomegalovirus infections.

—The most common route of infection is from the urethra to the bladder. Since the kidney receives about 25% of the cardiac output, systemic bacterial infection can lead to seeding of the kidneys with bacteria.

—UTIs can also result from infection through lymphatic channels and bladder distention (decreasing vascular circulation in the bladder wall increases the susceptibility to entering organisms). Recent studies suggest that infection results from a breakdown in local defense mechanisms in the bladder, allowing bacteria to invade the bladder mucosa and multiply. These bacteria cannot be readily eliminated by normal micturition.

3 Identify the relevant predisposing factors to UTI.

Common predisposing factors include vaginal and fecal contamination, use of urologic instruments, obstruction, suppression of the urge to void, and alkaline urine.

—Pregnant women are at especially high risk for UTIs.

—Other patients at high risk for UTIs include diabetics, men over age 50 with prostatitis, and patients who are catheterized, immunosuppressed, or debilitated.

—Women are prone to UTIs because the female urethra is short and close to the vagina, periurethral glands, and rectum. (In the male, the length of the urethra and the antibacterial properties of the prostatic secretions tend to ward off ascending urethral infections.)

4 List the most common signs and symptoms of UTI.

The classic symptoms of UTI are frequency, urgency, and dysuria (often described as a burning sensation during urination). Hematuria may also occur. The patient may also complain of back pain, fever, chills, nausea, and vomiting—all suggestive of an upper UTI.

5 Describe the medication regimen.

Uncomplicated UTIs (those not requiring surgical correction of an obstruction or congenital anomaly) can be treated with any of several different courses of antimicrobial therapy. (Some drugs commonly used for this disorder are ampicillin, co-trimoxazole, phenazopyridine hydrochloride, and sulfisoxazole. See Chapter 9, Drug Therapy, for specific medication instructions.)

6 Discuss ways to prevent recurrence of UTI.

Because women often experience recurring UTI, the following guidelines should be discussed with the female patient.

—She can reduce the concentrations of pathogens at the vaginal introitus by showering rather than bathing in a tub, since bacteria in the bath water may gain entrance to the urethra, and by cleansing around the perineum (from front to back), especially after each bowel movement.

—She should drink liberal amounts of fluid to flush out bacteria, unless her physician advises otherwise because of the medication prescribed.

—She should void every 2 to 3 hours during the day, completely emptying the bladder, and should not delay voiding.

—If sexual intercourse is the initiating event for the development of bacteriuria, she should void before and immediately after sexual intercourse.

—If bacteria continue to appear in the urine, long-term antimicrobial therapy may be required to prevent recurrence of infection. If so, the drug should be taken after emptying the bladder, just before going to bed, to ensure adequate concentration of the drug overnight.

—She must keep appointments for follow-up urine cultures and should seek prompt treatment of any vaginal discharge.

—She should wear cotton rather than nylon panties, because nylon tends to increase perineal moisture. Likewise, tight slacks and pantyhose should be avoided.

—She should not stay in a damp swimsuit once she has finished swimming.

—If the vaginal epithelium is dry, causing irritation during intercourse, she should use K-Y Lubricating Jelly.

—She should not use bubble bath, perfumed soaps, feminine hygiene sprays, or hexachlorophene. When washing clothes, she should avoid strong powders and bleaches and should rinse clothes until the water is clear.

INCONTINENCE

Patient objectives	*Teaching plan content*
1 Define incontinence.	Incontinence is a general term referring to the involuntary loss of urine.

2 Name the relevant type of incontinence.

The four types of incontinence include true, or total, incontinence (continuous urine leakage); stress incontinence (leakage of urine as a result of a sudden increase in intraabdominal pressure); urgency incontinence (incontinence that follows a sudden, strong desire to urinate); and paradoxical, or overflow, incontinence (dribbling as a result of obstruction or a flaccid bladder).

3 Identify the relevant causes of incontinence.

The most common causes of incontinence include neurogenic bladder resulting from neurologic disease, such as Parkinson's or Alzheimer's disease, or stroke; spinal cord lesions, such as injuries or tumors; urinary tract disease, such as urinary tract infections, bladder calculus, or benign prostatic hyperplasia; and traumatic or surgical urinary tract injury.

4 Identify the components of the treatment regimen for incontinence.

Treatment varies according to the type and cause of incontinence, but the program may include:
—Medications, which can improve urinary control by acting on the bladder to block uninhibited bladder contractions, relax the smooth muscle of the bladder, or increase the contractility of the bladder neck.
—Surgery to correct anatomic abnormalities, relieve obstruction, create a urinary diversion, or insert an artificial urinary sphincter.
—Intermittent self-catheterization to help gain some urinary control.
—A bladder-retraining program to help regain control.
—Pelvic floor exercises to strengthen perineal muscles and to help prevent incontinence.
—Long-term indwelling (Foley) catheter placement to prevent incontinence.
—Wearing an external urine collection device to prevent incontinence.

5 Describe the medication regimen.

Some drugs commonly used for this disorder are propantheline bromide, methantheline bromide, flavoxate hydrochloride, dicyclomine hydrochloride, ephedrine sulfate, and imipramine hydrochloride. See Chapter 9, Drug Therapy, for specific medication instructions.

6 Discuss relevant surgical procedures, such as prostatectomy.

See the "Prostatectomy" teaching plan in this chapter.

7 Demonstrate intermittent self-catheterization, if applicable.

See the "Intermittent Self-Catheterization" teaching plan in this chapter.

8 Demonstrate pelvic floor exercises, if applicable.

If necessary, female patients should learn to perform Kegel exercises, which consist of relaxing and contracting the perineal muscles 10 times or more, at least 4 times a day. The patient sits on a chair with her feet on the floor and her knees spread. Then she contracts the perineal muscles as though stopping the expulsion of urine. She should also try to stop and start her urinary stream several times whenever she voids.

9 Discuss and demonstrate long-term indwelling catheter care, if applicable.

See the "Long-Term Indwelling Catheter Care" teaching plan in this chapter.

10 Demonstrate the application and care of an external urine collection device.

The patient should learn to apply and care for an external urine collection device.

—Guidelines for female patients:

- The patient should be able to put on disposable waterproof pants (such as Attends) or sanitary pads with waterproof pants.
- She should change them frequently and wash her perineum thoroughly with mild soap and water at each change, drying the area gently and, if possible, exposing it to the air for a while.
- She should inspect her skin frequently for signs of irritation.

—Guidelines for male patients:

- The patient should be able to apply a condom catheter.
- He should wash his penis and perineal area with soap and water, dry the area thoroughly, prep the entire shaft of his penis with a skin-prep solution or swab, if available, and allow the penis to dry.
- Then, to tape the penis, he removes the covering from both sides of the elastic adhesive. Starting at the base of the penis, he winds the tape in a spiral toward the glans. The edges of the spiral should not overlap, and he should never apply the tape in a circle around the penis (doing so might cut off circulation). He must not stretch the elastic tape while he is applying it, or there will not be enough slack to accommodate an erection.
- Next he places the sheath on the end of his penis, making sure that the end of the sheath extends about ½" from the end of the penis—this gap serves as a urine reservoir so that the penis will not be in urine, even if the urine backs up.
- Then he unrolls the sheath along the penis, gently stretching the penis as he goes, and gently squeezes

the unrolled sheath along the length of the penis so it adheres to the tape.
• He connects the sheath to the leg bag, using extension tubing to join them, if necessary, and straps the leg bag to his thigh.
• He should wash his penis daily, as described previously, and empty the bag three or four times daily, or as needed, rinsing it with a vinegar and water solution to deodorize it. (See *Caring for Your Condom Catheter*, pp. 332-333.)

11 Demonstrate care of a urinary ostomy, if applicable.	See the "Ostomies" teaching plan in Chapter 6, Gastrointestinal Disorders, for a discussion of ostomy care.

CHRONIC RENAL FAILURE

Patient objectives	*Teaching plan content*
1 Define chronic renal failure.	Chronic renal failure, or uremia, is a clinical syndrome resulting from progressive loss of renal function.
2 Name the relevant causes of chronic renal failure.	The major causes of chronic renal failure include chronic glomerular disease, such as glomerulonephritis; chronic infections, such as pyelonephritis; congenital anomalies, such as polycystic kidneys; vascular diseases, such as hypertension; obstructive processes, such as calculi; collagen diseases, such as systemic lupus erythematosus; nephrotoxic agents, such as certain drugs or heavy metals; and endocrine diseases, such as diabetes mellitus.
3 Describe the disease process in chronic renal failure.	The conditions associated with chronic renal failure gradually destroy the functional units (nephrons) of the kidneys, and, as renal function declines, the products of protein metabolism that form the constituents of urine accumulate in the blood. Imbalances in body chemistry and in the cardiovascular, hematologic, GI, neurologic, and skeletal systems result. Skin and reproductive changes are also seen. —Chronic renal failure progresses through four stages, and the symptoms worsen and affect all body systems as the condition progresses. Death will occur without treatment. —The four stages of chronic renal failure are decreased renal reserve (no symptoms present), mild renal insufficiency, frank renal failure, and end-stage renal disease. —Symptoms the patient may have experienced before being diagnosed include fatigue; weakness; lethargy; headache; GI disturbances, such as anorexia, nausea,

vomiting, and diarrhea; bleeding tendencies; mental confusion; thirst; dry mouth; metallic taste in the mouth; loss of sense of smell or taste; inflammation of the salivary glands; and sore mouth.

4 Identify the components of the treatment regimen for chronic renal failure.

Treatment of chronic renal failure may include the following:
—Dietary restrictions to reduce the end products of protein metabolism and to regulate fluid and electrolyte balance.
—Medications to treat underlying conditions, prevent complications, or control symptoms.
—Scrupulous skin care and oral hygiene to relieve symptoms and prevent complications.
—Safety precautions to help compensate for any sensory loss.
—Dialysis therapy (either hemodialysis or peritoneal dialysis) to remove the end products of metabolism from the blood, thereby eliminating or markedly decreasing symptoms.
—Renal transplantation to provide the recipient with a functioning kidney and a more normal life-style.
—Continued medical follow-up to monitor blood chemistry.

5 Discuss the prescribed dietary restrictions for chronic renal failure.

The patient must restrict protein intake because a low-protein diet reduces the production of end products of metabolism that the kidneys cannot excrete. (If the patient is receiving dialysis, no protein restriction is necessary, since dialysis removes such end products.) The allowed protein must be of high biological value (dairy products, eggs, meat) to provide the essential amino acids. At least 25 g (but preferably 40 g) of high-biological-value protein are required daily. At the same time, adequate caloric intake and vitamin supplementation are required to prevent tissue wasting. Fluids may be restricted. Usually, the fluid allowance is 500 to 600 ml of fluid more than the 24-hour urine output. Sodium and potassium intake will be based on measurement of electrolytes in the serum and urine. The dietitian should provide specific instructions on the prescribed diet, and such instruction should be reinforced as needed.

6 Discuss the medication regimen for chronic renal failure.

The patient will probably need to take a variety of medications to relieve symptoms and to prevent or control complications. These medications may include diuretics and/or digitalis to mobilize edematous fluid, antihypertensives to control blood pressure, antiemetics taken before meals to relieve nausea and vomiting, medications to decrease gastric irritation, laxatives or stool softeners to prevent constipation, an antipruritic to relieve itching, aluminum hydroxide antacids to lower serum phosphorus levels, and supplementary vitamins. Some drugs commonly used for this disorder are hydrochlorothiazide, propranolol, methyldopa, captopril, cimetidine, aluminum hydroxide, vitamin D preparations (such as dihydrotachysterol), colace, and Kayexalate. (See Chapter 9, Drug Therapy, for specific instructions.)

7 Describe skin care and oral hygiene techniques.

The patient with chronic renal failure should bathe daily, using superfatted soaps, oatmeal baths, and a good skin lotion to ease pruritus and dryness. He should practice good perineal care, using mild soap and water, and should maintain good oral hygiene to reduce breath odor, prevent mouth soreness, and minimize bad taste. He should brush his teeth often with a soft brush or sponge tip. The use of a mouthwash and/or hard candy may help relieve any metallic taste in the mouth.

8 Explain safety precautions to help compensate for sensory loss.

See the "Cerebrovascular Accident" teaching plan in Chapter 4, Neurologic Disorders, for measures to prevent injury from sensory loss.

9 Discuss dialysis therapy used to treat chronic renal failure.

Two types of dialysis therapy may be used:

—In peritoneal dialysis, the peritoneum (the thin layer of tissue that lines the abdominal wall and covers the intestines) acts as a semipermeable membrane through which toxic substances, excess water, and body wastes move on their way out of the body.

- A dialysing fluid (dialysate) is run into the peritoneal cavity by a small tube inserted through the abdominal wall.
- The dialysate is left in the abdomen for a period of time, allowing the toxic substances, excess water, and body wastes to move out of the bloodstream and across the peritoneum and permitting any medications or electrolytes to move into the bloodstream.
- The fluid is then drained from the abdomen through the tube, and more solution is instilled (an exchange).
- Peritoneal dialysis is performed continuously and may be taught to the patient so he can continue treatment at home (continuous ambulatory peritoneal dialysis, or CAPD).

—In hemodialysis, a synthetic material is used as the semipermeable membrane through which excess water, nitrogenous wastes, and other toxins are removed from the blood. Access to the patient's circulation is achieved through an arteriovenous shunt (external Silastic tubing placed in an adjacent artery and vein), a fistula (internal access using the patient's own vessels), or a graft (internal access using a foreign material).

- The patient must be connected to a machine for hemodialysis.
- Waste-laden blood flows from the patient through an artery. Heparinized blood then passes, by means of a blood pump, through the machine to the semipermeable membrane, and the dialysate bath flows on the other side of the membrane.
- The toxins, wastes, and excess water move across the membrane into the dialysate bath. Electrolytes and medications may move from the bath into the blood. Purified blood is then returned to the patient through one of his veins.
- Hemodialysis requires going to the hospital or outpatient dialysis center for treatment, usually three or four times per week.

10 Demonstrate continuous ambulatory peritoneal dialysis (CAPD), if applicable.

See the "Continuous Ambulatory Peritoneal Dialysis (CAPD)" teaching plan in this chapter.

11 Discuss renal transplant surgery.

Kidney transplantation involves removing a kidney from a living donor or a human cadaver and surgically implanting it in a recipient with end-stage renal disease who requires dialysis to live. The patient's nonfunctional kidneys may or may not be removed. Dialysis is maintained until a suitable donor is found.

—The donor kidney is transplanted extraperitoneally in either iliac fossa, and the ureter of the newly transplanted kidney is transplanted into the bladder or anastomosed to the ureter of the recipient.

—After surgery, the patient may need dialysis temporarily if the new kidney does not function right away.

—He will receive immunosuppressive drugs to prevent rejection of the new kidney, but they will also make him more susceptible to infection. He must continue taking them for the rest of his life.

—Barring complications or adverse side effects from the medications, a patient with a transplanted kidney can look forward to improved general health and a lifestyle free from dialysis equipment. (See *Going Home After Renal Transplant Surgery,* pp. 336-337.)

12 Describe the need for continued medical follow-up in chronic renal failure.

Continued medical follow-up and monitoring are crucial to the patient's health. He will need to see his physician periodically for blood tests to monitor electrolytes and blood chemistry.

13 Discuss coping strategies for dealing with long-term dialysis therapy.	Feelings of anger and dismay are normal emotional reactions for patients and families in this situation. They should be given verbal and written instructions and informed of resources available for help. The patient and his family should be given a chance to express any feelings of anger and concern over the limitations imposed by the disease and treatment, as well as possible financial problems, job insecurity, pain, and discomfort. The patient needs a close relationship with someone to whom he can turn in times of stress and discouragement.

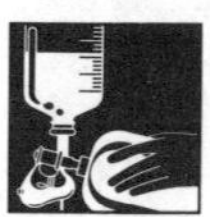

Explaining treatments

CONTINUOUS AMBULATORY PERITONEAL DIALYSIS (C.A.P.D.)

Patient objectives	*Teaching plan content*
1 Define CAPD.	CAPD is a treatment for end-stage renal disease in which the patient performs peritoneal dialysis continuously at home, providing himself with independence and control over his daily activities.
2 State the purpose of CAPD.	The purpose of CAPD is to maintain the life and well-being of the patient by removing toxic substances, excess water, and body wastes normally excreted by healthy kidneys.
3 Discuss the principles of CAPD.	In CAPD, the peritoneum (the thin layer of tissue that lines the abdominal wall and covers the intestines) acts as a semipermeable membrane through which toxic substances, excess water, and body wastes move on their way out of the body. A dialysing fluid (dialysate) is run into the peritoneal cavity by means of a small tube inserted through the abdominal wall. The dialysate remains in the abdomen for a period of time, allowing excess water, toxic substances, and wastes to move out of the bloodstream across the peritoneum and permitting any medications or electrolytes to move into the bloodstream across it. The fluid is then drained from the abdomen through the tube, and more solution is instilled (an exchange). This technique is continuous, 24 hours a day, 7 days a week.
4 Demonstrate the procedure for CAPD.	The patient should weigh himself at the same time each day. Then he should follow these guidelines:

—Gather the needed equipment: a bag of peritoneal dialysis solution of the correct volume and dextrose concentration; two outlet port clamps; a sterile CAPD prep kit, which includes povidone-iodine swabs, 4″ × 4″ sterile gauze pads, nonallergenic tape, and a mask; and, if medication must be injected into the dialysate, the necessary number of 25G needles, 10-cc syringes, and the medication itself.
—Arrange the work area so the bag can be hung above shoulder level. Warm the dialysate by placing it in a basin or sink full of warm water. Leave the protective wrap on the bag, and take care to keep the bag's ports dry. Remember to wash the hands thoroughly.
—Open the CAPD prep kit. Remove the empty dialysate bag from inside the clothing, and tape the bag's injection port so it is out of the way. Before opening the junction of the bag and the tubing spike, clean the junction by wrapping a povidone-iodine–soaked swab around it and then wrapping a dry gauze pad around the swab and taping the gauze pad into position.
—After placing the bag in the drainage position below the abdomen, open the clamp on the drainage tubing and allow about 15 to 20 minutes for the solution to drain into the bag. Meanwhile, remove the wrapping from the new dialysate bag. Make sure the solution is clear, not cloudy. Read the concentration information on the label to make sure it is the right solution, check the expiration date, and squeeze the bag firmly to test for leaks.
—If the physician has ordered it, add medication to the bag. To do so, put on a mask, draw up the medication, and then wipe the injection port with a povidone-iodine swab. After inserting the needle through the rubber stopper and into the injection port, mix the dialysate and the medication by upending the bag several times.
—When the dialysate has finished draining from the abdomen, close the clamp and place the drainage bag on a flat surface, next to the new bag. Position the used bag clear side up, and check the fluid for cloudiness or particles. (Cloudiness may indicate peritonitis, the most common complication of CAPD.) Position the new dialysate bag with its label side up, and double-check the dialysate concentration and the expiration date. Arrange the bags so that their ends extend over the edge of the work surface. Now put on a mask, if this was not done before. Tape the injection port of the new bag to keep it from touching the outlet port. Place a clamp on the outlet port to keep it stable during spike insertion.
—Remove the gauze pads from the outlet-port tubing junction. Clamp the outlet port, lining up the clamp

with the first step notch on the port. Remove the blue covering from the outlet port of the new bag without touching the port.
—To transfer the tubing spike, grasp its finger grip in the drainage-bag outlet port. With the free hand, hold the clamp on the outlet port. Twist and pull the spike to remove it from the port. Take care not to touch anything with the spike tip.
—Immediately insert the spike into the outlet port of the new bag. Unclamp the outlet port. Hang the new bag above shoulder level or on an I.V. pole, then open the clamp to allow the dialysate to drain into the abdomen. After about 5 minutes, when almost all the dialysate has drained from the bag, close the clamp. With a little fluid left in the bag, it will be easier to fold.
—Remove the bag from the pole (if used) and place it on the work surface. Fold over the spike-outlet port connection so it is centered on the bag. Coil the tubing over this connection. Then fold the other end of the bag over the connection and tubing, place the bag inside a pouch, if used, and put the pouch inside the clothing. If the physician has ordered a drainage sample, take the entire drainage bag of fluid to the hospital laboratory for analysis. Otherwise, carefully empty the used dialysate into the toilet, and discard the empty bag in a trash can.

5 Identify potential complications of CAPD requiring medical care.

Potential complications to look for include the following:
—Peritonitis: The symptoms of peritonitis may include fever, abdominal pain or tenderness, and cloudy dialysate drainage from the abdomen. The patient should notify his physician of such symptoms immediately; temporarily discontinue CAPD, as ordered by his physician; and save the entire bag of drained dialysate for laboratory analysis.
—Catheter exit-site infection: Symptoms of infection may include fever; redness, swelling, and drainage around the site; and tenderness at the site. The patient should notify his physician immediately if such symptoms occur.
—Dialysate leakage through the exit site: This complication may result from incomplete healing of the incision at the catheter exit site. The patient should notify his physician and withhold dialysis for several days, as ordered, until the incision heals. During this period, it is important to avoid or minimize factors that might delay healing, such as undue abdominal muscle activity and/or straining during bowel movements.
—Bleeding: A slightly bloody drainage may be noted during menstruation, after minor abdominal trauma, af-

ter placement of the catheter, or after an enema. Bleeding usually stops after a day or two and requires no specific intervention. The patient should notify the physician if the bleeding is profuse or does not stop spontaneously.

INTERMITTENT SELF-CATHETERIZATION

Patient objectives	*Teaching plan content*
1 Define intermittent self-catheterization.	Intermittent self-catheterization is the periodic insertion, by the patient, of a catheter through his urethra and into his bladder.
2 State the purpose of intermittent self-catheterization.	Intermittent self-catheterization provides periodic drainage of urine from the bladder when normal bladder function is impaired or absent.
3 Explain the procedure used in intermittent self-catheterization.	Although the patient will use clean technique for self-catheterization at home, he will need to use sterile technique while he is in the hospital, because there is much greater danger of infection. He must adhere strictly to his catheterization schedule, regardless of the circumstances. —The timing of catheterization is critical to prevent overdistention of the bladder, which may lead to infection. Intermittent self-catheterization is usually ordered every 4 to 6 hours, around the clock. (It may be ordered more frequently at first.) Even if the patient has no soap and water handy, he must catheterize himself when his schedule requires. —To perform this procedure, he must thoroughly cleanse the genital area and then insert a catheter through his urethra and into his bladder. (NOTE: Female patients must be able to identify the body parts involved in self-catheterization—labia majora, labia minora, vagina, and meatus.) —After the bladder has been completely emptied of urine, the patient should withdraw the catheter, clean it, and store it for future use. —The patient should keep careful records of the times of catheterization, the character of the urine, and any problems encountered during the procedure.
4 Demonstrate intermittent self-catheterization using sterile technique.	The patient should be given a sterile catheter kit, including a catheter, three cotton balls, forceps, a sterile waterproof drape, a povidone-iodine packet, a container for draining urine, and water-soluble lubricant. He should also be given sterile gloves if the kit does not

include them; a paper bag for discarding used equipment; and, for female patients, two sterile gauze pads.
—Male patients should follow these guidelines:

- Before inserting the catheter, try to urinate. To make this easier, press on the abdomen or stroke the inner thighs.
- Wash the hands thoroughly. Sit on the toilet or on a chair for the first few catheterizations. (You can stand over the toilet when you are more skilled.) Arrange clothing so it is out of the way. Place the catheter kit on a work surface, and open it without touching its contents.
- Put on one glove by grasping the folded edge of the cuff. Then place the fingers of the gloved hand into the cuff of the second glove and pull on the second glove, too. Then position the drape shiny (coated) side down, and lay out the equipment.
- Squirt the sterile lubricant onto the drape. Then open the povidone-iodine solution packet. Pour the solution on the cotton balls.
- Now clean the penis with the saturated cotton balls. With the nondominant hand, grasp the sides of the penis. (NOTE: The patient should not use this hand for anything else during the procedure.) An uncircumcised patient should pull back the foreskin with the same hand and hold it back during insertion. With the dominant hand, use the forceps to pick up a cotton ball. Begin cleaning at the opening of the penis. Move outward in a spiral motion to the edge of the penis head. Discard the cotton ball into the paper bag and repeat this step until all three of the cotton balls have been used. With the same hand, pick up the catheter and roll the first 7″ to 10″ (18 to 25 cm) of it in the lubricant. Now, using the nondominant hand, hold the penis at a right angle to the body. Holding the catheter like a pencil or a dart, gently advance it 7″ to 10″ into the urethra. Never force the catheter. However, when it is about halfway inserted, there may be resistance. Applying firm but gentle pressure on the catheter may help relax tight muscles and permit the catheter to pass.
- When urine begins to flow, gently push the catheter 1″ (3 cm) farther. Allow all urine to drain into the toilet or container; press down with the abdominal muscles to completely empty the bladder. When the urine stops draining, pinch the catheter near its tip and remove it slowly. Tilt the tip upward as it comes out of the meatus to avoid spilling urine. Discard the catheter in the paper bag. An uncircumcised patient should pull the foreskin forward again. Get

dressed, and discard the paper bag and used equipment in the trash can.

• Finally, if the physician requires it, document the amount, color, and odor of the urine. Also document whether the urine is clear or cloudy. Note any particles or blood, and tell the physician about them at once. Also let the physician know immediately if the amount of urine increases or decreases, if catheterization is difficult, or if pain or burning occurs during catheterization.

—Female patients should follow these guidelines:

• Before inserting the catheter, try to urinate. To make this easier, press on the abdomen or stroke the inner thighs.

• Wash the hands thoroughly. For the first few catheterizations, it may be convenient to sit on a bed with legs bent and knees apart. (You can sit on the toilet after you become more skilled.) Arrange clothing so it is out of the way. Place the kit on a work surface and open it without touching its contents.

• Put on one sterile glove by grasping the folded edge of the cuff. Then place the fingers of the gloved hand in the cuff of the second glove and pull on the second glove, too.

• Position the sterile drape with the shiny (coated) side down. Squirt sterile lubricant onto the drape. Open the povidone-iodine solution packet, and pour the solution on the cotton balls.

• Now use the gauze pads in the dominant hand to pick up the mirror. Touch only the gauze pads, not the mirror. Using the mirror, find the vaginal folds and urethral meatus. Hold the folds apart with the index and second fingers. Identify the meatus. That hand is now contaminated, so do not touch anything sterile with it. (After the first few catheterizations, the mirror should no longer be needed; do not become dependent on it.)

• Clean the vaginal area. To do this, pick up the soaked cotton balls with the forceps. Clean the area between the folds with three downward strokes, using one cotton ball on the right downstroke, one on the left downstroke, and one down the center. Throw the cotton balls into the trash bag.

• With the uncontaminated hand, pick up the catheter and roll the first 3″ (8 cm) of it in the lubricant. Holding the vaginal folds apart with the contaminated hand, use the other hand to grasp the catheter like a pencil or a dart. Insert it upward into the urethra. When urine begins to flow, gently push the catheter about 1″ (3 cm) farther. Then allow all urine to drain from the bladder. Press down with the abdominal muscles and move the catheter in and out once or twice to help drain the bladder completely.

• When the urine stops draining, pinch the catheter near its tip to prevent urine from leaking into the urethra. Remove the catheter slowly. Tilt the tip upward as it comes out of the meatus to avoid spilling urine. Throw the catheter into the trash bag. Get dressed, and dispose of the bag and the used equipment.

• Finally, if the physician requires it, document the amount, color, and odor of the urine. Also document whether the urine is clear or cloudy. Note any particles or blood in the urine, and tell the physician about them at once. Let the physician know immediately if the amount of urine increases or decreases, if catheterization is difficult, or if pain or burning occurs during catheterization.

5 Demonstrate intermittent self-catheterization using clean technique.

In most cases, the patient will use clean technique for self-catheterization.

—The female patient should follow these guidelines:

• Gather the needed equipment: a rubber catheter, a clean washcloth, soap and water, a small packet of water-soluble lubricant, and a plastic bag for used catheters. Obtain a container for draining urine if a toilet is not available or if urine must be measured. Make sure lighting is adequate.

• Before inserting the catheter, try to urinate. Wash the hands thoroughly.

• Separate the vaginal folds with one hand. Use downward strokes with the washcloth to wash the arca thoroughly. Lubricate the first 3″ (8 cm) of the catheter.

• Hold the catheter as if it were a pencil or a dart, about ½″ from its tip. Keeping the vaginal folds separated, slowly insert the lubricated catheter about 3″ into the urethra. Press down with the abdominal muscles to empty the bladder. Allow all urine to drain through the catheter.

• When the urine stops draining, remove the catheter slowly. Get dressed, and wash the catheter in warm, soapy water. Rinse it inside and out, and dry it with a clean towel. Place it in the plastic storage bag for used catheters.

• Finally, if the physician requires it, record information about the catheterization and urine, as indicated previously.

—The male patient should follow these guidelines:

• Gather the needed equipment: a rubber catheter, a clean washcloth, soap and water, a small package of lubricant, a paper towel, and a plastic bag. Obtain a container for draining urine if a toilet is not available or if urine must be measured.

- Before inserting the catheter, try to urinate.
- Arrange clothing so it is out of the way. Remember to wash the hands.
- Wash the end of the penis thoroughly with soap and water, pulling back the foreskin, if appropriate. The foreskin should be kept back throughout catheterization.
- Squeeze some lubricant onto the paper towel and lubricate the first 7″ to 10″ (18 to 25 cm) of the catheter. Then hold the penis at a right angle to the body. Grasp the catheter as if holding a pencil or a dart, and slowly insert it 7″ to 10″, until urine begins to flow. Then gently push the catheter 1″ (3 cm) farther. Allow all urine to drain into the toilet or container.
- When the urine stops draining, slowly remove the catheter. Pull the foreskin forward again. Get dressed, and wash the catheter in warm, soapy water. Rinse it inside and out, and dry it with a clean towel. Place the catheter in the plastic bag.
- Finally, if the physician requires it, record information about the catheterization and urine, as explained previously.

6 Discuss home-care guidelines to prevent urinary tract infection and incontinence.

The patient should follow these guidelines:

—The patient should buy a new supply of catheters when they become brittle. He should use each catheter only once, and when all but the last one has been used, he should boil the catheters for 20 minutes in a pan of water, drain the water, and store the catheters in the pan or in a freshly laundered towel.

—With external urine collection, he must first regulate his fluid intake, as ordered, to prevent incontinence while still maintaining a good hydration level. Second, he must take his medication, as ordered, to increase urine retention and to help prevent incontinence. Finally, he must avoid calcium-rich and phosphorus-rich foods, as ordered, to reduce the chance of kidney stone formation.

—Even though he is catheterizing himself intermittently, he may still experience incontinence. It will probably be a source of distress for him, and he will need emotional support. He and his family should develop a plan for managing incontinence, such as an increase or other change in the catheterization schedule, as discussed with the physician. A visit from a public health nurse can help in implementing the plan.

—The patient should wear some type of external collection device between catheterizations to control incontinence. If he has an incontinent episode, he must wash his skin with soap and water, pat it dry with a towel, and expose it to the air for as long as possible. He can reduce urine odor by putting methylbenzethonium chloride (Diaparene) or cornstarch on the skin. Bedding and furniture can be protected by covering them with rubber or plastic sheets and then covering the rubber or plastic with cloth.

BLADDER RETRAINING PROGRAM

Patient objectives	*Teaching plan content*
1 Define bladder retraining.	Bladder retraining (or training) is a method of overcoming incontinence by increasing the bladder's capacity to hold urine.
2 State the purpose of bladder retraining.	A bladder retraining program is instituted to overcome incontinence and to achieve successful urinary control.
3 Explain the procedure used in bladder retraining.	A schedule will be set up indicating times for the patient to try to empty his bladder. The interval between voidings in the early phase of the training program is fairly short (1½ to 2 hours), but as his bladder capacity increases, the interval is lengthened. A suggested procedure involves drinking a measured amount of fluid every 2 hours, then waiting 30 minutes and attempting to void. His goal is to gradually lengthen the period between voiding times. He should drink fluids during the day and restrict them in the evening. Certain medications may also be used in conjunction with a bladder retraining program. These medications improve urinary control by acting on the bladder to block uninhibited bladder contractions (decrease bladder contractility), relax the smooth muscle of the bladder, or increase the contractility of the bladder neck. See the "Incontinence" teaching plan in this chapter for specific medications used.
4 Discuss patient guidelines for bladder retraining.	The patient must thoroughly understand the procedure and adhere to the schedule. He should drink the prescribed amount of fluid at each interval and try to hold his urine until the specified voiding time. Usually, there is a relationship between eating, exercising, and voiding, and the alert patient can soon determine his own intake schedule. He should keep a written voiding schedule, which gives a continuous record of the time and amount of fluid ingested and the time and amount of each voiding. Regularity is the key to success. To assist voiding, the patient can stand or sit with his

thighs flexed and his feet and back supported. Increasing intraabdominal pressure by massage over the bladder or by leaning forward while sitting will help to initiate bladder evacuation. He should take his medications, as ordered, and wear an external urine collection device (condom catheter for men, sanitary pads or incontinence pants for women) between voidings until urinary control is achieved.

LONG-TERM INDWELLING CATHETER CARE

Patient objectives	*Teaching plan content*
1 Define an indwelling catheter.	An indwelling catheter (also known as a Foley, or retention, catheter) is a thin, flexible tube that is inserted through the urethra into the bladder to provide continuous urine drainage. After insertion of the catheter, a balloon is inflated to prevent it from slipping out. (The patient should be shown where the catheter connects to the drainage tubing and the drainage bag.)
2 State the purpose of long-term indwelling catheter care.	Daily catheter care is performed to maintain the patency of the catheter and to prevent complications.
3 Discuss patient guidelines for long-term indwelling catheter care.	The patient must wash his hands thoroughly before and after his routine. —He should wash the urinary meatus and the area around the catheter twice a day, using a clean washcloth and soap and water. He should begin at the meatus and gently proceed distally (away from himself), holding the distal end of the catheter to prevent pulling on the catheter while cleaning. He should remove any encrustations or blood from the outside of the catheter and dry the area well. He should not use powders or sprays. He should also wash around his rectal area twice a day (after washing the catheter) and after each bowel movement. If his physician has ordered an antibiotic or antiseptic ointment, he should apply it to the area where the meatus and catheter meet. The catheter must not be disconnected from the drainage bag. —The drainage bag should be emptied every 8 hours by unclamping the drain tube and removing it from its sleeve (without touching the tip) and letting the urine drain into the toilet or a measuring container, if ordered. (The patient should not let the drain tube touch the toilet or container.) When the bag is completely empty, he should swab the end of the drain tube with povidone-iodine solution, if recommended by his physician, and reclamp the tube and reinsert it into the

sleeve of the drainage bag. If the drainage bag accidentally becomes disconnected from the catheter, he should replace it with a sterile one.

4 Discuss care of the drainage bag.

If the patient wears a leg bag during the day, he must empty the bag every 3 to 4 hours, because it is smaller than the closed-drainage system he wears at night. In caring for a leg bag and a closed-drainage system, he should follow these guidelines:
—To empty the leg bag, first wash the hands. Then remove the stopper and drain all the urine. If requested by the physician, drain the urine into a measuring container and record the amount. Do not touch the drain port with the fingers or with the container.
—After the urine has drained completely, swab the drain port and the stopper with a povidone-iodine swab, as ordered. Replace the stopper.
—Before going to bed, replace the leg bag with a closed-system drainage bag. (Because the closed-system bag holds more urine, it will not need to be emptied during the night.) To replace the bag, first empty the leg bag. Then clamp the catheter and swab the connection between the catheter and the leg bag with povidone-iodine. Disconnect the leg bag, and connect the closed-system drainage tubing and bag. Finally, unclamp the catheter.
—Tape the drainage bag to the right thigh if it will hang on the right side of the bed or the left thigh if it will hang on the left. Use nonallergenic tape, and shave the skin in that area, if necessary. Leave some slack in the line so the catheter will not be pulled with leg movements. For men: Tape the drainage tubing to the inner thigh, opposite the base of the penis. For women: Tape the drainage tubing to the inner thigh, below the vaginal area.
—After disconnecting the leg bag, wash it with soap and water. Then mix white vinegar and water in these proportions: 1¼ cups of vinegar to 2 qt of water. Rinse the bag with this solution to reduce urine odor and to control bacterial growth. Allow the vinegar solution to remain in the bag until the bag is to be used again; then drain the excess.
—When getting into bed, arrange the drainage tubing so it does not kink or loop. Hang the drainage bag beside the bed. Be sure to keep the drainage bag below bladder level at all times, whether lying, sitting, or standing, to prevent urine flow back into the bladder; this decreases the risk of infection. When reconnecting the leg bag in the morning, empty the closed-system bag. Then repeat the steps used to connect the closed-system bag the night before, using the leg bag instead.

	Do not forget to empty the closed-system bag before disconnecting it. Wash the bag with soap and water, and rinse it with the vinegar and water solution. (NOTE: Both types of drainage bags can be reused for up to 1 month.) —Make sure the tubing is not kinked or looped so that urine is prevented from flowing freely into the bag. Drink plenty of fluids (unless contraindicated) to help maintain good urine flow. Never remove the catheter or irrigate it without specific instructions on how to do so. Report to the physician, as ordered, to have the catheter changed. (A visiting nurse may also do this.)
5 Discuss potential complications of long-term indwelling catheters.	The following complications may occur in patients with long-term indwelling catheters: —Urinary tract infection: The patient should contact his physician if he experiences fever, chills, low back or suprapubic pain, or persistent burning at the catheter site or if he notices cloudy urine, blood in the urine, or a strong odor to the urine. —Obstruction of the catheter: The patient should contact his physician if (despite changing his position or disentangling kinked tubing) he notices urine leakage around the catheter site, experiences pain and fullness in the abdomen, or finds that the urine level in the drainage bag has stopped rising.

PROSTATECTOMY

Patient objectives	*Teaching plan content*
1 Define prostatectomy.	A prostatectomy is the removal of all or part of the prostate gland.
2 State the purpose of a prostatectomy.	A prostatectomy is performed to relieve obstruction of the urethra or to rid the patient of cancer.
3 Explain the surgical procedure for prostatectomy.	The four types of prostatectomy are as follows: —Transurethral resection: The physician uses a resectoscope inserted through the urethra. This instrument has an electrically charged wire loop to trim or chip away the invading prostatic tissue from the walls of the urethra. —Suprapubic prostatectomy: The physician makes incisions above the pubis and in the bladder wall to expose the prostate and shells the obstructing prostatic tissue out of its bed with his finger. —Retropubic prostatectomy: The physician makes a suprapubic incision and approaches the prostate between

the bladder and the pubic arch. He then makes another incision in the prostatic capsule and removes the obstructing tissue.
—Radical perineal prostatectomy: The physician makes an incision in the perineum, between the anus and the scrotum, and removes the entire prostate and the seminal vesicles. Then he sutures the bladder to the urethra and closes the incision.

4 Describe the preoperative procedures for a prostatectomy.

Along with the routine preoperative tests, intravenous pyelography is usually performed to detect any anatomic abnormalities (see the "Intravenous Pyelography (IVP)" teaching plan in this chapter). The preoperative shave is from the umbilicus to midthigh. If the patient is to have a radical perineal prostatectomy, the preoperative shave will also include the perineum and scrotum. He will be placed on a low-residue diet for approximately 24 to 48 hours preoperatively and for 5 to 7 days postoperatively. He will also be placed on a regimen of enemas during the 24 hours before surgery, and a cathartic may be ordered. (See Chapter 1, Principles of Patient Teaching, for preoperative teaching instructions, and Appendix B, *Preoperative and Postoperative Teaching,* for guidelines.)

5 Describe what to expect following prostatectomy.

After prostatectomy, the patient can expect the following:
—An indwelling urethral catheter will be in place for several days after surgery. The catheter may need to be flushed or irrigated periodically to remove any blood clots that could obstruct urine flow. His urine will be bloody at first, but it will gradually return to normal.
—He will have an I.V. line in place and will be encouraged to drink fluids to maintain good urine flow. He will probably be able to have a light meal the evening after surgery.
—Depending on the type of prostatectomy performed, he may have an incision on his abdomen or perineum, and a drain may be left in place for several days. A dressing will be in place, and the nurse will check it frequently.
—He will experience some pain after surgery and should ask for pain medication when needed. (Upon discharge, the patient may need a copy of the patient-teaching aid *After Prostate Surgery: How to Care for Yourself,* p. 338.)

Patient-Teaching Aid

HOW TO PERFORM A CONTINUOUS AMBULATORY PERITONEAL DIALYSIS (C.A.P.D.) SOLUTION EXCHANGE

Dear Patient:

You and your physician have chosen continuous ambulatory peritoneal dialysis (CAPD) for your dialysis program. CAPD has an advantage over other forms of dialysis, because it is less expensive and easier to perform at home. But it has a big disadvantage, too. If you use CAPD, you may get an infection in your abdomen. So, when performing a CAPD solution exchange at home, you must guard against harmful bacteria entering the dialysis system. The following instructions will tell you how to drain the used dialysate and replace it with fresh dialysate, so you do not contaminate the system.

1

First, gather the equipment you will need: a 2-liter bag of peritoneal dialysis solution of the correct dextrose concentration; two outlet port clamps; and a sterile CAPD prep kit, which includes povidone-iodine swabs, 4″ × 4″ sterile gauze pads, nonallergenic tape, and a mask. If you must inject medication into the dialysate, you will also need the necessary number of 25G needles, 10-cc syringes, and the medication itself. Use an I.V. pole, if you have one.

Before you begin, warm the dialysate by placing it in a basin or sink full of warm water. Be sure the protective wrap remains on the bag, and take care to keep the bag's ports dry. Remember to wash your hands thoroughly.

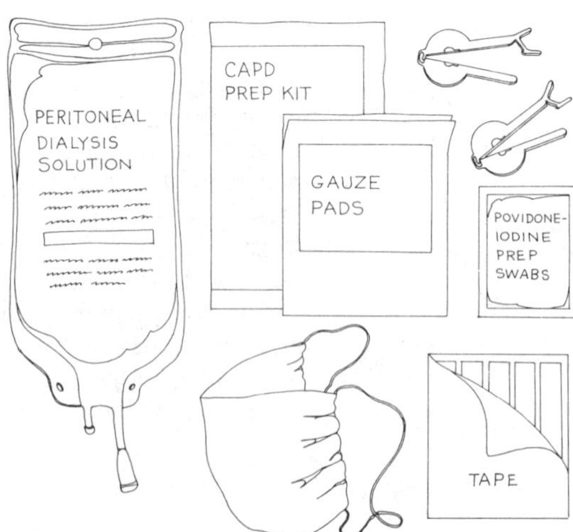

HOW TO PERFORM A CONTINUOUS AMBULATORY PERITONEAL DIALYSIS (C.A.P.D.) SOLUTION EXCHANGE—*continued*

2

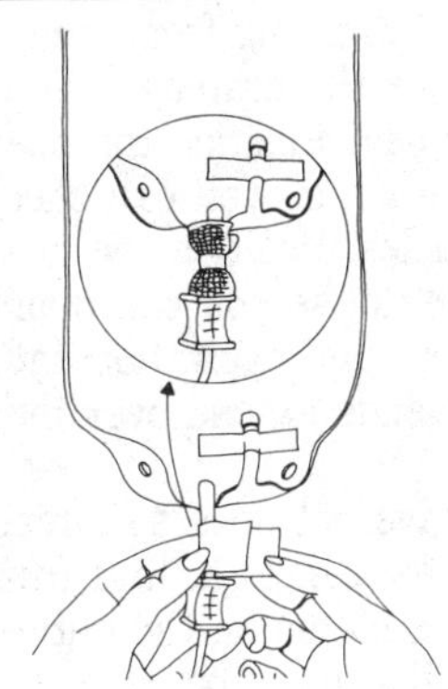

Open the CAPD prep kit. Then remove the empty dialysate bag from inside your clothing. Tape the bag's injection port so it is out of the way. Before you open the junction of the bag and tubing spike, you must clean the junction. To do so, wrap a povidone-iodine–soaked swab around it. Then wrap a dry gauze pad around the swab, and tape the gauze pad in position, as shown in the inset.

3

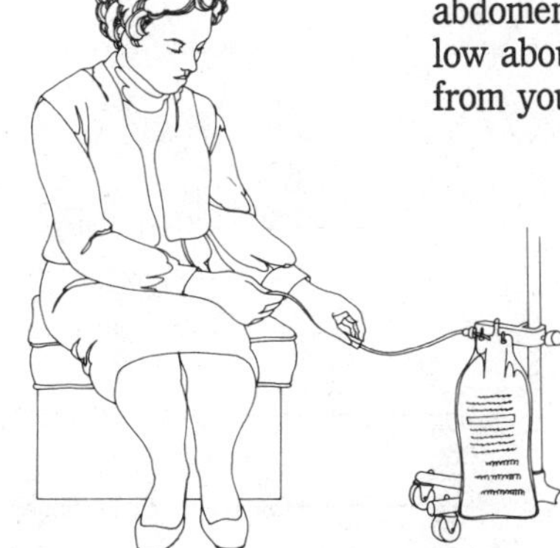

Now place the bag in the drainage position below your abdomen. Open the clamp on the drainage tubing. Allow about 15 to 20 minutes for the solution to drain from your abdomen into the bag.

4

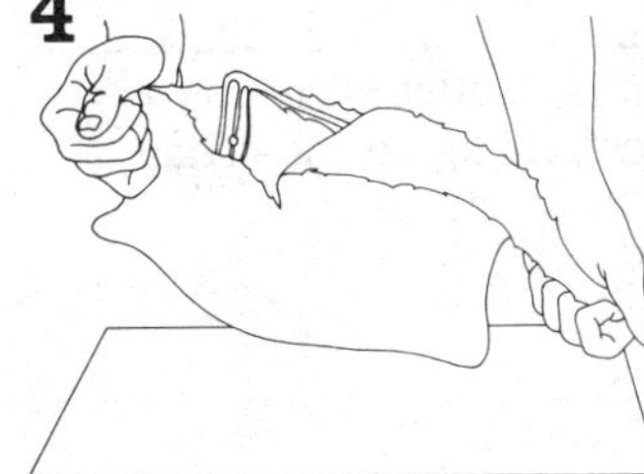

Meanwhile, remove the dialysate bag wrapping. Make sure the dialysate solution is clear, not cloudy. Read the concentration information on the label to make sure you have the right solution, and check the expiration date. Squeeze the bag firmly to test for leaks.

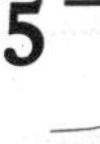

5

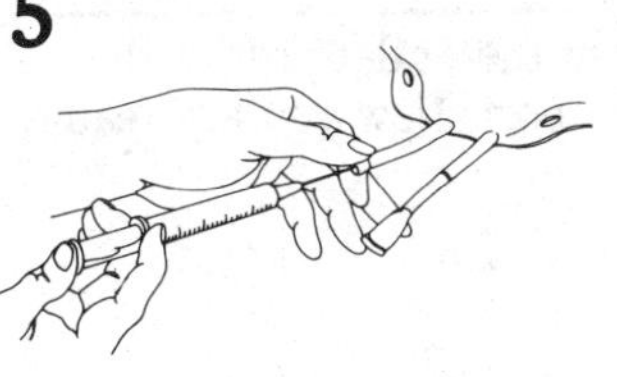

If your physician has ordered it, add medication to the bag. To do so, first put on your mask. Draw up the medication and wipe the injection port with a povidone-iodine swab. Inject the needle through the rubber stopper into the injection port. To mix the dialysate and the medication, upend the bag several times.

HOW TO PERFORM A CONTINUOUS AMBULATORY PERITONEAL DIALYSIS (C.A.P.D.) SOLUTION EXCHANGE—*continued*

6

When the dialysate has finished draining from your abdomen, close the clamp and place the drainage bag on a flat surface, next to the new bag. Position the used dialysate bag with its clear side up, so you can check the fluid for cloudiness or particles. Position the new dialysate bag with its label side up, so you can double-check the dialysate concentration and expiration date. Arrange the bags so that their ends extend over the edge of the work surface.

Now put on a mask, if you have not done so already. Tape the injection port of the new bag to keep it from touching the outlet port. Place a clamp on the outlet port to keep it stable during spike insertion.

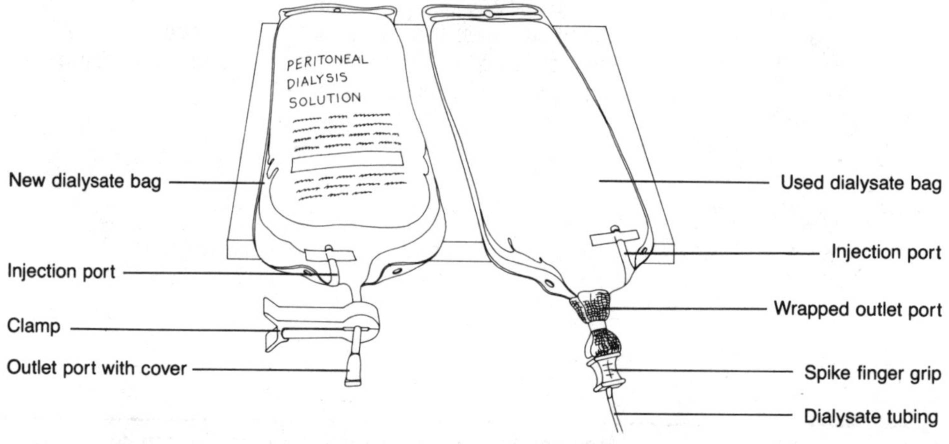

7

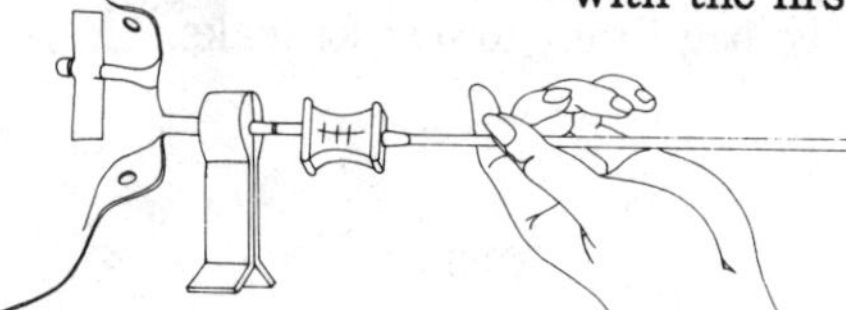

Remove the gauze pads from the outlet port tubing junction. Clamp the outlet port, lining up the clamp with the first step notch on the port.

8

Remove the blue covering from the outlet port of the new bag without touching the port. Now you are ready to transfer the tubing spike.

HOW TO PERFORM A CONTINUOUS AMBULATORY PERITONEAL DIALYSIS (C.A.P.D.) SOLUTION EXCHANGE—*continued*

9

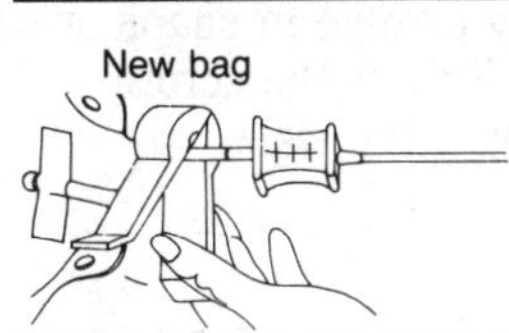

Grasp the finger grip on the tubing spike in the drainage-bag outlet port. With your free hand, hold the clamp on the outlet port. Twist and pull the spike to remove it from the port. Take care not to touch anything with the spike tip.

10

Immediately insert the spike into the outlet port of the new bag. Unclamp the outlet port.

11

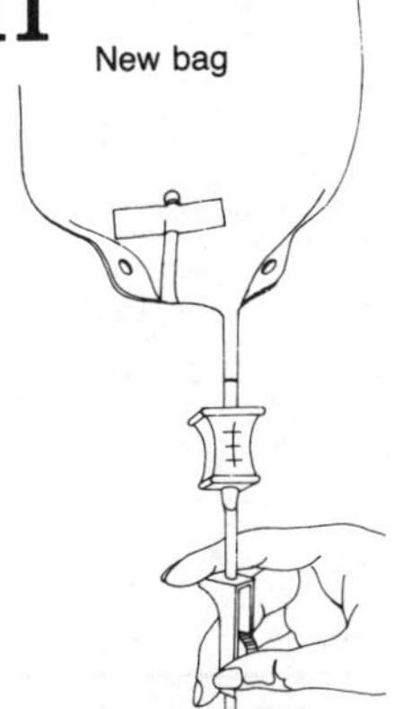

Hang the new bag on an I.V. pole. Then open the clamp to allow the dialysate to drain into your abdomen. After about 5 minutes, when almost all the dialysate has drained from the bag, close the clamp. Leaving a little fluid in the bag will make the bag easier to fold.

12

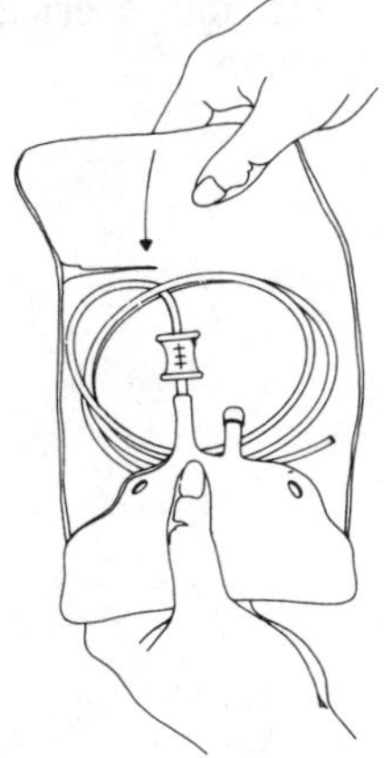

Remove the bag from the pole and place it in front of you. Fold over the spike-outlet port connection so it is centered on the bag. Coil the tubing over this connection. Then fold the other end of the bag over the connection and tubing and place the bag inside a pouch, if you use one. Put the pouch inside your clothing. If your physician has ordered a drainage sample, take the entire bag of fluid to the hospital laboratory for analysis. Otherwise, carefully empty the used dialysate into the toilet, and discard the empty bag in a trash can.

Patient-Teaching Aid

HOW TO EXAMINE YOUR TESTICLES

Dear Patient:
To help detect abnormalities early, you should examine your testicles once a month. Eventually, you will become familiar with them and will be able to recognize anything abnormal.

1

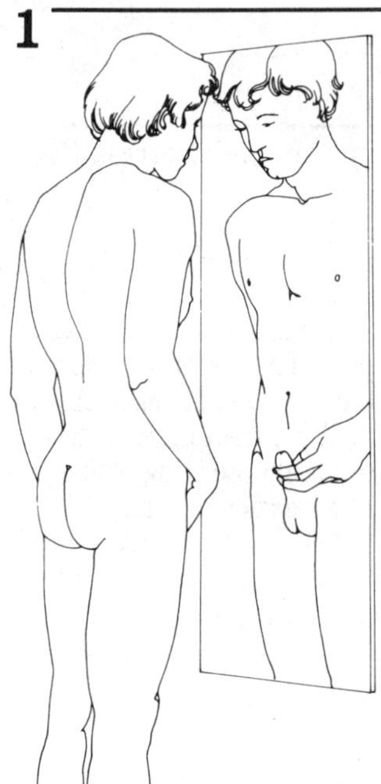

Here is how to examine your testicles: Remove your clothes and stand in front of a mirror. With one hand, lift your penis and check your scrotum (the sac containing your testicles) for any change in shape or size and for red, distended veins. Expect the scrotum's left side to hang slightly lower than the right.

2

Next you will feel your testicles for lumps and masses. First, locate the cordlike structure at the back of your testicles. This is called the epididymis. Your spermatic cord extends upward from the epididymis.

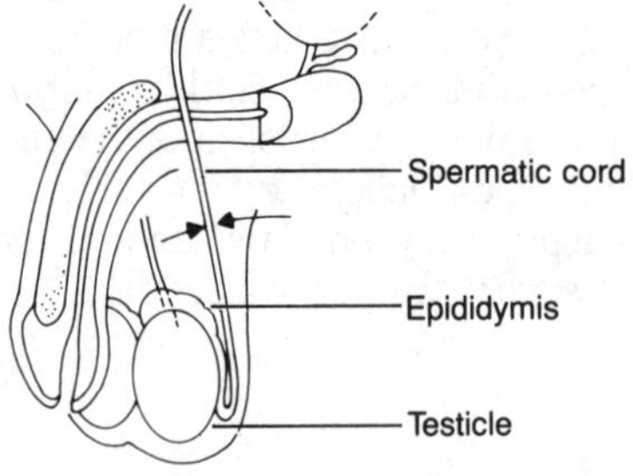

HOW TO EXAMINE YOUR TESTICLES—*continued*

3

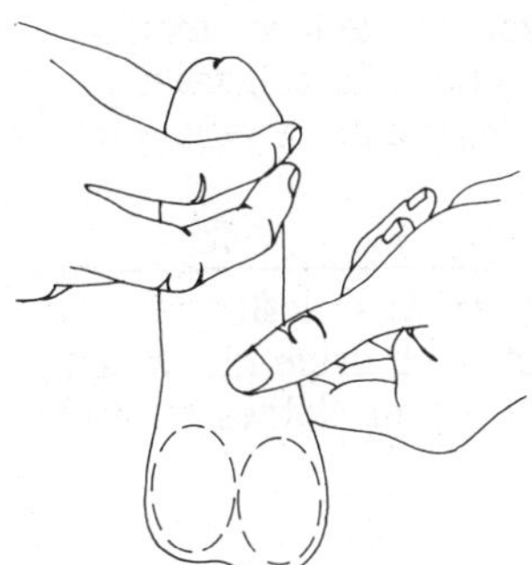
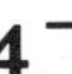

Gently squeeze the spermatic cord above your right testicle between the thumb and first two fingers of your right hand. Then, using the thumb and first two fingers of your left hand, examine the spermatic cord above your left testicle as shown here. Check for lumps and masses by squeezing along the entire length of the cords.

4

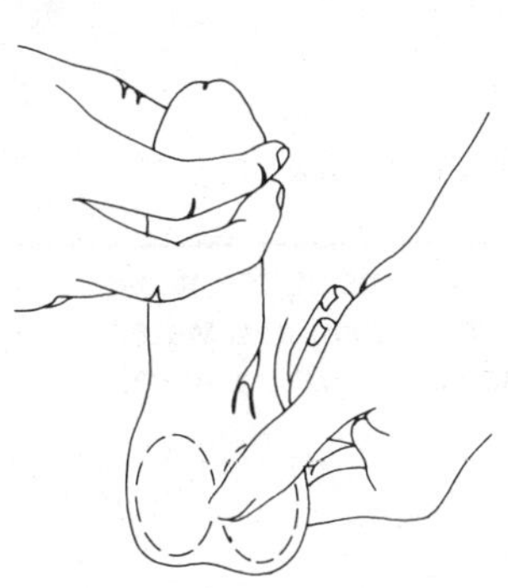

To examine your right testicle, place your right thumb on the front of the testicle and your index and middle fingers behind it. Gently press your thumb and fingers together. They should meet. Make sure you check your entire testicle. Then use your left hand to examine your left testicle in the same manner as shown here. Your testicles should feel smooth, rubbery, and slightly tender, and you should be able to move them.

If you notice any lumps, masses, or changes, notify your physician.

Patient-Teaching Aid

COLLECTING A URINE SPECIMEN (FOR THE FEMALE PATIENT)

Dear Patient:

The physician suspects you have a urinary tract infection. To confirm his diagnosis, he wants a specimen of your urine so it can be analyzed by the laboratory.

Carefully follow these instructions for collecting a urine specimen. Doing so will keep outside germs from contaminating the specimen.

1

First, make sure you have a clean washcloth and a towel, soap, water, and a clean-catch urine kit (which the nurse will give you). Remove your clothes from the waist down.

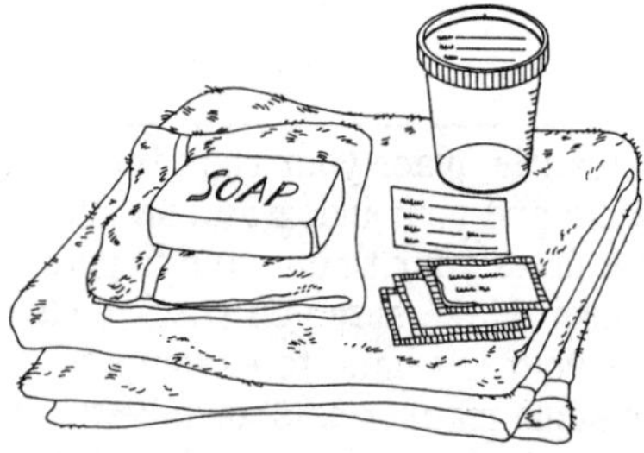

2

Wash your hands thoroughly. Then, using the washcloth, wash your genital area with soap and water. Rinse the area thoroughly and dry it with a towel.

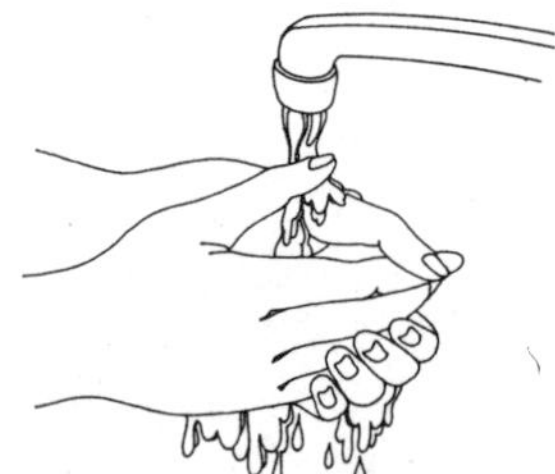

3

Next, place a clean paper towel on a nearby dry surface. Open the three disposable wipes from the clean-catch urine kit and place them on the paper towel.

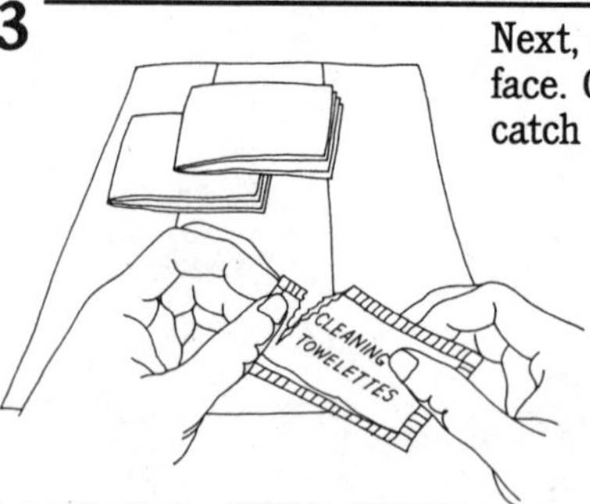

COLLECTING A URINE SPECIMEN (FOR THE FEMALE PATIENT)—*continued*

4

Remove the lid from the specimen cup. Place both the cup and the lid (flat side down) next to the wipes. Make sure you do not touch the inside of the lid or the cup.

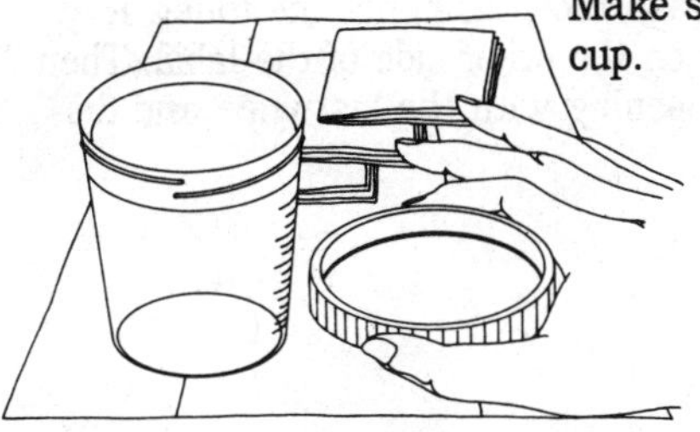

5

Sit as far back on the toilet as possible. Spread your legs apart.

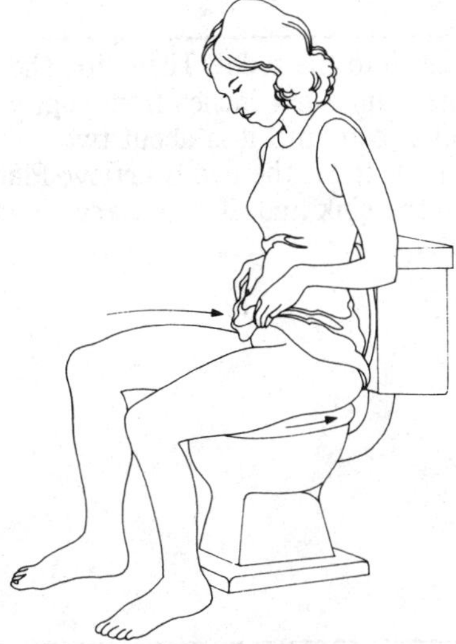

6

Using your fingertips, separate your labia. Keep the labia separated for the rest of the procedure.

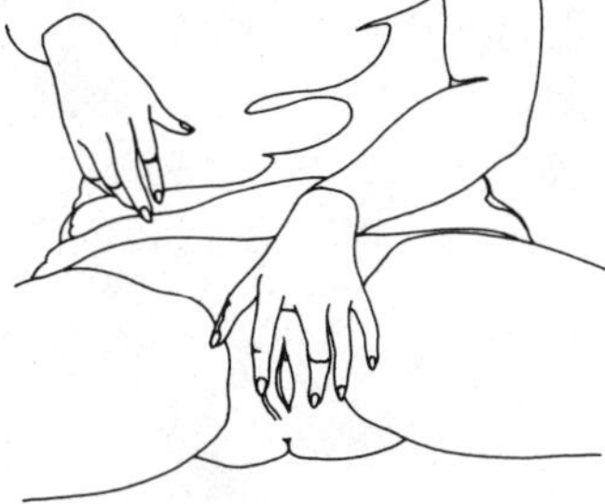

COLLECTING A URINE SPECIMEN (FOR THE FEMALE PATIENT)—*continued*

7

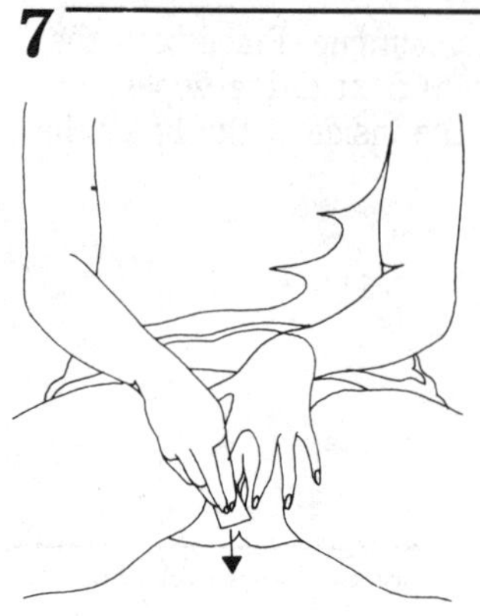

With the other hand, use a wipe to clean one side of your labia, using one top-to-bottom stroke. Discard the wipe in a covered trash receptacle, not the toilet. Repeat this procedure on the other side of the labia. Then clean the urethral opening with the last wipe and discard the wipe.

8

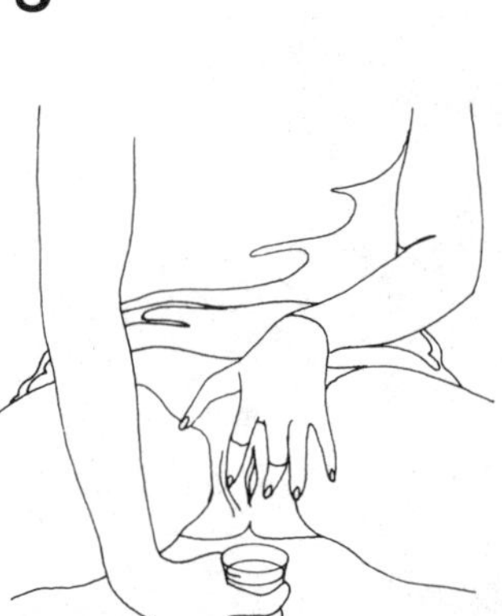

Urinate a small amount into the toilet. Then stop the flow. Hold the specimen cup a few inches from your urethra. Urinate into the cup until it is about two-thirds full. Be careful not to let the cup overflow. Place the filled cup back on the sink and, if necessary, finish urinating into the toilet.

9

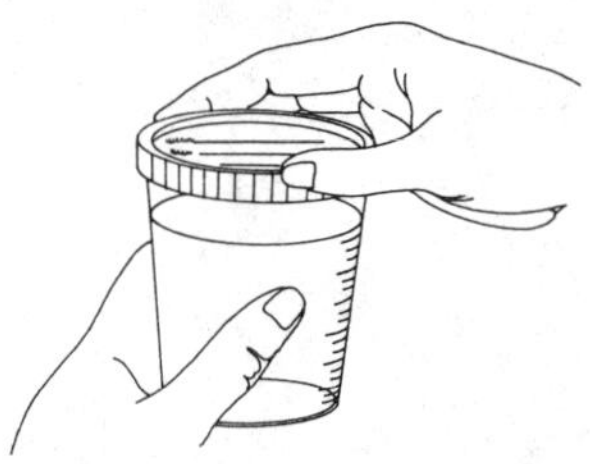

Place the lid on the cup, get dressed, and wash your hands thoroughly. Return the filled cup to the nurse.

Patient-Teaching Aid

PREVENTING URINARY TRACT INFECTIONS

Dear Patient:

To prevent recurrent urinary tract infections:

- Drink at least 10 glasses of fluid—especially water—daily. This helps flush bacteria from the urinary tract.
- Empty your bladder completely every 2 to 3 hours or as soon as you feel the urge to urinate.
- Wipe your perineum from front to back after urinating or defecating to prevent contamination with fecal material.
- Wear cotton underpants, which allow better ventilation and absorption than synthetic ones.
- Take showers instead of baths. If you must bathe, do not use bubble bath salts, bath oil, perfume, or other chemical irritants in the water. Also avoid using feminine deodorants, douches, and similar irritants.
- Urinate before and after intercourse.
- Eat an acid ash diet. Include meats, eggs, cheese, nuts, prunes, plums, whole grains, and especially cranberry juice in your daily intake. These foods acidify the urine, which helps decrease bacterial growth. Avoid foods containing baking soda or powder, such as most baked goods.
- Avoid coffee, tea, and alcohol, which tend to irritate the bladder.
- Seek medical help for any unusual vaginal discharge, which suggests infection.

Patient-Teaching Aid

COLLECTING A URINE SPECIMEN (FOR THE MALE PATIENT)

Dear Patient:

The physician suspects you have a urinary tract infection. To confirm his diagnosis, he wants a specimen of your urine cultured and analyzed by the laboratory.

Carefully follow these instructions for collecting a urine specimen. Doing so will keep you from contaminating it.

1

First, make sure you have a clean towel, soap, water, and a clean-catch urine kit (which the nurse will give you).

Wash your hands thoroughly. Place a clean paper towel on a nearby dry surface. Then open the three disposable wipes and place them on the paper towel.

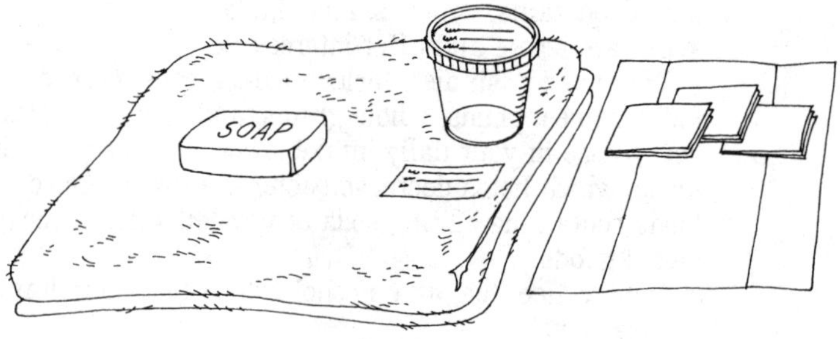

2

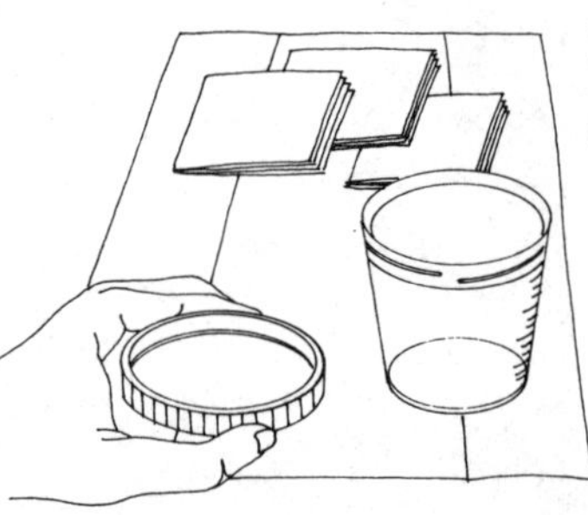

Remove the lid from the specimen cup. Place both the cup and the lid (flat side down) next to the wipes. Make sure you do not touch the inside of the lid or the cup.

3

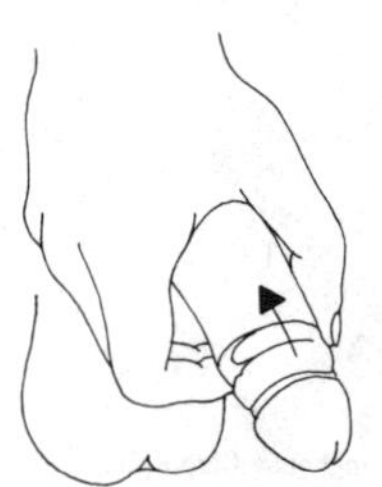

Prepare to urinate. (If you are uncircumcised, first pull back your foreskin.)

COLLECTING A URINE SPECIMEN (FOR THE MALE PATIENT)—*continued*

4

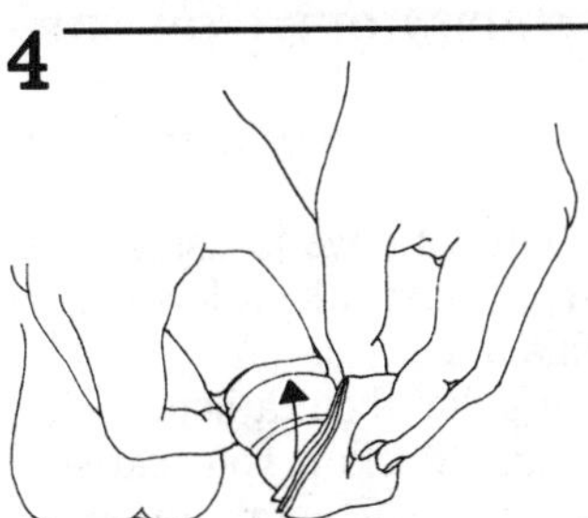

Using a wipe, clean the head of your penis. Clean from the urethral opening toward you, as shown. Then discard the wipe in a covered trash receptacle, not the toilet. Repeat this procedure with the other wipes.

5

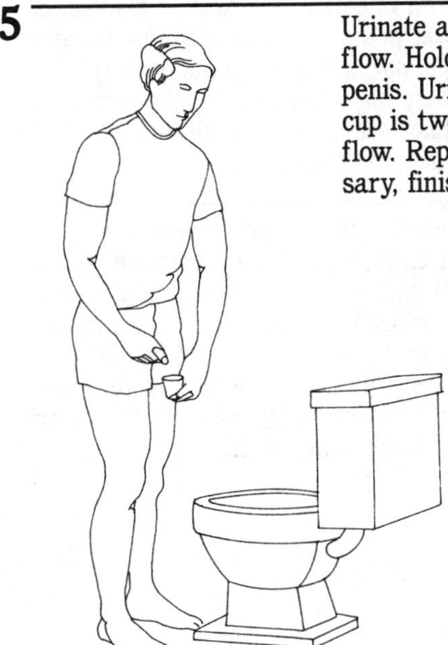

Urinate a small amount into the toilet, then stop the flow. Hold the specimen cup a few inches from your penis. Urinate into the cup until you are finished or the cup is two-thirds full. Be careful not to let the cup overflow. Replace the filled cup on the sink. Then, if necessary, finish urinating into the toilet.

6

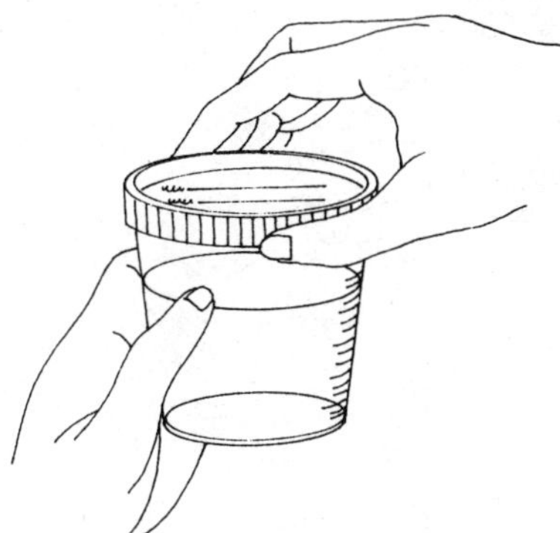

Put the lid on the cup. Remember to wash your hands thoroughly. Then return the cup to the nurse.

Patient-Teaching Aid

HOW TO CATHETERIZE YOURSELF USING CLEAN TECHNIQUE (FOR THE FEMALE PATIENT)

Dear Patient:

When you return home, you will not have to use sterile technique to catheterize yourself. Just take a few simple precautions outlined in this aid.

What is the most important point about a home self-catheterization program? To strictly follow your catheterization schedule. Otherwise, you will retain urine, which can lead to an infection, a stretched bladder, or urine leakage. Never postpone catheterization for any reason (for example, not having soap and water).

Cleanliness is very important, but on the rare occasion when you cannot wash, your bladder's natural resistance to bacteria will protect you.

1

To catheterize yourself using clean technique, you will need a rubber catheter, a clean washcloth, soap and water, a small package of water-soluble lubricant, and a plastic bag for used catheters. Also obtain a container for draining urine, if a toilet is not available or if you need to measure your urine. Make sure you have good lighting. Before catheterizing yourself, try to urinate. Remember to wash your hands.

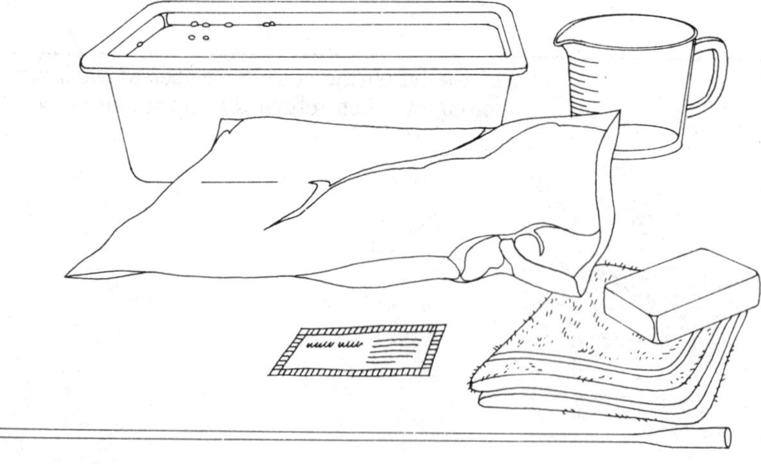

HOW TO CATHETERIZE YOURSELF USING CLEAN TECHNIQUE (FOR THE FEMALE PATIENT)—*continued*

2

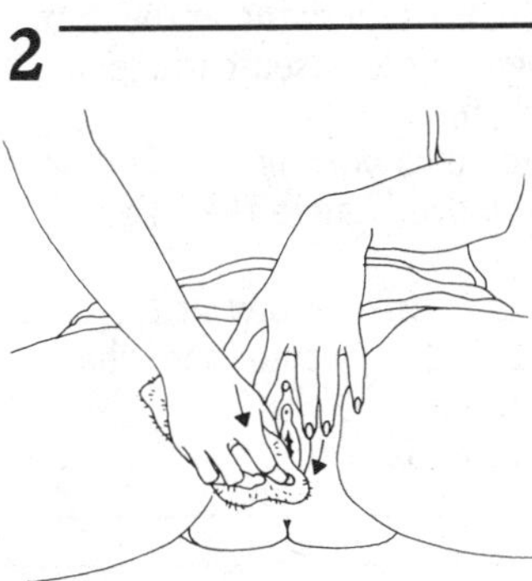

Now separate your vaginal folds with one hand. Use downward strokes with the washcloth to wash the area thoroughly.

3

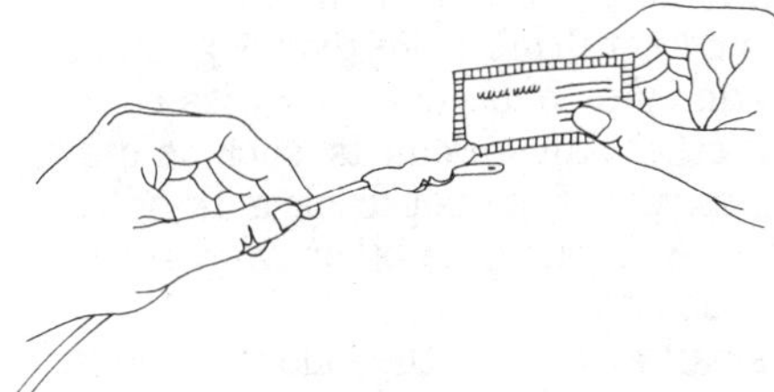

Lubricate the first 3″ (8 cm) of the catheter.

4

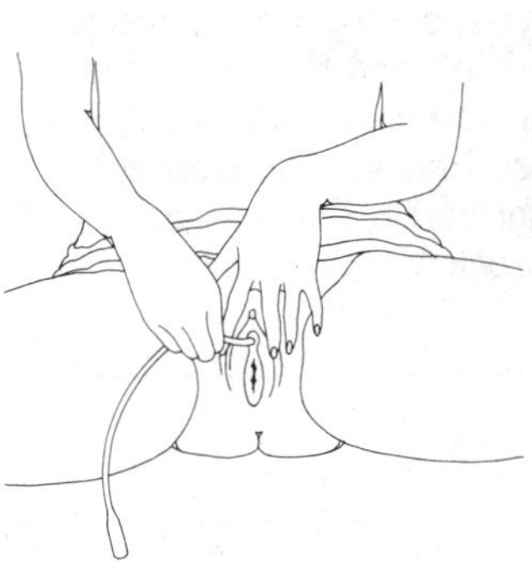

Hold the catheter as if it were a pencil or a dart, about ½″ from its tip. Keeping the vaginal folds separated, slowly insert the lubricated catheter about 3″ into your urethra. Press down with your abdominal muscles to empty your bladder. Allow all urine to drain through the catheter. When the urine stops draining, remove the catheter slowly. Dress yourself, and wash the catheter in warm, soapy water. Then rinse the catheter inside and out, and dry it with a clean towel. Place it in the plastic storage bag for used catheters.

Finally, if your physician requires it, write down the information about your urine, as indicated at the bottom of p. 324.

5

Buy a new supply of catheters each month or when the catheters become brittle. Use each catheter only once. When you have used all but the last catheter, boil the catheters for 20 minutes in a pan of water. Drain the water and store the catheters in the pan or in a freshly

HOW TO CATHETERIZE YOURSELF USING CLEAN TECHNIQUE (FOR THE FEMALE PATIENT)—*continued*

laundered towel. Each time you use a catheter, be sure to put it in the plastic storage bag for used catheters, not back with the clean catheters.

Here are instructions tailored to your needs. Follow them carefully. Be sure not to drink more than the amount indicated.

Catheterize yourself ________ times a day at ________.

Each day, drink at least ________ but no more than ________ 8-oz glasses of fluid.

The medication you are taking is:

____

____

This medication will help you control your bladder and prevent infection. Take all medication as directed.

Avoid calcium-rich and phosphorus-rich foods. This means that you should not drink more than 1 glass of milk or eat more than ½ oz of cheddar or Swiss cheese each day. If you eat other dairy products, such as other cheeses, ice cream, or yogurt, do not drink milk or eat hard cheese that day. And eat these other dairy products only in small amounts.

Also eat only a small amount of the following foods: organ meats (for example, liver), shellfish, cereals, beans, dried fruits, and dark green vegetables (for example, kale, brussels sprouts, and okra). Limit eggs to one each day.

The physician may want you to keep a daily record of the amount of liquid you drink and the amount of urine you excrete. Each time you drink any liquid, write down the amount. Each time you catheterize yourself, write down the information the physician wants by following the form below.

Amount of urine ________________________

This is (check one):

☐ increase ☐ decrease ☐ no change

Color ________________________

Odor ________________________

Clarity ________________________

Particles ________________________

Blood ________________________

Patient-Teaching Aid

HOW TO CATHETERIZE YOURSELF USING CLEAN TECHNIQUE (FOR THE MALE PATIENT)

Dear Patient:

When you return home, you will not have to use sterile technique to catheterize yourself. Just take a few simple precautions outlined in this aid.

What is the most important point about a home self-catheterization program? To strictly follow your catheterization schedule. Otherwise, you will retain urine, which can lead to an infection, a stretched bladder, or urine leakage. Never postpone catheterization for any reason (for example, not having soap and water). Cleanliness is very important, but on the rare occasion when you cannot wash, your bladder's natural resistance to bacteria will protect you.

1

To catheterize yourself using clean technique, you will need a rubber catheter, clean washcloths, soap and water, a small package of water-soluble lubricant, a paper towel (not shown), and a plastic bag. Also obtain a container for draining urine, if a toilet is not available or if you need to measure your urine.

Before catheterizing yourself, try to urinate. Now arrange your clothing so it is out of your way. Remember to wash your hands.

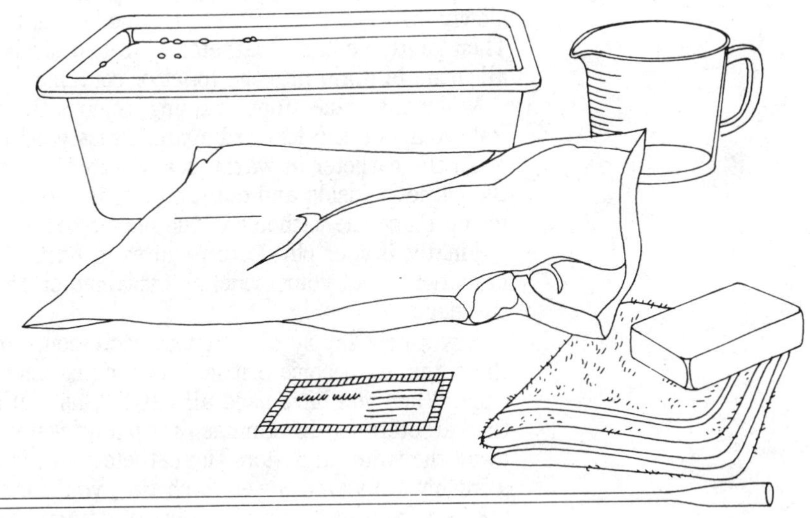

HOW TO CATHETERIZE YOURSELF USING CLEAN TECHNIQUE (FOR THE MALE PATIENT)—*continued*

2

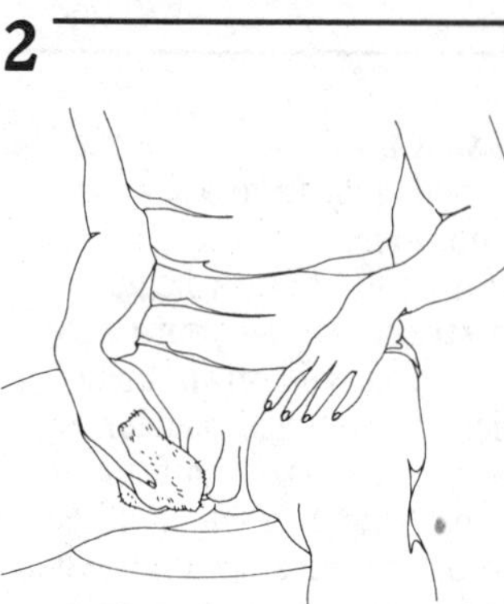

If you are uncircumcised, pull back your foreskin and keep it back throughout the catheterization. Then wash the end of your penis thoroughly with soap and water, as shown.

3

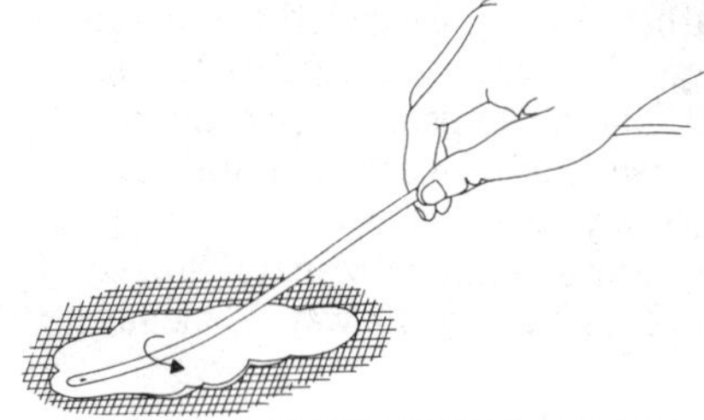

Squeeze some lubricant on the paper towel and lubricate the first 7″ to 10″ (18 to 25 cm) of the catheter.

4

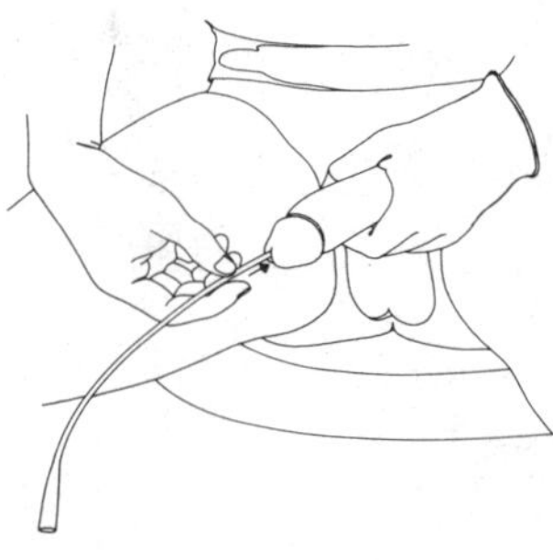

Then hold your penis at a right angle to your body. Grasp the catheter as you would a pencil or dart, and slowly insert it 7″ to 10″, until urine begins to flow. Then gently push the catheter 1″ (3 cm) farther. Allow all urine to drain into the toilet or container.

When the urine stops draining, remove the catheter. Pull your foreskin forward again. Dress yourself, and wash the catheter in warm, soapy water. Then rinse the catheter inside and out, and dry it with a clean towel. Place the catheter in the plastic bag.

Finally, if your physician requires it, write down information about your urine, as explained on the opposite page.

Buy a new supply of catheters each month or when the catheters become brittle. Use each catheter only once. When you have used all but the last catheter, boil the catheters for 20 minutes in a pan of water. Drain away the water and store the catheters in the pan or in a freshly laundered towel. Each time you use a catheter, be sure to put it in your plastic storage bag for used catheters, not back with the clean catheters.

HOW TO CATHETERIZE YOURSELF USING CLEAN TECHNIQUE (FOR THE MALE PATIENT)—*continued*

5

Here are instructions tailored to your needs. Follow them carefully. Be particularly cautious not to drink more than the amount indicated.

Catheterize yourself ______ times a day at ______.

Each day, drink at least ______ but no more than ______ 8-oz glasses of fluid.

The medication you are taking is:

____

____

This medication will help you control your bladder and prevent infection. Take all medication as directed.

Avoid calcium-rich and phosphorus-rich foods. This means you should not drink more than 1 glass of milk or eat more than ½ oz of cheddar or Swiss cheese each day. If you eat other dairy products, such as other cheeses, ice cream, or yogurt, do not drink milk or eat hard cheese that day. And eat these other dairy products only in small amounts.

Also eat only a small amount of the following foods: organ meats (for example, liver), shellfish, cereals, beans, dried fruits, and dark green vegetables (for example, kale, brussels sprouts, and okra). Limit eggs to one each day.

The physician may want you to keep a daily record of the amount of liquid you drink and the amount of urine you excrete. Each time you drink any liquid, write down the amount. Each time you catheterize yourself, write down the information the physician wants by following the form below.

Amount of urine ______________________

This is (check one):

☐ increase ☐ decrease ☐ no change

Color ______________________

Odor ______________________

Clarity ______________________

Particles ______________________

Blood ______________________

Patient-Teaching Aid

HOW TO CARE FOR A FOLEY CATHETER CONNECTED TO A LEG BAG

Dear Patient:

Your physician feels you can return home, but your Foley catheter will have to stay in your bladder for the next few weeks. This rubber tube allows for continuous urine drainage, so you will not need to use a bedpan or toilet. A balloon on one end of the tube holds it inside your bladder.

1

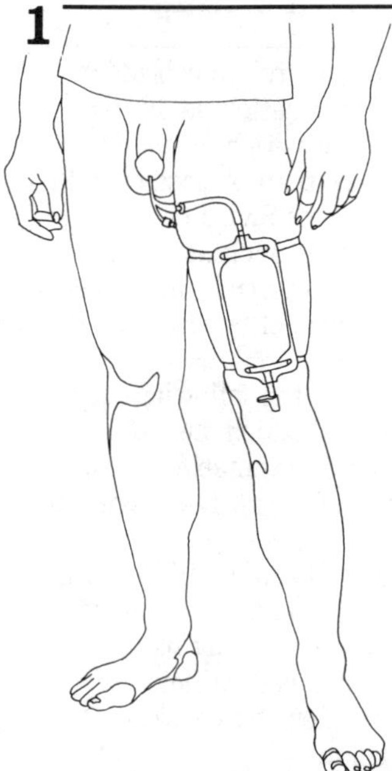

As you can see, your Foley catheter is connected to drainage tubing, which leads to a drainage bag. During the day, you will use a leg bag that straps around your thigh, as shown here. At night, you will connect the Foley catheter to a closed-system (hospital-type) drainage bag. Because the leg bag is smaller than the closed-system bag, it allows you to move around more easily. However, you must empty it every 3 to 4 hours.

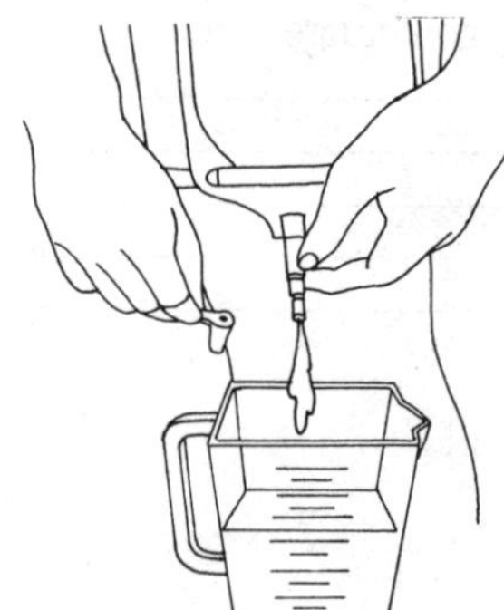

To empty the leg bag, first wash your hands. Then remove the stopper and drain all the urine. If requested by your physician, drain the urine into a measuring container, so you can record the amount. Do not touch the drain port with your fingers or with the container.

HOW TO CARE FOR A FOLEY CATHETER CONNECTED TO A LEG BAG—*continued*

3

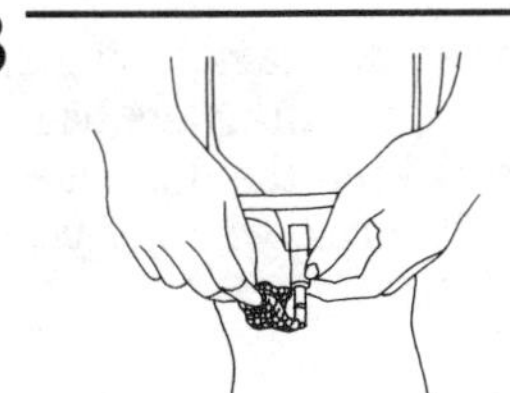

After the urine has drained completely, swab the drain port and the stopper with a povidone-iodine swab, as shown. Replace the stopper.

4

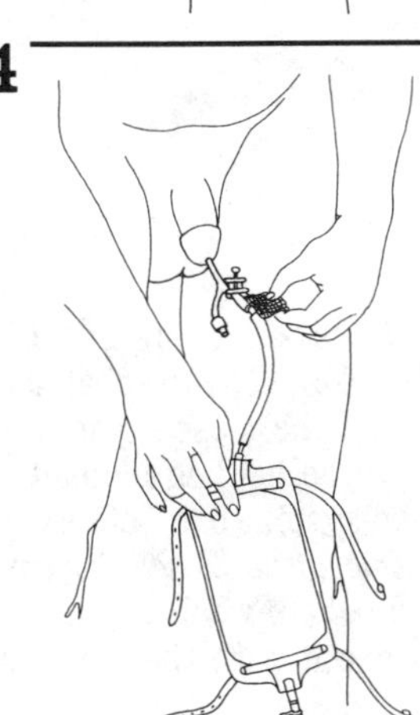

Before you go to bed, replace the leg bag with a closed-system drainage bag. Because the closed-system bag holds more urine, you will not have to worry about emptying the drainage bag during the night.

To replace the bag, first empty your leg bag. Now clamp the catheter and swab the connection between the catheter and the leg bag with povidone-iodine, as shown. Then disconnect the leg bag, and connect the closed-system drainage tubing and bag. Finally, unclamp the catheter.

5

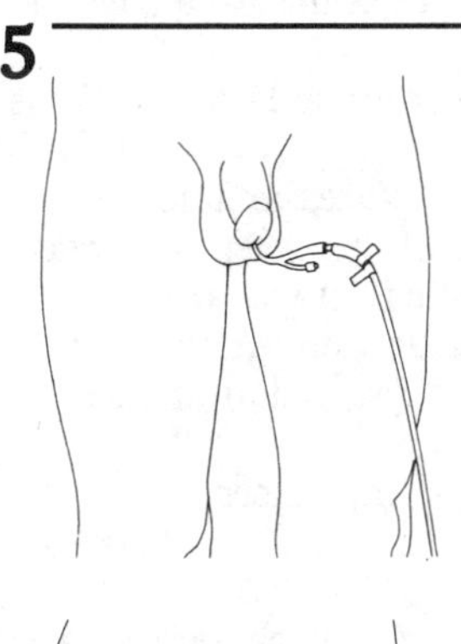

Now decide which side of the bed you want the drainage bag to hang from. Tape the drainage tubing to your thigh on that side, using nonallergenic tape. Shave your skin in that area, if needed. Leave some slack in the line so that you will not pull on the catheter when you move your leg. If you are a man, tape the drainage tubing to the inner thigh, opposite the base of your penis, as shown at left (top).

If you are a woman, tape the drainage tubing to the inner thigh below the vaginal area, as shown at left (bottom).

After you have disconnected the leg bag, wash it in soap and water. Then mix white vinegar and water in these proportions: 1¼ cups of vinegar to 2 qt of water. Rinse the bag with this solution to reduce urine odor.

HOW TO CARE FOR A FOLEY CATHETER CONNECTED TO A LEG BAG—*continued*

6

When you get into bed, arrange the drainage tubing so it does not kink or loop. Then hang the drainage bag on the side of your bed. Be sure to keep the drainage bag below your bladder level at all times, whether you are lying, sitting, or standing.

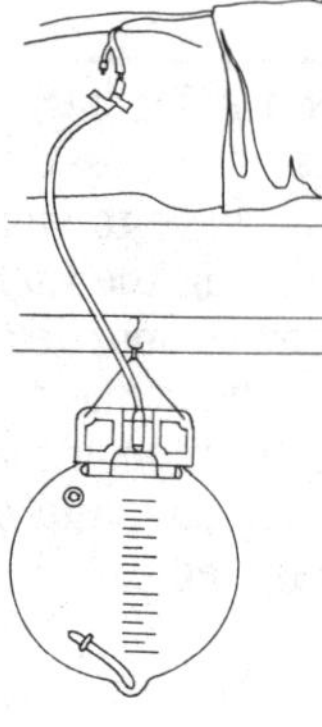

When you are ready to reconnect the leg bag in the morning, empty the closed-system bag. Then repeat the steps you took when you connected the closed-system bag last night. But, this time, use the leg bag instead. Do not forget to empty the closed-system bag before you disconnect it. (See *How to Empty the Closed-System Drainage Bag.*) When you have finished, wash out the bag with soap and water, and rinse it with the vinegar and water solution.

NOTE: You can reuse both types of drainage bags for up to 1 month.

To care for your Foley catheter properly, follow these guidelines:

- Use soap and water to wash the area around the catheter twice each day. This will help keep the area from becoming irritated or infected. (If you are a woman, wash your vaginal area as well.) Also wash your rectal area at least twice a day and after each bowel movement.
- Never pull on your catheter for any reason.
- Drink between _______ and _______ 8-oz. glasses of fluid each day.
- Take the medicine prescribed by your physician, as instructed on the label.
- Contact the physician immediately if you have any problems, such as urine leakage around the catheter, pain and fullness in your abdomen, scanty urine flow, or blood or particles in your urine.

Return to the physician on the following date ______ to have your catheter removed.

IMPORTANT: Don't try to remove the catheter yourself.

Patient-Teaching Aid

HOW TO EMPTY THE CLOSED-SYSTEM DRAINAGE BAG

Dear Patient:
To keep bacteria out of your drainage system, empty your drainage bag using the cleanest possible method.

1

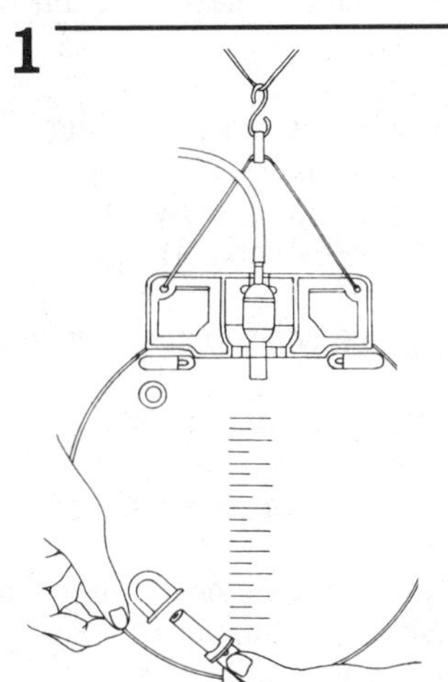

To do this, first unclamp the drain tube and remove it from its sleeve, without touching its tip.

2

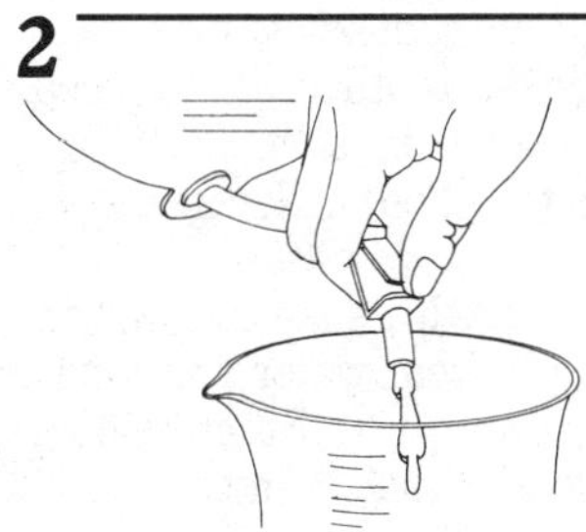

Then let the urine drain into the toilet. Or drain the urine into a measuring container, if required.

IMPORTANT: Do not let the drain tube touch the toilet or container.

3

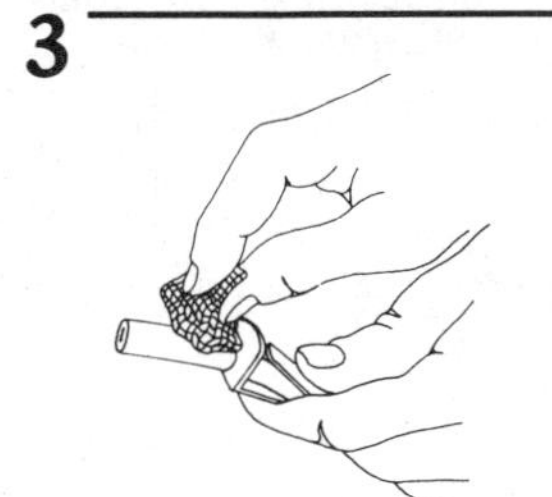

When the bag is completely empty, swab the end of the drain tube with povidone-iodine solution. Reclamp the tube and reinsert it into the sleeve of the drainage bag. Do not let anyone else empty your drainage bag, unless one member of your family performs your catheter care. If your physician has requested it, write down the amount of urine drained.

Patient-Teaching Aid

CARING FOR YOUR CONDOM CATHETER

Dear Patient:

When you go home from the hospital, you will need to care for your condom catheter. Use these illustrations when applying it. In addition, remember these very important points:

- Use a clean condom catheter every day.
- Wash and dry your hands before and after handling your condom catheter, tubing, or leg bag.
- Gently but thoroughly wash, rinse, and dry your penis before putting on the condom catheter. Do this again after removing it.
- To keep your urine flowing properly, keep your penis positioned downward.
- Check your penis every 2 hours for swelling or unusual color. If your penis feels uncomfortable or does not look normal, remove the condom catheter and call your physician.
- Also call your physician if you feel pain or burning when you urinate, feel the urge to urinate very frequently, smell an unpleasant odor from your urine, or see blood or pus in your urine.
- Do not go to bed with your condom catheter in place—you may injure yourself without knowing it. Ask your nurse or physician to suggest another way to keep urine from wetting your clothing or bed sheets.
- Empty your leg bag every 3 to 4 hours. Never allow it to fill to the top.
- Twice a day, wash your leg bag with soap and water, and rinse it with a solution made from water and vinegar. (Use one part vinegar to seven parts water.) Do not use the same leg bag for longer than 1 month.

1

Do you know what your catheter and leg bag will look like? If not, study this illustration. Then apply the catheter and leg bag according to the instructions in the following steps.

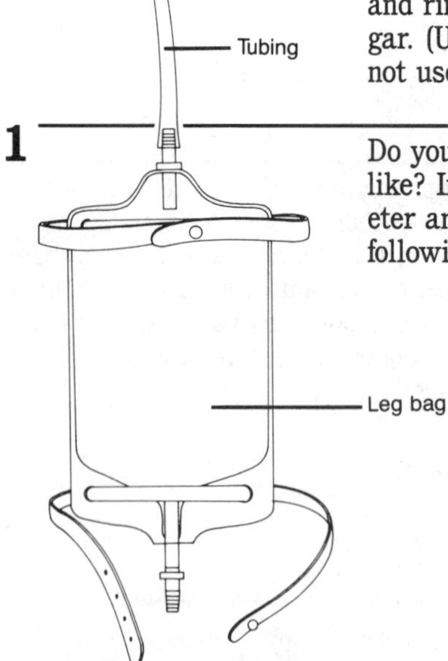

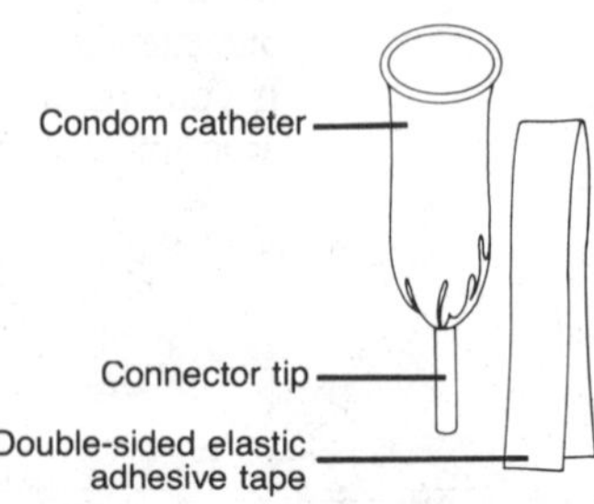

CARING FOR YOUR CONDOM CATHETER—*continued*

2

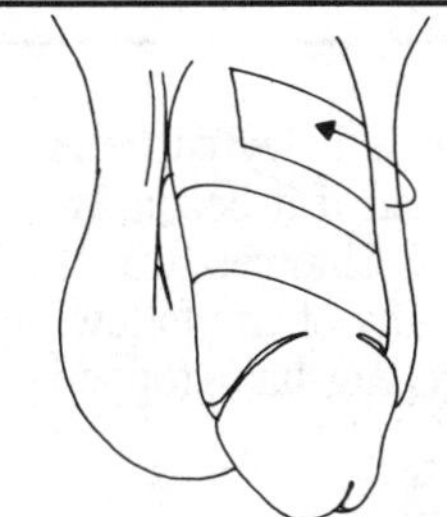

After washing, rinsing, and drying your penis, remove the covering from both sides of the double-sided elastic adhesive tape. Starting at the base of the penis, wind the tape in a spiral fashion (see arrow). Do not let the edges of the tape overlap at any point. IMPORTANT: Do not stretch the tape while applying it, or you will apply it too tightly. Also never apply tape in a circle around your penis, or you may cut off your blood circulation.

3

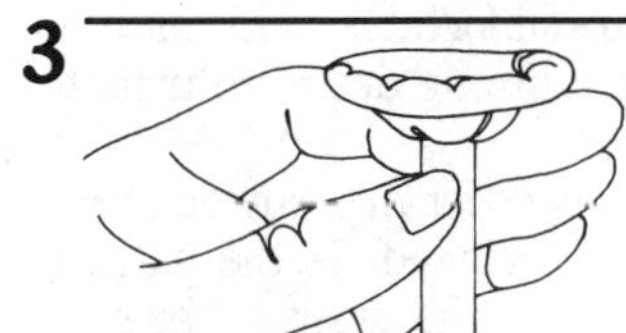

Now you are ready to apply the condom. Make sure the balloonlike part is tightly rolled up to the edge of the connector tip, as shown here.

4

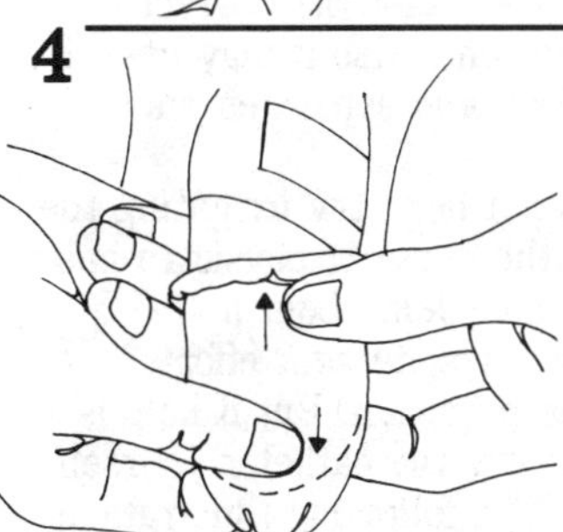

Place the sheath on the end of your penis. Leave about ½″ (1.3 cm) of space between the tip of your penis and the connector tip.

Unroll the condom along your penis, as shown here. Gently stretch the penis as you do so. Then, when the condom is fully unrolled, gently press it against the penis, so it sticks to the adhesive tape.

5

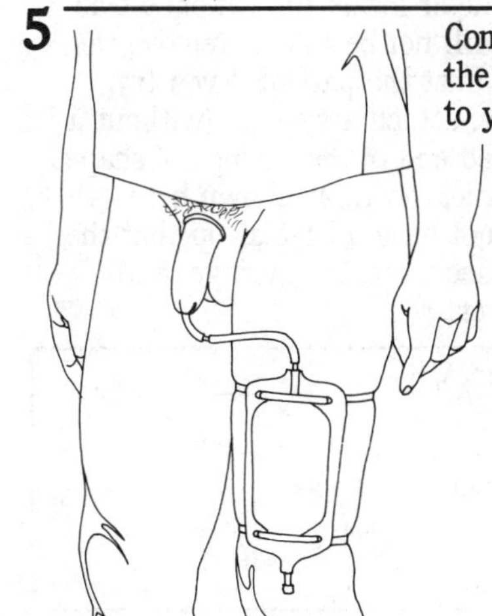

Connect one end of the tubing to the connector tip and the other end to the leg bag. Finally, strap the leg bag to your thigh.

Patient-Teaching Aid

WHAT TO DO ABOUT CATHETER PROBLEMS

Dear Patient:

Since someone in your family has a Foley catheter in place, you need to know how to tell if it becomes blocked—and what to do about it. Chances are, the catheter is blocked if you notice any of the following:

- The urine level in the drainage bag has stopped rising.
- The bed is wet with urine.
- The patient is restless or uncomfortable, with pain in his lower abdomen, or he has a strong desire to urinate (but cannot).

What should you do? First, look for any obvious reason for a blockage. Is the tubing kinked? Is the patient lying on the catheter or tubing? Is the drainage bag above his bladder level instead of below it? Correct these problems, if they are present. Also it may help if the patient changes his position and separates his thighs.

If doing these things does not help, try irrigating the catheter. But irrigate only if the nurse or physician has taught you how and you feel confident about it.

Is the catheter still blocked, despite your efforts? Contact your visiting nurse or physician. But if help is not immediately available, remove the catheter yourself, as the nurse has taught you. The following illustrations will remind you what steps to take.

As you know, you must first deflate the balloon that is on the end of the catheter inside the patient's bladder. If you do not, you will not be able to remove the catheter—and you will hurt the patient if you try.

To deflate the balloon, attach a syringe (without a needle) to the unattached end of the tubing's Y-shaped portion (called the inflation port), as shown here. (If the inflation port does not have a special tip that the syringe fits into, put a needle on the syringe, and puncture the inflation port.)

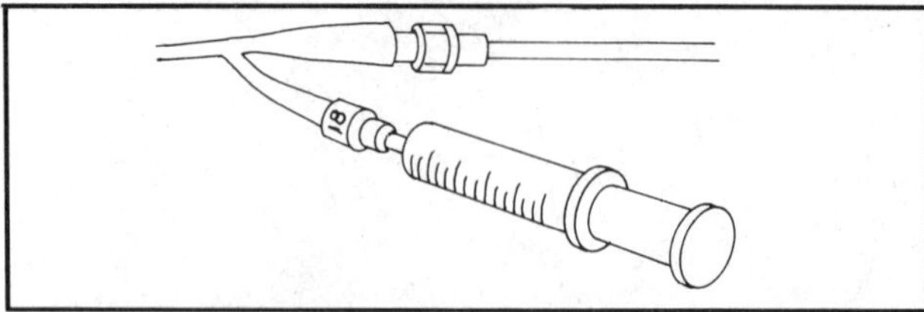

Gently pull back on the syringe plunger. The water in the balloon will flow into the syringe, deflating the balloon.

WHAT TO DO ABOUT CATHETER PROBLEMS—*continued*

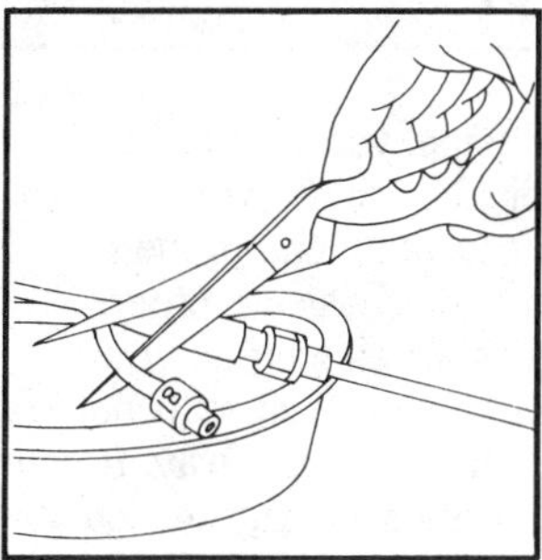

If you have trouble with this method, here is another way to deflate the balloon. (But do not use this way unless the first method does not work, because it destroys the catheter.) Place a small basin under the inflation port to protect the bed. Then, using scissors, cut the catheter in two just above the inflation port, as shown. Now the water in the balloon will escape into the basin.

When the balloon is deflated, pull gently on the catheter to remove it. IMPORTANT: If the catheter does not come out easily, do not force it. Wait for a nurse or physician to help you.

Keep the patient dry and comfortable until help arrives. If you cannot contact your nurse or physician, take the patient to a hospital emergency department.

Preventing problems

To prevent catheter blockage and other possible problems, you and the patient must follow these important directions:

- Never pull on the catheter. Disconnect it from the drainage tubing only to clean the bag.
- Always keep the drainage bag below the patient's bladder level.
- Empty the drainage bag every 8 hours.
- Twice a day, use soap and water to wash the patient's skin around the catheter. After washing his skin, dry it gently but thoroughly.
- If the patient is a woman, use a front-to-back motion for washing and drying. This way, you will not contaminate the catheter and her urinary tract with germs from her rectal area.
- Once a day, wash the drainage tubing and bag with soap and water. Rinse it with a solution made from water and white vinegar. (Use one part vinegar to seven parts water.)
- Unless the physician gives you different directions, the patient should drink at least 1½ qt (1.4 liters) of liquid each day. This simple precaution will help prevent bladder infection.

Patient-Teaching Aid

GOING HOME AFTER RENAL TRANSPLANT SURGERY

Dear Patient:

Now that you are ready to go home, you will need to follow these instructions to speed your recovery and to help ensure that your new kidney functions properly.

• Take medications exactly as your physician orders. You must take these medications for as long as you have your transplanted kidney, so your body will not reject it. Never skip a dose or alter it in any way. If you forget or cannot take your medication for any reason, call your physician at once. Follow these special instructions: ______________________________
____
____
____
____
____
____
____

Remember to take an antacid immediately before taking your medication. Avoid taking nonprescription drugs, such as aspirin or Tylenol, unless ordered by your physician.

• Avoid overeating, even if you find your appetite has increased because of the medication you are taking. Excessive weight can be harmful. For this reason, eat three well-balanced, calorie-controlled meals each day. Include high-protein foods, such as eggs, lean meats, fish, cheese, and skim milk. Avoid foods high in fat or carbohydrates. If you must snack, choose low-calorie, nutritious foods, such as fresh fruit.

• Drink four 8-oz glasses of fluid each day, unless your physician directs otherwise.

• Take your temperature every morning as soon as you awake. If your temperature goes above 100° F. (37.8° C.), call your physician.

• Weigh yourself every morning before dressing. If you gain more than 3 lb (1.4 kg) from one day to the next, call your physician.

• Take your blood pressure twice each day, or ask a family member to take it for you. To ensure an accurate measurement, take it at the same times of day. Be sure you are in the same position each time, either sitting, lying, or standing. Remember to rest for at least 5 minutes before taking the measurement so your blood pressure can stabilize.

• Measure and record the amount of urine you produce

GOING HOME AFTER RENAL TRANSPLANT SURGERY—*continued*

in a 24-hour period. To do this, urinate into a container. Measure and record the amount. Then discard the urine. If you urinate during the night, measure this, too. At the end of 24 hours, add up the amount of urine you produced. Notify the physician if your output is below 20 oz (600 ml) during any 24-hour period.

• In a notebook, record your daily temperature, weight, blood pressure, and urine output. Bring this record with you to the physician.

• See your physician as frequently as he directs. Keep each appointment and follow your physician's instructions exactly. Your next appointment is scheduled on ____________ at ________ o'clock.

You will need eye examinations every 6 months to check for glaucoma and cataracts. Before you schedule a visit to the dentist, contact your physician.

• Wait 6 weeks after surgery before engaging in sexual intercourse. Pregnancy poses an additional risk to your new kidney, so if you are female, practice a reliable birth-control method.

• Wait at least 2 weeks after returning home before you drive a car. Avoid wearing seat belts that may press on your new kidney. If you must wear a seat belt, wear it loosely.

• Exercise moderately. Begin slowly and increase the amount of exercise gradually. During the first 3 months after surgery, avoid excessive bending, heavy lifting, or contact sports, such as football.

• Avoid large groups of people during the first 3 months after surgery, to decrease the risk of contracting a contagious disease. Remember, your resistance to infection has been lowered by the medications you are taking.

Finally, call your physician immediately if you notice any of these signs:

• redness, swelling, warmth, or tenderness over the new kidney
• fever over 100° F. (37.8° C.)
• decreased urine output
• blood pressure above ____________________
• sudden weight gain of more than 3 lb (1.4 kg), or puffy eyelids and swollen ankles
• general feeling of uneasiness.

Patient-Teaching Aid

AFTER PROSTATE SURGERY: HOW TO CARE FOR YOURSELF

Dear Patient:

To speed your recovery after prostate surgery, observe these precautions:

- Restrict your activities. For example, take only short walks, and climb no more than two flights of stairs at a time. Ride in a car as little as possible during the first 3 weeks, because vehicle motion may strain your bladder. Do not lift heavy objects for at least 3 weeks.
- Drink 12 to 14 8-oz glasses of liquid each day, unless the physician orders otherwise.
- Do not become alarmed if you see blood in your urine during the first 2 weeks after surgery. If you do see blood, drink some fluid and lie down. The next time you urinate, the bleeding should decrease. If it does not, call your physician. If your urine stream diminishes or if you cannot urinate at all, notify your physician. Do not worry if you lose some control over urination, if you feel pain, or if you have a frequent need to urinate. These symptoms will disappear with time.
- To strengthen your perineal muscles, perform this exercise: Press your buttocks together. Hold this position a few seconds, then relax. Repeat 10 times in succession, ________ times a day.
- Do not strain to have a bowel movement. If you are constipated, take a laxative. Do not give yourself an enema or place anything—for example, a suppository—into your rectum for 4 weeks after surgery.
- Avoid sexual activity for 4 weeks after surgery, because it can cause bleeding. When you do engage in sex, most of the sperm will go into your bladder instead of out your penis. This will cause your urine to become cloudy and will decrease, though not end, your fertility. You will still experience orgasm.
- At your next physician's appointment, ask when you can return to work. This will vary, depending on your health, your job, and the type of surgery you have had.

8 Gynecologic Disorders

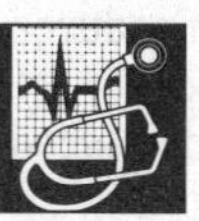

Patient-learner data base*

Areas of potential knowledge deficit

Anatomy/physiology of female reproductive system
Menstrual cycle
Contraception
Personal hygiene
Sexually transmitted diseases
Gynecologic disorder: Definition, causes, symptoms
Infertility: Definition, causes, symptoms
Treatment of gynecologic/reproductive disorders
—Medications
—Surgery
—Guidelines for daily living
—Prevention of complications
—Coping strategies (both patient and family)
—Other treatments used

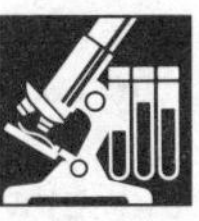

Explaining diagnostic tests

LAPAROSCOPY

Patient objectives	*Teaching plan content*
1 Define laparoscopy.	Laparoscopy is a procedure that permits inspection of the internal pelvic organs with an illuminated endoscope, an instrument used for looking into body cavities. (An illustration can be used to demonstrate the location of these organs in the body.)

* A general assessment should be done for all patients. For general asessment guidelines, see Chapter 1, Principles of Patient Teaching.

2 State the purpose of laparoscopy.

Laparoscopy is performed to diagnose a disorder or, in combination with a surgical procedure, to correct a problem. Indications for laparoscopy include evaluation of female infertility or pelvic pain, staging and follow-up of pelvic cancer, and detection of gynecologic disorders. It is also used during tubal ligation (tying the fallopian tubes) for sterilization.

3 Describe the procedure used in laparoscopy.

Just before the procedure, the patient will be given a general anesthetic.
—She will then be placed in the lithotomy position (supine, legs supported in stirrups, buttocks at the edge of the table). The physician will perform a bimanual examination to detect any abnormalities.
—The cervix will be stabilized with a clamplike instrument called a tenaculum.
—A small incision will be made at the lower rim of the navel or umbilicus.
—A special large-gauge needle will be inserted into the abdominal cavity, and 2 to 5 liters of carbon dioxide or nitrous oxide will flow into the peritoneal cavity. This distends the abdominal wall, providing an organ-free space for insertion of the trocar (a pointed rod that fits inside a tube).
—The trocar and a sleeve will be passed through the incision into the peritoneal cavity. The trocar then will be removed, and the endoscope passed through the sleeve.
—A fiberoptic light source will be attached to the endoscope for viewing the pelvic organs.
—Ancillary instruments, such as scissors, forceps, or probes, may be introduced through a suprapubic incision. In this case, the patient will have two small incisions.
—The patient should know who will perform the procedure and where it will be done. It takes 15 to 30 minutes.

4 Explain patient guidelines for laparoscopy.

These are the patient guidelines for laparoscopy:
—The patient should fast from midnight the night before the procedure or for at least 8 hours before surgery.
—She should know whether the procedure will be done during an outpatient visit or after overnight hospitalization.
—She will be asked to sign a consent form prior to the procedure. If she has any questions, she should ask them before signing the consent form.

—Following the procedure, she will be asked to walk around her room once to make sure she is fully recovered from the anesthetic.
—Some abdominal and/or shoulder pain is normal. It should disappear within 24 to 36 hours. Aspirin or Tylenol may be taken, as ordered, for pain.
—She may gradually resume her usual diet.
—She should restrict her activity for 4 to 7 days after the procedure, as ordered.
—She should return to her physician for a follow-up visit, as ordered.

PAPANICOLAOU TEST (Pap test, Pap smear)

Patient objectives	*Teaching plan content*
1 Define Pap test.	A Pap test is an analysis of secretions and cells taken from the cervix and vagina. (An illustration can be used to demonstrate the location of these structures in the body.)
2 State the purpose of a Pap test.	A Pap test is performed to detect malignant cells or inflammatory tissue changes, to assess response to chemotherapy, or to detect viral, fungal, and (occasionally) parasitic invasion.
3 Describe the procedure used in a Pap test.	Just before the procedure, the patient will be asked to disrobe from the waist down. She will then lie on the examination table, her feet in stirrups. A sheet will be provided to drape her. —A speculum will be placed in her vagina, and the blades will be spread. —Secretions from deep in her vagina and from her cervical canal will be obtained and applied to glass slides with a fixative. —After removal of the speculum, a bimanual examination will be performed. —The patient should know who will perform the test and where and when it will be done. It takes 5 to 15 minutes.
4 Explain patient guidelines for a Pap test.	These are the patient guidelines for a Pap test: —The patient should schedule the test preferably 5 to 6 days before or after her menstrual period. It should never be done during her menses, which will alter test results.

—She should not douche or insert vaginal medications for 24 hours before the examination, since doing so can alter the test results.
—She may experience discomfort, but no pain, when the speculum is inserted, and she should lie still during the procedure.
—She should return for her next Pap test as ordered.

HYSTEROSALPINGOGRAPHY

Patient objectives	*Teaching plan content*
1 **Define hysterosalpingography.**	Hysterosalpingography is a radiologic examination of the uterine cavity, the fallopian tubes, and the peritubal area. (An illustration can be used to demonstrate the position of these structures in the body.)
2 **State the purpose of hysterosalpingography.**	The purposes of hysterosalpingography include the following: —To confirm tubal abnormalities, such as adhesions and occlusion —To confirm uterine abnormalities, such as the presence of foreign bodies, congenital malformations, and traumatic injuries —To confirm the presence of fistulae or peritubal adhesions.
3 **Describe the procedure used in hysterosalpingography.**	Just before the procedure, the patient will be placed on a table with her legs up in stirrups, and a baseline X-ray of her pelvic area will be taken. —A speculum will be inserted into her vagina, its blades will be opened, and a clamplike instrument called a tenaculum will stabilize her cervix. —The cervix will be cleansed, and a cannula will be inserted. Dye, or contrast medium, then will be injected through the cannula into the uterus and fallopian tubes. —A fluoroscope (a device used for the immediate projection of an X-ray) then will be used to take pictures of the uterus and tubes, and permanent films will be made for future consultation. —The patient should know who will perform the test and where and when it will be done. It takes about 15 minutes.

4 Explain patient guidelines for hysterosalpingography.	These are the patient guidelines for hysterosalpingography: —The patient does not need to restrict food or fluids before the test. —The procedure involves some discomfort, and she may experience moderate cramping and a vagal reaction (nausea, dizziness) afterward. These symptoms will be transient.

PELVIC ULTRASONOGRAPHY (Ultrasound)

Patient objectives	*Teaching plan content*
1 Define pelvic ultrasonography.	Pelvic ultrasonography is a test that uses sound waves to produce images of the internal pelvic area on a special TV screen called an oscilloscope. (An illustration can be used to help explain the test.)
2 State the purpose of pelvic ultrasonography.	The purposes of pelvic ultrasonography include the following: —To detect foreign bodies and distinguish between cystic and solid masses (tumors) —To measure organ size —To measure the size and number of mature ova in patients who have taken fertility drugs.
3 Describe the procedure used in pelvic ultrasonography.	Pelvic ultrasonography requires a full bladder to be used as a landmark. A tap water enema may also be given to better define the bowel. —The patient's abdominal area will be covered with mineral oil or conductive jelly, and a transducer (an instrument that creates sound waves) will be guided over the area. —The images from the sound waves bouncing off the internal structures will be displayed on a screen and photographed. —The patient should know who will perform the test and where and when it will be done.
4 Explain patient guidelines for pelvic ultrasonography.	These are the patient guidelines for pelvic ultrasonography: —Before the test, the patient will have to drink large amounts of fluid to fill her bladder, or if the test is scheduled for early morning, she will not be allowed to urinate upon arising. —She will not be allowed to urinate until after the test is complete.

	—During the test, she will have to relax her abdominal muscles and lie as still as possible. She will experience no pain.

ENDOMETRIAL BIOPSY

Patient objectives	*Teaching plan content*
1 Define endometrial biopsy.	Endometrial biopsy is the removal of tissue from the endometrium (the mucosal uterine lining that sloughs off and regenerates during each menstrual cycle) for microscopic examination. (An illustration can be used to help explain the test.)
2 State the purpose of endometrial biopsy.	The purposes of endometrial biopsy include the following: —To screen for endometrial cancer —To diagnose a chronic inflammatory condition of the endometrium —To aid in diagnosing the cause of infertility.
3 Describe the jet-wash (Gravlee) procedure for endometrial biopsy, if applicable.	Just before the procedure, the patient will be asked to urinate and to remove all clothing from her waist down. A sheet will be provided to drape her, and she will be placed on the table in the lithotomy position. A bimanual examination and Pap test may also be performed during this procedure. (See the "Papanicolaou Test" teaching plan in this chapter.) —To begin the jet-wash procedure, a speculum will be inserted into her vagina. —The cannula (a flexible tube containing a pointed rod) of the jet-washer will be bent to fit the curvature of her uterine cavity. —With 30 ml of normal sterile saline solution (in a reservoir), the cannula will be gently inserted into her uterus, and a small rubber plug attached to the apparatus will be snugly fitted into her cervical os to prevent saline solution from leaking out during the irrigation. —When the physician retracts the plunger of the syringe, saline solution will be drawn into the uterus, will irrigate the endometrial tissue, and will return through the cannula to the syringe. When the syringe is filled, the physician will withdraw the device from her uterus, disconnect the syringe, and expel its contents into the reservoir, which will double as a specimen container. —The specimen will be sent to the laboratory for microscopic examination.

	—The biopsy is usually done in the physician's office during a gynecologic pelvic examination. It takes less than 15 minutes.
4 Describe the curettage method for endometrial biopsy, if applicable.	Just before the procedure, the patient will be asked to urinate and to remove all clothing from her waist down. A sheet will be provided to drape her, and then she will be placed in the lithotomy position. A bimanual examination and Pap test may be performed. (See the "Papanicolaou Test" teaching plan in this chapter.) —A speculum will be inserted into her vagina, and her cervix and vaginal vault will be cleansed with povidone-iodine solution, using a sterile sponge stick and gauze sponges. —Her cervix will be held still by a tenaculum (a clamplike instrument), and the depth of her uterus will be measured with a rounded rodlike instrument called a uterine sound. This is to prevent uterine perforation during curettage. —The curette, a spoonlike instrument, will be attached to the syringe and inserted into her uterus. It will be drawn from back to front in a single swipe, while the physician draws back on the plunger of the syringe. —The curette then will be removed, and the specimen will be mixed with formalin to preserve it. —The biopsy is usually done in the physician's office during a gynecologic pelvic examination. It takes less than 15 minutes.
5 Explain patient guidelines for endometrial biopsy.	These are the patient guidelines for endometrial biopsy: —The patient should rest for 24 hours after the biopsy. —The packing or tampon should be left in place for the recommended time—usually 8 to 24 hours. —A small amount of postprocedure bleeding is normal, but she should report excessive bleeding. —She should avoid sexual intercourse until the physician says it is safe. —She should check with the physician if any untoward symptoms occur, such as fever, pain, or heavy bleeding.

INTERNAL EXAMINATION (Vaginal examination, bimanual examination)

Patient objectives	*Teaching plan content*
1 Define internal examination.	An internal examination is a physical examination of the female reproductive organs using direct visual inspection and palpation techniques. (An illustration can be used to demonstrate the position of these organs.)

2 State the purpose of an internal examination.

An internal examination is performed for the following reasons:
—To detect abnormalities, such as cysts, tumors, a prolapsed uterus, or rectovaginal fissures
—To assess the size, shape, and position of reproductive organs before other procedures are done
—To assess the condition of the genitalia.

3 Describe the procedure used in an internal examination.

Just before the procedure, the patient will be asked to empty her bladder and to disrobe from the waist down. A gown or sheet will be provided to ensure her privacy. She will then be placed on the examination table in the lithotomy position. (See the "Laparoscopy" teaching plan in this chapter.)
—Her pubic hair, external genitalia (labia majora and labia minora), and perineum will be examined for symmetry, lacerations, fistulae, masses, or discharges.
—Her labia minora will be separated to observe her vestibule, clitoris, urethra, and vaginal opening.
—Her anal area will be checked for hemorrhoids.
—A vaginal speculum of the appropriate size will be warmed and inserted into her vagina. The blades of the speculum will be opened and locked to facilitate observation of her cervix. If a Pap smear is to be taken, it is done now. (See the "Papanicolaou Test" teaching plan in this chapter.)
—The speculum will be closed and removed, and a bimanual and rectovaginal examination will be performed.
—The examiner will insert the index and middle fingers of one hand into her vagina. Her vaginal walls, cervix, and urethra will be palpated for any abnormalities and for muscle tone. Mobility of her cervix will also be checked.
—The examiner will place the other hand on her abdomen and, by moving the internal and external hands simultaneously, will palpate her uterus and ovaries for position, size, and any abnormalities.
—The examiner will then remove his fingers from her vagina and perform a rectovaginal examination, after rinsing off his glove and relubricating it. When his middle finger is inserted into her rectum, she may feel like she is having a bowel movement.
—The examiner's index finger will be inserted into her vagina at the same time that his middle finger is inserted into her rectum. She will be asked to bear down with her rectal and vaginal muscles. This is done to check sphincter tone. Further palpation will be done to detect lumps, masses, abnormalities, or tenderness. This is not painful, but it may cause some discomfort.

	—The procedure is usually performed in the physician's office and is a fundamental portion of any gynecologic examination. It takes 5 to 10 minutes.
4 Explain patient guidelines for the examination.	The patient should relax her abdominal muscles during the examination by taking slow, deep breaths, with her hands across her chest.

MAMMOGRAPHY

Patient objectives	*Teaching plan content*
1 Define mammography.	Mammography is a radiographic technique that permits visualization of the soft tissue of the breast.
2 State the purpose of mammography.	The purpose of mammography is to detect breast cysts or tumors, especially those not palpable on physical examination.
3 Explain the procedure used in mammography.	The test is performed in a special section of the X-ray department. —The patient will be seated on a chair and asked to rest one of her breasts on a table above an X-ray cassette. —A compressor will then be placed on the breast, and an X-ray taken. The machine will be rotated, the breast compressed again, and another X-ray taken. —Then the procedure will be repeated on the other breast. —The patient should know who will perform the test and when it will be done. It takes only about 15 to 30 minutes, but she may be asked to wait while the mammograms are checked to make sure they are readable.
4 Explain patient guidelines for mammography.	The patient will be asked to hold her breath during the procedure when the X-ray is actually taken. Powders and salves on the breast or jewelry worn in the X-ray field may produce unsatisfactory films and should be removed prior to the test.

BREAST BIOPSY

Patient objectives	*Teaching plan content*
1 Define breast biopsy.	Breast biopsy is the removal of tissue from the breast for histologic examination.

2 State the purpose of a breast biopsy.	The purpose of a breast biopsy is to differentiate between benign and malignant breast tumors.
3 Explain the procedure used in breast biopsy.	There are two procedures for breast biopsy: needle biopsy and open biopsy. —If a needle biopsy is to be done, the patient will be asked to undress to the waist and to assume a sitting or recumbent position with her hands at her sides. • The biopsy site will be cleansed with an antiseptic solution, a local anesthetic administered, and a syringe inserted. • Fluid will be aspirated and sent to the laboratory for examination. • The needle will be removed and pressure will be exerted on the biopsy site; an adhesive bandage will then be applied. —If an open biopsy is to be performed, the patient will receive a general or local anesthetic, and an incision will be made in the breast to expose the tumor mass. • A portion of the tumor will then be excised or the entire mass will be excised if it is small and appears benign. • The wound will then be sutured, and an adhesive bandage will be applied. —The patient should know who will perform the procedure and where and when it will be done.
4 Explain patient guidelines for breast biopsy.	The patient must remain still during the procedure. Afterward, she should report any bleeding, tenderness, or redness at the biopsy site.

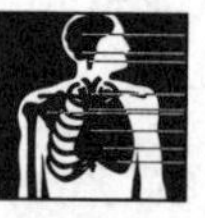

Explaining disorders

DYSFUNCTIONAL UTERINE BLEEDING (D.U.B.)

Patient objectives	*Teaching plan content*
1 Define DUB.	DUB refers to abnormal endometrial bleeding that occurs without recognizable organic lesions. (An illustration of the female reproductive system can be used to help explain normal menstrual function and DUB.)

2 Explain normal menstrual function.

Normal menstruation, or the menstrual period, is the vaginal discharge of blood and tissue from the endometrium (the uterine lining) at intervals of approximately 28 days. It is controlled by hormones.

—In a normal menstrual cycle, a structure in the brain, the hypothalamus, stimulates a second brain structure called the pituitary gland to secrete two hormones—follicle-stimulating hormone (FSH) and luteinizing hormone (LH). FSH is primarily responsible for the maturation of a follicle in the ovary. Follicles contain an ovum (egg).

—While the follicle is maturing, it is secreting a third hormone called estrogen. Estrogen helps the follicle continue to mature and grow. At the same time, the estrogen is also causing the lining of the uterus (the endometrium) to proliferate and build up.

—At the appropriate time in the cycle, LH helps the follicle totally mature and burst open, thereby releasing an ovum. This is called ovulation.

—The cells of the ruptured follicle now start to secrete a fourth hormone called progesterone. At this time, estrogen secretion is decreased.

—If the ovum is not fertilized and implanted into the uterine lining, the progesterone and estrogen secretions diminish and the endometrium breaks down. Menstruation follows this process.

3 Name the relevant cause of DUB.

The causes of DUB are disorders associated with sustained high estrogen levels. They include the following:

—Polycystic ovary syndrome

—Obesity

—Immaturity of the hypothalamic-pituitary ovarian mechanism (found in teens after puberty)

—Anovulation (found in women in their late 30s/early 40s).

4 Discuss the symptoms and diagnosis of DUB.

DUB usually occurs as metrorrhagia (episodes of bleeding between menses); it may also occur as hypermenorrhea (heavy or prolonged menses, longer than 8 days) or chronic polymenorrhea (menstrual cycles of less than 18 days). Such bleeding is unpredictable and can cause anemia.

—Diagnostic studies must rule out other causes of excessive bleeding, such as organic, systemic, psychogenic, and endocrine causes, including malignancy, polyps, incomplete abortion, pregnancy, and infection.

	—Dilatation and curettage (D & C) and biopsy results confirm the diagnosis by revealing endometrial hyperplasia (precancerous cells).
5 Explain the treatment for DUB.	Treatments for DUB include the following: —High-dose estrogen-progesterone combination therapy (oral contraceptives), the primary treatment, is designed to control endometrial growth and reestablish a normal cyclic pattern of menstruation. —If drug therapy is ineffective, a D & C can rule out other causes and can serve as a supplementary treatment by removing a large portion of the bleeding endometrium. Also, a D & C can help determine the original cause of hormonal imbalance and can aid in planning further therapy. (See the "Dilatation and Curettage" teaching plan in this chapter.) —Regardless of the primary treatment, the patient may need iron replacement or transfusions of packed cells or whole blood, as indicated, because of possible anemia caused by recurrent bleeding.
6 Describe the medication regimen.	Some drugs commonly used in this disorder are estrogen with progestogen combinations and medroxyprogesterone acetate. See Chapter 9, Drug Therapy, for specific medication instructions.
7 Explain the importance of routine medical follow-up.	Normal checkups are needed to assess treatment for DUB. If a D & C has been performed, a postoperative checkup may be required by the physician.

ENDOMETRIOSIS

Patient objectives	*Teaching plan content*
1 Define endometriosis.	Endometriosis is the presence of endometrial tissue outside the uterine cavity. (An illustration of the pelvic region can be used to demonstrate sites where the tissue becomes implanted.)
2 Explain the normal function of the endometrium in the menstrual cycle.	The menstrual cycle is divided into the following three distinct phases: —The menstrual phase starts on the first day of menstruation. The top layer of the endometrium (the tissue lining the uterus) breaks down and flows out the vagina. This flow, called the menses, or period, consists of blood, mucus, and unneeded tissue.

—During the proliferative phase, the endometrium begins to thicken, and the level of estrogen in the blood rises.
—In the secretory phase, the endometrium continues to thicken to nourish an embryo if fertilization were to occur. Without fertilization, the top layer of the endometrium breaks down, and the menstrual phase of the cycle begins again.

3 Explain the possible causes of endometriosis.

The direct cause of endometriosis is unknown, but research focuses on the following possible causes:
—During menstruation, the fallopian tubes may expel endometrial fragments that implant on the ovaries or pelvic peritoneum (sometimes called chocolate cysts).
—Inflammation or a hormonal change may trigger a change in the endometrial tissue of the uterus.
—The endometrium may chemically induce nonspecific tissue to change to endometrial tissue (a combination of the two causes listed above).

4 Identify the two types of endometriosis.

There are two types of endometriosis:
—Adenomyosis (sometimes called internal endometriosis) occurs within the uterus.
—In external endometriosis, endometrial tissue invades other pelvic or abdominal organs.

5 Describe the stages of external endometriosis.

These are the five stages of external endometriosis:
—In Stage I, one or more superficial implants of endometrial tissue are found on the pelvic peritoneum (the part of the membrane lining the abdominal cavity that is nearest the pelvic walls and organs).
—In Stage II, there are larger superficial implants on the uterosacral ligaments (those ligaments coming from the cervix and passing up and behind the rectum to the second sacral vertebra), the rectovaginal septum (the area separating the rectum and vagina), or ovaries.
—In Stage III, endometrial tumors (endometriomas) form on the ovary. These are more than 5 mm in diameter. There may be superficial implants on the broad ligaments (those ligaments connecting the sides of the uterus to the pelvic wall) and adjacent organs.
—In Stage IV, endometrial tissue penetrates the vagina, bowel, or urinary tract and spreads to lymph nodes, umbilicus (navel), or surgical wounds.
—In Stage V, endometriomas become adenocarcinomas (tumors arising from the outer tissue or epithelium of an organ).

6 Describe the signs and symptoms of endometriosis.

The classic symptom of endometriosis is acquired dysmenorrhea (painful periods or menses), which produces constant pain in the lower abdomen, vagina, posterior pelvis, and back. The pain usually begins 5 to 7 days before menses reaches its peak, and lasts for 2 to 3 days. This pain is different from primary dysmenorrheal pain, which is more cramplike and is concentrated in the abdominal midline. Depending on where the endometrial tissue implants itself, there will be other clinical features, such as the following:
—Infertility and heavy menses
—Painful sexual intercourse with deep penile thrust
—Bloody urine during menstruation
—Pain on moving bowels, rectal bleeding with menstruation, pain in the coccyx or sacrum
—Abdominal cramps, nausea, and vomiting that worsen before menstruation
—Bleeding from endometrial deposits in the cervix, vagina, and perineum during menstruation.

7 Discuss the diagnosis of endometriosis.

Many diagnostic tests, such as the following, may be performed to make a definite diagnosis of endometriosis.
—Pelvic examination may suggest diagnosis. There may be multiple tender nodules on palpation. Palpation may also uncover ovarian enlargement.
—Laparoscopy may be performed to confirm and determine the stage of the disease.
—Cul-de-sac aspiration may reveal abdominal bleeding, which indicates endometrial cyst rupture.
—A barium enema may be done to rule out malignant or inflammatory bowel disease.

8 Explain treatments used for endometriosis.

Treatment of endometriosis varies according to the stage of the disease, the patient's age, and her desire to have children.
—Conservative therapy for young women who want to have children includes administration of androgens, such as danazol, which produce a temporary remission in Stages I and II. Continuous progesterone therapy may induce similar remissions in Stages I and II by gradually producing pseudopregnancy, which results in amenorrhea (absence of menses) and possible relief of symptoms. Mild analgesics may be used to alleviate pain if the disease is not too severe.
—When ovarian masses are present (Stages III to V), surgery must be performed to rule out malignancy.

Conservative surgery for women in their childbearing years includes removal of the endometrial cysts and the adhesions they have caused.
—The treatment of choice for women who are past their childbearing years or who are not interested in having children is a total abdominal hysterectomy with bilateral salpingo-oophorectomy (the removal of the uterus, fallopian tubes, and ovaries through an abdominal incision).

9 Describe the medication regimen.

Some drugs commonly used for this disorder are danazol and medroxyprogesterone acetate. See Chapter 9, Drug Therapy, for specific medication instructions.

10 Explain the importance of routine medical follow-up.

An annual pelvic examination and Pap test are necessary for effective treatment of endometriosis.

GONORRHEA

Patient objectives	*Teaching plan content*

1 Define gonorrhea.

Gonorrhea, which is one of the most common sexually transmitted (or venereal) diseases, is an infection of the genitourinary tract (especially the urethra and cervix) and, occasionally, the rectum, pharynx, and eyes. Untreated gonorrhea can spread through the blood to the joints, tendons, meninges, and endocardium. In women it can also lead to pelvic inflammatory disease (PID) and sterility.

2 Explain the cause of gonorrhea.

The bacterium *Neisseria gonorrhoeae* causes gonorrhea.
—Transmission almost exclusively follows sexual contact with an infected person.
—Children born of infected mothers can contract gonococcal eye infection during passage through the birth canal.
—Children and adults with gonorrhea can contract gonococcal conjunctivitis by touching their eyes with contaminated hands.

3 Describe the signs and symptoms of gonorrhea.

The signs and symptoms of gonorrhea in women may not appear immediately after infection. When they do finally start to show, the most common ones are inflammation and a greenish yellow discharge from the cervix.

—Other common signs and symptoms, which vary according to the site involved, are as follows:
- Dysuria, urinary frequency and incontinence, purulent discharge, itching, red and edematous urethral meatus
- Occasional itching, burning, and pain due to discharge from an adjacent infected area (Vulval symptoms tend to be more severe before puberty or after menopause.)
- Engorgement, redness, swelling of the vagina (most common site in children over age 1), and profuse purulent vaginal discharge
- Severe pelvic and lower abdominal pain, muscular rigidity, tenderness, and abdominal distention (As the infection spreads, nausea, vomiting, fever, and tachycardia may develop in patients with infection of the fallopian tubes or PID.)
- Right upper quadrant pain in patients with perihepatitis.

—Other possible symptoms include pharyngitis, tonsillitis, and rectal burning, itching, and bloody mucopurulent discharge.
—Gonococcal septicemia is more common in females than in males. Its characteristic signs include tender papillary skin lesions on the hands and feet; these lesions may be pustular, hemorrhagic, or necrotic. Gonococcal septicemia may also produce migratory polyarthralgia, and polyarthritis and tenosynovitis of the wrists, fingers, knees, or ankles. Untreated septic arthritis leads to progressive joint destruction.
—Signs of gonococcal ophthalmia neonatorum (eye infection of newborns caused by the transmission of the gonococcal organism from the mother to the baby during birth) include lid edema, bilateral conjunctival infection, and abundant purulent discharge 2 to 3 days after birth.

---

4 Describe the procedure used in the diagnosis of gonorrhea.

The following procedure is used in diagnosing gonorrhea:
—A sterile swab is wiped over the infected area (urethra, cervix, rectum, pharynx, or conjunctiva).
—The swab is then passed across a dish containing culture medium.
—After a few days, the laboratory technician looks at the material in the dish through the microscope to check for the growth of the organism that causes gonorrhea.

5 Explain the treatment for gonorrhea.

The treatment of choice for uncomplicated gonorrhea is the administration of an antibiotic that will kill the gonorrhea organism. If the gonorrhea is complicated by PID or septicemia, then the antibiotic must be given intravenously (requiring hospitalization) rather than by mouth.

6 Describe the medication regimen.

Some drugs commonly used for this disorder are ampicillin, penicillin G benzathine, penicillin G procaine, probenecid, and spectinomycin hydrochloride. See Chapter 9, Drug Therapy, for specific medication instructions.

7 Explain the importance of routine medical follow-up.

To confirm that the patient is cured of gonococcal infection, follow-up cultures are necessary 7 to 14 days after treatment and again in 6 months, or, in pregnant females, before delivery.
—Until cultures prove negative, the patient is still infectious and can transmit gonococcal infection.
—She should inform her sexual contacts of her infection so they can seek treatment.

SYPHILIS

Patient objectives | *Teaching plan content*

1 Define syphilis.

Syphilis is a chronic, infectious, sexually transmitted (venereal) disease that begins in the mucous membranes and quickly becomes systemic, spreading to nearby lymph nodes and the bloodstream.

2 Explain the cause of syphilis.

The bacterial spirochete *Treponema pallidum* causes syphilis. Transmission occurs primarily through sexual contact. Prenatal transmission from an infected mother to the fetus is also possible.

3 Name the four stages of syphilis.

There are four stages of syphilis: primary, secondary, latent, and late.

4 Describe the signs and symptoms of the relevant stage of syphilis.

These are the signs and symptoms of the four stages of syphilis:
—Primary syphilis develops after an incubation period that generally lasts about 3 weeks.

- Initially, one or more chancres (small, fluid-filled lesions) erupt on the genitalia; others may erupt on the arms, fingers, lips, tongue, nipples, tonsils, or eyelids.

• The chancres, which are usually painless, start as papules (small, solid, raised skin lesions) and then erode. Even untreated chancres disappear after 3 to 6 weeks.
• Chancres are usually associated with regional swelling of lymph nodes (unilateral or bilateral).
• In females, chancres are often overlooked because they often develop on the cervix or vaginal wall.

—Symmetrical lesions (those of the skin and mucous membranes) and general swelling of the lymph nodes signal the start of secondary syphilis, which may develop within a few days or up to 8 weeks after the initial chancre.
• The rash of secondary syphilis can be macular, papular, pustular, or nodular. The lesions are of uniform size, well defined, and generalized.
• Macules often erupt between rolls of fat on the trunk and on the arms, palms, soles, face, and scalp. In warm, moist areas (perineum, vulva, between rolls of fat), the lesions enlarge and erode, producing highly contagious pink or grayish white lesions (condylomata lata).
• Mild constitutional symptoms of syphilis appear in this second stage and may include headache, malaise, anorexia, weight loss, nausea, vomiting, sore throat, and, possibly, slight fever. Alopecia (loss of hair) may occur, with or without treatment, and is usually temporary. Nails become brittle and pitted.

—Latent syphilis is characterized by an absence of clinical symptoms but a reactive serologic test for syphilis.
• Since infectious mucocutaneous lesions may reappear when infection is of less than 4 years' duration, early latent syphilis is considered contagious.
• Approximately two thirds of patients remain asymptomatic in the late latent stage, until death; the rest develop characteristic late-stage symptoms.

—Late syphilis is the final destructive but noninfectious stage of the disease. It has three subtypes, any or all of which may affect the patient: late benign syphilis, cardiovascular syphilis, and neurosyphilis.
• The lesions of late benign syphilis develop between 1 and 10 years after infection. They may appear on the skin, bones, mucous membranes, upper respiratory tract, liver, or stomach.
• Cardiovascular syphilis develops about 10 years after the initial infection in approximately 10% of patients with untreated late syphilis. It causes fibrosis of the elastic tissue of the aorta and leads to aorti-

tis, most often in the ascending and transverse sections of the aortic arch.

• Symptoms of neurosyphilis develop in about 8% of patients with untreated late syphilis and appear from 5 to 35 years after infection. These clinical effects consist of meningitis and widespread central nervous system damage that may include general paresis, personality changes, and arm and leg weakness.

5 Discuss the diagnosis of syphilis.	The diagnosis of syphilis is made by a blood test and examination of this serum under a microscope to identify the causative organism, *T. pallidum.* Fluid can also be taken from moist lesions, sputum specimens, ocular fluid, or cerebrospinal fluid.
6 Explain the treatment for syphilis.	Treatment for syphilis consists of injections of an antibiotic that will kill the responsible organism.
7 Describe the medication regimen.	Some drugs commonly used for this disorder are erythromycin, penicillin G benzathine, and penicillin G procaine. See Chapter 9, Drug Therapy, for specific medication instructions.
8 Explain the importance of routine medical follow-up.	Patients need Venereal Disease Research Laboratory testing after 1, 3, 9, and 12 months to detect possible relapse. Patients treated for latent or late syphilis should receive blood tests at 6-month intervals for 2 years. (Cases of syphilis are routinely reported to local public health authorities, and sexual partners of patients with syphilis are urged to receive treatment.)

TRICHOMONIASIS

Patient objectives	*Teaching plan content*
1 Define trichomoniasis.	Trichomoniasis is a protozoal infection of the lower genitourinary tract.
2 Explain the cause of trichomoniasis.	*Trichomonas vaginalis*—a motile, pear-shaped protozoan (single-celled animal)—causes trichomoniasis in females by infecting the vagina, the urethra, and, possibly, the endocervix, Bartholin's glands, Skene's glands, or the bladder. In males, it infects the lower urethra and, possibly, the prostate gland, seminal vesicles, or epididymis.

—*T. vaginalis* grows best when the vaginal mucosa is more alkaline than normal (pH about 5.5 to 5.8). Therefore, factors that raise the vaginal pH—use of oral contraceptives, pregnancy, bacterial overgrowth, exudative (pus-forming) cervical or vaginal lesions, or frequent douching (which disturbs the lactobacilli that normally live in the vagina and maintain acidity)—may predispose the patient to trichomoniasis.
—The infection is usually transmitted by intercourse; less often, by contaminated douche equipment or moist washcloths. Occasionally, the condition is transmitted to the newborn of an infected mother during vaginal delivery.

3 Describe the signs and symptoms of trichomoniasis.

Approximately 70% of females (including those with chronic infections) and most males with trichomoniasis are asymptomatic. In females, acute infection may produce variable signs, such as a gray or a greenish yellow and, possibly, profuse and frothy, malodorous vaginal discharge.
—Other effects include severe itching, redness, swelling, tenderness, dyspareunia (painful intercourse), dysuria, urinary frequency, and, occasionally, postcoital spotting, menorrhagia, or dysmenorrhea.
—Such signs and symptoms may persist for a week to several months and may be more pronounced just after menstruation or during pregnancy.
—If trichomoniasis is untreated, symptoms may subside, although *T. vaginalis* infection persists, possibly associated with an abnormal cytologic smear of the cervix.

4 Discuss the diagnosis of trichomoniasis.

Diagnosis is made by direct microscopic examination of vaginal discharge and is decisive when it reveals *T. vaginalis.*
—Physical examination of symptomatic females reveals vaginal redness; edema; frank excoriation; a frothy, malodorous, greenish yellow vaginal discharge; and, rarely, a thin, gray pseudomembrane over the vagina.
—Urine specimens may also reveal the *T. vaginalis* organism.
—A cervical examination may show small cervical hemorrhages, giving the cervix a characteristic strawberry appearance.

5 Explain the treatment for trichomoniasis.

A drug that effectively cures trichomoniasis is administered to the patient and her sexual partner(s).
—Acidifying or antiseptic douches are useful to relieve symptoms in pregnant females with trichomoniasis.

	Such douches may minimize the extent of infection, if used properly. —Oral administration of metronidazole, the drug of choice, has not been proven safe during pregnancy, especially in the first trimester.
6 Describe the medication regimen.	A drug commonly used for this disorder is metronidazole. See Chapter 9, Drug Therapy, for specific medication instructions.
7 Explain the importance of routine medical follow-up.	After treatment, the patient and her sexual partner(s) require a follow-up examination to check for residual signs of infection.

GENITAL HERPES

Patient objectives	*Teaching plan content*
1 Define genital herpes.	Genital herpes is an acute, inflammatory disease of the genitalia.
2 Explain the cause of genital herpes.	Genital herpes is caused by the herpes simplex II virus. —It is usually transmitted through sexual contact, but contamination from infected toilet seats, towels, and bathtubs also occurs. —Pregnant females may transmit the infection to newborns during vaginal delivery. Such transmitted infections may be localized (for instance, in the eyes) or disseminated and may be associated with central nervous system involvement.
3 Describe the signs and symptoms of genital herpes.	After a 3- to 7-day incubation period, fluid-filled vesicles appear, usually on the cervix (the primary infection site) and, possibly, on the labia, perianal skin, vulva, or vagina. Extragenital lesions may appear on the mouth or anus. —In both males and females, the vesicles, usually painless at first, may rupture and develop into extensive, shallow, painful ulcers, creating redness, marked edema, and tender, inguinal lymph nodes. —Other features of initial infection include fever, malaise, painful urination, and a whitish discharge. —Rare complications that generally arise from extragenital lesions include herpetic keratitis, which may lead to blindness, and potentially fatal herpetic encephalitis.

4 Discuss the diagnosis of genital herpes.

Diagnosis is based on physical examination and patient history.
—Helpful (but nondiagnostic) measures include laboratory data showing increased antibody titers (this shows that the body has been exposed to the virus and is trying to fight it off) and smears of genital lesions showing atypical cells.
—Diagnosis can be confirmed by using tissue culture techniques to demonstrate the presence of herpes simplex II virus in vesical fluid.

5 Explain the treatment for genital herpes.

Most antiviral agents are ineffective against herpes infection. Such medications as Burow's solution (aluminum acetate) and, occasionally, sulfonamide creams help reduce edema and may ease the discomfort of painful lesions. Also, two new drugs, 2-deoxy-D-glucose and acyclovir, promise to be beneficial by preventing multiplication of the virus. Antibacterial agents help combat secondary infections.
—Pain and fever may necessitate strict bed rest (sometimes hospitalization) and heat therapy.
—The patient should get adequate rest and nutrition and keep the lesions dry, except for applying prescribed medications, as directed, using aseptic technique (wearing gloves).
—She can maintain normal activity, but she should avoid sexual intercourse during the active stage of this disease (while lesions are present).

6 Describe the medication regimen.

A drug commonly used for this disorder is acyclovir. See Chapter 9, Drug Therapy, for specific medication instructions.

7 Explain the importance of routine medical follow-up.

Follow-up visits to the physician are important in order to keep a close watch on disease activity.
—If the patient is pregnant and at term, follow-up visits are important to ascertain if the lesions are active; if they are, a cesarean delivery will probably be performed to try to protect the newborn from contracting the virus.
—If she appears upset and unable to cope psychologically with the diagnosis, she may be referred to the Herpes Resource Center, an American Social Health Association group, for support. (Also, provide her with a copy of the patient-teaching aid *Coping with Genital Herpes*, p. 383.)

PELVIC INFLAMMATORY DISEASE (P.I.D.)

Patient objectives	*Teaching plan content*
1 Define PID.	PID is any acute, subacute, recurrent, or chronic infection of the fallopian tubes and ovaries with adjacent tissue involvement. It can also include inflammation of the cervix, uterus, and the connective tissue lying between the broad ligaments. (An illustration of these structures can be used to demonstrate their position in the body.)
2 Explain the causes of PID.	PID can result from infection with aerobic organisms (those that live with oxygen) or anaerobic organisms (those that live without oxygen). The aerobic bacterium *Neisseria gonorrhoeae* is its most common cause, because it most readily penetrates the bacteriostatic barrier of cervical mucus. —Normally, cervical secretions have a protective and defensive function. Procedures that alter or destroy cervical mucus (for example, conization or cauterization of the cervix) impair this bacteriostatic mechanism and allow bacteria present in the cervix or vagina to ascend into the uterine cavity. —Uterine infection can also follow the transfer of contaminated cervical mucus into the endometrial cavity by instrumentation. Consequently, PID can follow insertion of an intrauterine device, use of a biopsy curette or an irrigation catheter, or tubal insufflation (air injection of the tubes). —Other predisposing factors include abortion, pelvic surgery, and infection during or after pregnancy. —Bacteria may also enter the uterine cavity through the bloodstream or from drainage from a chronically infected fallopian tube, a pelvic abscess, a ruptured appendix, or other infectious foci. —The most common bacteria found in cervical mucus are staphylococci, streptococci, diphtheroids, and coliforms, including *Pseudomonas* and *Escherichia coli.* • Uterine infection can result from any one or several of these organisms or may follow the multiplication of normally nonpathogenic (non–disease-producing) bacteria in an altered endometrial environment. • Bacterial multiplication is most common postpartum because the endometrium is dormant, atrophic, and not stimulated by estrogen.

3 Identify the forms of PID.

There are three forms of PID:
—Salpingo-oophoritis is inflammation of the fallopian tubes and ovaries.
—Cervicitis is inflammation of the cervix.
—Endometritis is inflammation of the endometrium (lining of the uterus).

4 Describe the signs and symptoms of PID.

Signs and symptoms of PID vary with the affected area but generally include a profuse, purulent vaginal discharge, sometimes accompanied by low-grade fever and malaise (particularly if gonorrhea is the cause). The patient may experience lower abdominal pain; movement of the cervix or palpation of the adnexa may be extremely painful.
—In salpingo-oophoritis, symptoms include sudden onset of lower abdominal and pelvic pain, usually following menses; increased vaginal discharge; fever; malaise; lower abdominal pressure and tenderness; tachycardia; and pelvic peritonitis. The patient may experience recurring acute episodes.
—In cervicitis, signs and symptoms include purulent, foul-smelling vaginal discharge; vulvovaginitis with itching and/or burning; red, edematous cervix; pelvic discomfort; sexual dysfunction; metrorrhagia (uterine bleeding other than menses); infertility; and spontaneous abortion. The patient with chronic cervicitis may experience abnormal labor. Her cervix may be lacerated or everted. If cervicitis results from herpes simplex II virus, she may have ulcerative vesicular lesions.
—In acute endometritis (generally postpartum or postabortion), clinical features include mucopurulent or purulent vaginal discharge oozing from the cervix; edematous, hyperemic endometrium, possibly leading to ulceration and necrosis (with virulent organisms); lower abdominal pain and tenderness; fever; rebound pain; abdominal muscle spasm; and thrombophlebitis of uterine and pelvic vessels (in severe forms). The patient may experience recurring acute episodes (increasingly common because of the widespread use of intrauterine devices).

5 Discuss the diagnosis of PID.

Diagnosis is based on the patient's history and diagnostic tests.
—A Gram stain is used to stain secretions from the endocervix or cul-de-sac. Culture and sensitivity testing aids selection of the appropriate antibiotic. Urethral and rectal secretions may also be cultured.
—Ultrasonography may be used to identify an adnexal or uterine mass. (X-rays seldom identify pelvic masses.)

—Culdocentesis is used to obtain peritoneal fluid or pus for culture and sensitivity testing.

6 Explain the treatment for PID.

The goal of treatment for PID is to prevent its progression.
—Antibiotic therapy begins immediately after culture specimens are obtained. Such therapy can be reevaluated as soon as laboratory results are available (normally after 24 to 48 hours). Infection may become chronic if treated inadequately.
—The preferred antibiotic treatment for PID resulting from gonorrhea is penicillin G procaine administered intramuscularly in two injection sites, combined with oral administration of probenecid. If the patient is allergic to penicillin, tetracycline may be used.
—Supplemental treatment of PID may include bed rest, analgesics, and I.V. therapy.

7 Describe the medication regimen.

Some drugs commonly used for this disorder are ampicillin, penicillin G procaine, probenecid, and tetracycline. See Chapter 9, Drug Therapy, for specific medication instructions.

8 Explain the importance of routine medical follow-up.

Complying with the medication regimen and returning to the physician for regular checkups will help keep the patient's PID under control and may prevent it from worsening or spreading. If PID returns or worsens, her sexual partner should be examined and, if necessary, also treated for infection.

PREMENSTRUAL SYNDROME (P.M.S.)

Patient objectives	*Teaching plan content*
1 Define PMS.	PMS refers to a myriad of varying symptoms that appear 7 to 10 days before menses and usually subside with its onset. PMS can range from minimal discomfort to severe, disruptive symptoms. It usually occurs in women of ages 25 to 40, and its incidence rises with age and number of births.
2 Discuss the causes of PMS.	Although the direct cause of PMS is unknown, a known precipitating factor is the loss of intravascular fluid into body tissues, which triggers an increase in antidiuretic hormone and aldosterone secretion. This causes transient water retention, which in turn produces characteristic signs and symptoms, such as edema, bloating, weight gain, and breast tenderness.

Effects of edema include central nervous system changes, resulting in headaches and mood shifts. Other conditions that possibly contribute to PMS include estrogen-progesterone imbalance, progesterone allergy, and hypoglycemia, as well as psychogenic factors.

3 Identify the signs and symptoms of PMS.

The clinical effects of PMS vary widely and may include any combination of the following:
—Mild to severe personality changes, nervousness, irritability, agitation, sleep disturbances, fatigue, lethargy, and depression
—Headache, vertigo, syncope, paresthesia of the arms and legs, and exacerbation of epilepsy
—Increased incidence of colds and exacerbation of allergic rhinitis and/or asthma
—Abdominal bloating (the most common symptom), diarrhea or constipation, change in appetite, and exacerbation of spastic colitis
—Edema, temporary weight gain, palpitations, backache, exacerbation of skin problems (such as acne), breast changes (such as enlargement and/or tenderness), oliguria (decrease in urinary output), easy bruising (due to capillary fragility), and eye disorders (such as conjunctivitis).

4 Discuss the diagnosis of PMS.

The patient's history of complaints, unusual signs and symptoms, and physical problems may be the most important diagnostic tool for the physician. She should try to remember every menstruation-related symptom and to report all symptoms to the physician. In addition, her estrogen and progesterone blood levels may be evaluated to rule out hormonal imbalance.

5 Explain the treatment for PMS.

Treatment aims primarily to relieve symptoms. It may include tranquilizers and sedatives to relieve behavioral symptoms, and diuretics and decreased salt intake to relieve bloating and edema.
—Since the precipitating factor is often unknown, drug therapy should be avoided, when possible. Some physicians consider salt restriction or the use of diuretics unnecessary.
—Use of vitamin B_6 (pyridoxine) has been tried, but it is still very controversial.
—It has been demonstrated that exercise may be helpful. (See *How to Reduce Menstrual Discomfort: Some Exercises*, pp. 380-381.)

6 Discuss the medication regimen.	A drug commonly used for this disorder is progesterone. See Chapter 9, Drug Therapy, for specific medication instructions.

OVARIAN CYSTS

Patient objectives	*Teaching plan content*
1 Define ovarian cysts.	Ovarian cysts are sacs on the ovary that contain fluid or semisolid matter. They are usually noncancerous.
2 Discuss the types of ovarian cysts.	There are three types of ovarian cysts: —Follicular cysts, which are small, arise from follicles that overdistend instead of going through the retrogressive stage of the menstrual cycle. —Granulosa-lutein (corpus luteum) cysts are functional, noncancerous enlargements of the ovaries. (The corpus luteum is the small yellow body that develops after ovulation. If fertilization of an ovum took place, the corpus luteum would secrete progesterone to support the pregnancy.) —Theca-lutein cysts, which are commonly seen on both ovaries, are filled with a clear, straw-colored fluid. They are often associated with other conditions, such as hydatidiform mole (a degenerative process that transforms the placenta into a large number of swollen vesicles resembling a bunch of grapes); choriocarcinoma (an extremely rare neoplasm arising from the outer membrane enclosing an embryo); or hormone therapy.
3 Identify the causes of ovarian cysts.	The causes of ovarian cysts include the following: —Follicles that do not regress after ovulation —Excessive accumulation of blood in the follicle following ovulation —Neoplasms of the ovaries —Hormone therapy —Endocrine abnormalities —Polycystic ovarian syndrome.
4 Describe the signs and symptoms of ovarian cysts.	The signs and symptoms of ovarian cysts vary widely. —Small ovarian cysts (such as follicular cysts) usually do not produce symptoms, unless torsion or rupture causes signs of an acute abdomen (abdominal tenderness, distention, and rigidity). —Large or multiple cysts may induce mild pelvic discomfort, low back pain, dyspareunia (painful inter-

course), or abnormal uterine bleeding secondary to a disturbed ovulatory pattern.
—Ovarian cysts with torsion induce acute abdominal pain similar to that of appendicitis.
—Granulosa-lutein cysts that appear early in pregnancy may grow as large as 2″ to 2½″ (5 to 6 cm) in diameter and produce unilateral pelvic discomfort and, if rupture occurs, massive intraperitoneal hemorrhage. In nonpregnant women, these cysts may cause delayed menses, followed by prolonged or irregular bleeding.
—Polycystic ovarian disease may also produce secondary amenorrhea (no menses), oligomenorrhea (abnormally infrequent menses), or infertility.

5 Discuss the diagnosis of ovarian cysts.

Generally, characteristic clinical features suggest ovarian cysts.
—Visualization of the ovary through pelvic pneumoroentgenography, culdoscopy, culdotomy, laparoscopy, or surgery (often for another condition) confirms ovarian cysts.
—Extremely elevated human chorionic gonadotropin (HCG) titers strongly suggest theca-lutein cysts.
—In polycystic ovarian syndrome, physical examination demonstrates bilaterally enlarged polycystic ovaries. Tests reveal slight elevation of urinary 17-ketosteroids and anovulation (failure to ovulate), shown by basal body temperature graphs and endometrial biopsy. Direct visualization must rule out paraovarian cysts of the broad ligament, salpingitis, endometriosis, and neoplastic cysts.

6 Explain the treatment for ovarian cysts.

In general, treatment for ovarian cysts consists primarily of observation if the cyst is known to be nonmalignant. However, because a doubt often exists, surgery frequently becomes necessary for both diagnosis and treatment.
—Follicular cysts generally do not require treatment, since they tend to disappear spontaneously within 60 days. However, if they interfere with daily activities, oral administration of clomiphene citrate for 5 days, or intramuscular administration of progesterone for 5 days, reestablishes the ovarian hormonal cycle and induces ovulation. Oral contraceptives may also accelerate involution of functional cysts, including both types of lutein cysts and follicular cysts.
—Treatment for granulosa-lutein cysts that occur during pregnancy is symptomatic, since these cysts diminish during the third trimester and rarely require surgery. Theca-lutein cysts disappear spontaneously af-

ter elimination of the hydatidiform mole, the destruction of choriocarcinoma, or discontinuation of HCG or clomiphene citrate therapy.
—Treatment for polycystic ovarian disease varies. It may include administration of drugs, such as hydrocortisone or clomiphene citrate, to induce ovulation or surgical wedge resection of one half to one third of the ovary if drug therapy fails to induce ovulation.

7 Describe the medication regimen.	Some drugs used for this disorder are human chorionic gonadotropin, clomiphene citrate, hydrocortisone, and menotropins. See Chapter 9, Drug Therapy, for specific medication instructions.

UTERINE LEIOMYOMAS (Myomas, fibromyomas, fibroids)

Patient objectives	*Teaching plan content*
1 Define uterine leiomyomas.	Uterine leiomyomas are benign smooth muscle tumors. The most common benign tumors in women, usually they are multiple and occur within the body of the uterus, although they may appear on the cervix or on the round or broad ligaments.
2 Discuss the cause of uterine leiomyomas.	The cause of uterine leiomyomas is unknown, but estrogen and human growth hormone (GH) may influence tumor formation by stimulating susceptible fibromuscular elements. This theory seems likely, since tumor size and GH levels increase with large doses of estrogen and in the later stages of pregnancy. Leiomyomas usually shrink or disappear after menopause when estrogen production decreases.
3 Describe the signs and symptoms of uterine leiomyomas.	Usually, hypermenorrhea (an abnormal amount of menstrual bleeding) is the cardinal sign of uterine leiomyomas, although other forms of abnormal endometrial bleeding, as well as dysmenorrhea (painful menses) or leukorrhea (white or yellow discharge from the uterus), are possible. —Pain may occur if the tumors twist or degenerate after circulatory occlusion or infection or if the uterus contracts in an attempt to expel a pedunculated submucous leiomyoma (a tumor with a stalk). —Large tumors may produce a feeling of heaviness in the abdomen; pressure on surrounding organs may cause secondary pain, backache, intestinal obstruction, constipation, and urinary frequency or urgency. —Irregular uterine enlargement may occur, often asymptomatically.

4 Discuss the diagnosis of uterine leiomyomas.	Diagnosis is based on clinical findings and a thorough patient history. —Blood studies showing anemia may support the diagnosis, but palpation of the tumor, revealing a round mass, helps to confirm it. —Other diagnostic procedures include dilatation and curettage (D & C) to detect submucous leiomyomas in the endometrial cavity or laparoscopy to visualize subserous leiomyomas on the uterine surface. —Barium enema X-rays may rule out colonic tumors.
5 Explain the treatment for uterine leiomyomas.	Treatment depends on the severity of symptoms, size and location of the tumor(s), and the patient's age, parity, pregnancy status, desire to have children, and general health. —Only a pelvic examination every 6 to 12 months is required to monitor tumor growth patterns in a nonpregnant, asymptomatic woman. —If they have caused problems in the past, or if they are likely to threaten a future pregnancy, small leiomyomas may be surgically removed. This is the treatment of choice for a young woman who wants to have children. —Anemia caused by excessive bleeding may necessitate blood transfusions. —If the patient is pregnant, but her uterus is no larger than a 6-month normal uterus by the 16th week of pregnancy, the outlook for the pregnancy is favorable, and surgery is usually unnecessary. If surgery becomes necessary, a hysterectomy is usually performed 5 to 6 months after delivery when involution is complete (when the uterus shrinks to prepregnancy size). The ovaries are preserved, if possible. (See the "Hysterectomy" teaching plan in this chapter.)
6 Discuss the importance of routine medical follow-up.	Follow-up visits to the physician are an important part of therapy. At each visit, the subsequent growth and status of the tumor(s) can be ascertained. In pregnancy, they must be monitored carefully.

CHLAMYDIAL INFECTION

Patient objectives	*Teaching plan content*
1 Define chlamydial infection.	Chlamydial infection is an infection caused by the organism *Chlamydia trachomatis,* a microorganism that resembles a bacterium.

2 Name the conditions caused by *C. trachomatis*.	This organism may cause nongonococcal urethritis, cervicitis, pelvic inflammatory disease, ophthalmia neonatorum (eye infection in newborns), and newborn chlamydial pneumonia.
3 Discuss the diagnosis of chlamydial infections.	Until recently, chlamydial infections had gone undiagnosed, but now there is a test that cultures affected body fluid. The physician also takes a thorough patient health history.
4 Discuss criteria used to determine the specific treatment for chlamydial infection.	The specific treatment for chlamydial infection depends on the site of the infection, whether the patient is pregnant, and whether she is sensitive to the specific antibiotic used.
5 Describe the medication regimen.	Some drugs commonly used for this disorder are erythromycin and tetracycline. See Chapter 9, Drug Therapy, for specific medication instructions.
6 Discuss the importance of routine medical follow-up.	The patient is not free of the infection until cultures come back negative (that is, no *C. trachomatis* in the specimen). Follow-up visits are necessary to take specimens for these cultures. In addition, since chlamydial infection is a sexually transmitted disease, the patient's sexual partner(s) should also be examined and treated; otherwise, she will continue to be reinfected.

FEMALE INFERTILITY

Patient objectives	***Teaching plan content***
1 Define female infertility.	Infertility is the inability to achieve pregnancy after at least 1 year of unprotected intercourse on a regular basis.
2 Describe the causes of female infertility.	The causes of female infertility are primarily functional and structural. Psychological factors probably account for relatively few cases of infertility. —Functional disruptions in the complex hormonal interactions that regulate the female reproductive tract can cause infertility. • These interactions require an intact hypothalamic-pituitary-ovarian axis, a system that stimulates and regulates the production of hormones necessary for normal sexual development and reproductive function.

• Ovulation depends on secretion of luteinizing hormone (LH) and follicle-stimulating hormone (FSH) by the pituitary gland in response to stimulation by the hypothalamus.
• Any disorder that leads to insufficient levels of these hormones (such as infections, tumors, or neurologic disease of the hypothalamus or pituitary gland) can cause infertility.
• Hypothyroidism also impairs fertility.

—Ovarian factors are a major cause of infertility.
• Presumptive signs of ovulation include regular menses, cyclic changes reflected in basal body temperature readings, postovulatory progesterone levels, and endometrial changes due to the presence of progesterone. Absence of presumptive signs suggests anovulation.
• Ovarian failure, in which no ova are produced by the ovaries, may result from ovarian dysgenesis (impairment or loss of reproductive function) or premature menopause. Amenorrhea is often associated with ovarian failure.
• Infrequent ovulation, due to a mild hormonal imbalance, may be caused by polycystic disease of the ovary or abnormalities in the adrenal or thyroid gland that adversely affect hypothalamic-pituitary functioning.

—Uterine abnormalities that result in infertility include a congenitally absent uterus, a bicornuate or double uterus, leiomyomas, and Asherman's syndrome, in which the anterior and posterior uterine walls adhere because of scar tissue formation.

—Tubal and peritoneal factors that impair fertility include faulty tubal transport mechanisms and unfavorable environmental influences affecting the sperm, ova, or recently fertilized ovum. In many patients, infertility results from bilateral occlusion of the tubes due to salpingitis (resulting from gonorrhea, tuberculosis, or puerperal sepsis), peritubal adhesions (resulting from endometriosis, diverticulosis, or childhood rupture of the appendix), or uterotubal obstruction due to tubal spasm.

—A malfunctioning cervix that produces deficient or excessively viscous mucus that is impervious to sperm, preventing their entry into the uterus, is one of the cervical factors that may inhibit fertility. Also, in cervical infection, viscous mucus may contain spermicidal macrophages. The possible existence of cervical antibodies that immobilize sperm is also under investigation.

—Psychological problems more often result from infertility than cause it. Occasionally, ovulation may stop under stress because of the failure of LH release. Marital discord may affect the frequency of intercourse.

3 Discuss the diagnosis of female infertility.

Diagnosis requires a complete physical examination and health history, including answers to specific questions on the patient's reproductive and sexual function, past diseases, mental state, previous surgery, types of contraception used in the past, and family history. Irregular, painless menses may indicate anovulation. A history of pelvic inflammatory disease may suggest fallopian tube blockage.

—The following tests assess ovulation:

- Basal body temperature graphs show a sustained elevation in body temperature postovulation until just before onset of menses, indicating the approximate time of ovulation.
- Endometrial biopsy done on or about day 5 after the basal body temperature elevates provides histologic evidence that ovulation has occurred.
- Progesterone blood levels, measured when they should be highest, can show a luteal phase deficiency.

—The following procedures assess the structural integrity of the fallopian tubes, ovaries, and uterus:

- Rubin's test determines tubal patency by the uterotubal insufflation of carbon dioxide (CO_2). If one or both tubes are patent, the passage of CO_2 into the peritoneal cavity irritates the phrenic nerve, producing referred pain to the shoulder; if the patient feels no pain, the tubes are not patent, and intrauterine pressure of CO_2 rises rapidly.
- Hysterosalpingography provides radiologic evidence of tubal obstruction and abnormalities of the uterine cavity after an injection of radiopaque contrast fluid through the cervix.
- Endoscopy confirms the results of hysterosalpingography. It allows visualization of the endometrial cavity by hysteroscopy or exploration of the posterior surface of the uterus, fallopian tubes, and ovaries by culdoscopy. Laparoscopy allows the visualization of the abdominal and pelvic areas.

—The following tests assess postcoital conditions in the reproductive tract:

- The Sims'-Huhner test determines if sperm can penetrate the cervical mucus. The couple has coitus just before the patient's expected time of ovulation (predicted from basal body temperature), using no precoital lubricants. Following coitus, the patient lies on her back for at least 30 minutes to ensure that spermatozoa will reach the cervix. She uses no postcoital douche and reports to the health care facility within 2 to 8 hours following coitus.
- Immunologic or antibody testing detects spermici-

dal antibodies in the sera of the female. (Further research is being conducted in this area.)

4 Discuss the treatment for female infertility.

Treatment depends on identifying the underlying abnormality or dysfunction of the hypothalamic-pituitary-ovarian axis.
—In overactivity or underactivity of the adrenal or thyroid gland, hormone therapy is necessary; progesterone deficiency requires progesterone replacement.
—Anovulation necessitates treatment with clomiphene, human menopausal gonadotropins, or human chorionic gonadotropin. Ovulation usually occurs several days after these drugs are given. If mucous production decreases (a side effect of clomiphene), small doses of estrogen may be given concomitantly to improve the quality of the cervical mucus.
—Surgical restoration may correct certain structural causes of infertility, such as fallopian tube obstruction. Surgery may also be necessary to remove tumors located within or near the hypothalamus or pituitary gland.
—Endometriosis requires drug therapy (danazol or medroxyprogesterone, or noncyclic administration of oral contraceptives), surgical removal of areas of endometriosis, or a combination of both.
—In vitro (test tube) fertilization has been successful in a few instances and has been widely publicized. However, this procedure is still experimental, and not all patients qualify for it.

5 Describe the medication regimen.

Some drugs commonly used for this disorder are human chorionic gonadotropin, clomiphene citrate, danazol, estrogen, medroxyprogesterone, menotropins, progesterone, and thyroid USP. See Chapter 9, Drug Therapy, for specific medication instructions.

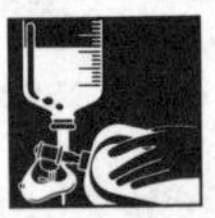

Explaining treatments

HYSTERECTOMY

Patient objectives	*Teaching plan content*
1 State the purpose of a hysterectomy.	The purpose of a hysterectomy is to surgically remove a diseased, ruptured, or cancerous uterus (or uterus, fallopian tubes, ovaries, cervix, and/or vagina).

2 Describe the surgical procedure to be used.

Just before the procedure, the patient will be taken to the operating room and anesthetized.

—Either a vaginal or an abdominal incision will be made, depending on the surgeon's assessment, his discussions with the patient, and the type of hysterectomy to be done.

- If a vaginal procedure is to be done, the incision will be made above and around the cervix.
- Pfannenstiel's (bikini) incision extends transversely across the lower abdomen. Because it leaves a less noticeable scar than a vertical abdominal incision, it is often chosen for cosmetic reasons. However, it may cause more postoperative discomfort.
- The vertical incision extends along the patient's midline from her upper to lower abdomen. This incision takes longer to heal and may be weaker after healing.

The procedures used in a hysterectomy include the following:

—A subtotal, or partial, hysterectomy is removal of the uterus only. It may be done vaginally.

—A total hysterectomy is removal of the uterus and cervix. It may be done vaginally.

—A panhysterectomy, or total abdominal hysterectomy (TAH), with bilateral salpingo-oophorectomy (BSO) is removal of the uterus, cervix, fallopian tubes, and ovaries. This must be done abdominally.

—Wertheim's operation is removal of the uterus, cervix, fallopian tubes, and ovaries as well as partial removal of the vagina and pelvic lymph node dissection. This must be done abdominally.

3 Describe preoperative procedures for a hysterectomy.

In addition to routine preoperative procedures, the patient can expect the following (see Appendix B, *Preoperative and Postoperative Teaching*):

—An anesthesiologist or anesthetist will visit her the day before surgery to discuss what type of anesthetic she will have. Almost all hysterectomies are performed under a general anesthetic; however, if the patient has a breathing problem, a spinal anesthetic may be used. If a general anesthetic is used, she will not awaken during surgery, and if a spinal is used, she will not feel any pain.

—The surgeon will also visit the day before surgery to explain the hysterectomy procedure to be used and the risks involved. The patient should ask questions if she does not understand something. She should write her questions down so she does not forget them.

—She will be asked to sign the operative permit at that time, giving her consent for the procedure. She should not sign the permit until all her questions are answered and she understands everything that is going to happen.
—She will be shaved from her nipple line down to and including her perineum and rectum to prevent infection in the incision from bacteria in the hair.
—A medicated douche may be administered to cleanse her vagina of any discharge or secretions that might harbor bacteria.
—It may also be necessary for her to have an enema to clear her lower bowel and flatten it out, thus lessening the risk of trauma during the operation.
—She will receive a sleeping pill the night before the surgery to help her relax and sleep. She will receive one or two intramuscular injections to sedate her shortly before going to the operating room.
—On the morning of the operation, a nurse will start an I.V. infusion. This is done routinely for the purpose of administering medications or blood during the operation. The I.V. infusion will also provide her with nourishment until she can resume solid foods.
—A urinary catheter (indwelling [Foley] catheter) will be placed into her bladder the morning of surgery. This is to keep the bladder empty so she will not have to worry about getting up to go to the bathroom postoperatively and so the bladder will not be traumatized by instruments during surgery.
—After midnight the night before surgery she should not eat or drink anything. This is to prevent her from vomiting during surgery.

4 Explain postoperative procedures for a hysterectomy.

The patient can expect the following after surgery:
—She will wake up in the recovery room with unfamiliar equipment and sounds, and a nurse will check her frequently.
—When her pulse, breathing, and blood pressure are stable and she is awake and oriented, she will be taken back to her room.
—She will have a large bandage on her abdomen (if she had an abdominal incision) and will be wearing a sanitary pad in case of any vaginal bleeding or drainage.
—Medication will be available for pain and she should ask for it as needed.
—She will sleep most of the first day, and she may experience nausea from the anesthetic.
—She will have sutures or staples on her incision.

5 Discuss patient guidelines for discharge after a hysterectomy.	Once the urinary catheter and I.V. line have been removed and the patient can keep her food down and walk in the hall, the physician will write her discharge. This is usually 4 to 6 days after surgery. —She should take medications as ordered and continue to follow any dietary restrictions or instructions the physician has given her. (See Chapter 9, Drug Therapy, for specific medication instructions.) —She should obtain specific instructions about activity from the physician. Usually, light activity will be allowed at first; more strenuous exercises and increased amounts of activity are acceptable as time progresses. —The sutures or staples may be removed from her incision before she is discharged. The incision must be kept clean and dry. She should expect itching and discomfort as it heals. She should call her physician if the incision becomes red or very tender, starts draining, or opens. —She should also call her physician if she develops a fever, nausea, malaise, or other signs of systemic infection. —Once the vaginal discharge from the operation has stopped, the patient will no longer menstruate. She may begin to experience symptoms of menopause. If she cannot identify them, she should learn them at this time. —In follow-up visits, the physician will want to check her healing and check for any signs of complications. (Provide her with the patient-teaching aid *After a Hysterectomy: How to Care for Yourself,* pp. 392-394.)

DILATATION AND CURETTAGE (D. & C.)

Patient objectives	*Teaching plan content*
1 State the purpose of a D & C.	The purpose of a D & C is to remove the endometrial lining of the uterus to correct dysfunctional bleeding problems.
2 Explain the surgical procedure used in a D & C.	Just before the procedure, the patient will be taken to the operating room and anesthetized. —She will be placed in the lithotomy position, with her feet in stirrups. —Her cervix will be slowly dilated by the insertion of instruments called cervical sounds, which are rods of graduated sizes. —The endometrial lining of the uterus will then be scraped away with a curette, a spoonlike instrument.

3 Describe preoperative procedures for a D & C.

In addition to routine preoperative procedures, the patient can expect the following (see Appendix B, *Preoperative and Postoperative Teaching*):
—An anesthesiologist or anesthetist will visit her the day before surgery to discuss what type of anesthetic she will be given. Either a general or a spinal anesthetic will be used.
—The surgeon will also visit her the day before surgery to explain the procedure. At that time, she will be asked to sign the operative permit. She should not sign it until her questions about the risks of surgery have been answered by her physician. She should write her questions down so she can remember them.
—She may have a preoperative enema to cleanse her bowels and deflate her colon to make surgery easier.
—She will receive a sleeping pill the night before surgery to help her relax and sleep. She will receive a sedative by intramuscular injection just before going to the operating room to help her relax.
—She must not eat or drink anything after midnight the night before surgery or on the morning of surgery.
—On the morning of surgery a nurse will start an I.V. infusion. This is done in case medications and/or blood need to be administered during the operation.

4 Explain postoperative procedures for a D & C.

The patient can expect the following after surgery:
—She will wake up in the recovery room with unfamiliar equipment and sounds, and a nurse will check her often.
—When she is awake enough to respond to her name and her pulse, blood pressure, and breathing are stable, she will be taken to her room.
—She will be wearing a sanitary pad in case of vaginal discharge and/or bleeding.

5 Discuss patient guidelines for discharge after a D & C.

As soon as the patient is awake and able to keep clear liquids down, her I.V. line will be discontinued. That night, she will be expected to walk in her room and use the bathroom; if all goes well, she will be discharged the morning following surgery.
—Pain medication will be provided for cramps.
—She will experience bleeding for a few days, similar to her menses.
—She will have to avoid strenuous activity for 1 or 2 weeks, then will be able to resume her normal activities.
—In her postoperative follow-up appointment at her physician's office, she will be checked for infection or any other complications.

MASTECTOMY

Patient objectives	*Teaching plan content*
1 Define a mastectomy.	A mastectomy is the surgical removal of the breast (simple), the removal of the breast and axillary lymph nodes (modified radical), or the removal of the breast, axillary lymph nodes, and muscle (radical).
2 State the purpose of a mastectomy.	The purpose of a mastectomy is to remove a malignant tumor.
3 Describe preoperative procedures for a mastectomy.	The patient should expect routine preoperative procedures (see Appendix B, *Preoperative and Postoperative Teaching*). Based on discussions with the surgeon, she should be familiar with the procedure and the pros and cons of the alternatives, as well as the possibilities of breast reconstruction if the disease is not advanced.
4 Explain postoperative procedures for a mastectomy.	The patient can expect the following after surgery: —She will wake up in the recovery room with unfamiliar equipment and sounds, and a nurse will check her frequently. —After she is awake and oriented, she will return to her room, where a nurse will check her frequently. —An incisional drain or some type of suction (Hemovac) will be used to remove accumulated fluid and to keep tension off the suture line, promoting healing. —She may move about and get out of bed as soon as possible (even as soon as the anesthetic wears off or the first evening after surgery). —She will receive pain medication and should let the nurse know when she is experiencing pain. She can ease the pain by lying on the affected side or by placing a hand or a pillow on the incision site. A small pillow under the arm may also provide comfort. —She will be expected to deep-breathe and cough periodically to prevent pulmonary problems. She should not suppress full inhalation to avoid pain at the incision site. —She should rotate her ankles periodically to help prevent thromboembolism (blood clots).
5 Demonstrate postoperative arm and hand exercises, if applicable.	If lymph node resection is part of the mastectomy, fluid normally drained by the lymph nodes may accumulate in the affected arm (a condition called lymphedema) if the arm is not exercised. The following exercises (planned with the surgeon to avoid problems with the suture line) prevent this.

—Open the hand on the affected side and close it tightly six to eight times every 3 hours while awake.
—Elevate the arm on the affected side on a pillow above heart level.
—Washing the face and combing the hair are also effective exercises.

6 Discuss patient guidelines for discharge after a mastectomy.

The patient should be able to demonstrate exercises to strengthen her muscles on the affected side (see *Strengthening Exercises: Postmastectomy,* pp. 390-391). She should also know how to prevent complications (see *How to Prevent Complications After a Mastectomy,* pp. 388-389). Her surgeon will schedule a follow-up visit to check for complications and assess healing. The American Cancer Society's Reach for Recovery program can provide instructions, emotional support, and a list of nearby stores that sell prostheses.

Patient-Teaching Aid

MENSTRUAL CYCLE

Dear Patient:

Your menstrual cycle is divided into three distinct phases:

- The menstrual phase starts on the first day of menstruation. The top layer of the endometrium (the material lining the uterus) breaks down and flows out of the body. This flow, called the menses, consists of blood, mucus, and unneeded tissue.
- During the proliferative phase, the endometrium begins to thicken, and the level of estrogen in the blood rises.
- In the secretory phase, the endometrium continues to thicken to nourish an embryo should fertilization occur. Without fertilization, the top layer of the endometrium breaks down, and the menstrual phase of the cycle begins again.

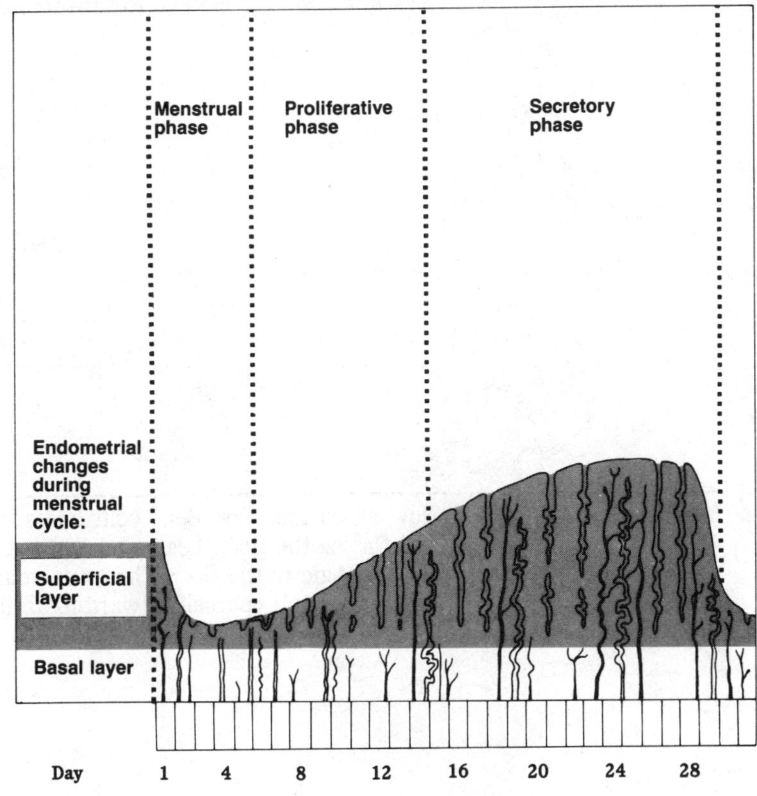

Patient-Teaching Aid

HOW TO REDUCE MENSTRUAL DISCOMFORT: SOME EXERCISES

Dear Patient:

You can help relieve menstrual discomfort by exercising several times a day. Try to repeat each exercise one time and gradually work up to ten times. But if you feel severe pain when performing any of these exercises, stop immediately. If the pain persists, notify the physician. And remember, to get maximum benefit from these exercises, perform each one slowly. Try working the exercises into your daily routine; for example, exercise first thing in the morning, before dinner, or whenever you feel discomfort.

Use these instructions as a guide:

1 Bicycling exercise

Swing your legs up to raise your hips and lower back off the floor. Support your hips with your hands, as shown. The soles of your feet should be facing the ceiling. Now, bend your knees and alternately move your legs in a pedaling motion. Return to starting position.

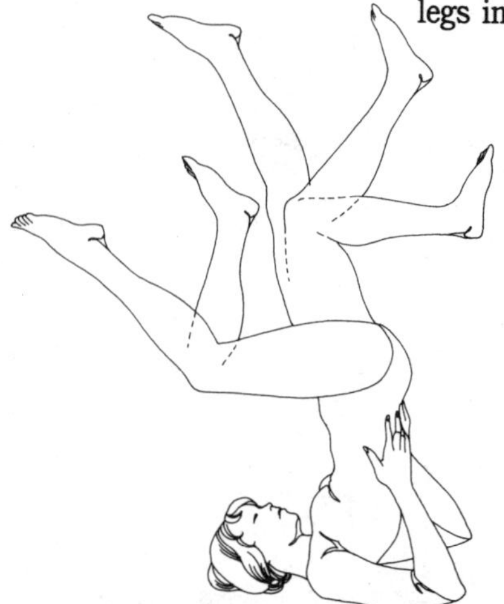

2 Modified sit-ups

Now, sit on the floor. Bend your knees, and place your feet flat on the floor. Lean back until you are at a 45-degree angle to the floor. Then, use your abdominal muscles to pull yourself forward to an upright position.

HOW TO REDUCE MENSTRUAL DISCOMFORT: SOME EXERCISES—*continued*

3 Trunk bends

Next, stand with your legs about 12″ (30 cm) apart. Position your hands on your hips. Bend forward as far as possible. Return to starting position. Now, bend to the right as far as possible. Return to starting position. Bend backward as far as possible. Return to starting position. And finally, bend to the left as far as possible. Return to starting position.

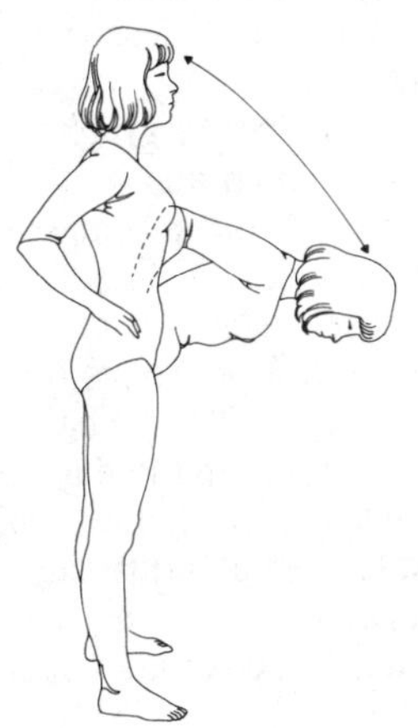

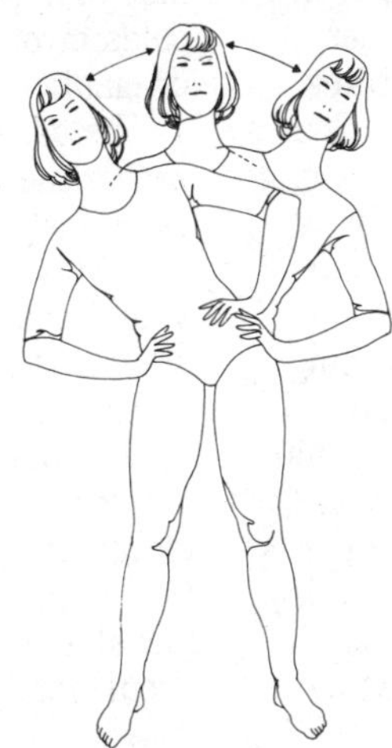

4 Elbow-to-knee stretch

Stand, and clasp your hands behind your head. Lift your right knee to your left elbow, or as close as possible. Lower your leg. Then, lift your left knee to your right elbow, or as close as possible. Lower your leg.

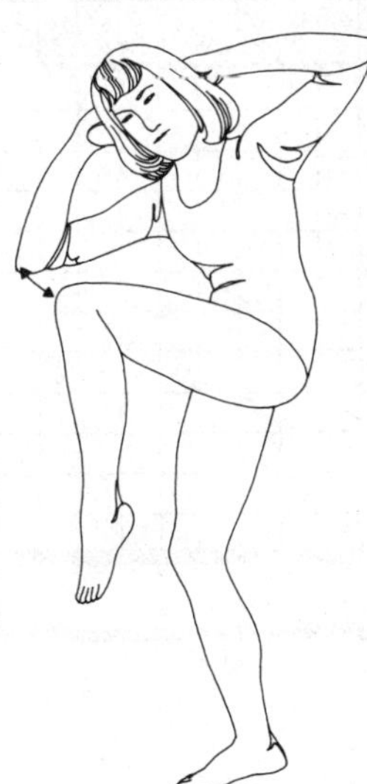

Patient-Teaching Aid

HOW TO TAKE YOUR BASAL BODY TEMPERATURE

Dear Patient:

You are currently taking clomiphene to induce ovulation. Knowing when ovulation has occurred is helpful in both planning and avoiding pregnancy. You can determine when your ovulatory (fertile) period is by taking your basal body temperature every morning. To do so:

- Use a basal body temperature thermometer. This measures temperatures between 96° F. and 100° F. (35.6° C. and 37.8° C.) and is calibrated by tenths of a degree, enabling easier identification of slight temperature changes that occur during your cycle.
- Take your temperature each morning before getting out of bed, since physical activity changes basal temperature. You may take your temperature by the oral, rectal, vaginal, or axillary route. But you should use the same route each day.
- After taking your temperature, shake down the thermometer for the next day. Even shaking the thermometer when you awake can change your basal body temperature.
- Plot your daily temperatures on a monthly graph, like the one shown below. Note any conditions that might affect your basal temperature, such as colds or other infections, sleeplessness, or emotional upset.

The basal body temperature graph shows the time of ovulation and indicates your fertile period. Basal temperature dips slightly at ovulation, then rises approximately 1 degree. The temperature stays at this level until 3 or 4 days before the next cycle begins. The probable time of ovulation in this graph is day 13; note the drop in temperature followed by elevation. An elevated temperature sustained past the time of the next normal menstrual flow suggests pregnancy has occurred.

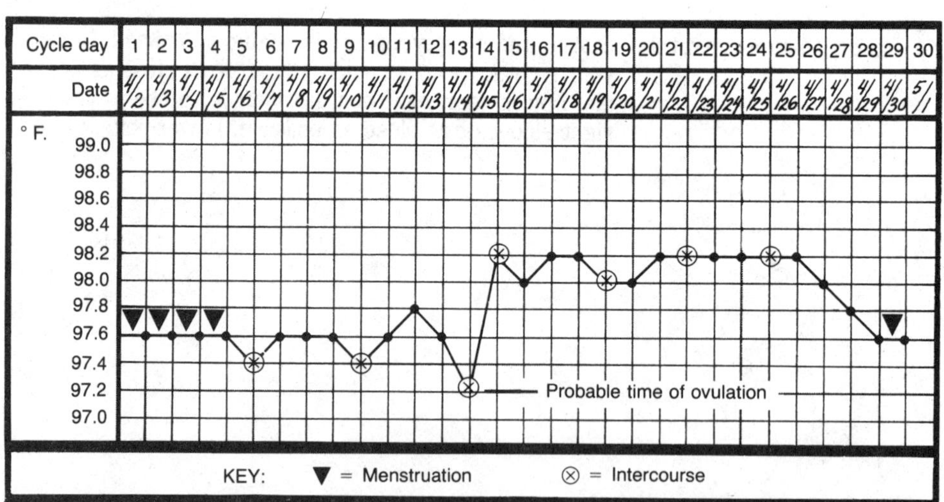

Patient-Teaching Aid

COPING WITH GENITAL HERPES

Dear Patient:

This aid is meant to supplement, not replace, the instructions from your nurse and physician. Use it as a written reminder of what they have taught you.

As you know, genital herpes is contagious in the active stage—in other words, when you have open, draining sores. Keep in mind that after your initial attack, you may have four or more recurrences a year. Be alert for early signs and symptoms that signal an attack, such as itching, redness, or irritation in your genital area; fever; chills; or a tingling or burning sensation in your thighs or buttocks. Keep track of the active attacks and try to figure out what caused them. Emotional stress or exposure to sunlight, for example, may cause an attack.

Routinely check your genital area with a hand-held mirror. Check for reddened or swollen areas. If you see any, consider yourself in the early contagious stage. After you check yourself, wash your hands and dry them. Try to avoid *any* type of sexual contact during this stage. If you choose to engage in sexual intercourse, have your partner wear a condom. But remember, even the condom may not prevent the disease from spreading to your partner.

You can help your lesions heal more quickly by keeping them clean and dry. To help absorb excess moisture, wear cotton underpants. Also, try sprinkling a little cornstarch into your underpants. Wash the lesions several times a day with mild, unscented soap and warm water. Pat your skin dry. Be careful not to scratch the sores.

Because herpes spreads easily, wash your clothes and bed linens separately from those of other family members. If possible, transfer the laundry directly to a dryer. Otherwise, hang the clothing or bed linens in the sun and iron them later. If this is inconvenient, you may want to send the articles to a professional dry cleaner.

When the herpes virus is in its active stage, take special precautions to avoid spreading the infection. Using soap and hot water, separately wash any eating utensils you use, including your plate, cup, and glasses. To dry the utensils, wrap them in aluminum foil and place them for 10 minutes in an oven warmed to 200° F. (93.3° C.). Or use disposable utensils, cups, and plates. NOTE: If you wash and dry your utensils in a mechanical dishwasher, these precautions are not necessary. But set the dishwasher at its high temperature setting (usually 160° F. [71.1° C.]).

Keep your towel, washcloth, toothbrush, toothpaste, soap, and bathroom cup in your bedroom. That way, other family members will be less likely to use these personal articles.

Patient-Teaching Aid

HOW TO EXAMINE YOUR BREASTS

Dear Patient:
To help detect abnormalities early, you should examine your breasts once a month. If you have gone through menopause, examine your breasts on the same date each month. If you have not gone through menopause, do the examination a few days after your menstrual period ends, since your breasts may swell or harden during your period. Also, try to do each examination the same number of days after your period ends, so you can more easily recognize any changes. Eventually, you will become very familiar with your breasts and will be able to recognize anything abnormal.

1

Here is how to examine your breasts: First, stand or sit at a slight angle in front of a mirror, with your left side closer to the mirror than your right. Raise your arms above your head and check your breasts for any change in their shape or size and any puckering or dimpling of the skin.

Now, turn so your right side is closer to the mirror. With your arms raised, repeat the procedure.

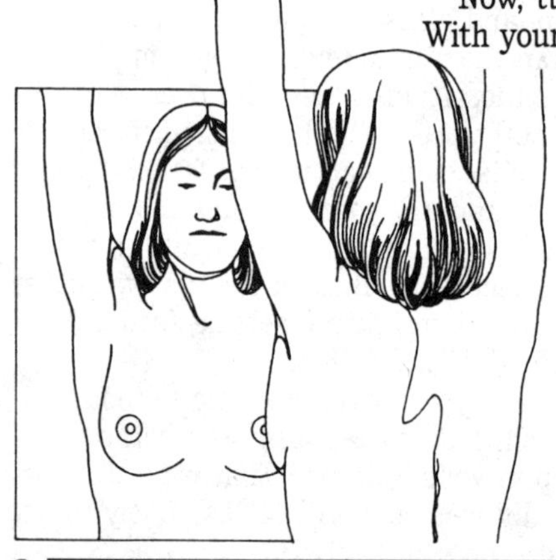

2

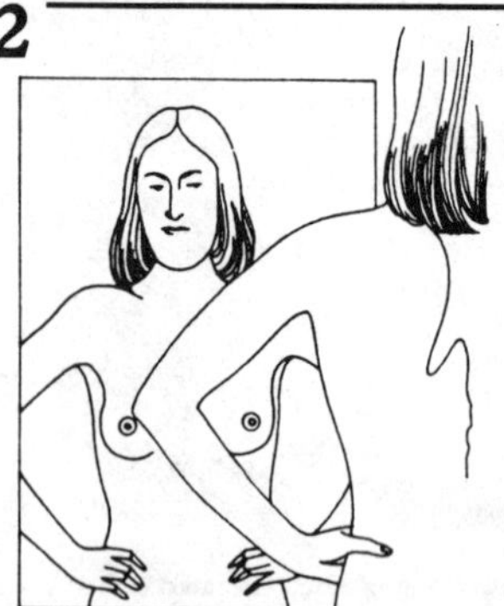

Directly face the mirror. Place your hands on your hips and press downward, while holding your shoulders back. Then, slowly turn your body from side to side, and look for any changes in either breast's appearance.

HOW TO EXAMINE YOUR BREASTS—*continued*

3

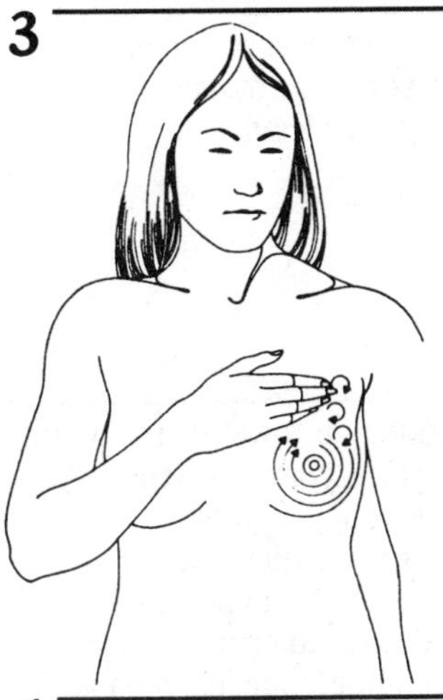

Now, place your arms at your sides, and prepare to feel your breasts for lumps or thickenings. First place your right hand on the very top part of your left breast, directly in line with the nipple. Moving your fingertips in a small, circular, clockwise motion, feel the top part of your breast. Repeat this motion on the side of your breast; then, on the underside of your breast. (If you have large breasts, you may have to lift each breast slightly to check its underside.) Continue until you have covered a circle around the outside of your breast. Now move your fingertips slightly closer to the nipple and repeat this step. Continue repeating this step until you have covered your entire breast, including the area immediately surrounding your nipple. Repeat this step on your right breast, using your left hand.

4

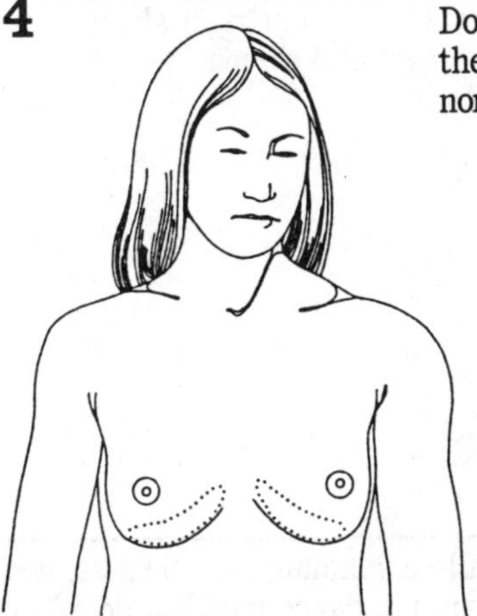

Do not worry if you feel a hard ridge of tissue along the lower part of your breast, as illustrated here. It is normal.

5

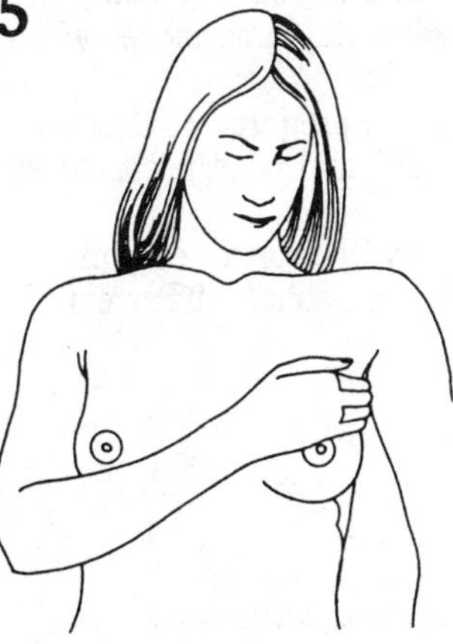

Remain standing. Using your right hand, feel the area beneath your left armpit with your left arm raised. Check it again with your arm at your side. Then, use your left hand to check under your right armpit, following the same procedure.

If you feel a small lump under your armpit that moves freely, do not be alarmed. This area contains your lymph glands, which may become swollen when you are sick. Check the size of the lump daily. Call the physician if it does not go away in a few days or if it gets larger.

HOW TO EXAMINE YOUR BREASTS—*continued*

6

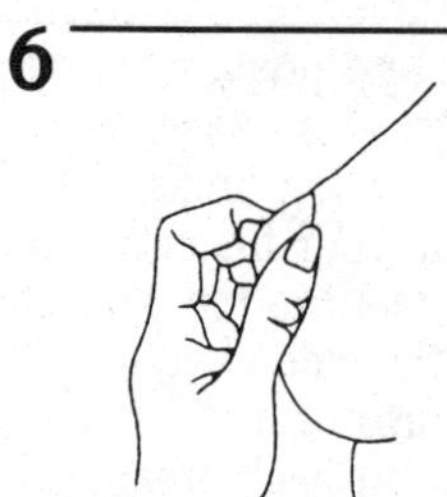

Gently squeeze your nipples between your fingers to check for liquid secretions. If you see any, note the color and amount, and call the physician.

7

Now, lie down, and place a rolled-up towel or pillow under your left shoulder. Then, place your left arm beneath your head, and examine your left breast and armpit with your right hand in the same manner you did while standing. Again, feel for any lumps or thickenings in your breast or under your armpit.

After you are finished examining your left breast, place the towel or pillow beneath your right shoulder, and examine your right breast and armpit.

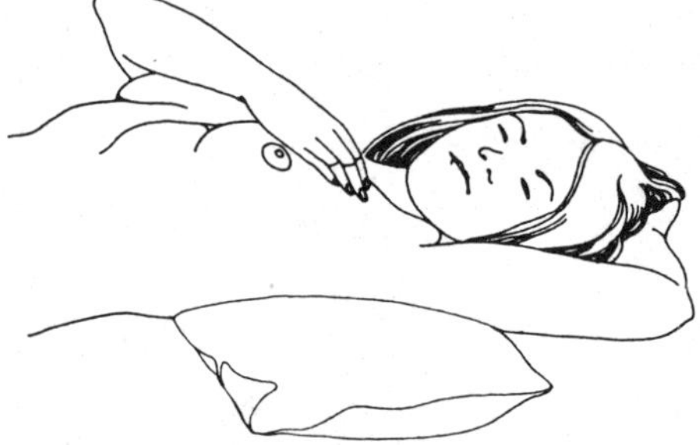

8

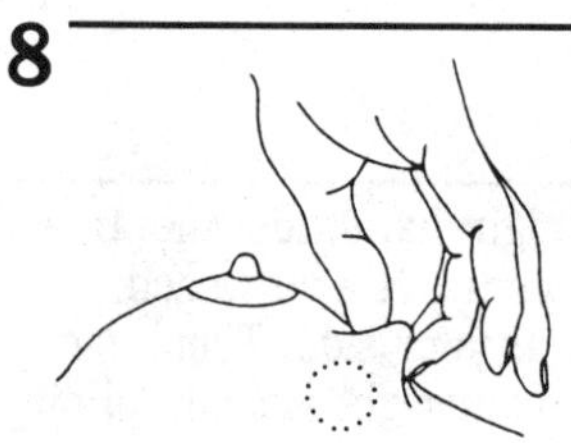

If you do feel a lump while examining your breasts, do not panic—most lumps are not cancerous. But do follow these steps. First, note whether you can easily lift the skin covering it and whether the lump moves when you do so.

Next, notify your physician. Be prepared to describe how the lump feels (hard or soft) and whether it moves easily under the skin.

Chances are, your physician will want to examine the lump. Then, he can advise you about what treatment (if any) you need.

Patient-Teaching Aid

HOW TO DO KEGEL EXERCISES

Dear Patient:

Repeated painful intercourse may cause involuntary contraction of a muscle called the pubococcygeus (PC), which encircles your urinary opening and vagina. When this happens, intercourse becomes even more difficult.

Below are some isometric exercises—called Kegel exercises—that can strengthen and help you gain voluntary control of the PC muscle.

- Begin by sitting on the toilet with your legs spread. Then, without moving your legs, start and stop the flow of urine. The PC muscle is the one that contracts to help control urine flow.
- Now that you have identified the PC muscle, you can exercise it regularly. Like most isometric exercises, Kegel exercises can be performed almost anywhere—while sitting at your desk, lying in bed, standing in line, and especially while urinating. As you perform these exercises, remember to breathe naturally—do not hold your breath.

Now, periodically contract the PC muscle as you did to stop the urine flow. Count slowly to three, then relax the muscle.

- Next, contract and relax the PC muscle as quickly as possible, without using your stomach or buttock muscles.
- Finally, slowly contract the entire vaginal area. Then bear down, using your abdominal muscles as well as your PC muscle.

For the first week, repeat each exercise 10 times (1 set) for 5 sets daily. Then, each week add 5 repetitions to each exercise (15, 20, and so forth). Keep doing 5 sets daily.

After a week or two of practice, you will notice improvement. To monitor your progress, insert one or two well-lubricated fingers into your vagina so you can feel the PC muscle contract.

Patient-Teaching Aid

HOW TO PREVENT COMPLICATIONS AFTER A MASTECTOMY

Dear Patient:

Now that you are ready to return home, you will want to avoid complications, such as infection. Check both the arm affected by surgery and the incision site twice each day. If an area looks red, feels warm, or is unusually hard or swollen, notify the physician immediately. Also notify him if you see drainage (fluid) from the incision or if you develop a fever.

Here are a few simple guidelines to follow during your recovery:

- Do not put heavy lotions, creams, or medications on or near the incision site (unless the physician tells you to do so).
- If you cut or scratch your affected arm, immediately wash the area with soap and warm water. Apply an antiseptic ointment, if needed.

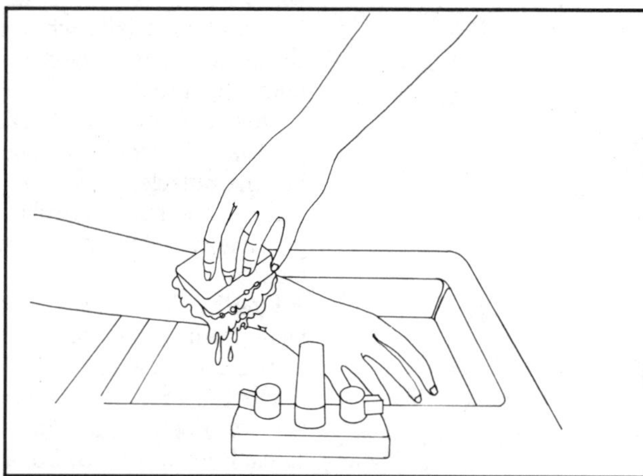

- Do not pick or cut cuticles or hangnails on your affected hand. Use lanolin hand cream to keep cuticles soft.
- Do not carry your pocketbook in the crook of your affected arm. To protect this arm, get into the habit of using your other arm to carry your pocketbook or articles weighing more than 10 lb (4.5 kg).
- If you wear a wristwatch or other jewelry on the affected arm, make sure it fits loosely. Wear clothing with loose-fitting sleeves.
- If you sew, use a thimble to avoid pinpricks.
- Avoid exposing your affected side to excessive sunlight.

HOW TO PREVENT COMPLICATIONS AFTER A MASTECTOMY—*continued*

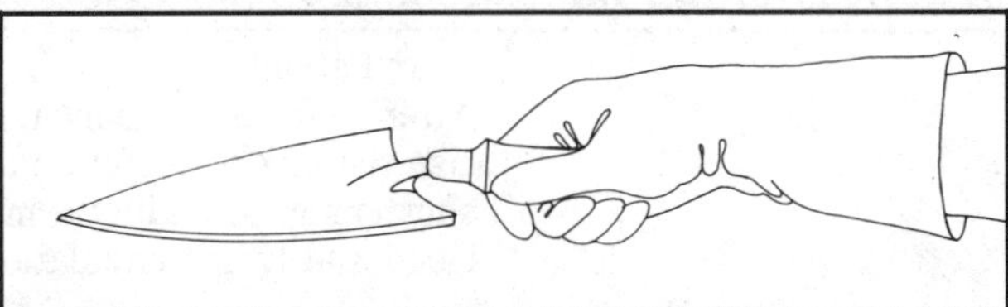

- Wear heavy gloves when gardening.
- Apply protective insect repellent before going to areas with biting insects.
- Do not let anyone give you an injection or vaccinate you in your affected arm—unless specifically recommended by a physician who knows you have had breast surgery.
- Similarly, make sure your blood pressure is taken on your unaffected arm. And, if you must give blood samples for any reason, give them from your unaffected arm.
- Regularly perform strengthening exercises, as instructed.
- Every other day, record the amount of swelling (if any) in your affected arm. To do this, measure the circumference of your upper arm, about 5″ (12.7 cm) above your elbow. Then, measure the circumference of the largest part of your forearm, about 5″ above your wrist. Record your findings. If you detect swelling, use a few pillows to elevate your arm above heart level. If the swelling does not go away, notify the physician.

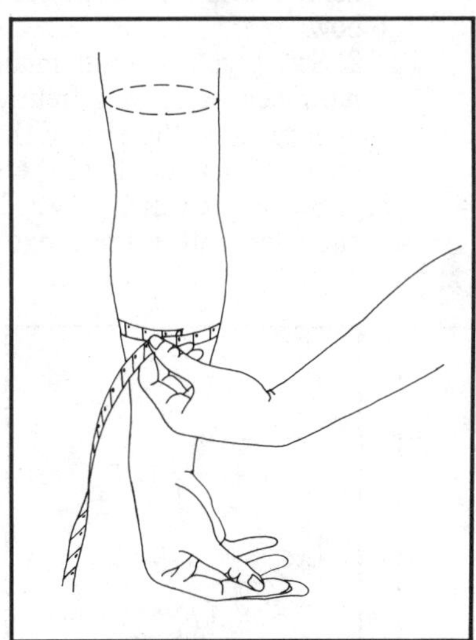

Patient-Teaching Aid

STRENGTHENING EXERCISES: POSTMASTECTOMY

Dear Patient:

After your mastectomy, it is important that you exercise the involved arm and shoulder to prevent muscle shortening, to maintain muscle tone, and to improve blood and lymph circulation.

Wall climbing

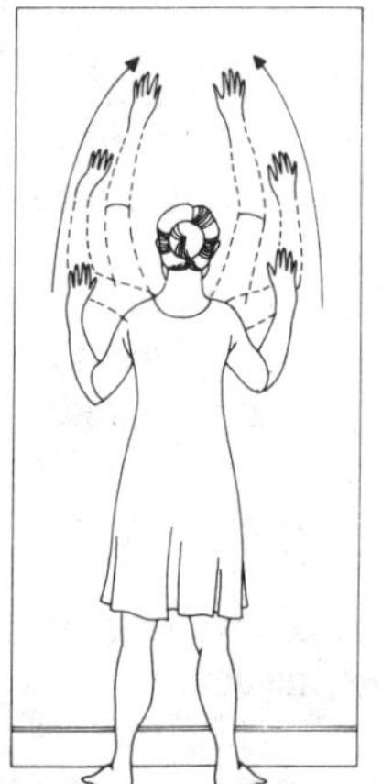

Stand facing a wall, with your toes as close to the wall as possible and your feet apart. Bending your elbows slightly, place your palms against the wall at shoulder level. Then, flexing your fingers, work your hands up the wall until your arms are fully extended. Work your hands back down to the starting point.

Pendulum swing

Place your uninvolved arm on the back of a chair. Let your involved (free) arm hang loosely.

1. Swing your arm from left to right. Be sure the movement comes from your shoulder joint and not your elbow.
2. Swing your arm in small circles. Again, be sure the movement is coming from your shoulder joint. As your arm relaxes, the size of the circle will probably increase. Then, circle in the opposite direction.
3. Swing your arm forward and backward from your shoulder, within the range of comfort.

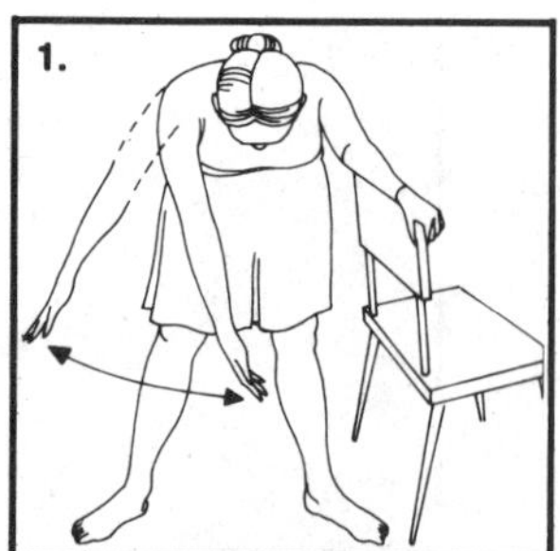

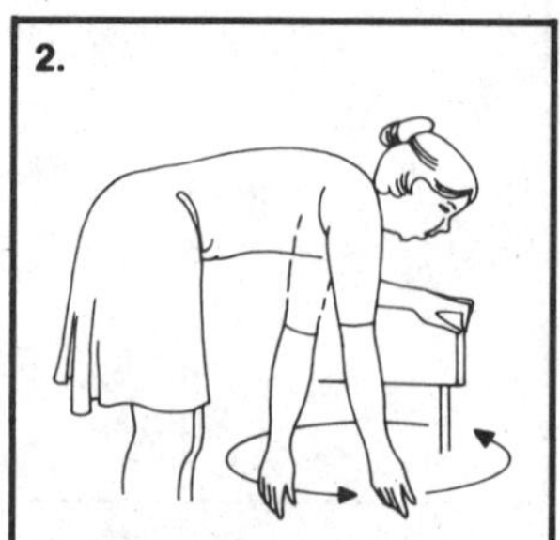

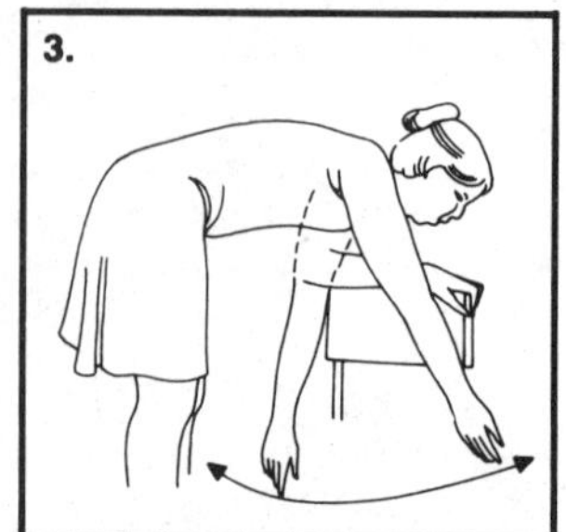

STRENGTHENING EXERCISES: POSTMASTECTOMY—*continued*

Pulley

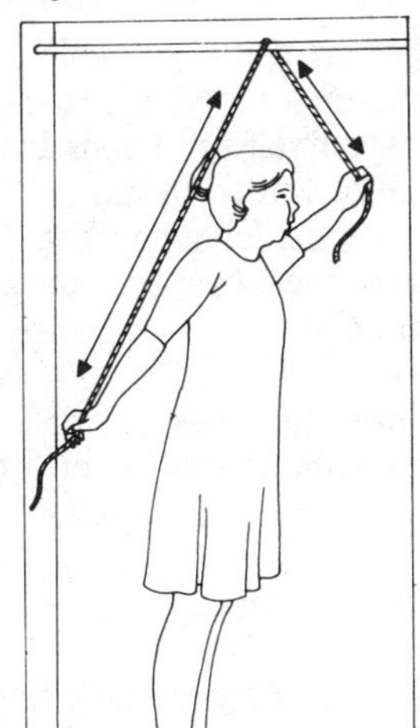

Toss a rope over your shower curtain rod and hold an end of the rope in each hand. Using a seesaw motion and with your arms outstretched, slide the rope up and down over the rod.

Rope turning

Stand facing the door. Take the free end of a rope in the hand of the operated side. Place your other hand on your hip. With your arm extended and held away from your body, turn the rope, making as wide a swing as possible. Start slowly, and increase your speed as your arm gets stronger.

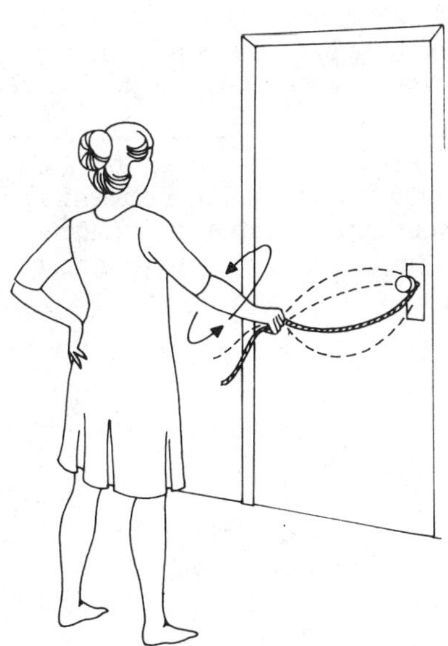

Patient-Teaching Aid

AFTER A HYSTERECTOMY: HOW TO CARE FOR YOURSELF

Dear Patient:

Because you have just had a hysterectomy, you will want to take special precautions to speed your recovery. Take care not to overexert yourself until your incision heals completely. The nurse has filled in the physician's specific instructions on the following list. Read it carefully. If you have any questions, talk to your nurse. Then, when you go home, make a special effort to follow these guidelines:

- Restrict your activities. For example, avoid heavy lifting and cleaning, as well as vigorous sports, for 6 to 8 weeks. Also wait at least ________ weeks before driving a car.
- Avoid sexual activity and douching for ____________ weeks after surgery.
- Take a shower ________ days after surgery. Before taking a tub bath, get your physician's okay.
- Call your physician if you have heavy bleeding, abnormal cramps, hot flashes, or changes in your bowel habits.

Now here are some exercises to help strengthen your abdomen. You can begin this exercise program ________ days after surgery. Add a new exercise each day. Repeat each exercise four times, twice a day, in the morning and in the evening. Continue this program for _____ weeks, or as ordered by your physician.

IMPORTANT: If any of these exercises is painful, stop it immediately. If the pain persists, notify the physician.

1

Sit at the edge of your bed or chair. Take a slow deep breath. Breathe in through your nose, and concentrate on fully expanding your chest. Breathe out through your mouth and concentrate on drawing in your abdominal muscles.

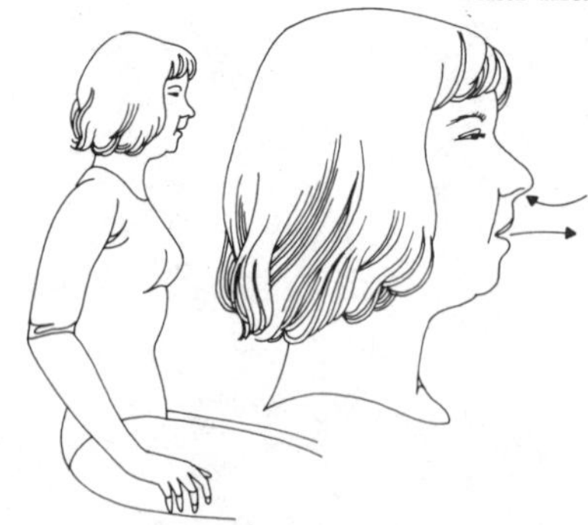

AFTER A HYSTERECTOMY: HOW TO CARE FOR YOURSELF—*continued*

2

Now, lie on your back, on the bed or floor, with your legs slightly apart. Extend your arms straight out at shoulder level. Without bending your elbows, slowly raise your arms above your chest until your hands touch. Slowly lower your arms.

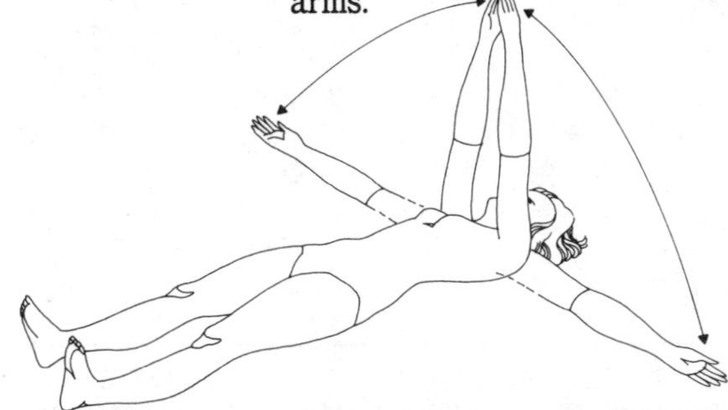

3

Maintaining the same position, place your arms at your sides. Bend your knees slightly; then arch your back. Return to starting position.

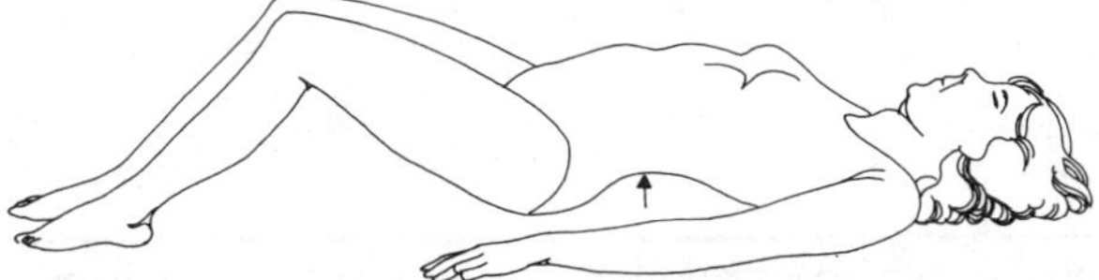

4

Lie with your knees bent and your feet on the bed or floor, as shown. Now, lift your head and contract your buttocks at the same time. Concentrate on rolling your pelvis toward your abdomen (see arrow). Return to starting position.

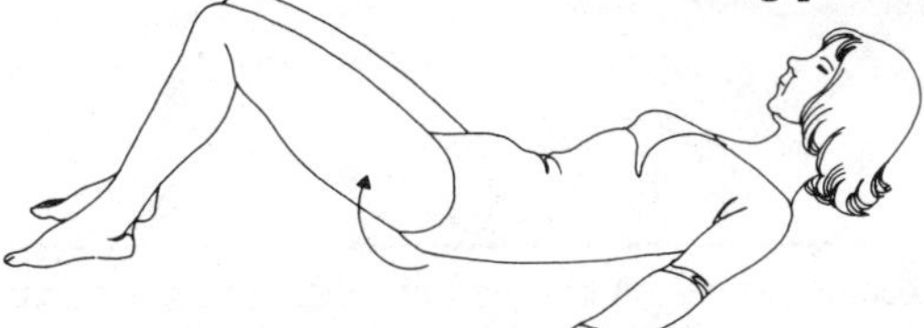

5

Next, lie on your back, with your legs straight. Slightly raise your head and your right knee. Then reach for—but do not touch—your right knee with your left hand. Return to starting position. Repeat with your left knee and right hand.

AFTER A HYSTERECTOMY: HOW TO CARE FOR YOURSELF—*continued*

6

Now, bend your right knee and bring it toward your chest, as close as possible. Straighten and lower your right leg, until your right foot again rests on the bed or floor. Repeat with your left leg.

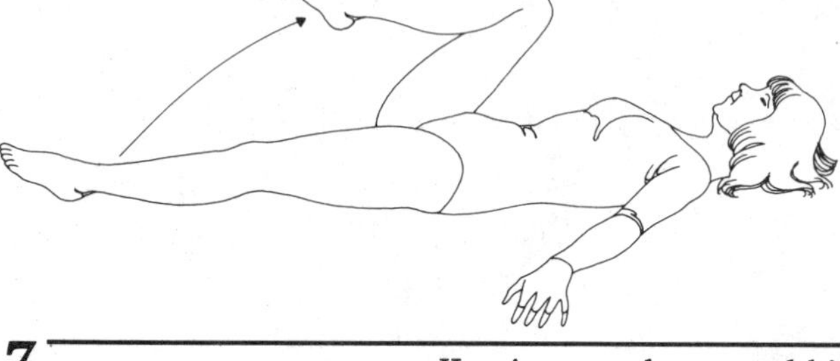

7

Keeping your knees and hips straight and toes pointed upward, raise your right leg as high as possible. Return to starting position, and repeat with your left leg.

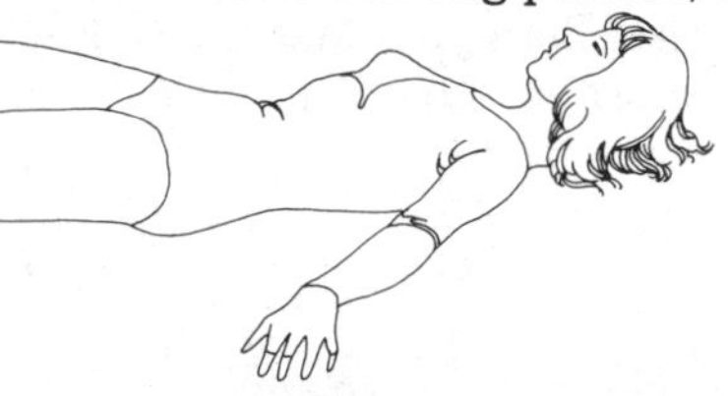

8

Keeping your knees and hips straight and toes pointed upward, raise both legs as high as possible. Return to starting position.

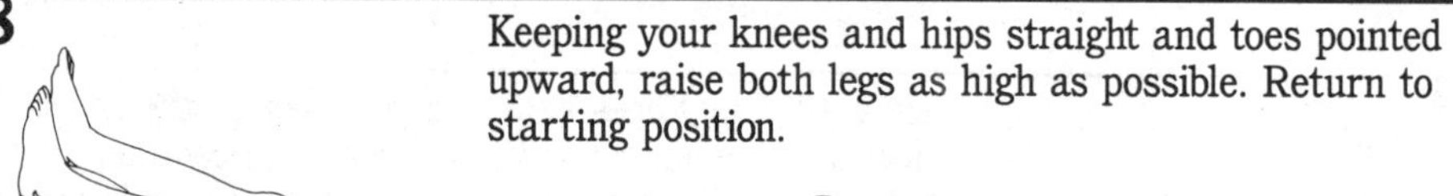

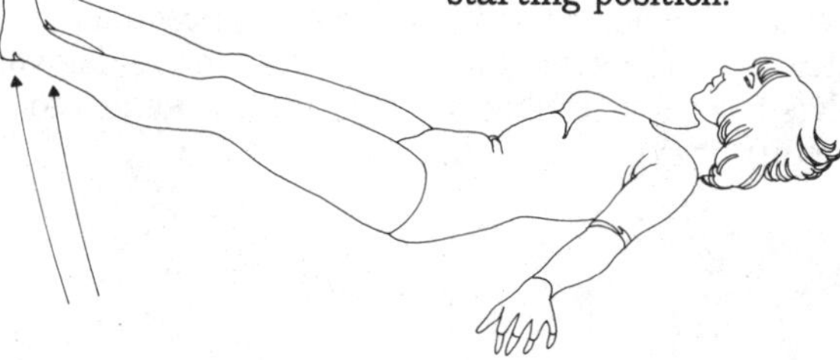

9

For this exercise, kneel on the bed or floor and support your weight on your elbows and knees, as shown. Hump your back upward as you contract your buttocks and pull in your abdomen. Then relax and breathe deeply.

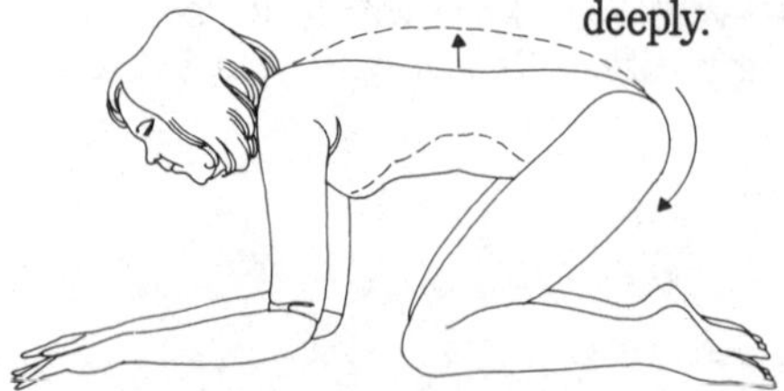

Patient-Teaching Aid

STRENGTHENING THE PELVIC FLOOR MUSCLES

Dear Patient:

Many women suffer from stress incontinence—urine leakage during a sudden physical strain, such as a cough or sneeze. You can prevent or minimize this problem by doing simple exercises that will strengthen your pelvic floor muscles. You can perform them sitting or standing and during a variety of activities, such as reading, watching TV, waiting in a line, and especially while urinating.

Here is how to do the exercises:

- Tense the muscles around your anus. This tightens the posterior muscles of the pelvic floor.
- While urinating, stop the flow of urine and then restart it. This tightens the anterior muscles of the pelvic floor.
- Now that you have identified these muscles, you can exercise them anywhere at any time. As you perform the exercises, slowly tighten each group of muscles and then release them.

Patient-Teaching Aid

GIVING YOURSELF A SITZ BATH

Dear Patient:
For a few days after you go home, your perineum (the area near your vagina) may feel uncomfortable, especially if you had stitches or if you have hemorrhoids. To make yourself more comfortable, take warm-water sitz baths, as shown in this aid.

1

Take a sitz bath at these times: ____________________

____

If the physician orders, add this medication to the warm water: ____________________

____

For your convenience, we have provided you with a sitz bath kit. It contains a plastic pan and a plastic bag with attached tubing. Here is how to use it.

First, raise the toilet seat and fit the plastic pan onto the toilet bowl. Position the pan so its drainage holes are along the back of the bowl, as shown here. If you have placed the pan correctly, you will see a single slot in front.

2

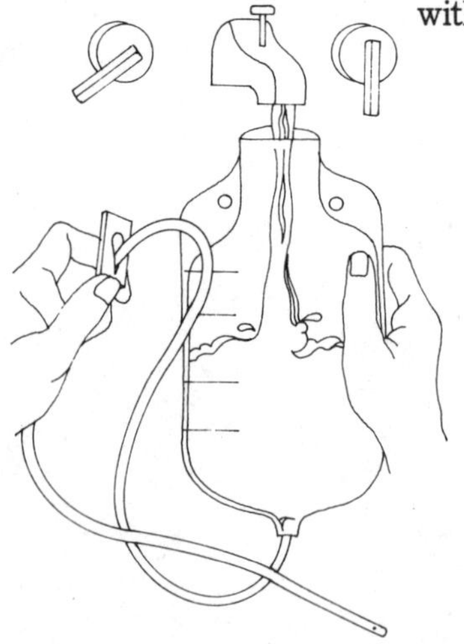

Next, close the clamp on the bag's tubing. Fill the bag with warm water and medication (if ordered).

GIVING YOURSELF A SITZ BATH—*continued*

3

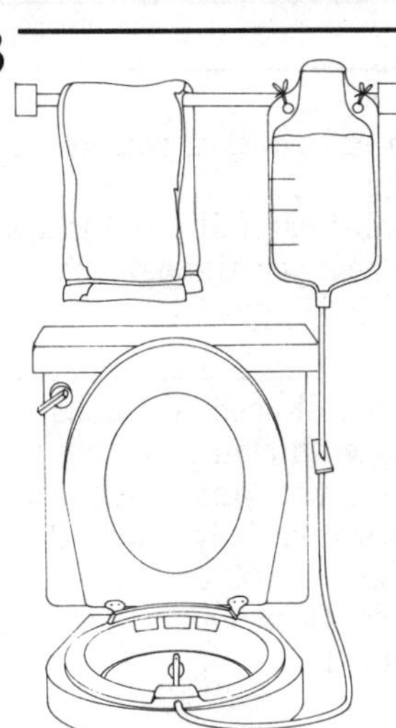

Snap the free end of the tubing into the slot at the front of the pan. Then, hang the bag on the doorknob or towel bar. Make sure the bag is higher than the toilet.

4

Now, you are ready for your sitz bath. Sit in the pan and open the clamp on the tubing. Let the warm water flow from the bag and fill the pan. (Do not worry about it overflowing, because excess water will flow out the drainage holes.) Continue sitting in the pan until the water begins to cool.

After your sitz bath, dry yourself completely. Use a front-to-back motion to avoid contaminating your vagina with rectal bacteria. If ordered, apply an ointment or dressing.

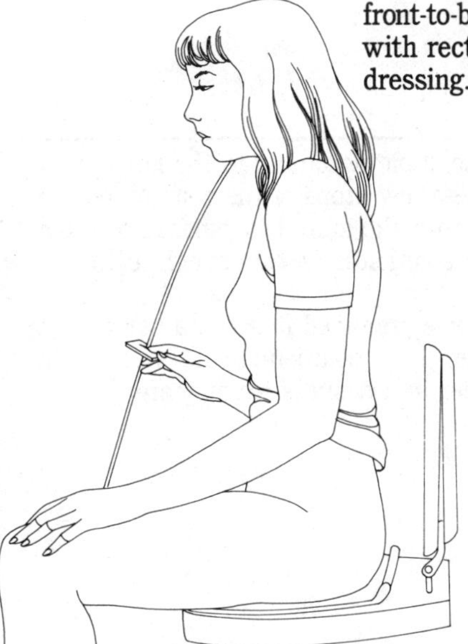

Patient-Teaching Aid

LEARNING HOW TO DOUCHE

Dear Patient:
To treat your vaginal infection or irritation, your physician has prescribed this douche: ________________.
Read the instructions on the label carefully, and follow them. Use these guidelines to help you through the procedure.

1

First, gather the equipment you will need: a douche bag; about 3′ (90 cm) of tubing with clamp and hard-rubber douche nozzle; douche solution; and water-soluble lubricant, such as K-Y Lubricating Jelly. You will also need a hook positioned about 2′ (60 cm) above your bathtub to hang the bag on. Or use a straight-backed chair, as shown in this aid.

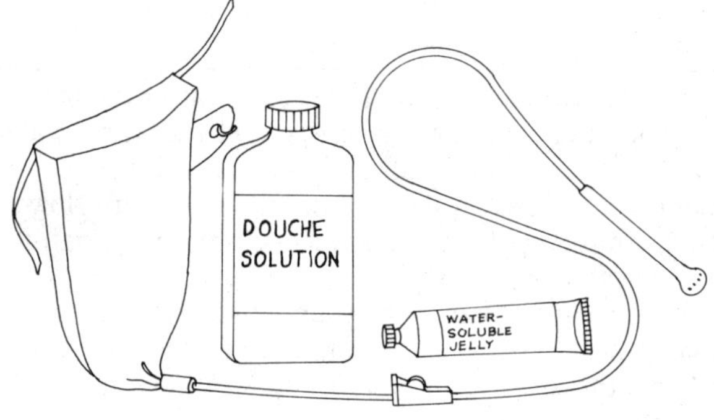

2

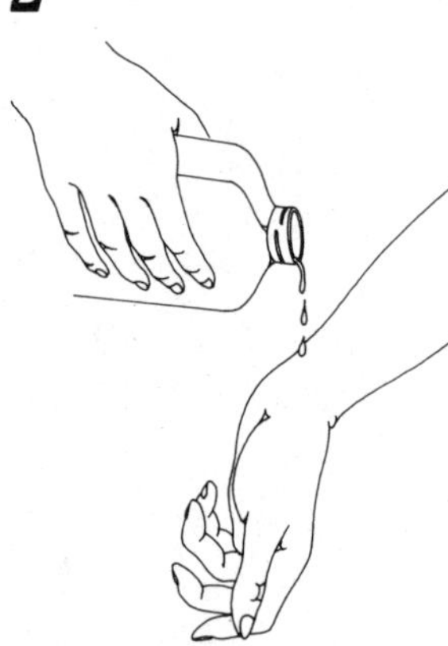

Now, prepare the solution, according to the label instructions. Sprinkle a few drops of the solution on the inside of your arm to make sure it is warmed to room temperature. If the solution is warm enough, fill the douche bag with it.

Some douches come premixed in a container with a prelubricated nozzle. If the solution is cold, warm it by placing the container in a basin of warm water for about 20 minutes.

LEARNING HOW TO DOUCHE—*continued*

3

Next, hang the douche bag on the chair. Place the chair as close to the bathtub as possible. Lubricate the nozzle with water-soluble jelly.

Recline in the bathtub with your feet toward the drain. Prop your back against the bathtub's slanting portion. Flex your knees and spread apart your legs, as shown here.

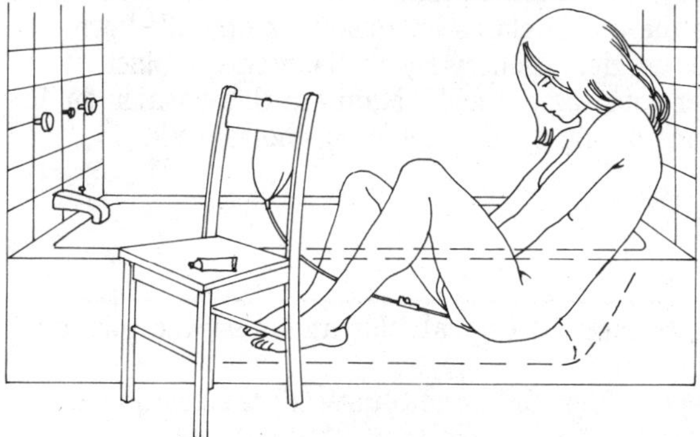

4

Suppose you have a shower stall instead of a bathtub. Position yourself on the floor of the stall with your back against the side at a 45-degee angle, as shown here. Flex your knees and spread your legs.

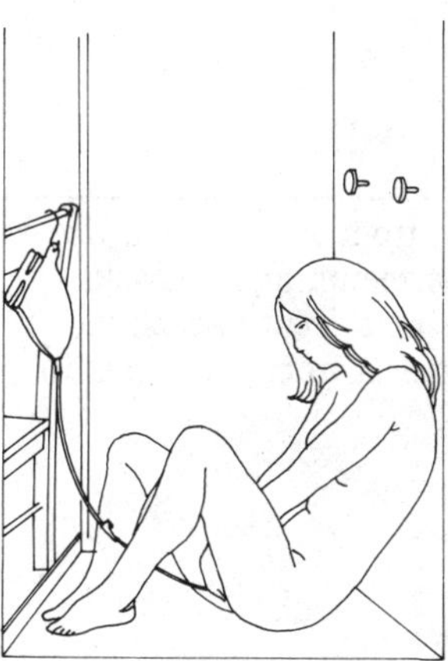

5

Using your fingertips, spread your vaginal folds (labia). With your other hand, gently insert the nozzle a short way into your vagina. To do this, angle it slightly up toward the base of your spine, as shown in this illustration.

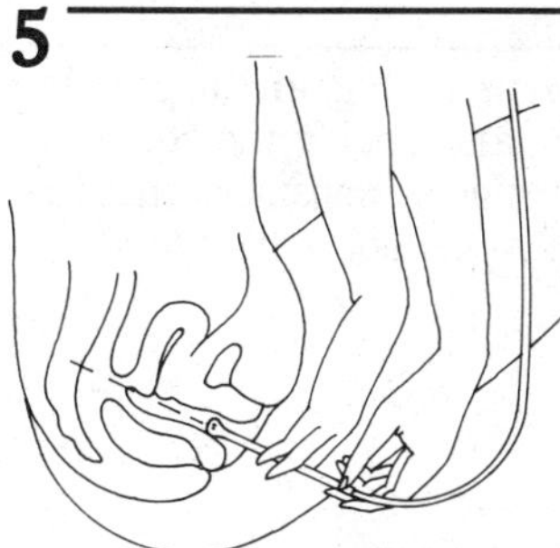

LEARNING HOW TO DOUCHE—*continued*

6

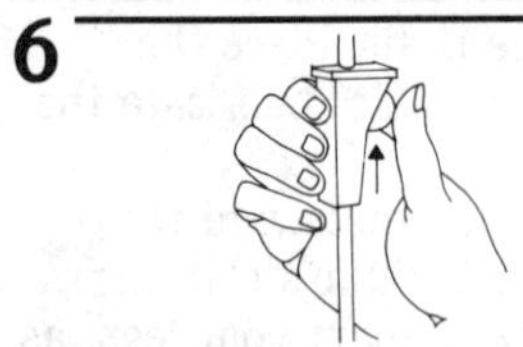

Now, open the clamp and allow gravity to draw the solution into your vagina. Slowly rotate the nozzle, advancing it 1″ to 2″ (2.5 to 5 cm) as you do.

7

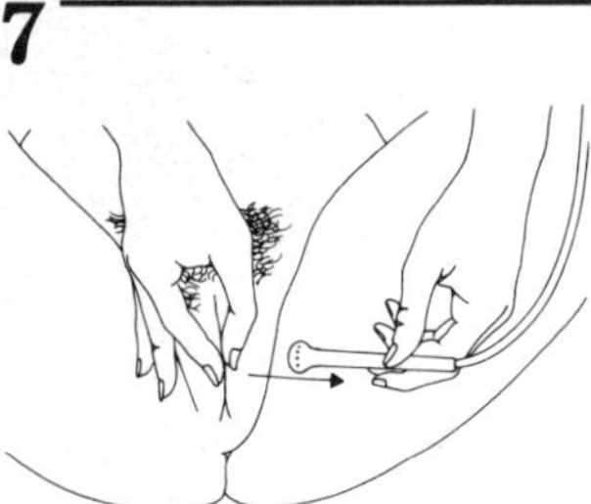

When you feel fullness or pressure on your bladder, close the tubing clamp (or remove the prefilled container nozzle). Then, use your fingertips to pinch together your vaginal folds. Maintain this position for 15 seconds. Doing so allows the douche to work.

8

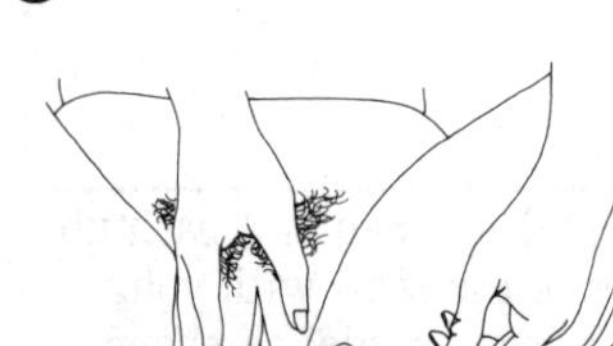

Next, release the vaginal folds and allow the solution to gush out.

Repeat steps 6, 7, and 8 until all the solution is gone.

9

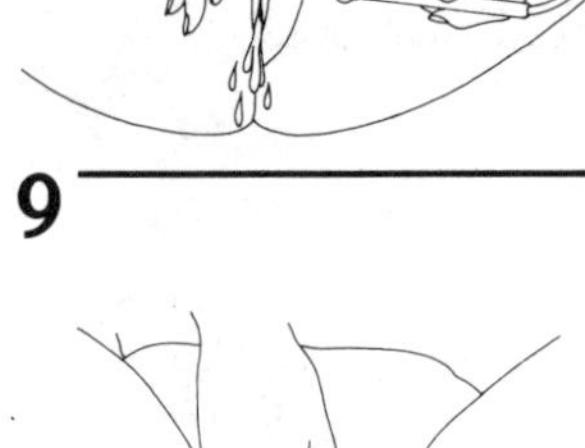

Now, gently remove the nozzle from your vagina. Use a clean towel to pat dry your perineum and buttocks. (Remember to dry yourself using a front-to-back motion, so you do not spread bacteria from your anus to your vagina.)

10

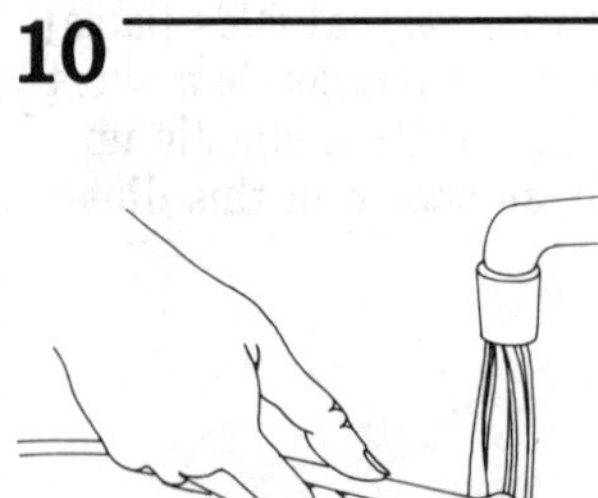

Finally, wash the douche nozzle, tubing, and bag with soap and water. After rinsing and drying the equipment, store it in a clean, dry place. Remember that the equipment is for your use only—do not loan it to anyone.

Drug Therapy

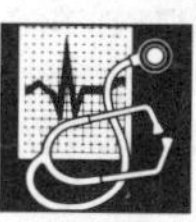

Patient-learner data base*

Areas of potential knowledge deficit

Risk factors (for noncompliance with medication regime)
—Fear of addiction
—Misconceptions about medication
—Unpleasant side effects
—Multiple drug regimen
—Presence of administration difficulty
—Presence of financial difficulty
—Previous medication teaching inadequate/ineffective

Specific level of knowledge about his medication
—Name of medication
—Dosage prescribed
—Ordered frequency of administration
—Medication action
—Side effects of medication
—Administration guidelines

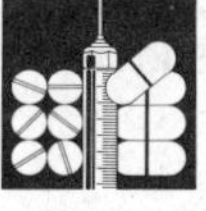

Explaining medications

ACETOHEXAMIDE (Dimelor, Dymelor)

Patient objectives	*Teaching plan content*
1 State the name of the medication, the dose prescribed, and the ordered frequency of administration.	This information should be obtained from the patient's physician.

*A general assessment should be done for all patients. For general assessment guidelines, see Chapter 1, Principles of Patient Teaching.

2 Explain the use of acetohexamide.	Acetohexamide is used to treat Type II diabetes (uncontrolled by diet alone) because of its ability to lower blood sugar levels by stimulating the release of insulin from the pancreas.
3 Identify potential side effects of acetohexamide.	Acetohexamide has the following side effects: —Blood: bone marrow aplasia (underdevelopment of bone marrow) —GI: nausea, heartburn, vomiting —Metabolic: sodium loss, hypoglycemia —Skin: rash, pruritus (itching), facial flushing —Other: hypersensitivity reactions.
4 Discuss patient guidelines for taking acetohexamide.	The patient should follow these guidelines while taking acetohexamide: —Take the drug only as directed. Do not adjust the dose or stop taking it without the physician's approval. —Maintain the diabetic diet, as ordered. This drug does not replace dietary means to control blood sugar levels. —Be aware that hypoglycemia may occur. (See the "Diabetes Mellitus" teaching plan in Chapter 5, Endocrine Disorders, for further instructions.) —Avoid moderate to large intake of alcohol, as unpleasant side effects may occur with acetohexamide. —Do not take over-the-counter medications in conjunction with acetohexamide without first consulting the physician.

ACYCLOVIR (Zovirax)

Patient objectives	*Teaching plan content*
1 State the name of the medication, the dose prescribed, and the ordered frequency of administration.	This information should be obtained from the patient's physician.
2 Explain the use of acyclovir.	Acyclovir is a local anti-infective used to treat herpes simplex virus infections.
3 Identify potential side effects of acyclovir.	Acyclovir has the following side effects: —Skin: transient burning and stinging, rash, pruritus (itching).

4 Discuss patient guidelines for using acyclovir.	The patient should follow these guidelines while using acyclovir: —Use the ointment on cutaneous areas only. Do not apply it to the eye. —Although the dose size for each application may vary, depending on the total lesion area, use approximately a ½″ ribbon of ointment on each 4″ of surface area. —Thoroughly cover all lesions with ointment. —Use a finger cot or rubber glove when applying the ointment to prevent the transmission of infection to other body sites and to other people.

ALBUTEROL (Proventil, Ventolin)

Patient objectives	*Teaching plan content*
1 State the name of the medication, the dose prescribed, and the ordered frequency of administration.	This information should be obtained from the patient's physician.
2 Explain the use of albuterol.	Albuterol is used to treat obstructive airway disease because of its ability to relax the smooth muscle of the respiratory tract, thus enhancing breathing.
3 Identify potential side effects of albuterol.	Albuterol has the following side effects: —CNS: tremor, nervousness, dizziness, insomnia, headache —CV: tachycardia, palpitations, hypertension —EENT: drying and irritation of nose and throat (with inhaled form) —GI: heartburn, nausea, vomiting —Other: muscle cramps.
4 Discuss patient guidelines for using albuterol.	The patient should follow these guidelines while using albuterol: —Use the drug exactly as prescribed. —Use both tablets and aerosol if ordered by the physician. —Allow 2 minutes between inhalations. Use the inhaler correctly to obtain the maximum effect. (See Appendix D, *Medication Administration,* for further instructions.) —Store in a light-resistant container. —If breathing difficulty occurs after the drug has been used, discontinue use and seek medical attention. —If breathing does not improve, or worsens, also seek medical attention immediately.

ALUMINUM HYDROXIDE (AlternaGEL, Alu-Cap, Al-U-Creme, Alugel, Aluminett, Amphojel, Basaljel, Dialume, Hydroxal, No-Co-Gel, Nutrajel)

Patient objectives	*Teaching plan content*
1 State the name of the medication, the dose prescribed, and the ordered frequency of administration.	This information should be obtained from the patient's physician.
2 Explain the use of aluminum hydroxide.	Aluminum hydroxide is used primarily as an antacid to relieve heartburn, sour stomach, acid indigestion, or discomfort associated with certain GI disorders, such as peptic ulcer, gastritis, esophagitis, and hiatal hernia. It is also used in renal failure to treat hypophosphatemia because of its ability to bond phosphate in the GI tract.
3 Identify potential side effects of aluminum hydroxide.	Aluminum hydroxide has the following side effects: —GI: constipation, intestinal obstruction.
4 Discuss patient guidelines for taking aluminum hydroxide.	The patient should follow these guidelines while taking aluminum hydroxide: —Shake the suspension well. Take it with a small amount of milk or water to ensure passage to the stomach. —Do not use it indiscriminately. —Do not switch to another antacid without the physician's advice. —If constipation occurs, consult the physician for instructions on managing it. —If enteric-coated medication is also prescribed, take it 1 hour before or after taking the antacid.

AMANTADINE HYDROCHLORIDE (Symmetrel)

Patient objectives	*Teaching plan content*
1 State the name of the medication, the dose prescribed, and the ordered frequency of administration.	This information should be obtained from the patient's physician.

2 Explain the use of amantadine hydrochloride.	Amantadine hydrochloride is used to relieve the symptoms of Parkinson's disease. It may also be used in the prophylactic or symptomatic treatment of the flu caused by influenza type A virus and of respiratory tract illnesses.
3 Identify potential side effects of amantadine hydrochloride.	Amantadine hydrochloride has the following side effects: —CNS: depression, fatigue, confusion, dizziness, psychosis, hallucinations, anxiety, irritability, ataxia (unsteady gait), insomnia, weakness, headache, lightheadedness, difficulty in concentrating —CV: peripheral edema, orthostatic hypotension (drop in blood pressure on arising), congestive heart failure —GI: anorexia, nausea, constipation, vomiting, dry mouth —GU: urinary retention —Skin: livedo reticularis (reddish blue netlike mottling of the skin), with prolonged use.
4 Discuss patient guidelines for taking amantadine hydrochloride.	The patient should follow these guidelines while taking amantadine hydrochloride: —Take the drug only as directed. Do not stop taking it abruptly, as this might precipitate a parkinsonian crisis. Adjust the dose only under the guidance of the physician. —To minimize dizziness, change positions slowly, dangle the legs before getting up, and lie down if faintness or dizziness occurs. —Be aware that elderly male patients should sit down to urinate, especially at night. —Take the last daily dose as early in the evening as possible to avoid insomnia. —Resume activities that require mental alertness gradually. —Be aware that the drug may produce dizziness, blurred vision, and impaired coordination.

AMINOPHYLLINE (Aminophyllin, Corophyllin)

Patient objectives	*Teaching plan content*
1 State the name of the medication, the dose prescribed, and the ordered frequency of administration.	This information should be obtained from the patient's physician.

2 Explain the use of aminophylline.	Aminophylline is used to treat acute and chronic bronchial asthma because of its ability to relax the smooth muscle of the respiratory tract, thus enhancing breathing.
3 Identify potential side effects of aminophylline.	Aminophylline has the following side effects: —CNS: restlessness, dizziness, headache, insomnia, light-headedness, convulsions —CV: palpitations, sinus tachycardia, extrasystoles, flushing, marked hypotension, increase in respiratory rate —GI: nausea, vomiting, anorexia, bitter aftertaste, dyspepsia, heavy feeling in stomach, diarrhea —Local: rectal suppositories may cause irritation —Skin: urticaria (hives).
4 Discuss patient guidelines for using aminophylline.	The patient should follow these guidelines while using aminophylline: —Use the drug exactly as directed. Do not alter the dose without first consulting the physician. —Take the oral drug with a full glass of water at meals to relieve GI symptoms. —Use the suppository form of the drug after evacuation, if possible. It may be retained better if taken before a meal. Remain recumbent for 15 to 20 minutes after insertion. —Avoid over-the-counter remedies that contain ephedrine in combination with theophylline salts, as excessive nervous system stimulation may result.

AMPICILLIN (Amcill, Ampilean, Omnipen, Omnipen-N, Pfizerpen A, Polycillin-N, Principen, Roampicillin, Totacillin-N)

Patient objectives	*Teaching plan content*
1 State the name of the medication, the dose prescribed, and the ordered frequency of administration.	This information should be obtained from the patient's physician.
2 Explain the use of ampicillin.	Ampicillin is an antibiotic used to treat infections, particularly urinary tract infections and uncomplicated gonorrhea.
3 Identify potential side effects of ampicillin.	Ampicillin has the following side effects: —Blood: anemia, thrombocytopenia (decrease in the

	number of platelets), thrombocytopenic purpura (bruising of the skin due to a decrease in the number of platelets), eosinophilia (increase in the number of eosinophils in the blood), leukopenia (decrease in the number of white blood cells) —GI: nausea, vomiting, diarrhea, glossitis (inflammation of the tongue), stomatitis (inflammation of the mouth) —Local: pain at injection site, vein irritation, thrombophlebitis —Other: hypersensitivity, reddened, raised rash, urticaria (hives), anaphylaxis, overgrowth of nonsusceptible organisms.
4 Discuss patient guidelines for taking ampicillin.	The patient should follow these guidelines while taking ampicillin: —Inform the physician of any known penicillin allergic reactions before taking ampicillin. —Take it exactly as prescribed, and take the entire quantity prescribed even after symptoms are gone. —Report skin rash, fever, or chills immediately to the physician. —Take doses 1 to 2 hours before meals or 2 to 3 hours after meals. —Never use leftover ampicillin for a new illness or share it with family or friends.

ASPIRIN (A.S.A., Aspergum, Aspirin, Bayer Timed-Release, Buffinol, Easprin, Ecotrin, Empirin, Measurin, Zorprin)

Patient objectives	*Teaching plan content*
1 State the name of the medication, the dose prescribed, and the ordered frequency of administration.	This information should be obtained from the patient's physician.
2 Explain the use of aspirin.	Aspirin is used to relieve mild to moderate pain; alleviate inflammation of rheumatoid arthritis, osteoarthritis, gout, and other conditions; and reduce fever. Aspirin also inhibits platelet aggregation, hindering coagulation.
3 Identify potential side effects of aspirin.	Aspirin has the following side effects: —Blood: prolonged bleeding time —EENT: tinnitus and hearing loss —GI: nausea, vomiting, GI distress, occult bleeding —Hepatic: abnormal liver function studies, hepatitis

	—Skin: rash, bruising —Other: hypersensitivity manifested by anaphylaxis and/or asthma.
4 Discuss patient guidelines for taking aspirin.	The patient should follow these guidelines while taking aspirin: —Be aware that because of epidemiologic association with Reye's syndrome, the Centers for Disease Control recommends that children with chicken pox or an influenza-like illness should not be given salicylates. —Keep out of reach of children—aspirin is one of the leading causes of poisoning in children. Encourage use of child-resistant containers. —Be aware that febrile, dehydrated children can develop toxicity rapidly. —When receiving large doses of aspirin for an extended period of time, watch for petechiae, bleeding gums, and signs of GI bleeding, and maintain adequate fluid intake. —Take with food, milk, an antacid, or a large glass of water to reduce GI side effects. —Check with the physician or pharmacist before taking over-the-counter combinations containing aspirin. —If possible, stop aspirin dosage 1 week before elective surgery.

ATENOLOL (Tenormin)

Patient objectives	*Teaching plan content*
1 State the name of the medication, the dose prescribed, and the ordered frequency of administration.	This information should be obtained from the patient's physician.
2 Explain the use of atenolol.	Atenolol is used to manage hypertension because of its ability to lower blood pressure. It is also used to treat angina pectoris because of its ability to block certain types of nervous stimulation of the heart muscle.
3 Identify potential side effects of atenolol.	Atenolol has the following side effects: —CNS: fatigue, lethargy —CV: bradycardia, hypotension, congestive heart failure, peripheral vascular disease —GI: nausea, vomiting, diarrhea —Skin: rash —Other: fever.

4 Discuss patient guidelines for taking atenolol.	The patient should follow these guidelines while taking atenolol: —Take atenolol at a regular time every day. Do not stop taking it abruptly or adjust the dose without the advice of the physician. —For diabetics who are on antidiabetic medications: Monitor blood sugar levels closely, through blood glucose self-monitoring, if necessary, because this drug masks common signs of hypoglycemia.

ATROPINE SULFATE

Patient objectives	*Teaching plan content*
1 State the name of the medication, the dose prescribed, and the ordered frequency of administration.	This information should be obtained from the patient's physician.
2 Explain the use of atropine sulfate.	Atropine sulfate is used as adjunctive therapy in the treatment of peptic ulcers, irritable bowel syndrome, bowel disturbances caused by nervous system dysfunction, and functional GI disorders because of its ability to decrease GI motility and inhibit gastric acid secretion.
3 Identify potential side effects of atropine sulfate.	Atropine sulfate has the following side effects: (NOTE: Overdosage may cause symptoms similar to those of curare toxicity [muscle paralysis].) —CNS: headache, insomnia, drowsiness, dizziness, confusion or excitement in elderly patients, nervousness, weakness —CV: palpitations, tachycardia —EENT: blurred vision, mydriasis (dilation of the pupil), increased ocular tension, cycloplegia (paralysis of the ciliary muscle of the eye), photophobia (increased visual sensitivity to light) —GI: dry mouth, dysphagia (difficulty swallowing), heartburn, loss of taste, nausea, vomiting, paralytic ileus —GU: urinary hesitancy and retention, impotence —Skin: urticaria (hives), decreased sweating or anhidrosis, other dermal manifestations —Other: fever, allergic reactions.

4 Discuss patient guidelines for taking atropine sulfate.	The patient should follow these guidelines while taking atropine sulfate: —Take the drug only as directed. Do not adjust the dose without consulting the physician. —Report rapid heartbeat, skin rash, or urinary retention to the physician immediately. —Take doses 30 minutes to 1 hour before meals and at bedtime. The bedtime dose should be taken at least 2 hours after the last meal of the day. —Avoid activities that require alertness if drowsiness, dizziness, or blurred vision occurs. —Drink plenty of liquids to help prevent constipation. —Use sugarless gum or hard candy to relieve mouth dryness. —Be aware that drug-induced heatstroke can develop in hot or humid environments, and take precautions.

BACLOFEN (Lioresal, Lioresal DS)

Patient objectives	*Teaching plan content*
1 State the name of the medication, the dose prescribed, and the ordered frequency of administration.	This information should be obtained from the patient's physician.
2 Explain the use of baclofen.	Baclofen is a skeletal muscle relaxant used to treat spasticity found in spinal cord injury and multiple sclerosis.
3 Identify potential side effects of baclofen.	Baclofen has the following side effects: —CNS: drowsiness, dizziness, headache, weakness, fatigue, confusion, insomnia —CV: hypotension —EENT: nasal congestion —GI: nausea, constipation —GU: urinary frequency —Hepatic: increased SGOT, alkaline phosphatase —Metabolic: hyperglycemia —Skin: rash, pruritus (itching) —Other: ankle edema, excessive perspiration, weight gain.
4 Discuss patient guidelines for taking baclofen.	The patient should follow these guidelines while taking baclofen: —Take the drug only as directed. Do not adjust the

dose or stop taking it abruptly without the physician's recommendation.
—Take it with meals or milk.
—Avoid activities that require alertness until the nervous system response is known.
—Report seizures, fever, skin eruptions, or difficulty breathing to the physician immediately.

BISACODYL (Biscolax, Codylax, Dulcolax, Fleet Bisacodyl, Rolax)

Patient objectives	*Teaching plan content*
1 State the name of the medication, the dose prescribed, and the ordered frequency of administration.	This information should be obtained from the patient's physician.
2 Explain the use of bisacodyl.	Bisacodyl is a laxative used to treat chronic constipation. It may also be used as a bowel preparation for delivery, surgery, or rectal or bowel examinations.
3 Identify potential side effects of bisacodyl.	Bisacodyl has the following side effects: —CNS: muscle weakness with excessive use —GI: nausea, vomiting, abdominal cramps, diarrhea in high doses, burning sensation in rectum with suppositories —Metabolic: alkalosis, hypokalemia, tetany, protein loss through the bowels with excessive use, fluid and electrolyte imbalance —Other: laxative dependence with long-term or excessive use.
4 Discuss patient guidelines for using bisacodyl.	The patient should follow these guidelines while using bisacodyl: —Use the drug only as directed. Avoid excessive use. —Swallow enteric-coated tablets whole to avoid stomach upset. —Do not take it with milk or antacids. —Expect results 6 to 12 hours after oral administration and 15 to 60 minutes after rectal administration. —Time the administration of the drug so as not to interfere with scheduled activities or sleep. —To avoid future constipation, be sure to have adequate fluid intake, exercise, and dietary bulk. Sources of bulk include bran and other cereals and fresh fruits and vegetables.

CAPTOPRIL (Capoten)

Patient objectives	*Teaching plan content*
1 State the name of the medication, the dose prescribed, and the ordered frequency of administration.	This information should be obtained from the patient's physician.
2 Explain the use of captopril.	Captopril is used to treat severe hypertension and also to treat heart failure that is inadequately controlled by other medications, such as digitalis and diuretics.
3 Identify potential side effects of captopril.	Captopril has the following side effects: —Blood: leukopenia (reduction of white blood cells), agranulocytosis (a symptom complex characterized by a decrease in granulocytes), pancytopenia (deficiency of all cell products of the blood) —CNS: dizziness, fainting —CV: tachycardia, hypotension, angina pectoris, congestive heart failure, pericarditis —EENT: dysgeusia (loss of taste) —GU: proteinuria, nephrotic syndrome, membranous glomerulopathy, renal failure, urinary frequency —GI: anorexia —Metabolic: hyperkalemia —Skin: urticaria (hives), pruritus (itching) —Other: fever, subcutaneous swelling of the face (angioedema) and extremities, transient increases in liver enzymes.
4 Discuss patient guidelines for taking captopril.	The patient should follow these guidelines while taking captopril: —Take the drug only as directed. Never adjust the dose or abruptly stop taking it without consulting the physician. —Take doses 1 hour before meals, because food may reduce absorption. —Avoid sudden postural changes, as this drug may cause dizziness or fainting. —Report to the physician any sign of infection (sore throat, fever) or fluid retention (puffiness, swelling in hands or feet, shortness of breath), as well as an impaired sense of taste. —Expect to have blood drawn for white blood cell counts on a regular basis.

CARBAMAZEPINE (Tegretol)

Patient objectives	*Teaching plan content*
1 State the name of the medication, the dose prescribed, and the ordered frequency of administration.	This information should be obtained from the patient's physician.
2 Explain the use of carbamazepine.	Carbamazepine is used to control seizure activity.
3 Identify potential side effects of carbamazepine.	Carbamazepine has the following side effects: —Blood: aplastic anemia (type of anemia in which the bone marrow fails to produce adequate numbers of peripheral blood cells), agranulocytosis (a symptom complex characterized by a decrease in granulocytes), eosinophilia (increase in the number of eosinophils), leukocytosis (increase in the number of white blood cells), thrombocytopenia (decrease in the number of platelets) —CNS: dizziness, vertigo, drowsiness, fatigue, ataxia (unsteady gait) —CV: congestive heart failure, hypertension, hypotension, aggravation of coronary artery disease —EENT: conjunctivitis, dry mouth and pharynx, blurred vision, diplopia (double vision), nystagmus (a rapid, involuntary movement of the eyeball) —GI: nausea, vomiting, abdominal pain, diarrhea, anorexia, stomatitis (inflammation of the mouth), glossitis (inflammation of the tongue), dry mouth —GU: urinary frequency or retention, impotence, albuminuria, glycosuria, elevated BUN —Hepatic: abnormal liver function test results, hepatitis —Metabolic: water intoxication —Skin: rash, urticaria (hives), Stevens-Johnson syndrome (erythema multiforme) —Other: diaphoresis, fever, chills, pulmonary hypersensitivity.
4 Discuss patient guidelines for taking carbamazepine.	The patient should follow these guidelines while taking carbamazepine: —Take the drug only as directed. Do not adjust the dose or stop taking the drug abruptly without the physician's recommendation. —Avoid activities that require alertness.

—Be aware that this drug may cause dizziness when first taken. This effect usually disappears within 3 to 4 days.
—Notify the physician immediately if fever, sore throat, mouth ulcers, or easy bruising occurs.

CHLORPROPAMIDE (Diabinese, Novopropamide)

Patient objectives	*Teaching plan content*
1 State the name of the medication, the dose prescribed, and the ordered frequency of administration.	This information should be obtained from the patient's physician.
2 Explain the use of chlorpropamide.	Chlorpropamide is used to treat Type II diabetes (uncontrolled by diet alone) because of its ability to lower blood sugar levels by stimulating the release of insulin from the pancreas.
3 Identify potential side effects of chlorpropamide.	Chlorpropamide has the following side effects: —Blood: bone marrow aplasia (underdevelopment of bone marrow) —GI: nausea, heartburn, vomiting —GU: tea-colored urine —Metabolic: prolonged hypoglycemia, dilutional hyponatremia —Skin: rash, pruritus (itching), facial flushing —Other: hypersensitivity reactions.
4 Discuss patient guidelines for taking chlorpropamide.	The patient should follow these guidelines while taking chlorpropamide: —Take the drug only as directed. Do not adjust the dose or stop taking it without the physician's approval. —Maintain the diabetic diet, as ordered. This drug does not replace dietary means to control blood sugar levels. —Be aware that hypoglycemia may occur. (See the "Diabetes Mellitus" teaching plan in Chapter 5, Endocrine Disorders, for further instructions.) —Avoid drinking alcohol, as unpleasant side effects may occur with chlorpropamide. —Do not take over-the-counter medications without first consulting the physician, because they can affect blood sugar levels.

CHORIONIC GONADOTROPIN, HUMAN (Android HCG, A.P.L., Chorex, Follutein, Glukor, Libigen, Pregnyl, Profasi HP, Stemutrolin)

Patient objectives	*Teaching plan content*
1 State the name of the medication, the dose prescribed, and the ordered frequency of administration.	This information should be obtained from the patient's physician.
2 Explain the use of human chorionic gonadotropin.	Human chorionic gonadotropin is used to treat anovulation and infertility. It may also be used to treat hypogonadism and nonobstructive cryptorchidism (undescended testicles) in boys aged 4 to 9.
3 Identify potential side effects of human chorionic gonadotropin.	Human chorionic gonadotropin has the following side effects: —CNS: headache, fatigue, irritability, restlessness, depression —GU: early puberty —Local: pain at injection site —Other: gynecomastia (enlargement of the breasts in the male), edema.
4 Discuss patient guidelines for human chorionic gonadotropin administration.	The patient should follow these guidelines while human chorionic gonadotropin is being administered: —Be aware that the nurse will administer the drug as an injection. —If the drug is used for infertility, have daily intercourse from the day before it is administered until ovulation occurs. —Be aware that multiple births are possible if this drug is used in conjunction with menotropins (Pergonal) to induce ovulation. —If the drug is used for nonobstructive cryptorchidism, notify the physician if signs of early puberty occur (growth of testes, penis, pubic and axillary hair; voice change; downy hair on upper lip; growth of body hair).

CIMETIDINE (Tagamet)

Patient objectives	*Teaching plan content*
1 State the name of the medication, the dose prescribed, and the ordered frequency of administration.	This information should be obtained from the patient's physician.

2 Explain the use of cimetidine.	Cimetidine is used to prevent or treat duodenal ulcers of hypersecretory conditions, such as Zollinger-Ellison syndrome, systemic mastocytosis (accumulation of mast cells in the tissues), and multiple endocrine adenomas, because of its ability to decrease gastric acid secretion in the GI tract.
3 Identify potential side effects of cimetidine.	Cimetidine has the following side effects: —Blood: agranulocytosis (a symptom complex characterized by a decrease in granulocytes), neutropenia (deficiency of neutrophils), thrombocytopenia (deficiency of platelets), aplastic anemia (type of anemia in which the bone marrow fails to produce adequate numbers of peripheral blood cells) —CNS: mental confusion, dizziness, headaches, depression —CV: bradycardia —GI: mild and transient diarrhea, perforation of chronic peptic ulcers after abrupt cessation of the drug, phytobezoars (gastric secretions composed of vegetable matter) in the elderly —GU: interstitial nephritis, transient elevations in BUN and serum creatinine, reduced sperm count, impotence —Hepatic: jaundice —Skin: acnelike rash, urticaria (hives), exfoliative dermatitis (severe inflammation of the skin accompanied by peeling) —Other: hypersensitivity, muscle pain, mild gynecomastia (enlargement of the breasts in the male) after using longer than 1 month, hypospermia.
4 Discuss patient guidelines for taking cimetidine.	The patient should follow these guidelines while taking cimetidine: —Take the drug only as directed. Do not adjust the dose without consulting the physician. —Take it with meals. —Report any episodes of mental confusion to the physician at once. —Be aware that smoking decreases the efficiency of cimetidine.

CLINDAMYCIN (Cleocin, Dalacin C)

Patient objectives	*Teaching plan content*
1 State the name of the medication, the dose prescribed, and the ordered frequency of administration.	This information should be obtained from the patient's physician.

2 Explain the use of clindamycin.	Clindamycin is an antibiotic used to treat a variety of infections.
3 Identify potential side effects of clindamycin.	Clindamycin has the following side effects: —Blood: transient leukopenia (deficiency of white blood cells), eosinophilia (increase in the number of eosinophils), thrombocytopenia (deficiency of platelets) —GI: nausea, vomiting, abdominal pain, diarrhea, pseudomembranous enterocolitis (necrosis of the mucosa of the small intestine and colon), esophagitis (inflammation of the esophagus), flatulence, anorexia, bloody or tarry stools, dysphagia (difficulty swallowing) —Hepatic: elevated SGOT, alkaline phosphatase, bilirubin —Local: pain, induration, sterile abscess with I.M. injection; thrombophlebitis, erythema, pain after I.V. administration —Skin: maculopapular rash, urticaria (hives) —Other: unpleasant or bitter taste, anaphylaxis.
4 Discuss patient guidelines for taking clindamycin.	The patient should follow these guidelines while taking clindamycin: —Take the drug exactly as directed. Do not adjust the dose or stop taking the drug without first consulting the physician. —Take the capsule with a full glass of water to prevent dysphagia (difficulty swallowing). —Report any side effects, especially diarrhea, to the physician. Do not treat diarrhea without consulting the physician.

CLOFIBRATE (Atromid-S)

Patient objectives	*Teaching plan content*
1 State the name of the medication, the dose prescribed, and the ordered frequency of administration.	This information should be obtained from the patient's physician.
2 Explain the use of clofibrate.	Clofibrate is used when triglyceride levels are high and cholesterol levels are moderately elevated, because it inhibits the production of cholesterol.
3 Identify potential side effects of clofibrate.	Clofibrate has the following side effects: —Blood: leukopenia (decrease in white blood cells)

	—CNS: fatigue, weakness —GI: nausea, diarrhea, vomiting, stomatitis (inflammation of the mouth), dyspepsia, flatulence —GU: decreased libido —Hepatic: gallstones, transient and reversible elevations of liver function test results —Skin: rashes, urticaria (hives), pruritus, dry skin and hair —Other: myalgias (aching muscles) and arthralgias (aching joints), resembling a flulike syndrome; weight gain; polyphagia (excessive eating); fever.
4 Discuss patient guidelines for taking clofibrate.	The patient should follow these guidelines while taking clofibrate: —Report any flulike symptoms to the physician immediately. —Continue to adhere to the prescribed diet.

CLOMIPHENE CITRATE (Clomid)

Patient objectives	*Teaching plan content*
1 State the name of the medication, the dose prescribed, and the ordered frequency of administration.	This information should be obtained from the patient's physician.
2 Explain the use of clomiphene citrate.	Clomiphene citrate is used in the treatment of infertility caused by anovulation because of its ability to induce ovulation.
3 Identify potential side effects of clomiphene citrate.	Clomiphene citrate has the following side effects: —CNS: headache, restlessness, insomnia, dizziness, light-headedness, depression, fatigue, tension —CV: hypertension —EENT: signs of impending visual toxicity, such as blurred vision, diplopia (double vision), scotoma (area of depressed vision), photophobia —GI: nausea, vomiting, bloating, distention, increased appetite, weight gain —GU: urinary frequency and polyuria, ovarian enlargement and cyst formation that regress spontaneously when the drug is stopped —Metabolic: hyperglycemia —Skin: urticaria (hives), rash, dermatitis —Other: hot flashes, reversible alopecia (hair loss), breast discomfort.

4 Discuss patient guidelines for taking clomiphene citrate.	The patient should follow these guidelines while taking clomiphene citrate: —Take the drug exactly as prescribed. —Take the basal body temperature daily, and chart it on a graph to ascertain if ovulation has occurred. —Avoid performing hazardous tasks until the effects of the drug are known. —Stop taking the drug and contact the physician immediately if visual disturbances, abdominal symptoms, or pain occurs or if pregnancy is suspected. —Be aware of the possibility of multiple births; the risk increases with higher doses.

CLONIDINE HYDROCHLORIDE (Catapres)

Patient objectives	*Teaching plan content*
1 State the name of the medication, the dose prescribed, and the ordered frequency of administration.	This information should be obtained from the patient's physician.
2 Explain the use of clonidine hydrochloride.	Clonidine hydrochloride is used to treat hypertension because of its ability to lower blood pressure. It is also used to suppress abstinence symptoms during narcotic withdrawal.
3 Identify potential side effects of clonidine hydrochloride.	Clonidine hydrochloride has the following side effects: —CNS: drowsiness, dizziness, fatigue, sedation, nervousness, headache —CV: orthostatic hypotension (drop in blood pressure on arising), bradycardia —EENT: mouth dryness —GI: constipation —GU: urinary retention —Metabolic: glucose intolerance —Other: impotence.
4 Discuss patient guidelines for taking clonidine hydrochloride.	The patient should follow these guidelines while taking clonidine hydrochloride: —Take the drug only as directed. Never stop taking it abruptly. If necessary, the dosage should be reduced gradually over 2 to 4 days under the direction of the physician. —Be aware that tolerance to drowsiness will develop.

—Rise slowly and avoid sudden posture changes to minimize dizziness.
—Relieve mouth dryness with sugarless gum or candy or ice chips.
—Take the last dose of the day immediately before retiring.

CODEINE

Patient objectives	*Teaching plan content*
1 State the name of the medication, the dose prescribed, and the ordered frequency of administration.	This information should be obtained from the patient's physician.
2 Explain the use of codeine.	Codeine is used to relieve pain and/or suppress coughing.
3 Identify potential side effects of codeine.	Codeine has the following side effects: —CNS: sedation, clouded sensorium, euphoria, convulsions with large doses —CV: hypotension, bradycardia —GI: nausea, vomiting, constipation, ileus —GU: urinary retention —Other: respiratory depression, physical dependence.
4 Discuss patient guidelines for taking codeine.	The patient should follow these guidelines while taking codeine: —Take the drug only as directed. It may become addictive if it is used on a prolonged basis. —Avoid activities that require alertness. —For full analgesic effect, take the drug before intense pain develops. —For maximum pain relief, take codeine and aspirin together, if ordered.

CO-TRIMOXAZOLE (Bactrim, Cotrim, Septra)

Patient objectives	*Teaching plan content*
1 State the name of the medication, the dose prescribed, and the ordered frequency of administration.	This information should be obtained from the patient's physician.

2 Explain the use of co-trimoxazole.	Co-trimoxazole is an antibiotic used to treat infections of the urinary tract and shigellosis. It may also be used to treat chronic bacterial prostatitis.
3 Identify potential side effects of co-trimoxazole.	Co-trimoxazole has the following side effects: —Blood: agranulocytosis (symptom complex characterized by a decrease in granulocytes), aplastic anemia (type of anemia in which the bone marrow fails to produce adequate numbers of peripheral blood cells), thrombocytopenia (decrease in the number of platelets), leukopenia (deficiency of white blood cells), hemolytic anemia —CNS: headache, mental depression, convulsions, hallucinations —GI: nausea, vomiting, diarrhea, abdominal pain, anorexia, stomatitis (inflammation of the mouth) —GU: toxic nephrosis with oliguria and anuria, crystalluria (crystals of uric acid in the urine), hematuria —Hepatic: jaundice —Skin: generalized skin eruption, exfoliative dermatitis (inflammation of the skin characterized by peeling), photosensitivity, urticaria (hives), pruritus —Other: hypersensitivity, serum sickness (allergic reaction following an injection of a foreign serum), drug fever, anaphylaxis.
4 Discuss patient guidelines for taking co-trimoxazole.	The patient should follow these guidelines while taking co-trimoxazole: —Take co-trimoxazole for as long as prescribed, even after symptoms are gone. —If skin rash, sore throat, fever, or mouth sores develop, promptly report them to the physician. —Be aware that if swallowing large tablets is difficult, an oral suspension is available. Check with the pharmacist.

CROMOLYN SODIUM (Intal, Nasalcrom, Rynacrom)

Patient objectives	*Teaching plan content*
1 State the name of the medication, the dose prescribed, and the ordered frequency of administration.	This information should be obtained from the patient's physician.

2 Explain the use of cromolyn sodium.	Cromolyn sodium is used to prevent acute attacks of perennial bronchial asthma by interfering with the allergic reaction responsible for asthma development.
3 Identify potential side effects of cromolyn sodium.	Cromolyn sodium has the following side effects: —CNS: dizziness, headache —EENT: irritation of the throat and trachea, cough, and bronchospasm following inhalation of dry powder; esophagitis (inflammation of the esophagus), nasal congestion; pharyngeal irritation; wheezing —GI: nausea —GU: dysuria, urinary frequency —Skin: rash, urticaria (hives) —Other: joint swelling and pain, lacrimation (tear formation), swollen parotid gland, angioedema (generalized subcutaneous edema of the face).
4 Discuss patient guidelines for using cromolyn sodium.	The patient should follow these guidelines while using cromolyn sodium: —Use the drug exactly as directed. To use a Spinhaler correctly, insert the capsule in the device properly, exhale completely before placing the mouthpiece between the lips, then inhale deeply and rapidly with a steady, even breath; remove the inhaler from the mouth, hold the breath a few seconds, and exhale. Repeat until all of the powder has been inhaled. —Never swallow the capsule; it is for inhalation use only. —Store the capsules at room temperature in a tightly closed container; protect them from moisture and temperatures higher than 104° F. (40° C.). —Avoid excessive handling of the capsules. —If discomfort in the esophagus occurs (pain or burning), take an antacid or a glass of milk.

CYCLANDELATE (Cyclospasmol)

Patient objectives	*Teaching plan content*
1 State the name of the medication, the dose prescribed, and the ordered frequency of administration.	This information should be obtained from the patient's physician.
2 Explain the use of cyclandelate.	Cyclandelate is used to treat peripheral vascular disease because of its ability to relax blood vessel walls, which increases the blood supply to the extremities. It

	may also be used for selected cases of ischemic cerebrovascular disease to increase blood flow to the brain.
3 Identify potential side effects of cyclandelate.	Cyclandelate has the following side effects: —CNS: headache, tingling of extremities, dizziness —CV: mild flushing, tachycardia —GI: eructation (belching), nausea, heartburn —Other: sweating.
4 Discuss patient guidelines for taking cyclandelate.	The patient should follow these guidelines while taking cyclandelate: —Take the drug exactly as directed. —Take it with food or antacids to lessen GI distress. —Anticipate long-term treatment with cyclandelate. —Be aware that side effects usually disappear after several weeks of therapy.

DANAZOL (Cyclomen, Danocrine)

Patient objectives	*Teaching plan content*
1 State the name of the medication, the dose prescribed, and the ordered frequency of administration.	This information should be obtained from the patient's physician.
2 Explain the use of danazol.	Danazol is used to treat endometriosis and fibrocystic breast disease by inhibiting the release of pituitary hormones that influence ovary or breast activity. It may also be used to prevent hereditary angioedema.
3 Identify potential side effects of danazol.	Danazol has the following side effects: —Androgenic: acne, edema, weight gain, hirsutism (masculinization of the female), hoarseness, clitoral enlargement, decrease in breast size, changes in libido, male-pattern baldness, oiliness of skin and hair —CNS: dizziness, headache, sleep disorders, fatigue, tremor, irritability, excitation, lethargy, mental depression, chills, paresthesias (numbness and tingling) —CV: elevated blood pressure —EENT: visual disturbances —GI: gastric irritation, nausea, vomiting, diarrhea, constipation, appetite change —GU: hematuria —Hepatic: reversible jaundice

—Hypoestrogenic: flushing; sweating; vaginitis, including itching, dryness, burning, and vaginal bleeding; nervousness, emotional lability, menstrual irregularities
—Other: muscle cramps or spasms.

4 Discuss patient guidelines for taking danazol.

The patient should follow these guidelines while taking danazol:
—Take the drug exactly as directed. Do not adjust the dose without first consulting the physician.
—Watch closely for signs of masculine traits, such as a deepening of the voice. If this occurs, report it to the physician immediately.
—Examine the breasts regularly. If the breast nodule being treated enlarges during treatment, call the physician immediately.
—Eat a diet high in calories and protein, unless contraindicated.
—Wear cotton underwear only.
—Wash after intercourse to decrease the risk of vaginitis.

DANTROLENE SODIUM (Dantrium)

Patient objectives	*Teaching plan content*
1 State the name of the medication, the dose prescribed, and the ordered frequency of administration.	This information should be obtained from the patient's physician.
2 Explain the use of dantrolene sodium.	Dantrolene sodium is a skeletal muscle relaxant used to treat spasticity found in spinal cord injury, stroke, cerebral palsy, and multiple sclerosis.
3 Identify potential side effects of dantrolene sodium.	Dantrolene sodium has the following side effects: —Blood: eosinophilia (increase in the number of eosinophils) —CNS: muscle weakness, drowsiness, dizziness, lightheadedness, malaise, headache, confusion, nervousness, insomnia —CV: tachycardia, blood pressure changes —EENT: excessive tearing, visual disturbances —GI: anorexia, constipation, cramping, dysphagia (difficulty swallowing), severe diarrhea —GU: urinary frequency, incontinence, nocturia, dys-

	uria, crystalluria (uric acid crystals in the urine), difficulty achieving erection —Hepatic: hepatitis —Skin: eczematoid eruption (eczema-type skin rash), pruritus, urticaria (hives), photosensitivity —Other: abnormal hair growth, drooling, sweating, pleural effusion (fluid in the pleural space), myalgia (pain in the muscles), chills, fever.
4 Discuss patient guidelines for taking dantrolene sodium.	The patient should follow these guidelines while taking dantrolene sodium: —Take the drug only as directed. Do not adjust the dose without the physician's recommendation. —Take it with meals or milk. —Avoid activities requiring alertness. —Avoid combining the drug with alcohol or other depressants. —Avoid photosensitivity reactions by using sunscreening agents and protective clothing. —Report abdominal discomfort or GI problems immediately to the physician. —Follow the physician's orders regarding rest and physical therapy.

DIAZEPAM (Valium)

Patient objectives	*Teaching plan content*
1 State the name of the medication, the dose prescribed, and the ordered frequency of administration.	This information should be obtained from the patient's physician.
2 Explain the use of diazepam.	Diazepam is used to treat anxiety and tension and as an adjunct for the relief of skeletal muscle spasm present in spinal cord and musculoskeletal injury and in seizure disorders.
3 Identify potential side effects of diazepam.	Diazepam has the following side effects: —CNS: fatigue, drowsiness, ataxia (unsteady gait), dizziness, headache, dysarthria (speech difficulties), slurred speech, tremor —CV: hypotension, bradycardia, cardiovascular collapse —EENT: diplopia (double vision), blurred vision, nystagmus (uncontrolled movements of the eyeball) —GI: nausea, constipation, change in salivation

	—GU: incontinence, urinary retention —Local: pain, phlebitis at injection site —Skin: rash, urticaria (hives) —Other: respiratory depression.
4 Discuss patient guidelines for taking diazepam.	The patient should follow these guidelines while taking diazepam: —Take the drug only as directed. Do not adjust the dose or discontinue the drug suddenly. Addiction may occur with prolonged use. —Avoid activities that require alertness. —Avoid using alcohol or other nervous system depressants while taking diazepam.

DICYCLOMINE HYDROCHLORIDE (Antispas, Bentyl, Bentylol, Dibent, Dicen, Formulex, Neoquess, Nospaz, Or-Tyl, Rocyclo, Rotyl HCl, Stannitol, Viscerol)

Patient objectives	*Teaching plan content*
1 State the name of the medication, the dose prescribed, and the ordered frequency of administration.	This information should be obtained from the patient's physician.
2 Explain the use of dicyclomine hydrochloride.	Dicyclomine hydrochloride is used as adjunctive therapy for peptic ulcers and other functional GI disorders because of its ability to decrease GI motility.
3 Identify potential side effects of dicyclomine hydrochloride.	Dicyclomine hydrochloride has the following side effects: (NOTE: Overdosage may cause symptoms similar to those of curare toxicity [muscle paralysis].) —CNS: headache, insomnia, drowsiness, dizziness —CV: palpitations, tachycardia —GI: nausea, constipation, vomiting, paralytic ileus —GU: urinary hesitancy and retention, impotence —Skin: urticaria (hives), decreased sweating or anhidrosis (no sweat formation), other dermal manifestations —Other: fever, allergic reactions.
4 Discuss patient guidelines for taking dicyclomine hydrochloride.	The patient should follow these guidelines while taking dicyclomine hydrochloride: —Take the drug only as directed. Do not adjust the dose without consulting the physician.

—Avoid strenuous work or exercise during hot and humid weather, as drug-induced heatstroke may occur.
—Take doses 30 minutes to 1 hour before meals and at bedtime. The bedtime dose should be taken at least 2 hours after the last meal of the day.
—Report any skin rash or urinary hesitancy and retention to the physician.
—Avoid driving and other hazardous activities if drowsiness, dizziness, or blurred vision occurs.
—Drink plenty of fluids to help prevent constipation.
—Take sugarless gum or hard candy to relieve mouth dryness.

DIGOXIN (Lanoxicaps, Lanoxin)

Patient objectives	*Teaching plan content*
1 State the name of the medication, the dose prescribed, and the ordered frequency of administration.	This information should be obtained from the patient's physician.
2 Explain the use of digoxin.	Digoxin regulates and strengthens the heart's pumping action so that it can send needed blood to other parts of the body.
3 Identify potential side effects of digoxin.	Digoxin has the following side effects: (NOTE: The following are signs of toxicity that may occur with all cardiac glycosides. Toxic effects on the heart may be life-threatening and require immediate attention.) —CNS: fatigue, generalized muscle weakness, agitation, hallucinations, headache, malaise, dizziness, vertigo, stupor, paresthesias (numbness and tingling) —CV: increased severity of congestive heart failure, dysrhythmias (most commonly conduction disturbances with or without AV block, premature ventricular contractions, and supraventricular dysrhythmias), hypotension —EENT: yellow-green halos around visual images, blurred vision, light flashes, photophobia, diplopia (double vision) —GI: anorexia, nausea, vomiting, diarrhea.
4 Discuss patient guidelines for taking digoxin.	The patient should follow these guidelines while taking digoxin: —Always take digoxin at the same time every day.

Take it only as prescribed. Never skip a dose or take extra doses without first checking with the physician.
—Take a pulse reading for 1 full minute daily before taking digoxin. (See Chapter 2, Cardiovascular Disorders, for patient instructions on how to take a pulse.) If the pulse rate is irregular or falls below 60, call the physician before taking any more pills.
—Do not substitute one brand for another.
—Do not take any other drugs, including nonprescription drugs, without first asking the physician.

DIHYDROTACHYSTEROL (DHT Intensol, DHT Oral Solution, Hytakerol)

Patient objectives	*Teaching plan content*
1 State the name of the medication, the dose prescribed, and the ordered frequency of administration.	This information should be obtained from the patient's physician.
2 Explain the use of dihydrotachysterol.	Dihydrotachysterol is used to stimulate calcium absorption from the GI tract and to promote secretion of calcium from bone into the blood in the treatment of renal osteodystrophy in chronic renal failure.
3 Identify potential side effects of dihydrotachysterol.	Dihydrotachysterol has the following side effects: Vitamin D intoxication associated with hypercalcemia: —CNS: headache, somnolence —EENT: conjunctivitis, photophobia, rhinorrhea —GI: nausea, vomiting, constipation, metallic taste, dry mouth, anorexia, diarrhea —GU: polyuria —Other: weakness, bone and muscle pain.
4 Discuss patient guidelines for taking dihydrotachysterol.	The patient should follow these guidelines while taking dihydrotachysterol: —Be aware that adequate dietary calcium intake is necessary. —Report hypercalcemia reactions to the physician. Early signs of hypercalcemia include thirst, headache, vertigo (dizziness), tinnitus (ringing in the ears), anorexia. —Store in tightly closed, light-resistant containers. Don't refrigerate.

DILTIAZEM (Cardizem)

Patient objectives	*Teaching plan content*
1 State the name of the medication, the dose prescribed, and the ordered frequency of administration.	This information should be obtained from the patient's physician.
2 Explain the use of diltiazem.	Diltiazem reduces the oxygen demand of the heart and is used in the management of angina pectoris.
3 Identify potential side effects of diltiazem.	Diltiazem has the following side effects: —CNS: headache, fatigue, drowsiness, dizziness, nervousness, depression, insomnia, confusion —CV: edema, dysrhythmia, flushing, bradycardia, hypotension, conduction abnormalities —GI: nausea, vomiting, diarrhea —GU: nocturia, polyuria —Hepatic: transient elevation of liver enzymes —Skin: rash, pruritus —Other: photosensitivity.
4 Discuss patient guidelines for taking diltiazem.	The patient should follow these guidelines while taking diltiazem: —Take the drug as directed. Never adjust the dose without the physician's recommendation. —Take sublingual nitroglycerin in addition, as ordered, when anginal symptoms are acute.

DIPHENHYDRAMINE HYDROCHLORIDE (Benadryl)

Patient objectives	*Teaching plan content*
1 State the name of the medication, the dose prescribed, and the ordered frequency of administration.	This information should be obtained from the patient's physician.
2 Explain the use of diphenhydramine.	Diphenhydramine is a multipurpose medication used to suppress a nonproductive cough, aid nighttime sleep, treat allergic reactions, treat motion sickness, and aid in the relief of symptoms produced by Parkinson's disease.

3 Identify potential side effects of diphenhydramine.	Diphenhydramine has the following side effects: —CNS: (especially in the elderly) drowsiness, confusion, insomnia, headache, vertigo (dizziness) —CV: palpitations —EENT: photosensitivity, diplopia (double vision), nasal stuffiness —GI: nausea, vomiting, diarrhea, dry mouth, constipation —GU: dysuria, urinary retention —Skin: urticaria (hives).
4 Discuss patient guidelines for taking diphenhydramine.	The patient should follow these guidelines while taking diphenhydramine: —Take the drug only as directed. Tolerance may develop with prolonged use. —Avoid activities that require alertness until the nervous system response is known. —Do not drink alcoholic beverages while taking diphenhydramine. —Take it with food or milk. —Be aware that coffee or tea may reduce drowsiness. —Relieve dry mouth with ice chips or sugarless gum.

DIPYRIDAMOLE (Persantine)

Patient objectives	*Teaching plan content*
1 State the name of the medication, the dose prescribed, and the ordered frequency of administration.	This information should be obtained from the patient's physician.
2 Explain the use of dipyridamole.	Dipyridamole is a vasodilator (that is, it increases the diameter of blood vessels) used to treat angina pectoris and transient ischemic attacks by increasing the amount of blood and oxygen delivered to the heart and brain. It is also used in combination with warfarin to inhibit platelet adhesion to prosthetic heart valves.
3 Identify potential side effects of dipyridamole.	Dipyridamole has the following side effects: —CNS: headache, dizziness, weakness —CV: flushing, fainting, hypotension —GI: nausea, vomiting, diarrhea —Skin: rash.

4 Discuss patient guidelines for taking dipyridamole.

The patient should follow these guidelines while taking dipyridamole:
—Take the drug 1 hour before meals.
—Watch for signs of bleeding (easy bruising, bleeding gums, blood in stool or urine) and report them to the physician.
—Be aware that clinical response to dipyridamole may not be evident before the 2nd or 3rd month. It is important to continue taking the drug despite the lack of observable response.

DISOPYRAMIDE PHOSPHATE (Norpace, Norpace CR)

Patient objectives	*Teaching plan content*
1 State the name of the medication, the dose prescribed, and the ordered frequency of administration.	This information should be obtained from the patient's physician.
2 Explain the use of disopyramide phosphate.	Disopyramide phosphate suppresses extra heartbeats to regulate the rhythm of the heart.
3 Identify potential side effects of disopyramide phosphate.	Disopyramide phosphate has the following side effects: —CNS: dizziness, agitation, depression, fatigue, muscle weakness, syncope —CV: hypotension, congestive heart failure, heart block —EENT: blurred vision, dry eyes, dry nose —GI: nausea, vomiting, anorexia, bloating, abdominal pain, constipation, dry mouth —GU: urinary retention and hesitancy —Hepatic: cholestatic jaundice (jaundice resulting from an abnormal flow of bile) —Metabolic: hypoglycemia —Skin: rash in 1% to 3% of patients.
4 Discuss patient guidelines for taking disopyramide phosphate.	The patient should follow these guidelines while taking disopyramide phosphate: —Take the drug as prescribed. It must be taken at regular intervals on schedule. —Manage constipation with proper diet and/or bulk laxatives. —Relieve dry mouth with sugarless gum or hard candy. —Notify the physician immediately if urinary retention

or hesitancy occurs.
—Stand up slowly to prevent dizziness.
—For diabetics on antidiabetic medication: Be alert for the signs and symptoms of low blood sugar.

DOCUSATE (Colace [sodium salt], Kasof [potassium salt], Surfak [calcium salt])

Patient objectives	*Teaching plan content*
1 State the name of the medication, the dose prescribed, and the ordered frequency of administration.	This information should be obtained from the patient's physician.
2 Explain the use of docusate.	Docusate is a stool softener used to prevent constipation.
3 Identify potential side effects of docusate.	Docusate has the following side effects: —EENT: throat irritation —GI: bitter taste, mild abdominal cramping, diarrhea —Other: laxative dependence with long-term or excessive use.
4 Discuss patient guidelines for taking docusate.	The patient should follow these guidelines while taking docusate: —Use docusate only occasionally. Do not use it for more than 1 week without the physician's knowledge. —Mix the liquid form in milk, fruit juice, or infant formula to mask the bitter taste. —Be aware that the drug acts within 24 to 48 hours to produce a firm, semisolid stool. —Be aware that dietary sources of bulk include bran and other cereals and fresh fruits and vegetables. —Protect the liquid form from light. —Store at 59° to 86° F. (15° to 30° C.).

EPHEDRINE SULFATE

Patient objectives	*Teaching plan content*
1 State the name of the medication, the dose prescribed, and the ordered frequency of administration.	This information should be obtained from the patient's physician.

2 Explain the use of ephedrine sulfate.	Ephedrine sulfate is used in the prevention and symptomatic treatment of bronchial asthma. It is also used to relieve congestion of the nasal passages.
3 Identify potential side effects of ephedrine sulfate.	Ephedrine sulfate has the following side effects: —CNS: insomnia, nervousness, dizziness, headache, muscle weakness, sweating, euphoria, confusion, delirium —CV: palpitations, tachycardia, hypertension —EENT: dryness of mouth and throat —GI: nausea, vomiting, anorexia —GU: urinary retention, painful urination due to sphincter spasm.
4 Discuss patient guidelines for taking ephedrine sulfate.	The patient should follow these guidelines while taking ephedrine sulfate: —Take the drug only as directed. Do not adjust the dose without first consulting the physician. —Be aware that the effectiveness decreases after 2 to 3 weeks and an increased dosage may be required. Although tolerance develops, the drug is not known to cause addiction. —To prevent insomnia, avoid taking it within 2 hours of bedtime. —Do not take over-the-counter drugs that contain ephedrine without informing the physician.

EPINEPHRINE INHALANT (AsthmaHaler, Bronkaid Mist, Medihaler-Epi, Primatene Mist)

Patient objectives	*Teaching plan content*
1 State the name of the medication, the dose prescribed, and the ordered frequency of administration.	This information should be obtained from the patient's physician.
2 Explain the use of an epinephrine inhalant.	An epinephrine inhalant is used to treat acute asthmatic attacks by relaxing the smooth muscle of the respiratory tract, thus enhancing breathing.
3 Identify potential side effects of an epinephrine inhalant.	An epinephrine inhalant has the following side effects: —CNS: nervousness, tremor, euphoria, anxiety, coldness of extremities, vertigo (dizziness), headache, sweating, cerebral hemorrhage, disorientation, agitation. In patients with Parkinson's disease, the drug in-

	creases rigidity and tremor. —CV: palpitations, widened pulse pressure, hypertension, tachycardia, ventricular fibrillation, CVA, anginal pain, EKG changes —Metabolic: hyperglycemia, glycosuria —Other: pulmonary edema, dyspnea, pallor.
4 Discuss patient guidelines for using an epinephrine inhalant.	Provide your patient with these guidelines to follow while using an epinephrine inhalant: —Use the drug exactly as directed. —Use the inhaler correctly to obtain the maximum effect. (See Appendix D, *Medication Administration,* for further instructions, if needed.) —Report any side effects to the physician immediately. —If breathing does not improve or if it worsens, seek medical attention immediately.

ERYTHRITYL TETRANITRATE (Cardilate)

Patient objectives	*Teaching plan content*
1 State the name of the medication, the dose prescribed, and the ordered frequency of administration.	This information should be obtained from the patient's physician.
2 Explain the use of erythrityl tetranitrate.	Erythrityl tetranitrate is used to manage or prevent frequent or recurrent anginal pain because of its ability to reduce the heart's oxygen demand as well as to increase blood flow through the coronary vessels.
3 Identify potential side effects of erythrityl tetranitrate.	Erythrityl tetranitrate has the following side effects: —CNS: headache, sometimes with throbbing; dizziness; weakness —CV: orthostatic hypotension (drop in blood pressure on arising), tachycardia, flushing, palpitations, fainting —GI: nausea, vomiting —Local: sublingual burning —Skin: cutaneous vasodilation —Other: hypersensitivity reactions.
4 Discuss patient guidelines for taking erythrityl tetranitrate.	The patient should follow these guidelines while taking erythrityl tetranitrate: —Take the drug exactly as directed. Do not stop taking it abruptly, as chest pain may occur. Keep the medi-

cation easily accessible at all times. Be aware that although it is physiologically necessary, it is not habit-forming.
—Headaches may occur initially. Treat them with a mild analgesic, such as aspirin or acetaminophen. Tolerance usually develops with usage of the drug, and the headaches will stop.
—Be aware that an additional dose may be taken before anticipated stress or at bedtime if angina is nocturnal, if approved by the physician.
—Avoid alcoholic beverages, as they may produce unpleasant side effects.
—To minimize dizziness, change to an upright position slowly, go up and down stairs carefully, and lie down at the first sign of dizziness.
—If taking a sublingual tablet, wet it with saliva, place it under the tongue until it is completely absorbed, and sit down and rest. Be aware that a burning sensation indicates potency.
—Take the oral tablet on an empty stomach, either ½ hour before or 1 to 2 hours after meals.
—Chew the chewable tablets thoroughly before swallowing.
—Store the medication in a cool place and in a tightly closed container, away from light. To ensure freshness, replace the supply every 3 months. Remove the cotton from the container, since it absorbs the drug.

ERYTHROMYCIN (E-Mycin, Erythrocin, Ilosone, Ilotycin)

Patient objectives	*Teaching plan content*
1 State the name of the medication, the dose prescribed, and the ordered frequency of administration.	This information should be obtained from the patient's physician.
2 Explain the use of erythromycin.	Erythromycin is an antibiotic used to treat a wide variety of infections. It may also be used prophylactically to prevent endocarditis after dental procedures.
3 Identify potential side effects of erythromycin.	Erythromycin has the following side effects: —EENT: slowed corneal wound healing —Other: overgrowth of nonsusceptible organisms with long-term use; hypersensitivity, including itching and burning eyes, urticaria (hives), dermatitis, angioedema (generalized facial swelling).

4 Discuss patient guidelines for taking erythromycin.	The patient should follow these guidelines while taking erythromycin: —Take the medication for as long as prescribed, even after symptoms are gone. —Take doses with a full glass of water 1 hour before or 2 hours after meals. If the tablets are coated, they may be taken with meals. Do not drink fruit juice with erythromycin. Chewable erythromycin tablets should not be swallowed whole. —Watch for signs of other infections, such as vaginal, urinary, or respiratory discomfort, and report them to the physician. In addition, report any nausea, abdominal pain, or fever.

ESTROGEN WITH PROGESTOGEN (Brevicon, Demulen, Enovid, Enovid-E, Loestrin 1/20, Loestrin 1.5/30, Lo/Ovral, Min-Ovral, Modicon, Norinyl 1 + 35, Norinyl 1 + 50, Norinyl 1 + 80, Norinyl 2 mg, Norlestrin, Ortho-Novum 1/50, Ortho-Novum 1/80, Ortho-Novum 2 mg, Ortho-Novum 10/11, Ovcon 35, Ovcon 50, Ovral, Ovulen)

Patient objectives	*Teaching plan content*
1 State the name of the medication, the dose prescribed, and the ordered frequency of administration.	This information should be obtained from the patient's physician.
2 Explain the use of estrogen with progestogen.	Estrogen with progestogen inhibits ovulation and is used to prevent conception and to treat a variety of menstrual disorders.
3 Identify potential side effects of estrogen with progestogen.	Estrogen with progestogen has the following side effects: (NOTE: Adverse effects may be more serious, frequent, and rapid in onset with high-dose than with low-dose combinations.) —CNS: headache, dizziness, depression, libido changes, lethargy, migraine —CV: thromboembolism, hypertension, edema —EENT: worsening of myopia (nearsightedness) or astigmatism (unequal curvature of the eye in which a ray of light is not sharply focused), intolerance to contact lenses —GI: nausea, vomiting, abdominal cramps, bloating, diarrhea, constipation, anorexia, change in appetite, weight gain, bowel ischemia, pancreatitis

—GU: breakthrough bleeding, dysmenorrhea (painful menstruation), amenorrhea (lack of menstrual flow), cervical erosion or abnormal secretions, enlargement of uterine fibromas, vaginal candidiasis
—Hepatic: gallbladder disease, cholestatic jaundice (jaundice resulting from abnormal flow of bile), liver tumors
—Metabolic: hyperglycemia, hypercalcemia, folic acid deficiency
—Skin: rash, acne, seborrhea, oily skin, erythema multiforme, hyperpigmentation
—Other: breast tenderness, enlargement, secretion.

4 Discuss patient guidelines for taking estrogen with progestogen.

The patient should follow these guidelines while taking estrogen with progestogen:
—Take the drug exactly as prescribed. Missed doses in midcycle greatly increase the likelihood of pregnancy. If one tablet is missed, take it as soon as it is remembered or take two tablets the next day, and continue the regular schedule. If the medication is missed two consecutive days, take two tablets daily for 2 days, and resume the normal schedule. Use an additional method of birth control for 7 days after two missed doses.
—Be aware that headache, nausea, dizziness, breast tenderness, spotting, and breakthrough bleeding are common at first; these should diminish after 3 to 6 cycles (months). However, breakthrough bleeding may necessitate a dosage adjustment if estrogen with progestogen is being used to treat menstrual disorders.
—Use an additional method of birth control for the first week of administration in the initial cycle.
—Take the tablets at the same time each day; nighttime dosing may reduce nausea and headaches.
—Immediately report any of the following symptoms: abdominal pain; numbness, stiffness, or pain in legs, buttocks, or chest; shortness of breath; severe headache; visual disturbances, such as blind spots, blurriness, or flashing lights; unusual vaginal bleeding or discharge; two consecutive missed menstrual periods; lumps in the breast; swelling of hands or feet.
—If one menstrual period is missed and the tablets have been taken on schedule, continue taking the medication. If two consecutive menstrual periods are missed, stop the drug and have a pregnancy test performed, as progestogens may cause birth defects if taken early in pregnancy.
—Perform monthly breast examinations, and have a semiannual Pap test and an annual gynecologic examination.

—Check your weight at least twice a week, and report any sudden weight gain or edema (swelling) to the physician.
—Avoid exposure to ultraviolet light or prolonged exposure to sunlight.
—Do not take the same drug for longer than 18 months without consulting the physician.
—Be aware that a delay in achieving pregnancy may occur when the pill is discontinued and that many physicians recommend waiting 2 months after stopping the pill before attempting pregnancy. Check with the physician about how soon pregnancy may be attempted after stopping the pill.
—Read the package insert carefully. If it is missing, request one from the pharmacist.
—Be aware that smoking increases the risks associated with oral contraceptives.

FLAVOXATE HYDROCHLORIDE (Urispas)

Patient objectives	*Teaching plan content*
1 State the name of the medication, the dose prescribed, and the ordered frequency of administration.	This information should be obtained from the patient's physician.
2 Explain the use of flavoxate hydrochloride.	Flavoxate hydrochloride is used for the symptomatic relief of dysuria (painful urination), urinary frequency or urgency, nocturia (nighttime urination), incontinence, and lower abdominal pain related to urologic disorders.
3 Identify potential side effects of flavoxate hydrochloride.	Flavoxate hydrochloride has the following side effects: —CNS: restlessness, dizziness, headache, insomnia, light-headedness, convulsions —CV: palpitations, sinus tachycardia, extrasystoles, flushing, marked hypotension, increase in respiratory rate —GI: nausea, vomiting, anorexia, bitter aftertaste, dyspepsia, heavy feeling in the stomach —Skin: urticaria (hives).
4 Discuss patient guidelines for taking flavoxate hydrochloride.	The patient should follow these guidelines while taking flavoxate hydrochloride: —Take the drug only as directed. Do not adjust the dose without first consulting the physician.

—Watch for possible drowsiness, mental confusion, or blurred vision.
—Report any of the above side effects, or a lack of response, to the physician.

FLUDROCORTISONE ACETATE (Florinef Acetate)

Patient objectives	*Teaching plan content*
1 State the name of the medication, the dose prescribed, and the ordered frequency of administration.	This information should be obtained from the patient's physician.
2 Explain the use of fludrocortisone acetate.	Fludrocortisone acetate is used in the treatment of adrenal insufficiency to prevent sodium and water from being excreted in excessive amounts.
3 Identify potential side effects of fludrocortisone acetate.	Fludrocortisone acetate has the following side effects: —CV: sodium and water retention, hypertension, cardiac hypertrophy (enlarged heart), edema —Metabolic: hypokalemia.
4 Discuss patient guidelines for taking fludrocortisone acetate.	The patient should follow these guidelines while taking fludrocortisone acetate: —Take the drug only as directed. —Check your weight daily, and report any sudden weight gain to the physician. —Be aware that mild swelling of the extremities may occur from fluid retention. —Adhere to a salt-restricted diet, rich in potassium and protein, if ordered. (See the dietitian, if necessary.)

FUROSEMIDE (Lasix, Novosemide, SK-Furosemide, Uritol)

Patient objectives	*Teaching plan content*
1 State the name of the medication, the dose prescribed, and the ordered frequency of administration.	This information should be obtained from the patient's physician.
2 Explain the use of furosemide.	Furosemide is a diuretic used to remove excess water from the body by increasing the frequency and volume

of urination. It is useful in treating heart failure. Because excess fluid can elevate blood pressure, this drug may also be useful in controlling high blood pressure.

3 Identify potential side effects of furosemide.

Furosemide has the following side effects:
—Blood: agranulocytosis (a symptom complex characterized by a decrease in granulocytes), leukopenia (deficiency of white blood cells), thrombocytopenia (deficiency of platelets)
—CV: volume depletion and dehydration, orthostatic hypotension (drop in blood pressure on arising)
—EENT: transient deafness with too-rapid I.V. injection
—GI: abdominal discomfort and pain, diarrhea (with oral solution)
—Metabolic: hypokalemia; hypochloremic alkalosis (increase in basic substances in the blood due to decrease in blood chloride); asymptomatic hyperuricemia (increased serum uric acid); fluid and electrolyte imbalances, including dilutional hyponatremia, hypocalcemia, hypomagnesemia, hyperglycemia, and impairment of glucose tolerance
—Skin: dermatitis.

4 Discuss patient guidelines for taking furosemide.

The patient should follow these guidelines while taking furosemide:
—Take the drug exactly as prescribed. Never skip a dose or change the dosage without first asking the physician.
—Because furosemide will increase the need to urinate, take the pill(s) in the morning or before 6 p.m. to avoid nighttime trips to the bathroom.
—Stay on the prescribed diet, and check your weight in similar clothing at the same time each day.
—Be aware that this drug may cause a loss of potassium, an important element in the body. If the physician has prescribed a potassium supplement to replace this loss, be sure to take it as directed. (He may also suggest a diet rich in potassium—citrus fruits, tomatoes, bananas, dates, and apricots.)
—Stand up slowly to prevent dizziness, and limit alcohol intake and strenuous exercise in hot weather to avoid a drop in blood pressure.
—Tell all other physicians about taking this drug.

GLIPIZIDE (Glucotrol)

Patient objectives	*Teaching plan content*
1 State the name of the medication, the dose prescribed, and the ordered frequency of administration.	This information should be obtained from the patient's physician.
2 Explain the use of glipizide.	Glipizide is used to treat Type II diabetes (uncontrolled by diet alone) because of its ability to lower blood sugar levels by stimulating the release of insulin from the pancreas.
3 Identify potential side effects of glipizide.	Glipizide has the following side effects: —CNS: dizziness —Blood: bone marrow aplasia (underdevelopment of bone marrow) —GI: nausea, vomiting, constipation —Hepatic: cholestatic jaundice (jaundice resulting from an abnormality in the flow of bile) —Metabolic: hypoglycemia —Skin: rash, pruritus (itching), facial flushing.
4 Discuss patient guidelines for taking glipizide.	The patient should follow these guidelines while taking glipizide: —Take the drug only as directed. Do not adjust the dose or stop taking it without the physician's approval. —Take doses approximately 30 minutes before eating. —Maintain the diabetic diet, as ordered. This drug does not replace dietary means to control blood sugar levels. —Be aware that hypoglycemia may occur. (See the "Diabetes Mellitus" teaching plan in Chapter 5, Endocrine Disorders, for further instructions.) —Do not take over-the-counter medications in conjunction with glipizide without first consulting the physician.

GLUCAGON

Patient objectives	*Teaching plan content*
1 State the name of the medication, the dose prescribed, and the ordered frequency of administration.	This information should be obtained from the patient's physician.

2 Explain the use of glucagon.	Glucagon is used to increase the blood glucose level when it has fallen to dangerously low levels or to treat coma from insulin shock.
3 Identify potential side effects of glucagon.	Glucagon has the following side effects: —GI: nausea, vomiting —Other: hypersensitivity.
4 Discuss patient guidelines for using glucagon.	The patient should follow these guidelines while using glucagon: —Use the drug only as directed. Obtain clear guidelines from the physician as to when and how it should be used. —Have family members learn how to administer glucagon subcutaneously because it is vital to arouse a diabetic from a coma as quickly as possible. (See *How to Give Yourself a Subcutaneous Injection,* pp. 536-537.) —Tell them they must call for emergency help if a glucagon injection is unsuccessful in restoring consciousness. —Tell family members that if glucagon is successful in restoring consciousness, they should give additional carbohydrates orally to prevent another hypoglycemic reaction. (See the "Diabetes Mellitus" teaching plan in Chapter 5, Endocrine Disorders, for further instructions.)

GLYBURIDE (Diaβeta, Micronase)

Patient objectives	*Teaching plan content*
1 State the name of the medication, the dose prescribed, and the ordered frequency of administration.	This information should be obtained from the patient's physician.
2 Explain the use of glyburide.	Glyburide is used to treat Type II diabetes (uncontrolled by diet alone) because of its ability to lower blood sugar levels by stimulating the release of insulin from the pancreas.
3 Identify potential side effects of glyburide.	Glyburide has the following side effects: —Blood: bone marrow aplasia (underdevelopment of bone marrow) —GI: nausea, epigastric fullness, heartburn —Hepatic: cholestatic jaundice (jaundice resulting from

	an abnormality in the flow of bile) —Metabolic: hypoglycemia —Skin: rash, pruritus (itching), facial flushing.
4 Discuss patient guidelines for taking glyburide.	The patient should follow these guidelines while taking glyburide: —Take the drug only as directed. Do not adjust the dose or stop taking it without the physician's approval. —Maintain the diabetic diet, as ordered. This drug does not replace dietary means to control blood sugar levels. —Be aware that hypoglycemia may occur. (See the "Diabetes Mellitus" teaching plan in Chapter 5, Endocrine Disorders, for further instructions.) —Do not take over-the-counter medications in conjunction with glyburide without first consulting the physician.

HEPARIN (Hepalean, Liquaemin Sodium)

Patient objectives	*Teaching plan content*
1 State the name of the medication, the dose prescribed, and the ordered frequency of administration.	This information should be obtained from the patient's physician.
2 Explain the use of heparin.	Heparin is a blood thinner used in the treatment of deep-vein thrombosis, myocardial infarction, and pulmonary embolism because of its action to reduce the blood's ability to clot.
3 Identify potential side effects of heparin.	Heparin has the following side effects: —Blood: hemorrhage with excessive dosage, overly prolonged clotting time, thrombocytopenia (decrease in platelets) —Local: irritation, mild pain —Other: hypersensitivity reactions—chills, fever, pruritus (itching), rhinitis (inflammation of the mucous membrane of the nose), burning of feet, conjunctivitis (inflammation of conjunctiva of the eyes), lacrimation (tearing), arthralgia (pain in joints), urticaria (hives).
4 Discuss patient guidelines for using heparin.	The patient should follow these guidelines while using heparin: —Use the drug exactly as prescribed. Do not skip a

dose or try to catch up on missed doses.
—Give injections subcutaneously, between the iliac crests in the lower abdomen, deep into subcutaneous fat. (See *How to Give Yourself a Subcutaneous Injection*, pp. 536-537.)
—Slowly inject the drug into the fat pad. Leave the needle in place for 10 seconds after injection; then, withdraw it. Do not massage the site after the injection.
—Rotate injection sites.
—Notify the physician immediately if bleeding gums, bruises on arms or legs, petechiae, nosebleeds, bloody urine, or black, tarry stools develop.
—Avoid over-the-counter medications containing aspirin and other salicylates.
—Expect to have blood drawn on a regular basis. Do not miss an appointment; if possible, have the physician make arrangements for blood to be drawn at home.

HYDRALAZINE (Apresoline)

Patient objectives	*Teaching plan content*
1 State the name of the medication, the dose prescribed, and the ordered frequency of administration.	This information should be obtained from the patient's physician.
2 Explain the use of hydralazine.	Hydralazine is used to treat hypertension because of its ability to lower blood pressure.
3 Identify potential side effects of hydralazine.	Hydralazine has the following side effects: —CNS: peripheral neuritis, headache, dizziness —CV: orthostatic hypotension (drop in blood pressure on arising), tachycardia, dysrhythmias, angina, palpitations, sodium retention —GI: nausea, vomiting, diarrhea, anorexia —Skin: rash —Other: lupus erythematosus–like syndrome, weight gain.
4 Discuss patient guidelines for taking hydralazine.	The patient should follow these guidelines while taking hydralazine: —Take the drug only as directed. Never adjust the dose or stop taking it abruptly. —Take it with meals to increase absorption.

	—Rise slowly and avoid sudden position changes to minimize dizziness. —Call the physician immediately if a sore throat, fever, muscle or joint aches, or skin rashes develop. —Expect to have blood drawn periodically to monitor adverse effects (complete blood count, lupus erythematosus cell preparation, and antinuclear antibody titer determinations).

HYDROCHLOROTHIAZIDE (Chlorzide, Diaqua, Diu-Scrip, Esidrix, HydroDIURIL, Hydromal, Hydro-Z-50, Oretic, SK-Hydrochlorothiazide, Zide)

Patient objectives	*Teaching plan content*
1 State the name of the medication, the dose prescribed, and the ordered frequency of administration.	This information should be obtained from the patient's physician.
2 Explain the use of hydrochlorothiazide.	Hydrochlorothiazide is a diuretic used to treat essential hypertension and also to treat edema associated with congestive heart failure, cirrhosis of the liver, and renal disease.
3 Identify potential side effects of hydrochlorothiazide.	Hydrochlorothiazide has the following side effects: —Blood: aplastic anemia, agranulocytosis, leukopenia, thrombocytopenia —CV: volume depletion and dehydration, orthostatic hypotension —GI: anorexia, nausea, pancreatitis —Hepatic: hepatic encephalopathy —Metabolic: hypokalemia; asymptomatic hyperuricemia; hyperglycemia and impairment of glucose tolerance; fluid and electrolyte imbalances, including dilutional hyponatremia and hypochloremia, metabolic alkalosis, hypercalcemia; gout —Skin: dermatitis, photosensitivity, rash —Other: hypersensitivity reactions, such as pneumonitis and vasculitis.
4 Discuss patient guidelines for taking hydrochlorothiazide.	The patient should follow these guidelines while taking hydrochlorothiazide: —Check your weight regularly. —Include potassium-rich foods in the diet daily; foods rich in potassium include citrus fruits, tomatoes, ba-

nanas, dates, and apricots.
—Report signs of hypokalemia (for example, muscle weakness, cramps) to the physician immediately.
—For patients taking digitalis, be especially alert to signs of digitalis toxicity (nausea, vomiting, anorexia, dysrhythmias, yellow-green halos around visual images, blurred vision, increased severity of congestive heart failure, fatigue, generalized muscle weakness) due to the potassium-depleting effect of this diuretic.
—Take the medication in the morning to prevent nocturia.
—For diabetics who are on insulin, monitor blood sugar levels, through blood glucose self-monitoring, if necessary, and adjust the dose accordingly, because this medication may cause hyperglycemia.

HYDROCORTISONE (Cortef, Hydrocortone, Solu-Cortef)

Patient objectives	*Teaching plan content*
1 State the name of the medication, the dose prescribed, and the ordered frequency of administration.	This information should be obtained from the patient's physician.
2 Explain the use of hydrocortisone.	Hydrocortisone is used for hormone replacement in the treatment of Addison's disease. It may also be used to treat severe inflammation in conditions such as ulcerative colitis because of its ability to hinder the inflammatory process.
3 Identify potential side effects of hydrocortisone.	Hydrocortisone has the following side effects: (NOTE: Most side effects of corticosteroids are dose- or duration-dependent, but acute adrenal insufficiency may occur with increased stress [infection, surgery, trauma] or abrupt withdrawal after long-term therapy. Sudden withdrawal may be fatal.) —CNS: euphoria, insomnia, psychotic behavior —CV: congestive heart failure, hypertension, edema —EENT: cataracts, glaucoma —GI: peptic ulcer, gastrointestinal irritation, increased appetite —Metabolic: possible hypokalemia, hyperglycemia, and carbohydrate intolerance; growth suppression in children

—Skin: delayed wound healing, acne, various skin eruptions
—Other: muscle weakness, pancreatitis, hirsutism (masculinization of the female), susceptibility to infections
—Withdrawal symptoms: rebound inflammation, fatigue, weakness, arthralgia (joint pain), fever, dizziness, lethargy, depression, fainting, orthostatic hypotension (fall in blood pressure on arising), dyspnea, anorexia, hypoglycemia.

4 Discuss patient guidelines for taking hydrocortisone.	The patient should follow these guidelines while taking hydrocortisone: —Take the drug only as directed. Do not adjust the dose or stop taking it abruptly without the physician's approval. —Always carry an I.D. card identifying the need for supplemental systemic glucocorticoids during periods of stress, including times of illness. —Inspect the skin frequently for signs of bruising. Be aware that easy bruising may occur. —For diabetics on antidiabetic medication: Watch for hyperglycemia, as hydrocortisone may increase blood sugar levels. —Take this drug with food. —Be alert for Cushing's syndrome (facial puffiness, hirsutism, thinning of extremities with abdominal obesity, amenorrhea in females, and edema) or early adrenal insufficiency (fatigue, muscular weakness, joint pain, fever, anorexia, nausea, shortness of breath, dizziness, fainting). —Adhere to a salt-restricted diet, rich in potassium and protein, if ordered. (See the dietitian, if necessary.)

IMIPRAMINE HYDROCHLORIDE (Impril, Janimine, Novopramine, Presamine, Ropramine, SK-Pramine, Tofranil)

Patient objectives	*Teaching plan content*
1 State the name of the medication, the dose prescribed, and the ordered frequency of administration.	This information should be obtained from the patient's physician.
2 Explain the use of imipramine hydrochloride.	Imipramine hydrochloride is used to treat childhood enuresis (bed wetting). It may also be used to treat depression.

3 Identify potential side effects of imipramine hydrochloride.	Imipramine hydrochloride has the following side effects: (NOTE: With abrupt withdrawal of long-term therapy, nausea, headache, and malaise may occur. These effects do not indicate addiction.) —CNS: drowsiness, dizziness, excitation, tremors, weakness, confusion, headache, nervousness —CV: orthostatic hypotension (fall in blood pressure on arising), tachycardia, EKG changes, hypertension —EENT: blurred vision, tinnitus (ringing in the ears), mydriasis (dilation of the pupil) —GI: dry mouth, constipation, nausea, vomiting, anorexia, paralytic ileus —GU: urinary retention —Skin: rash, urticaria (hives) —Other: sweating, allergy.
4 Discuss patient guidelines for taking imipramine hydrochloride.	The patient should follow these guidelines while taking imipramine hydrochloride: —Take the drug only as directed. Do not adjust the dose or stop taking it abruptly without first consulting the physician. —Whenever possible, take the full dose at bedtime. —Avoid taking over-the-counter drugs without first consulting the physician. —Inform all other physicians that this drug is being taken. —Avoid alcohol or other depressants. —Relieve dry mouth with sugarless hard candy or gum. —Expect to wait 10 to 14 days for noticeable effects. The full effect usually appears in 30 days. —Avoid activities that require alertness and good psychomotor coordination until the nervous system response is known. Drowsiness and dizziness will usually subside after a few weeks. —Be alert for signs of urinary retention and constipation, and report them to the physician if they occur. Increase fluid intake to lessen constipation.

INSULIN

Patient objectives	*Teaching plan content*
1 State the name of the medication, the dose prescribed, and the ordered frequency of administration.	This information should be obtained from the patient's physician.

2 Explain the use of insulin.

Insulin is used in the treatment of diabetes to increase glucose transport to body cells, thus reducing blood glucose levels.

3 Identify potential side effects of insulin.

Insulin has the following side effects:
—Metabolic: hypoglycemia, rebound hyperglycemia
—Skin: urticaria (hives)
—Local: lipoatrophy (diminishing subcutaneous fat), lipohypertrophy (increasing subcutaneous fat), itching, swelling, redness, stinging, warmth at injection site
—Other: anaphylaxis.

4 Discuss patient guidelines for using insulin.

The patient should follow these guidelines while using insulin:
—Use insulin as directed. Do not adjust the dose or stop using it without the physician's approval.
—Be aware that accurate measurement is very important to prevent complications.
—Since regular, intermediate, and long-acting insulins may be mixed, be sure that all insulins to be mixed are of the same concentration. Use mixtures promptly (within 15 minutes of mixing) to avoid bonding.
—Do not alter the order of mixing insulins or change the model or brand of syringe or needle. To mix insulins as ordered, observe the following:

- Draw air into the syringe by pulling the plunger out to the dose of the longer-acting (cloudy) insulin. Insert the needle into the cleansed rubber stopper of the upright bottle of cloudy insulin. Inject the air into the bottle by pushing the plunger. Pull the needle out of the bottle without drawing up the insulin (keep the plunger down).
- Draw up air into the same syringe equal to the dose of the short-acting (clear) insulin. Insert the needle into the cleansed rubber stopper of the upright bottle of short-acting insulin, and push down on the plunger to inject the air into the bottle.
- Turn over the bottle and syringe, and slowly pull the plunger back to draw up the short-acting insulin to the prescribed dose; then draw 10 extra units. Remove any air bubbles by flicking or tapping the syringe. When the bubbles go to the top of the syringe, push the plunger tip up to the prescribed dose of regular insulin. If bubbles remain, push the plunger until they disappear into the bottle, then slowly pull back the plunger to the correct dose. Withdraw the needle.
- Insert the needle into the upside-down bottle of

the longer-acting insulin, and slowly draw out only the required dose. Never pull out any extra units, or you will contaminate the bottle when adjusting the dose. (If you see air bubbles now, you will need to start over with a new syringe.) Remove the syringe from the bottle. Now, administer the insulin. (See *How to Give Yourself a Subcutaneous Injection,* pp. 536-537.)

—Store the insulin in a cool area. Refrigeration is desirable but not essential, except with regular insulin concentrate. If insulin is stored in the refrigerator, allow it to warm to room temperature for 30 minutes before mixing or administering.

—Never use insulin that has changed color or become clumped or granular in appearance.

—Always check the expiration date on the vial.

—Press, but do not rub, the site after injection. Rotate injection sites. Chart the sites to avoid overusing one area.

—Mix the insulin suspension before drawing it up into the syringe by swirling the vial gently or rotating between palms. Do not shake it.

—Remember that meals must not be omitted. Blood glucose self-monitoring is recommended to monitor blood sugar levels as an aid in determining daily insulin requirements. (See the "Diabetes Mellitus" teaching plan in Chapter 5, Endocrine Disorders, for further instructions.)

—Watch closely for signs of hypoglycemia or hyperglycemia. (See the "Diabetes Mellitus" teaching plan in Chapter 5, Endocrine Disorders, for further instructions, if needed.)

—Always wear a medical I.D., carry ample insulin supplies on trips, and take note of time zone changes for dose scheduling when traveling.

—Always carry a form of quick-acting carbohydrate (a lump of sugar or hard candy) for treating insulin reactions. (See the "Diabetes Mellitus" teaching plan in Chapter 5, Endocrine Disorders, for further instructions on the treatment of hypoglycemia.)

—Note that marijuana use may increase insulin requirements.

—Note that cigarette smoking decreases the amount of insulin absorbed when administered subcutaneously.

—Do not interchange single-source beef, pork, or human insulins.

—Discuss any exercise regimen with the physician before undertaking it, as the insulin dose may need adjustment.

ISOSORBIDE DINITRATE (Coronex, Dilatrate-SR, Iso-Bid, Iso-D, Isordil, Isosorb, Onset, Sorate, Sorbitrate)

Patient objectives	*Teaching plan content*
1 State the name of the medication, dose prescribed, and ordered frequency of administration.	This information should be obtained from the patient's physician.
2 Explain the use of isosorbide dinitrate.	Isosorbide dinitrate is a vasodilator (that is, it increases the diameter of blood vessels) used to treat angina pectoris by increasing the amount of oxygen and blood delivered to the heart muscle.
3 Identify potential side effects of isosorbide dinitrate.	Isosorbide dinitrate has the following side effects: —CNS: headache, sometimes with throbbing; dizziness; weakness —CV: orthostatic hypotension (drop in blood pressure on arising), tachycardia, palpitations, ankle edema, fainting —GI: nausea, vomiting —Local: sublingual burning —Skin: cutaneous vasodilation, flushing —Other: hypersensitivity reactions.
4 Discuss patient guidelines for taking isosorbide dinitrate.	The patient should follow these guidelines while taking isosorbide dinitrate: —Take the drug only as prescribed. It must be taken regularly, and on a long-term basis, if ordered. Keep it easily accessible at all times. —Be aware that, if approved by the physician, an additional dose may be taken before anticipated stress or at bedtime if angina is nocturnal. —Avoid alcoholic beverages, as they may produce unpleasant side effects in combination with isosorbide dinitrate. —Change to an upright position slowly to minimize dizziness. Go up and down stairs slowly and carefully, and lie down at the first sign of dizziness. —Do not confuse the sublingual form of the drug with the oral form. —Take a sublingual tablet at the first sign of angina by wetting the tablet with saliva, then placing it under the tongue until it is completely absorbed. A burning sensation indicates potency. Repeat the dose every 10 to 15 minutes, for a maximum of three doses, if needed. If no relief is noted, call the physician or go to the hospital emergency department.

—Take the oral tablet on an empty stomach, either ½ hour before or 1 to 2 hours after meals. Swallow oral tablets whole. Chew chewable tablets thoroughly before swallowing.
—Never discontinue isosorbide dinitrate abruptly.
—Store in a cool place, in a tightly closed container, away from light.

ISOXSUPRINE HYDROCHLORIDE (Rolisox, Vasodilan, Vasoprine)

Patient objectives	*Teaching plan content*
1 State the name of the medication, dose prescribed, and ordered frequency of administration.	This information should be obtained from the patient's physician.
2 Explain the use of isoxsuprine hydrochloride.	Isoxsuprine hydrochloride is used in the treatment of peripheral vascular disease and cerebrovascular insufficiency to relieve symptoms of ischemia because of its ability to increase blood flow to the extremities and the brain.
3 Identify potential side effects of isoxsuprine hydrochloride.	Isoxsuprine hydrochloride has the following side effects: —CNS: dizziness, nervousness, weakness, trembling, light-headedness —CV: hypotension, tachycardia, transient palpitations —GI: vomiting, abdominal distress, intestinal distention —Skin: severe rash.
4 Discuss patient guidelines for taking isoxsuprine hydrochloride.	The patient should follow these guidelines while taking isoxsuprine hydrochloride: —Take the drug exactly as directed. —Stop taking it if a rash develops, and notify the physician.

KAOLIN AND PECTIN MIXTURES (Baropectin, Kaoparin, Kaopectate, Kapectin, Keotin, Pectokay)

Patient objectives	*Teaching plan content*
1 State the name of the medication, the dose prescribed, and the ordered frequency of administration.	This information should be obtained from the patient's physician.

2 Explain the use of kaolin and pectin mixtures.	Kaolin and pectin mixtures are used to treat mild diarrhea by decreasing the stool's fluid content.
3 Identify potential side effects of kaolin and pectin mixtures.	Kaolin and pectin mixtures have the following side effects: —GI: absorption of nutrients, drugs, and enzymes; fecal impaction or ulceration in infants, elderly, and debilitated patients after chronic use; constipation.
4 Discuss patient guidelines for taking kaolin and pectin mixtures.	The patient should follow these guidelines while taking kaolin and pectin mixtures: —Take the drug only as directed. Do not use it for more than 2 days. —Be aware that reduced absorption of other oral medications may occur, requiring dosage adjustments. Consult with the physician before taking kaolin and pectin mixtures.

LEVODOPA (Dopar, Larodopa)

Patient objectives	*Teaching plan content*
1 State the name of the medication, dose prescribed, and ordered frequency of administration.	This information should be obtained from the patient's physician.
2 Explain the use of levodopa.	Levodopa is used to reduce the rigidity, tremor, sluggish movement, and gait disturbances of Parkinson's disease.
3 Identify potential side effects of levodopa.	Levodopa has the following side effects: —Blood: hemolytic anemia, leukopenia (decrease in the number of white blood cells) —CNS: choreiform (rapid, jerky), dystonic (disordered tone to the muscles), dyskinetic (difficulty moving) movements; involuntary grimacing, head movements, myoclonic (shocklike contractions of the muscle) body jerks, ataxia (uneven gait), tremors, muscle twitching; bradykinetic (slow movement) episodes; psychiatric disturbances, memory loss, nervousness, anxiety, disturbing dreams, euphoria, malaise, fatigue; severe depression, suicidal tendencies, dementia, delirium, hallucinations (may necessitate reduction or withdrawal of the drug) —CV: orthostatic hypotension (drop in blood pressure on arising), cardiac irregularities, flushing, hypertension, phlebitis

—EENT: blepharospasm (twitching of the eyelid), blurred vision, diplopia (double vision), mydriasis (extreme dilation of the pupil) or miosis (contraction of the pupil), widening of palpebral fissures, oculogyric crises (movement of the eye about the anteroposterior axis), nasal discharge
—GI: nausea, vomiting, anorexia; possible weight loss at the start of therapy; constipation; flatulence; diarrhea, epigastric pain; hiccups; sialorrhea (excessive saliva production); dry mouth; bitter taste
—GU: urinary frequency, retention, incontinence; darkened urine; excessive and inappropriate sexual behavior; priapism (sustained, inappropriate erection of the penis)
—Hepatic: hepatotoxicity
—Other: dark perspiration, hyperventilation.

4 Discuss patient guidelines for taking levodopa.

The patient should follow these guidelines while taking levodopa:
—Take the drug only as directed. Do not adjust the dose without the physician's approval.
—Rise slowly and avoid sudden position changes to minimize dizziness.
—Watch for muscle and eyelid twitching. If present, notify the physician.
—Be aware that multivitamin preparations, fortified cereals, and certain over-the-counter medications may contain vitamin B_6, which can reverse the effects of levodopa.
—Be aware that pills may be crushed and mixed with applesauce.

LEVODOPA-CARBIDOPA (Sinemet)

Patient objectives	*Teaching plan content*
1 State the name of the medication, the dose prescribed, and the ordered frequency of administration.	This information should be obtained from the patient's physician.
2 Explain the use of levodopa-carbidopa.	Levodopa-carbidopa is used to reduce the rigidity, tremor, sluggish movement, and gait disturbances of Parkinson's disease.
3 Identify potential side effects of levodopa-carbidopa.	Levodopa-carbidopa has the following side effects: —Blood: hemolytic anemia —CNS: choreiform (rapid, jerky), dystonic (disordered

tone of the muscles), dyskinetic (difficulty moving) movements; involuntary grimacing, head movements, myoclonic (shocklike contractions of the muscle) body jerks, ataxia (uneven gait), tremors, muscle twitching; bradykinetic (slow movement) episodes; psychiatric disturbances, memory loss, nervousness, anxiety, disturbing dreams, euphoria, malaise, fatigue; severe depression, suicidal tendencies, dementia, delirium, hallucinations (may necessitate reduction or withdrawal of the drug)
—CV: orthostatic hypotension (drop in blood pressure on arising), cardiac irregularities, flushing, hypertension, phlebitis
—EENT: blepharospasm (twitching of the eyelid), blurred vision, diplopia (double vision), mydriasis (extreme dilation of the pupil) or miosis (contraction of the pupil), widening of palpebral fissures, oculogyric crises (movement of the eye about the anteroposterior axis), nasal discharge
—GI: nausea, vomiting, anorexia, possible weight loss at the start of therapy; constipation; flatulence; diarrhea; epigastric pain; hiccups; sialorrhea (excessive saliva production); dry mouth; bitter taste
—GU: urinary frequency, retention, incontinence; darkened urine; excessive and inappropriate sexual behavior; priapism (sustained, inappropriate erection of the penis)
—Hepatic: hepatotoxicity
—Other: dark perspiration, hyperventilation.

4 Discuss patient guidelines for taking levodopa-carbidopa.

The patient should follow these guidelines while taking levodopa-carbidopa:
—Take the drug only as directed. Do not adjust the dose without the physician's approval.
—Rise slowly and avoid sudden position changes to minimize dizziness.
—Watch for muscle and eyelid twitching. If present, notify the physician.
—Report any adverse effects to the physician at once.

LEVOTHYROXINE SODIUM (T_4, OR L-THYROXINE SODIUM) (Eltroxin, Levoid, Levothroid, Noroxine, Synthroid)

Patient objectives	*Teaching plan content*
1 State the name of the medication, the dose prescribed, and the ordered frequency of administration.	This information should be obtained from the patient's physician.

2 Explain the use of levothyroxine sodium.	Levothyroxine sodium is used to replace thyroid hormone in the treatment of hypothyroidism.
3 Identify potential side effects of levothyroxine sodium.	Levothyroxine sodium has the following side effects: —CNS: nervousness, insomnia, tremor —CV: tachycardia, palpitations, dysrhythmias, angina pectoris, hypertension —GI: change in appetite, nausea, diarrhea —Other: headache, leg cramps, weight loss, sweating, heat intolerance, fever, menstrual irregularities.
4 Discuss patient guidelines for taking levothyroxine sodium.	The patient should follow these guidelines while taking levothyroxine sodium: —Take the drug only as directed. Do not adjust the dose or stop taking it without the physician's approval. —Take it at the same time each day (preferably in the morning) to maintain constant hormone levels. —Once stabilized on one brand, do not switch to another. Avoid generic levothyroxine sodium. —Call the physician at once if chest pain, palpitations, sweating, nervousness, or any signs of aggravated heart disease (chest pain, rapid heartbeat, difficulty breathing) occur. Also report unusual bleeding or bruising. —Be aware that, during the first few months of therapy, children may suffer temporary partial hair loss. —Be aware that this drug will alter thyroid function test results. Inform any new physician that this medication is being taken.

LIOTHYRONINE SODIUM (T_3) (Cytomel, Cytomine)

Patient objectives	*Teaching plan content*
1 State the name of the medication, the dose prescribed, and the ordered frequency of administration.	This information should be obtained from the patient's physician.
2 Explain the use of liothyronine sodium.	Liothyronine sodium is used to replace thyroid hormone in the treatment of hypothyroidism.
3 Identify potential side effects of liothyronine sodium.	Liothyronine sodium has the following side effects: —CNS: hyperirritability, nervousness, insomnia, twitching, tremors, headache

	—CV: increased cardiac output, tachycardia, cardiac dysrhythmias, angina pectoris, increased blood pressure, cardiac decompensation and collapse —GI: diarrhea, abdominal cramps, vomiting —Other: weight loss, heat intolerance, hyperhidrosis (excessive sweating), menstrual irregularities; in infants and children—accelerated rate of bone maturation.
4 Discuss patient guidelines for taking liothyronine sodium.	The patient should follow these guidelines while taking liothyronine sodium: —Take the drug only as directed. Do not adjust the dose or stop taking it without the physician's approval. —Take it at the same time each day (preferably in the morning) to maintain constant hormone levels. —Call the physician at once if chest pain, palpitations, difficulty breathing, sweating, or nervousness occurs. Also report unusual bleeding or bruising. —Be aware that, during the first few months of therapy, children may suffer temporary partial hair loss. —Be aware that this drug will alter thyroid function test results. Inform any new physician that liothyronine sodium is being taken.

MAALOX (Maalox No. 1, Maalox No. 2, Maalox Plus)

Patient objectives	***Teaching plan content***
1 State the name of the medication, the dose prescribed, and the ordered frequency of administration.	This information should be obtained from the patient's physician.
2 Explain the use of Maalox.	Maalox is an antacid composed of aluminum and magnesium hydroxide that is used to provide relief from the discomfort associated with peptic ulcer disease, gastritis, peptic esophagitis, gastric hyperacidity, heartburn, or hiatal hernia.
3 Identify potential side effects of Maalox.	Maalox has the following side effects: —GI: diarrhea, abdominal cramps.
4 Discuss patient guidelines for taking Maalox.	The patient should follow these guidelines while taking Maalox:

—Take the drug exactly as directed. Do not overuse it.
—Take doses 20 minutes to 1 hour after meals and at bedtime, as directed by the physician.
—Chew chewable tablets completely before swallowing.
—Be aware that the doses may be followed by milk or water.
—Do not use Maalox if taking an antibiotic containing tetracycline.
—Shake the suspension well.

MAGNESIUM SALTS (Concentrated Milk of Magnesia, Magnesium Citrate, Magnesium Sulfate, Milk of Magnesia)

Patient objectives	*Teaching plan content*
1 State the name of the medication, the dose prescribed, and the ordered frequency of administration.	This information should be obtained from the patient's physician.
2 Explain the use of magnesium salts.	Magnesium salts are used as laxatives to treat constipation. Milk of Magnesia may also be used as an antacid.
3 Identify potential side effects of magnesium salts.	Magnesium salts have the following side effects: —GI: abdominal cramping, nausea —Metabolic: fluid and electrolyte disturbances with daily use —Other: laxative dependence with long-term or excessive use.
4 Discuss patient guidelines for taking magnesium salts.	The patient should follow these guidelines while taking magnesium salts: —Take these drugs only as directed. They are meant only for short-term therapy; do not use them for longer than 1 week. Frequent or prolonged use may cause dependence. —When taking magnesium salts as a laxative, do not take oral drugs for 1 to 2 hours before or after. —Shake the suspension well. —Take the drugs with a large amount of water when used as a laxative. —Time drug administration so it does not interfere with scheduled activities or sleep. —Be aware that chilling before use may make magnesium citrate more palatable.

—To avoid future constipation, be sure to have adequate fluid intake, exercise, and dietary bulk. Sources of bulk include bran and other cereals and fresh fruits and vegetables.

MEDROXYPROGESTERONE ACETATE (MPA) (Amen, Depo-Provera, Provera)

Patient objectives	*Teaching plan content*
1 State the name of the medication, the dose prescribed, and the ordered frequency of administration.	This information should be obtained from the patient's physician.
2 Explain the use of medroxyprogesterone acetate.	Medroxyprogesterone acetate is used to treat abnormal uterine bleeding due to hormonal imbalance and to treat secondary amenorrhea because of its ability to mimic the body's production of progesterone—a hormone that influences the menstrual cycle.
3 Identify potential side effects of medroxyprogesterone acetate.	Medroxyprogesterone acetate has the following side effects: —CNS: dizziness, migraine headache, lethargy, depression —CV: hypertension, thrombophlebitis, pulmonary embolism, edema —GI: nausea, vomiting, abdominal cramps —GU: breakthrough bleeding, dysmenorrhea (painful menstruation), amenorrhea (lack of menstrual flow); cervical erosion or abnormal secretions; uterine fibromas, vaginal candidiasis —Hepatic: cholestatic jaundice (jaundice resulting from an abnormality in the flow of bile) —Metabolic: hyperglycemia, decreased libido —Skin: melasma (blotchy, brown spots on forehead, cheeks, and temples), rash —Other: breast tenderness, enlargement, secretion.
4 Discuss patient guidelines for taking medroxyprogesterone acetate.	The patient should follow these guidelines while taking medroxyprogesterone acetate: —Take the drug exactly as directed. Do not adjust the dose without first consulting the physician. —Report any unusual symptoms immediately; stop the drug and call the physician. —Perform a monthly breast self-examination.

MENOTROPINS (Pergonal)

Patient objectives	*Teaching plan content*
1 State the name of the medication, the dose prescribed, and the ordered frequency of administration.	This information should be obtained from the patient's physician.
2 Explain the use of menotropins.	Menotropins is used to treat anovulation and infertility in conjunction with human chorionic gonadotropin.
3 Identify potential side effects of menotropins.	Menotropins has the following side effects: —Blood: hemoconcentration with fluid loss into abdomen —GI: nausea, vomiting, diarrhea —GU (women): ovarian enlargement with pain and abdominal distention, multiple births, ovarian hyperstimulation syndrome (sudden ovarian enlargement, ascites with or without pain, or pleural effusion [fluid in the pleura]) —GU (men): gynecomastia (breast enlargement in the male) —Other: fever.
4 Discuss patient guidelines for menotropins administration.	The patient should follow these guidelines while menotropins is being administered: —Be aware that the nurse will administer the medication as an injection. —If menotropins is being used for infertility, have daily intercourse from the day before human chorionic gonadotropin is given until ovulation occurs. —Be aware of the possibility of multiple births.

METHANTHELINE BROMIDE (Banthine)

Patient objectives	*Teaching plan content*
1 State the name of the medication, the dose prescribed, and the ordered frequency of administration.	This information should be obtained from the patient's physician.
2 Explain the use of methantheline bromide.	Methantheline bromide is used as adjunctive therapy in peptic ulcer, pylorospasm, spastic colon, biliary dyski-

	nesia (abnormal movement of bile), pancreatitis, and certain forms of gastritis because of its ability to decrease GI motility and inhibit gastric acid secretion.
3 Identify potential side effects of methantheline bromide.	Methantheline bromide has the following side effects: (NOTE: Overdosage may cause symptoms similar to those of curare toxicity [muscle paralysis].) —CNS: headache, insomnia, dizziness, confusion or excitement in elderly patients, nervousness, weakness —CV: palpitations, tachycardia —EENT: blurred vision, mydriasis (extreme dilation of the pupil), increased ocular tension, cycloplegia (paralysis of the ciliary muscle of the eye), photophobia —GI: dry mouth, dysphagia, constipation, heartburn, loss of taste, nausea, vomiting, paralytic ileus —GU: urinary hesitancy and retention, impotence —Skin: urticaria (hives), decreased sweating or anhidrosis (inability to sweat), other dermal manifestations —Other: fever, allergic reactions.
4 Discuss patient guidelines for taking methantheline bromide.	The patient should follow these guidelines while taking methantheline bromide: —Take the drug only as directed. Do not adjust the dose without consulting the physician. —Do not take over-the-counter cough medicines or hay fever preparations in conjunction with methantheline bromide without first consulting the physician. —Avoid strenuous work or exercise during hot and humid weather, as drug-induced heatstroke may develop. —Take doses 30 minutes to 1 hour before meals and at bedtime. The bedtime dose should be taken at least 2 hours after the last meal of the day. —Report any skin rash or urinary hesitancy and retention immediately to the physician. —Avoid driving and other hazardous activities if drowsiness, dizziness, or blurred vision occurs. —Drink plenty of fluids to help prevent constipation. —Take sugarless gum or hard candy to relieve mouth dryness.

METHIMAZOLE (Tapazole)

Patient objectives	*Teaching plan content*
1 State the name of the medication, dose prescribed, and ordered frequency of administration.	This information should be obtained from the patient's physician.

2 Explain the use of methimazole.	Methimazole is used to treat hyperthyroidism by interfering with the production of thyroid hormone. It may also be used to ameliorate hyperthyroidism prior to subtotal thyroidectomy or radioactive iodine therapy.
3 Identify potential side effects of methimazole.	Methimazole has the following side effects: —Blood: agranulocytosis (a symptom complex characterized by a decrease in granulocytes), leukopenia (deficiency of white blood cells), granulocytopenia (deficiency of granulocytes), thrombocytopenia (deficiency of platelets). These side effects appear to be dose-related. —CNS: headache, drowsiness, vertigo —GI: diarrhea, nausea, vomiting (may be dose-related) —Hepatic: jaundice —Skin: rash, urticaria (hives), skin discoloration —Other: arthralgia (pain in joints), myalgia (pain in muscles), salivary gland enlargement, loss of taste, drug fever, lymphadenopathy.
4 Discuss patient guidelines for taking methimazole.	The patient should follow these guidelines while taking methimazole: —Take the drug only as directed. Do not adjust the dose or stop taking it without the physician's approval. —Be aware that a loss of taste may occur while taking methimazole. —Watch for signs of hypothyroidism (mental depression, cold intolerance, swelling of legs that feels hard when pressed). —Notify the physician immediately if fever, sore throat, unusual bleeding or bruising, headache, or skin rashes occur. —Avoid using iodized salt and/or eating shellfish, if ordered by the physician. —Take the drug with meals. —Store methimazole in the original container or in a light-resistant container. —Do not take over-the-counter cough medicines, as many contain iodine.

METHYLDOPA (Aldomet, Dopamet, Medimet-250, Novomedopa)

Patient objectives	*Teaching plan content*
1 State the name of the medication, the dose prescribed, and the ordered frequency of administration.	This information should be obtained from the patient's physician.

2 Explain the use of methyldopa.	Methyldopa is used to manage hypertension because of its ability to lower blood pressure.
3 Identify potential side effects of methyldopa.	Methyldopa has the following side effects: —Blood: hemolytic anemia, reversible granulocytopenia (decrease in granulocytes), thrombocytopenia (decrease in platelets) —CNS: sedation, headache, asthenia, weakness, dizziness, decreased mental acuity, involuntary choreoathetotic movements (jerky, slow movements), psychic disturbances, depression, nightmares —CV: bradycardia (unusually slow heart rate), orthostatic hypotension (drop in blood pressure on arising), aggravated angina, myocarditis (inflammation of the cardiac muscle), edema, weight gain —EENT: dry mouth, nasal stuffiness —GI: diarrhea, pancreatitis —Hepatic: hepatic necrosis —Other: gynecomastia (breast enlargement in the male), lactation, skin rash, drug-induced fever, impotence.
4 Discuss patient guidelines for taking methyldopa.	The patient should follow these guidelines while taking methyldopa: —Take methyldopa as directed. Never adjust the dose, and do not stop taking it abruptly without the physician's recommendation. —Check the weight daily. Notify the physician of any weight increase or swelling of the hands or feet. —Be aware that urine may turn dark in toilet bowls treated with bleach. —Rise slowly and avoid sudden position changes to minimize dizziness. —Relieve mouth dryness with sugarless gum or candy or ice chips. —If drowsiness is a problem, ask the physician about taking a once-daily dose at bedtime.

METOPROLOL TARTRATE (Betaloc, Lopresor, Lopressor)

Patient objectives	*Teaching plan content*
1 State the name of the medication, the dose prescribed, and the ordered frequency of administration.	This information should be obtained from the patient's physician.

2 Explain the use of metoprolol tartrate.	Metoprolol tartrate is used to treat hypertension because of its ability to lower blood pressure. It may also be used for early intervention in heart attack.
3 Identify potential side effects of metoprolol tartrate.	Metoprolol tartrate has the following side effects: —CNS: fatigue, lethargy —CV: bradycardia, hypotension, congestive heart failure, peripheral vascular disease —GI: nausea, vomiting, diarrhea —Skin: rash —Other: fever.
4 Discuss patient guidelines for taking metoprolol tartrate.	The patient should follow these guidelines while taking metoprolol tartrate: —Take the drug only as directed. Never adjust the dose or stop taking it abruptly without consulting the physician. —Take it with meals, as food may enhance its absorption. —For diabetics on antidiabetic medication: Be aware that this drug masks common signs of hypoglycemia. Monitor blood sugar levels closely.

METRONIDAZOLE (Flagyl, Metryl, Neo-Tric)

Patient objectives	*Teaching plan content*
1 State the name of the medication, the dose prescribed, and the ordered frequency of administration.	This information should be obtained from the patient's physician.
2 Explain the use of metronidazole.	Metronidazole is used to treat liver or intestinal infections caused by amebiasis or vaginal infections caused by trichomoniasis. It may also be used to treat certain bacterial infections.
3 Identify potential side effects of metronidazole.	Metronidazole has the following side effects: —Blood: transient leukopenia (decrease in white blood cells), neutropenia (decrease in neutrophils) —CNS: vertigo, headache, ataxia (unsteady gait), incoordination, confusion, irritability, depression, restlessness, weakness, fatigue, drowsiness, insomnia, sensory neuropathy, paresthesias (numbness and tingling) of extremities, psychic stimulation, neuromyopathy —CV: EKG change (flattened T wave)

—GI: abdominal cramping, stomatitis (inflammation of the mouth), nausea, vomiting, anorexia, diarrhea, constipation, proctitis (inflammation of the rectum), dry mouth
—GU: darkened urine, polyuria, dysuria, pyuria (pus in the urine), incontinence, cystitis, decreased libido, dyspareunia (painful intercourse), dryness of vagina and vulva, sense of pelvic pressure
—Skin: pruritus (itching), flushing
—Local: thrombophlebitis after I.V. infusion
—Other: overgrowth of nonsusceptible organisms, especially *Candida* (glossitis, furry tongue); metallic taste; fever.

4 Discuss patient guidelines for taking metronidazole.

The patient should follow these guidelines while taking metronidazole:
—Take the drug exactly as directed. Do not adjust the dose or stop taking it without first consulting the physician.
—Take it with meals to minimize GI distress.
—Avoid alcohol or alcohol-containing medications for 48 hours after therapy is complete.
—Be aware that a metallic taste and dark or red-brown urine are possible but harmless side effects.
—If the drug is being taken to treat amebiasis, record the number and character of stools.
—If it is being taken to treat a vaginal infection, inform asymptomatic sexual partners that they should be treated simultaneously to avoid reinfection.
—Practice good hygiene.

MINOXIDIL (Loniten)

Patient objectives	*Teaching plan content*
1 State the name of the medication, the dose prescribed, and the ordered frequency of administration.	This information should be obtained from the patient's physician.
2 Explain the use of minoxidil.	Minoxidil is used to treat hypertension because of its ability to lower blood pressure.
3 Identify potential side effects of minoxidil.	Minoxidil has the following side effects: —CV: edema, tachycardia, pericardial effusion and

	tamponade, congestive heart failure, EKG changes —Skin: rash, Stevens-Johnson syndrome (erythema multiforme) —Other: hypertrichosis (elongation, thickening, and enhanced pigmentation of fine body hair), breast tenderness.
4 Discuss patient guidelines for taking minoxidil.	The patient should follow these guidelines while taking minoxidil: —Take the drug exactly as directed. Do not adjust the dose or stop taking it without the physician's consent. —Be aware that unwanted hair can be controlled with a depilatory or by shaving. Extra hair will disappear within 1 to 6 months after the drug is discontinued. —Read the package insert carefully.

MYLANTA (Mylanta, Mylanta-II)

Patient objectives	*Teaching plan content*
1 State the name of the medication, the dose prescribed, and the ordered frequency of administration.	This information should be obtained from the patient's physician.
2 Explain the use of Mylanta.	Mylanta is an antacid composed of aluminum hydroxide, magnesium hydroxide, and simethicone that is used to provide relief from the discomfort associated with heartburn, hiatal hernia, peptic esophagitis, gastritis, and peptic ulcer disease. It may also be used to provide relief from entrapped air, or gas, because of its antiflatulent property.
3 Identify potential side effects of Mylanta.	Mylanta has the following side effects: —GI: diarrhea, abdominal cramps, bloating.
4 Discuss patient guidelines for taking Mylanta.	The patient should follow these guidelines while taking Mylanta: —Use the drug exactly as directed. Do not overuse it. —Take doses between meals and at bedtime. —Do not use Mylanta if taking an antibiotic containing tetracycline. —Shake the suspension well.

NADOLOL (Corgard)

Patient objectives	*Teaching plan content*
1 State the name of the medication, the dose prescribed, and the ordered frequency of administration.	This information should be obtained from the patient's physician.
2 Explain the use of nadolol.	Nadolol is used to manage angina pectoris by reducing the heart's oxygen demand. It is also used to manage hypertension because it blocks certain mechanisms that increase blood pressure.
3 Identify potential side effects of nadolol.	Nadolol has the following side effects: —CNS: fatigue, lethargy —CV: bradycardia, hypotension, congestive heart failure, peripheral vascular disease —GI: nausea, vomiting, diarrhea —Metabolic: hypoglycemia without tachycardia —Skin: rash —Other: increased airway resistance, fever.
4 Discuss patient guidelines for taking nadolol.	The patient should follow these guidelines while taking nadolol: —Take nadolol as directed. Never adjust the dose, and do not abruptly stop taking the drug without the physician's recommendation. —Swallow the capsule whole, without breaking, crushing, or chewing it. —Be aware that angina may worsen at the start of therapy or with dosage increases. This effect is temporary. Continue to take sublingual nitroglycerin, as ordered, when anginal symptoms are acute.

NIFEDIPINE (Adalat, Procardia)

Patient objectives	*Teaching plan content*
1 State the name of the medication, the dose prescribed, and the ordered frequency of administration.	This information should be obtained from the patient's physician.
2 Explain the use of nifedipine.	Nifedipine reduces the oxygen demand of the heart and is used in the management of angina pectoris.

3 Identify potential side effects of nifedipine.	Nifedipine has the following side effects: —CNS: dizziness, light-headedness, flushing, headache, weakness, syncope (fainting) —CV: peripheral edema, hypotension, palpitations —EENT: nasal congestion —GI: nausea, heartburn, diarrhea —Other: muscle cramps, dyspnea.
4 Discuss patient guidelines for taking nifedipine.	The patient should follow these guidelines while taking nifedipine: —Take the drug only as directed. Never adjust the dosage without the physician's recommendation. —Be aware that angina may worsen at the start of therapy or with dosage increases. This effect is temporary. Continue to take sublingual nitroglycerin, as ordered. —Swallow the capsule whole, without breaking, crushing, or chewing it.

NITROFURANTOIN (Furadantin, Novofuran)
NITROFURANTOIN MACROCRYSTALS (Macrodantin)

Patient objectives	***Teaching plan content***
1 State the name of the medication, the dose prescribed, and the ordered frequency of administration.	This information should be obtained from the patient's physician.
2 Explain the use of nitrofurantoin.	Nitrofurantoin is an antibiotic used to treat urinary tract infections.
3 Identify potential side effects of nitrofurantoin.	Nitrofurantoin has the following side effects: —Blood: hemolysis in patients with G-6-PD deficiency (reversed after stopping the drug), agranulocytosis (a symptom complex characterized by a decrease in granulocytes), thrombocytopenia (decrease in the number of platelets) —CNS: peripheral neuropathy, headache, dizziness, drowsiness, ascending polyneuropathy with high doses or renal impairment —GI: anorexia, nausea, vomiting, abdominal pain, diarrhea —Hepatic: hepatitis —Skin: maculopapular, erythematous, or eczematous

	eruption; pruritus (itching); urticaria (hives); exfoliative dermatitis (severe inflammation of the skin accompanied by peeling); Stevens-Johnson syndrome (erythema multiforme) —Other: asthmatic attacks in patients with a history of asthma; anaphylaxis; hypersensitivity; transient alopecia (hair loss); drug fever; overgrowth of nonsusceptible organisms in the urinary tract; pulmonary sensitivity reactions, such as cough, chest pain, fever, chills, and dyspnea.
4 Discuss patient guidelines for taking nitrofurantoin.	The patient should follow these guidelines while taking nitrofurantoin: —Take the drug exactly as prescribed, even after symptoms are gone. —Take it with food or milk to minimize GI distress. —Be aware that a harmless side effect of this drug is brown or darker urine. —Store the drug in an amber container. To avoid precipitate formation, do not keep it in pillboxes made of metal other than stainless steel or aluminum. —For diabetics: Because nitrofurantoin may cause false-positive results with Clinitest, use a different product to test urine sugar.

NITROGLYCERIN (Ang-O-Span, Cardabid, Corobid, Glyceryl Trinitrate, Gly-Trate, NitroBid, Nitrocap, Nitrocels, Nitro-Dial, Nitrodisc, Nitro-Dur, Nitroglyn, Nitrol, Nitro-Lyn, Nitrong, Nitrospan, Nitrostabilin, Transderm-Nitro, Trates, Tridil)

Patient objectives	***Teaching plan content***
1 State the name of the medication, the dose prescribed, and the ordered frequency of administration.	This information should be obtained from the patient's physician.
2 Explain the use of nitroglycerin.	Nitroglycerin is a vasodilator (that is, it increases the diameter of blood vessels) used to treat angina pectoris by increasing the amount of oxygen and blood delivered to the heart muscle.
3 Identify potential side effects of nitroglycerin.	Nitroglycerin has the following side effects: —CNS: headache, sometimes with throbbing; dizziness; weakness

—CV: orthostatic hypotension (drop in blood pressure on arising), tachycardia, flushing, palpitations, syncope (fainting)
—GI: nausea, vomiting
—Local: sublingual burning
—Skin: cutaneous vasodilation
—Other: hypersensitivity reactions.

4 Discuss patient guidelines for using nitroglycerin.

The patient should follow these guidelines while using nitroglycerin:
—Use the medication exactly as directed. Use the sublingual form to relieve acute attacks, and have it easily accessible at all times.
—To use the sublingual tablets: At the first sign of attack, wet a tablet with saliva and place it under the tongue until it is completely absorbed. During this time, sit down and rest. If no relief is noted after a second dose, call the physician or go to the hospital emergency department.
—To take the oral or chewable tablets: Take them on an empty stomach, either ½ hour before or 1 to 2 hours after a meal. Swallow oral tablets whole; chew chewable tablets thoroughly before swallowing.
—To use buccal tablets: Let a buccal sustained-release tablet dissolve between cheek and gum. The tablet should dissolve within 3 to 5 minutes.
—To apply the ointment: Spread a uniformly thin layer of ointment on any nonhairy area (except the distal parts of the arms or legs) or on the face and neck. Do not rub it in. Cover it with plastic film to aid absorption and to protect clothing.
—Avoid drinking alcoholic beverages, which may cause unpleasant side effects in combination with nitroglycerin.
—Change to an upright position slowly, as nitroglycerin can affect the blood pressure. In addition, go up and down stairs carefully, and lie down at the first sign of dizziness.
—Store this drug in a cool, dark place in a tightly closed container. To ensure freshness, replace the supply every 3 months. Remove cotton from the container, as it absorbs the drug.
—Do not use the sublingual nitroglycerin tablets if you opened the original container more than 60 days ago. With repeated exposure to air, sublingual nitroglycerin tablets gradually lose their strength and become ineffective.

PENICILLIN G BENZATHINE (Bicillin L-A, Megacillin Suspension, Permapen)

Patient objectives	*Teaching plan content*
1 State the name of the medication, the dose prescribed, and the ordered frequency of administration.	This information should be obtained from the patient's physician.
2 Explain the use of penicillin G benzathine.	Penicillin G benzathine is an antibiotic used to treat syphilis and upper respiratory infections caused by a streptococcal agent. It may also be used as a prophylactic in poststreptococcal rheumatic fever.
3 Identify potential side effects of penicillin G benzathine.	Penicillin G benzathine has the following side effects: —Blood: eosinophilia (increase in the number of eosinophils in the blood), hemolytic anemia, thrombocytopenia (decrease in the number of platelets), leukopenia (decrease in the number of white blood cells) —CNS: neuropathy, convulsions with high doses —Local: pain and sterile abscess at injection site —Other: hypersensitivity (maculopapular and exfoliative dermatitis, chills, fever, edema, anaphylaxis).
4 Discuss patient guidelines for penicillin G benzathine administration.	The patient should follow these guidelines while penicillin G benzathine is being administered: —Tell the physician of any previous allergic reaction to this drug. —Call the physician if rash, fever, or chills develop. —Be aware that a nurse or physician will administer this drug as an injection, in the buttocks in adults and in the thigh in infants and small children.

PENICILLIN G PROCAINE (Ayercillin, Crysticillin A.S., Duracillin A.S., Pfizerpen A.S., Wycillin)

Patient objectives	*Teaching plan content*
1 State the name of the medication, the dose prescribed, and the ordered frequency of administration.	This information should be obtained from the patient's physician.

2 Explain the use of penicillin G procaine.	Penicillin G procaine is an antibiotic used to treat a variety of moderate to severe infections. It is particularly effective in the treatment of uncomplicated gonorrhea and pneumococcal pneumonia.
3 Identify potential side effects of penicillin G procaine.	Penicillin G procaine has the following side effects: —Blood: thrombocytopenia (decrease in the number of platelets), hemolytic anemia, leukopenia (decrease in the number of white blood cells) —CNS: arthralgia (aching joints), convulsions —Other: hypersensitivity (rash, urticaria, chills, fever, edema, prostration, anaphylaxis), overgrowth of nonsusceptible organisms.
4 Discuss patient guidelines for penicillin G procaine administration.	The patient should follow these guidelines while penicillin G procaine is being administered: —Tell the physician of any previous allergic reactions to this drug before receiving the first dose. —Call the physician if rash, fever, or chills develop. —Be aware that a nurse or physician will administer this drug as an injection, in the buttocks in adults or in the thigh in infants or children. —With prolonged therapy, other infections may occur. Report any vaginal, urinary, or respiratory discomfort to the physician.

PENTOXIFYLLINE (Trental)

Patient objectives	*Teaching plan content*
1 State the name of the medication, the dose prescribed, and the ordered frequency of administration.	This information should be obtained from the patient's physician.
2 Explain the use of pentoxifylline.	Pentoxifylline is used in the treatment of intermittent claudication due to chronic occlusive vascular disease.
3 Identify potential side effects of pentoxifylline.	Pentoxifylline has the following side effects: —CNS: headache, dizziness —GI: dyspepsia, nausea, vomiting.
4 Discuss patient guidelines for taking pentoxifylline.	The patient should follow these guidelines while taking pentoxifylline: —Do not discontinue taking this drug during the first

8 weeks of treatment unless ordered to do so by the physician; this drug should be taken for a minimum of 8 weeks to achieve clinical effects.
—Take with meals to minimize gastrointestinal upset.
—Report any gastrointestinal or CNS adverse reactions; the physician may reduce the dose.

PHENAZOPYRIDINE HYDROCHLORIDE (Phenazo, Pyridium)

Patient objectives	*Teaching plan content*
1 State the name of the medication, the dose prescribed, and the ordered frequency of administration.	This information should be obtained from the patient's physician.
2 Explain the use of phenazopyridine hydrochloride.	Phenazopyridine hydrochloride is a urinary tract analgesic used to relieve pain caused by urinary tract irritation or infection.
3 Identify potential side effects of phenazopyridine hydrochloride.	Phenazopyridine hydrochloride has the following side effects: —CNS: headache —GI: nausea.
4 Discuss patient guidelines for taking phenazopyridine hydrochloride.	The patient should follow these guidelines while taking phenazopyridine hydrochloride: —Take the drug as directed. It may be stopped in 3 days if the pain is relieved. —Be aware that a harmless side effect of this drug is that it colors urine red or orange, staining fabrics. —Notify the physician immediately and stop taking the drug if the skin or the white portion of the eyes become yellow-tinged. —For diabetics: Because phenazopyridine hydrochloride may alter Clinistix or Tes-Tape results, use a different product to test urine for glucose.

PHENOBARBITAL

Patient objectives	*Teaching plan content*
1 State the name of the medication, the dose prescribed, and the ordered frequency of administration.	This information should be obtained from the patient's physician.

2 Explain the use of phenobarbital.	Phenobarbital is used to control seizures. It may also be ordered for sedation.
3 Identify potential side effects of phenobarbital.	Phenobarbital has the following side effects: —CNS: drowsiness, lethargy, hangover, paradoxical excitement in elderly patients —GI: nausea, vomiting —Skin: rash, urticaria (hives) —Local: pain, swelling, thrombophlebitis, necrosis, nerve injury —Other: Stevens-Johnson syndrome (erythema multiforme), angioedema.
4 Discuss patient guidelines for taking phenobarbital.	The patient should follow these guidelines while taking phenobarbital: —Take the drug only as directed. Do not adjust the dose or stop taking it abruptly. —Because of its sedative effect, avoid activities that require alertness. —Avoid drinking alcohol. —Be aware that full therapeutic effects may not be seen for 2 to 3 weeks. —Be aware that phenobarbital may become addictive if used on a prolonged basis.

PHENYTOIN (Dilantin)

Patient objectives	*Teaching plan content*
1 State the name of the medication, the dose prescribed, and the ordered frequency of administration.	This information should be obtained from the patient's physician.
2 Explain the use of phenytoin.	Phenytoin is used to control seizures. It is also sometimes used to regulate the rhythm of the heart.
3 Identify potential side effects of phenytoin.	Phenytoin has the following side effects: —Blood: thrombocytopenia (decrease in the number of platelets), leukopenia (decrease in the number of white blood cells), agranulocytosis (a symptom complex characterized by a decrease in granulocytes), pancytopenia (deficiency of all cell products of blood), lymphadenopathy (enlargement of lymph nodes), megaloblastic anemia —CNS: ataxia, slurred speech, insomnia, headache,

	muscle twitching, lethargy —CV: severe hypotension, vascular collapse (with rapid I.V. infusions greater than 50 mg/minute), vasodilation, asystole, ventricular fibrillation, AV block —EENT: nystagmus (rapid, involuntary movement of the eyeball), diplopia (double vision), blurred vision —GI: gingival hyperplasia, nausea, vomiting, constipation —Metabolic: hyperglycemia —Skin: rash (morbilliform most common), dermatitis (bullous, exfoliative, purpuric), lupus erythematosus, Stevens-Johnson syndrome (erythema multiforme).
4 Discuss patient guidelines for taking phenytoin.	The patient should follow these guidelines while taking phenytoin: —Take the drug only as ordered. Do not adjust the dose or stop taking it abruptly. —Because of potential drowsiness, avoid activities that require alertness. —Take phenytoin with food or a large glass of water. —Always take the drug on time. —Maintain good oral hygiene. —Do not drink alcohol.

POTASSIUM IODIDE (Potassium Iodide Solution, USP; Strong Iodine Solution, USP [Lugol's Solution])

Patient objectives	*Teaching plan content*
1 State the name of the medication, the dose prescribed, and the ordered frequency of administration.	This information should be obtained from the patient's physician.
2 Explain the use of potassium iodide.	Potassium iodide is used to ameliorate hyperthyroidism prior to subtotal thyroidectomy by inhibiting thyroid hormone formation.
3 Identify potential side effects of potassium iodide.	Potassium iodide has the following side effects: —EENT: acute rhinitis (inflammation of the nasal passages), inflammation of salivary glands, periorbital edema, conjunctivitis, hyperemia —GI: burning, irritation, nausea, vomiting, metallic taste —Skin: acneiform rash, mucous membrane ulceration —Other: fever, frontal headache; acute iodism, shock, pulmonary edema with I.V. use.

4 Discuss patient guidelines for taking potassium iodide.	The patient should follow these guidelines while taking potassium iodide: —Take the drug only as directed. Do not adjust the dose or stop taking it without the physician's approval. —Dilute it in water, milk, or fruit juice to mask the salty taste. —Take it after meals, and use a straw to drink the solution to avoid tooth discoloration. —Avoid iodized salt, shellfish, or iodine-rich foods, if ordered by the physician. —Store potassium iodide in the original container or in a light-resistant container.

PRAZOSIN HYDROCHLORIDE (Minipress)

Patient objectives	*Teaching plan content*
1 State the name of the medication, the dose prescribed, and the ordered frequency of administration.	This information should be obtained from the patient's physician.
2 Explain the use of prazosin hydrochloride.	Prazosin hydrochloride is used primarily to manage hypertension because of its ability to lower blood pressure. It may also be used in severe chronic congestive heart failure because of its ability to reduce vascular resistance and decrease the work of the heart muscle in pumping blood into the vessels.
3 Identify potential side effects of prazosin hydrochloride.	Prazosin hydrochloride has the following side effects: —CNS: dizziness, headache, drowsiness, weakness, "first-dose syncope" (fainting), depression —CV: orthostatic hypotension (a drop in blood pressure upon arising), palpitations —EENT: blurred vision, dry mouth —GI: vomiting, diarrhea, abdominal cramps, constipation, nausea —GU: priapism (sustained, inappropriate erection of the penis).
4 Discuss patient guidelines for taking prazosin hydrochloride.	The patient should follow these guidelines while taking prazosin hydrochloride: —Take the drug as directed. Never adjust the dose or stop taking it without the physician's recommendation. —Rise slowly and avoid sudden position changes to

minimize dizziness. If dizziness occurs, sit or lie down.
—Relieve mouth dryness with sugarless gum or candy or ice chips.

PREDNISONE (Colisone, Deltasone, Liquid Pred, Meticorten, Orasone, Prednicen-M, SK-Prednisone, Wojtab)

Patient objectives	*Teaching plan content*
1 State the name of the medication, the dose prescribed, and the ordered frequency of administration.	This information should be obtained from the patient's physician.
2 Explain the use of prednisone.	Prednisone is used to treat severe inflammatory conditions (for example, ulcerative colitis). Its mode of action is unknown.
3 Identify potential side effects of prednisone.	Prednisone has the following side effects: (NOTE: Acute adrenal insufficiency may occur with increased stress [infection, surgery, trauma] or abrupt withdrawal after long-term therapy. Sudden withdrawal may be fatal.) —CNS: euphoria, insomnia, psychotic behavior, pseudotumor cerebri (a condition caused by cerebral edema, marked by increased intracranial pressure) —CV: congestive heart failure, hypertension, edema —EENT: cataracts, glaucoma —GI: peptic ulcer, gastrointestinal irritation, increased appetite —Metabolic: possible hypokalemia, hyperglycemia, and carbohydrate intolerance; growth suppression in children —Skin: delayed wound healing, acne, various skin eruptions —Other: muscle weakness, pancreatitis, hirsutism (masculinization of the female), susceptibility to infections. Withdrawal symptoms: rebound inflammation, fatigue, weakness, arthralgia, fever, dizziness, lethargy, depression, fainting, orthostatic hypotension, dyspnea, anorexia, hypoglycemia.
4 Discuss patient guidelines for taking prednisone.	The patient should follow these guidelines while taking prednisone: —Take the drug only as directed. Do not adjust the

dose or stop taking it abruptly without first consulting the physician.
—Take once-daily doses in the morning for better results.
—Always carry an I.D. card identifying the need for supplemental systemic glucocorticoids during periods of stress, including times of illness.
—For diabetics: Watch for signs of hyperglycemia.
—Take prednisone with food.
—Be alert for cushingoid symptoms (facial puffiness, hirsutism, thinning of the extremities with abdominal obesity, amenorrhea in females, and edema).
—Adhere to a salt-restricted diet, rich in potassium and protein, if ordered. (See the dietitian, if necessary.)
—Check your weight daily, and report any sudden weight gain to the physician.

PRIMIDONE (Mysoline, Sertan)

Patient objectives	*Teaching plan content*
1 State the name of the medication, the dose prescribed, and the ordered frequency of administration.	This information should be obtained from the patient's physician.
2 Explain the use of primidone.	Primidone is used to control seizure activity.
3 Identify potential side effects of primidone.	Primidone has the following side effects: —Blood: leukopenia (decrease in the number of white blood cells), eosinophilia (increase in the number of eosinophils) —CNS: drowsiness, ataxia (unsteady gait), emotional disturbances, vertigo (dizziness), hyperirritability, fatigue —EENT: diplopia (double vision), nystagmus (rapid, involuntary movement of the eyeball), edema of the eyelids —GI: anorexia, nausea, vomiting —GU: impotence, polyuria —Skin: morbilliform rash, alopecia (hair loss) —Other: edema, thirst.
4 Discuss patient guidelines for taking primidone.	The patient should follow these guidelines while taking primidone: —Take the drug only as directed. Do not adjust the

dose or stop taking it abruptly without the physician's recommendation.
—Avoid activities that require alertness and good psychomotor coordination until the nervous system response has been determined.
—Shake the liquid suspension well.

PROBENECID (Benemid, Benuryl)

Patient objectives	*Teaching plan content*
1 State the name of the medication, the dose prescribed, and the ordered frequency of administration.	This information should be obtained from the patient's physician.
2 Explain the use of probenecid.	Probenecid is used as adjunctive therapy with penicillin in the treatment of gonorrhea because of its ability to hinder the excretion of penicillin in the urine. It is also used to treat gout or gouty arthritis because of its ability to promote the excretion of uric acid in the urine.
3 Identify potential side effects of probenecid.	Probenecid has the following side effects: —Blood: hemolytic anemia —CNS: headache, dizziness —CV: hypotension —GI: anorexia, nausea, vomiting, gastric distress —GU: urinary frequency —Skin: dermatitis, pruritus (itching) —Other: flushing, sore gums, fever.
4 Discuss patient guidelines for taking probenecid.	The patient should follow these guidelines while taking probenecid: —Take the drug exactly as prescribed. If it is not taken regularly, gout attacks may result. —Take it with milk, food, or antacids to minimize GI distress. —Drink enough fluids to maintain a minimum daily urinary output of 2 to 3 qt (2 to 3 liters). —Avoid drinking alcohol. —Avoid all medications that contain aspirin, as these may precipitate gout. —Restrict foods high in purine—anchovies, liver, sardines, kidneys, sweetbreads, peas, and lentils. —Visit the physician regularly. Expect periodic urine

and blood tests for BUN and renal function studies.
—For diabetics: Because this drug may produce false-positive glucose tests with Clinitest, use a glucose-oxidase method, such as Clinistix, Diastix, or Tes-Tape, instead.

PROCAINAMIDE HYDROCHLORIDE (Procan SR, Pronestyl, Pronestyl-SR, Sub-Quin)

Patient objectives	*Teaching plan content*
1 State the name of the medication, the dose prescribed, and the ordered frequency of administration.	This information should be obtained from the patient's physician.
2 Explain the use of procainamide hydrochloride.	Procainamide hydrochloride is used to regulate the rhythm of the heart.
3 Identify potential side effects of procainamide hydrochloride.	Procainamide hydrochloride has the following side effects: —Blood: thrombocytopenia (decreased number of platelets); neutropenia (decreased number of neutrophils), especially with sustained-release forms; agranulocytosis (a symptom complex characterized by a decrease in granulocytes); hemolytic anemia; increased ANA titer —CNS: hallucinations, confusion, convulsions, depression —CV: severe hypotension, bradycardia, AV block, ventricular fibrillation (after parenteral use) —GI: nausea, vomiting, anorexia, diarrhea, bitter taste —Skin: maculopapular rash —Other: fever, lupus erythematosus syndrome (especially after prolonged administration), myalgia (muscle aches).
4 Discuss patient guidelines for taking procainamide hydrochloride.	The patient should follow these guidelines while taking procainamide hydrochloride: —Take the drug exactly as prescribed. It must be taken at regular intervals, on schedule. —Because procainamide hydrochloride can sometimes cause stomach distress, take it with milk or food. —Store the drug in a tightly closed container, at room temperature.

PROCHLORPERAZINE (Compazine, Stemetil)

Patient objectives	*Teaching plan content*
1 State the name of the medication, the dose prescribed, and the ordered frequency of administration.	This information should be obtained from the patient's physician.
2 Explain the use of prochlorperazine.	Prochlorperazine is used to inhibit nausea and vomiting.
3 Identify potential side effects of prochlorperazine.	Prochlorperazine has the following side effects: —Blood: transient leukopenia (decrease in the number of white blood cells), agranulocytosis (a symptom complex characterized by a decrease in granulocytes) —CNS: extrapyramidal reactions (high incidence), sedation (low incidence), pseudoparkinsonism, EEG changes, dizziness —CF: orthostatic hypotension (a drop in blood pressure upon arising), tachycardia, EKG changes —EENT: ocular changes, blurred vision —GI: dry mouth, constipation —GU: urinary retention, dark urine, menstrual irregularities, gynecomastia (breast enlargement in the male), inhibited ejaculation —Hepatic: cholestatic jaundice (jaundice caused by an abnormal flow of bile) —Metabolic: hyperprolactinemia —Skin: mild photosensitivity, dermal allergic reactions, exfoliative dermatitis (severe inflammation of the skin accompanied by peeling) —Other: weight gain, increased appetite.
4 Discuss patient guidelines for taking prochlorperazine.	The patient should follow these guidelines while taking prochlorperazine: —Take the drug only as directed. If more than four doses are needed in a 24-hour period, notify the physician. —Dilute the oral concentrate with tomato or fruit juice, milk, coffee, a carbonated beverage, tea, water, soup, or pudding. —Wear protective clothing when exposed to sunlight. —Change positions slowly to minimize dizziness.

PROGESTERONE (Profac-O, Progelan, Progestasert)

Patient objectives	*Teaching plan content*
1 State the name of the medication, the dose prescribed, and the ordered frequency of administration.	This information should be obtained from the patient's physician.
2 Explain the use of progesterone.	Progesterone is used to treat amenorrhea and uterine bleeding or as a contraceptive (as an intrauterine device, or IUD) because of its effect on the menstrual cycle.
3 Identify potential side effects of progesterone.	Progesterone has the following side effects: —CNS: dizziness, migraine headache, lethargy, depression —CV: hypertension, thrombophlebitis, pulmonary embolism, edema —GI: nausea, vomiting, abdominal cramps —GU: breakthrough bleeding, dysmenorrhea (painful menstruation), amenorrhea (lack of menstrual flow); cervical erosion or abnormal secretions; uterine fibromas; vaginal candidiasis —Hepatic: cholestatic jaundice (jaundice caused by an abnormal flow of bile) —Local: pain at injection site —Metabolic: hyperglycemia, decreased libido —Skin: melasma (blotchy brown macules on cheeks, forehead, and temples), rash —Other: breast tenderness, enlargement, or secretion.
4 Discuss patient guidelines for using progesterone.	The patient should follow these guidelines while using progesterone: —Use the drug exactly as directed. —Read the package insert carefully about possible progesterone side effects. —Report any unusual symptoms immediately; stop the drug and call the physician if visual disturbances or migraine headaches occur. —Perform monthly breast self-examination. —With the Progestasert IUD, be aware of the following: • Cramps may occur for several days after insertion, and menstrual periods may be heavier. Report excessively heavy menses or bleeding between menses to the physician.

• The device must be changed at the end of 1 year. Pregnancy risks increase after 1 year when a progesterone device is used for contraception.
• IUD placement must be checked prior to intercourse.

PROPANTHELINE BROMIDE (Banlin, Norpanth, Pro-Banthine, Propanthel, Robantaline, SK-Propantheline Bromide)

Patient objectives	*Teaching plan content*
1 State the name of the medication, the dose prescribed, and the ordered frequency of administration.	This information should be obtained from the patient's physician.
2 Explain the use of propantheline bromide.	Propantheline bromide is used as adjunctive treatment of peptic ulcer, irritable bowel syndrome, and other GI disorders because of its ability to decrease GI motility and inhibit gastric acid secretion.
3 Identify potential side effects of propantheline bromide.	Propantheline bromide has the following side effects: (NOTE: Overdosage may cause symptoms similar to those of curare toxicity [muscle paralysis].) —CNS: headache, insomnia, drowsiness, dizziness, confusion or excitement in elderly patients, nervousness, weakness —CV: palpitations, tachycardia —EENT: blurred vision, mydriasis (dilation of the pupil), increased ocular tension, cycloplegia (paralysis of the eye muscles), photophobia —GI: dry mouth, dysphagia, constipation, heartburn, loss of taste, nausea, vomiting, paralytic ileus —GU: urinary hesitancy and retention, impotence —Skin: urticaria, decreased sweating or anhidrosis, other dermal manifestations —Other: fever, allergic reactions.
4 Discuss patient guidelines for taking propantheline bromide.	The patient should follow these guidelines while taking propantheline bromide: —Take the drug only as directed. Do not adjust the dose without consulting the physician. —Do not take over-the-counter cough or hay fever preparations in conjunction with propantheline bromide without consulting the physician. —Avoid strenuous work or exercise during hot and hu-

mid weather, as drug-induced heatstroke can develop.
—Take doses 30 minutes to 1 hour before meals and at bedtime. The bedtime dose should be taken at least 2 hours after the last meal of the day.
—Report any skin rash or urinary hesitancy or retention to the physician immediately.
—Avoid driving and other hazardous activities if drowsiness, dizziness, or blurred vision are present.
—Drink plenty of liquids to help prevent constipation.
—Take sugarless gum or hard candy to relieve mouth dryness.

PROPRANOLOL HYDROCHLORIDE (Inderal)

Patient objectives	*Teaching plan content*
1 State the name of the medication, the dose prescribed, and the ordered frequency of administration.	This information should be obtained from the patient's physician.
2 Explain the use of propranolol hydrochloride.	Propranolol hydrochloride blocks certain actions of the sympathetic nervous system that regulate contraction of cardiac and smooth muscle. —It is used to reduce angina attacks because of its ability to decrease the rate and contraction force of the heart, thereby reducing the oxygen needs of the heart muscle. —It is used to manage heart rhythm disturbances because of its ability to lengthen conduction time of nerve impulses through the heart. —It is used to lower blood pressure because of its ability to expand the diameter of blood vessels.
3 Identify potential side effects of propranolol hydrochloride.	Propranolol hydrochloride has the following side effects: —CNS: fatigue, lethargy, vivid dreams, hallucinations —CV: bradycardia, hypotension, congestive heart failure, peripheral vascular disease —GI: nausea, vomiting, diarrhea —Metabolic: hypoglycemia without tachycardia —Skin: rash —Other: increased airway resistance, fever.
4 Discuss patient guidelines for taking propranolol hydrochloride.	The patient should follow these guidelines while taking propranolol hydrochloride: —Always take the drug as directed, and do not stop

taking it unless advised by the physician. Gradual withdrawal is necessary to prevent serious problems, such as an increased risk of heart attack or angina attacks.
—Keep propranolol hydrochloride in a dry, tightly closed container.
—For diabetics: Monitor blood sugar levels carefully or watch for evidence of hypoglycemia. If hypoglycemia occurs, treat it as directed, and notify the physician prior to the next scheduled dose of propranolol hydrochloride.

PROPYLTHIOURACIL (PTU)

Patient objectives	*Teaching plan content*
1 State the name of the medication, the dose prescribed, and the ordered frequency of administration.	This information should be obtained from the patient's physician.
2 Explain the use of propylthiouracil.	Propylthiouracil is used to treat hyperthyroidism by interfering with the production of thyroid hormone. It may also be used to ameliorate hyperthyroidism prior to subtotal thyroidectomy or radioactive iodine therapy.
3 Identify potential side effects of propylthiouracil.	Propylthiouracil has the following side effects: —Blood: agranulocytosis (a symptom complex characterized by a decrease in granulocytes), leukopenia (decrease in the number of white blood cells), thromobocytopenia (decrease in the number of platelets) (these appear to be dose-related) —CNS: headache, drowsiness, vertigo —EENT: visual disturbances —GI: diarrhea, nausea, vomiting (may be dose-related) —Hepatic: jaundice —Skin: rash, urticaria (hives), skin discoloration, pruritus (itching) —Other: arthralgia (joint pain), myalgia (muscle pain), salivary gland enlargement, loss of taste, drug fever, lymphadenopathy (lymph node enlargement).
4 Discuss patient guidelines for taking propylthiouracil.	The patient should follow these guidelines while taking propylthiouracil: —Take the drug only as directed. Do not adjust the

dose or stop taking it without the physician's approval.
—Be aware that a loss of taste may occur while taking propylthiouracil.
—Watch for signs of hypothyroidism (mental depression, cold intolerance, swelling of legs that feels hard when pressed).
—Notify the physician immediately if fever, sore throat, unusual bleeding or bruising, headache, or skin rashes occur.
—Avoid eating iodized salt and shellfish, if ordered by the physician.
—Take the drug with meals.
—Store it in the original container or in a light-resistant container.
—Do not take over-the-counter cough medicines, as many contain iodine.

PYRIDOXINE HYDROCHLORIDE (VITAMIN B_6) (Beesix, Hexa-Betalin, Hexacrest)

Patient objectives	*Teaching plan content*
1 State the name of the medication, the dose prescribed, and the ordered frequency of administration.	This information should be obtained from the patient's physician.
2 Explain the use of pyridoxine hydrochloride.	Pyridoxine hydrochloride is used to treat vitamin B_6 deficiency.
3 Identify potential side effects of pyridoxine hydrochloride.	Pyridoxine hydrochloride has the following side effects: —CNS: drowsiness, paresthesias (numbness and tingling in the extremities).
4 Discuss patient guidelines for taking pyridoxine hydrochloride.	The patient should follow these guidelines while taking pyridoxine hydrochloride: —Take the drug exactly as directed. —Avoid excessive protein intake, as it increases daily pyridoxine hydrochloride requirements. —Maintain a well-balanced diet. —Alert the physician if levodopa is being used, as pyridoxine hydrochloride should not be used with it.

QUINIDINE SULFATE (CinQuin, Quine, Quinidex Extentabs, Quinora, SK-Quinidine Sulfate)

Patient objectives	*Teaching plan content*
1 State the name of the medication, the dose prescribed, and the ordered frequency of administration.	This information should be obtained from the patient's physician.
2 Explain the use of quinidine sulfate.	Quinidine sulfate is used to regulate the rhythm of the heart.
3 Identify potential side effects of quinidine sulfate.	Quinidine sulfate has the following side effects: —Blood: hemolytic anemia, thrombocytopenia (decrease in the number of platelets), agranulocytosis (a symptom complex characterized by a decrease in granulocytes) —CNS: vertigo (dizziness), headache, light-headedness, confusion, restlessness, cold sweat, pallor, fainting —CV: premature ventricular contractions; severe hypotension; SA and AV block; ventricular fibrillation, tachycardia; aggravated congestive heart failure; EKG changes (particularly widening of QRS complex, notched P waves, widened Q-T interval, ST segment depression) —EENT: tinnitus (ringing in the ears), excessive salivation, blurred vision —GI: diarrhea, nausea, vomiting, anorexia, abdominal pains —Hepatic: hepatotoxicity including granulomatous hepatitis —Skin: rash, petechial hemorrhage of buccal mucosa, pruritus —Other: angioedema (facial edema), acute asthmatic attack, respiratory arrest, fever.
4 Discuss patient guidelines for taking quinidine sulfate.	The patient should follow these guidelines while taking quinidine sulfate: —Take the drug as directed. Never adjust the dose. —Use caffeine-containing beverages (such as cocoa, coffee, tea, and cola drinks) sparingly. —Store the drug in a tightly closed container, and protect it from light. —Because quinidine sulfate can sometimes cause stomach distress, take it with milk or food.

RANITIDINE (Zantac)

Patient objectives	*Teaching plan content*
1 State the name of the medication, the dose prescribed, and the ordered frequency of administration.	This information should be obtained from the patient's physician.
2 Explain the use of ranitidine.	Ranitidine is used to treat duodenal ulcers of hypersecretory conditions, such as Zollinger-Ellison syndrome, systemic mastocytosis, and multiple endocrine adenomas, because of its ability to decrease gastric acid secretion.
3 Identify potential side effects of ranitidine.	Ranitidine has the following side effects: —Blood: neutropenia (decrease in the number of neutrophils), thrombocytopenia (decrease in the number of platelets) —CNS: headache, malaise, dizziness —GI: nausea, constipation —Hepatic: increases in liver enzymes, jaundice —Skin: rash.
4 Discuss patient guidelines for taking ranitidine.	The patient should follow these guidelines while taking ranitidine: —Take the drug only as directed. Do not adjust the dose without first consulting the physician. —Avoid smoking, which impairs the effectiveness of ranitidine.

SODIUM POLYSTYRENE SULFONATE (Kayexalate)

Patient objectives	*Teaching plan content*
1 State the name of the medication, the dose prescribed, and the ordered frequency of administration.	This information should be obtained from the patient's physician.
2 Explain the use of Kayexalate.	Kayexalate is used to treat hyperkalemia; it exchanges sodium ions for potassium ions in the intestine, ultimately reducing serum potassium levels.

3 Identify the potential side effects of Kayexalate.	Kayexalate has the following side effects: —GI: constipation, fecal impaction (in elderly), anorexia, gastric irritation, nausea, vomiting, diarrhea (with sorbitol emulsions) —Other: hypokalemia, hypocalcemia, hypomagnesemia, sodium retention.
4 Discuss patient guidelines for taking Kayexalate.	The patient should follow these guidelines while taking Kayexalate: —Watch for other signs of hypokalemia: irritability, confusion, palpitations, severe muscle weakness and sometimes paralysis, and digitalis toxicity (anorexia, nausea, vomiting) in digitalized patients. —Do not heat resin. This will impair the drug's effectiveness. Mix resin only with water or sorbitol for P.O. administration. Above all, never mix with orange juice (high potassium content) to disguise taste. —Chill oral suspension for greater palatability. —If sorbitol is given, it may be mixed with resin suspension. —Consider the solid form. Resin cookie and candy recipes are available; perhaps the pharmacist or dietitian can supply them. —Watch for constipation in oral or nasogastric administration. Use sorbitol (10 to 20 ml of 70% syrup every 2 hours as needed) to produce one or two watery stools daily.

SPECTINOMYCIN DIHYDROCHLORIDE (Trobicin)

Patient objectives	*Teaching plan content*
1 State the name of the medication, the dose prescribed, and the ordered frequency of administration.	This information should be obtained from the patient's physician.
2 Explain the use of spectinomycin dihydrochloride.	Spectinomycin dihydrochloride is an antibiotic used to treat gonorrhea.
3 Identify potential side effects of spectinomycin dihydrochloride.	Spectinomycin dihydrochloride has the following side effects: —CNS: insomnia, dizziness —GI: nausea

	—GU: decreased urine output —Local: pain at injection site —Skin: urticaria (hives) —Other: fever, chills (may mask or delay symptoms of incubating syphilis).
4 Discuss patient guidelines for spectinomycin dihydrochloride administration.	The patient should follow these guidelines while spectinomycin dihydrochloride is being administered: —Be aware that a physician or nurse will administer this drug as an injection into the buttocks. If a large dose is prescribed, two injections, one in each buttock, will be given. —Return to the physician in 3 months for a blood test for syphilis. —Report any side effects to the physician.

SULFASALAZINE (Azulfidine, Azulfidine En-Tabs, SAS-500)

Patient objectives	*Teaching plan content*
1 State the name of the medication, the dose prescribed, and the ordered frequency of administration.	This information should be obtained from the patient's physician.
2 Explain the use of sulfasalazine.	Sulfasalazine is used to treat ulcerative colitis because of its antibacterial action.
3 Identify potential side effects of sulfasalazine.	Sulfasalazine has the following side effects: —Blood: agranulocytosis (a symptom complex characterized by a decrease in granulocytes), aplastic anemia, megaloblastic anemia, thrombocytopenia (decrease in number of platelets), leukopenia (decrease in number of white blood cells), hemolytic anemia —CNS: headache, mental depression, convulsions, hallucinations —GI: nausea, vomiting, diarrhea, abdominal pain, anorexia, stomatitis (inflammation of the mouth) —GU: toxic nephrosis with oliguria and anuria, crystalluria (uric acid crystals in urine), hematuria —Hepatic: jaundice, hepatotoxicity —Skin: Stevens-Johnson syndrome (erythema multiforme), generalized skin eruption, epidermal necrolysis, exfoliative dermatitis (inflammation of the skin accompanied by peeling), photosensitivity, urticaria (hives), pruritus (itching)

	—Other: hypersensitivity, serum sickness, drug fever, anaphylaxis, oligospermia (deficiency in the number of spermatozoa in the semen), infertility.
4 Discuss patient guidelines for taking sulfasalazine.	The patient should follow these guidelines while taking sulfasalazine: —Take the medication for as long as prescribed, even after symptoms are gone. —Avoid direct sunlight and ultraviolet light to prevent a photosensitivity reaction. —Be aware that urine may turn orange-yellow (a harmless side effect). —Take the drug after food intake, and space daily doses evenly to minimize GI discomfort.

SULFISOXAZOLE (Barazole, Gantrisin, G-Sox, J-Sul, Lipo Gantrisin, Novosoxazole, Rosoxol, Sosol, Soxa, Soxomide, Sulfagan, Urisoxin, Urizole, Velmatrol)

Patient objectives	*Teaching plan content*
1 State the name of the medication, the dose prescribed, and the ordered frequency of administration.	This information should be obtained from the patient's physician.
2 Explain the use of sulfisoxazole.	Sulfisoxazole is an antibiotic used to treat infections, particularly urinary tract infections.
3 Identify potential side effects of sulfisoxazole.	Sulfisoxazole has the following side effects: —Blood: agranulocytosis (a symptom complex characterized by a decrease in granulocytes), aplastic anemia, megaloblastic anemia, thrombocytopenia (decrease in number of platelets), leukopenia (decrease in number of white blood cells), hemolytic anemia —CNS: headache, mental depression, convulsions, hallucinations —GI: nausea, vomiting, diarrhea, abdominal pain, anorexia, stomatitis (inflammation of the mouth) —GU: toxic nephrosis with oliguria and anuria, crystalluria (uric acid crystals in urine), hematuria —Hepatic: jaundice —Skin: Stevens-Johnson syndrome (erythema multiforme), generalized skin eruption, epidermal necrolysis, exfoliative dermatitis, photosensitivity, urticaria (hives), pruritus (itching)

	—Other: hypersensitivity, serum sickness, drug fever, anaphylaxis.
4 Discuss patient guidelines for taking sulfisoxazole.	The patient should follow these guidelines while taking sulfisoxazole: —Take sulfisoxazole for as long as prescribed, even after symptoms are gone. —If a sore throat, fever, or pallor (pale skin color) develops, stop taking sulfisoxazole and notify the physician immediately. —Avoid direct sunlight and ultraviolet light to prevent a photosensitivity reaction. —Drink a full glass of water with each dose, and drink 3 to 4 qt (3 to 4 liters) of water throughout the day.

TERBUTALINE SULFATE (Brethine, Bricanyl)

Patient objectives	*Teaching plan content*
1 State the name of the medication, the dose prescribed, and the ordered frequency of administration.	This information should be obtained from the patient's physician.
2 Explain the use of terbutaline sulfate.	Terbutaline sulfate is used in respiratory disease to relax bronchial smooth muscle, thus enhancing breathing.
3 Identify potential side effects of terbutaline sulfate.	Terbutaline sulfate has the following side effects: —CNS: nervousness, tremors, headache, drowsiness, sweating —CV: palpitations, increased heart rate —GI: vomiting, nausea.
4 Discuss patient guidelines for taking terbutaline sulfate.	The patient should follow these guidelines while taking terbutaline sulfate: —Take the drug exactly as directed. —Be aware that tolerance may develop with prolonged use. —If the drug is to be administered subcutaneously at home, the patient should be taught how to give himself a subcutaneous injection. (See *How to Give Yourself a Subcutaneous Injection,* pp. 536-537.)

TETRACYCLINE (Achromycin, Novotetra, Sumycin)

Patient objectives	*Teaching plan content*
1 State the name of the medication, the dose prescribed, and the ordered frequency of administration.	This information should be obtained from the patient's physician.
2 Explain the use of tetracycline.	Tetracycline is an antibiotic used to treat a variety of infections.
3 Identify potential side effects of tetracycline.	Tetracycline has the following side effects: —Blood: neutropenia (decrease in the number of neutrophils), eosinophilia (increase in the number of eosinophils) —CNS: dizziness, headache, intracranial hypertension —CV: pericarditis —EENT: sore throat, glossitis (inflammation of the tongue), dysphagia (difficulty swallowing) —GI: anorexia, epigastric distress, nausea, vomiting, diarrhea, stomatitis (inflammation of the mouth), enterocolitis, inflammatory lesions in anogenital region —Hepatic: hepatotoxicity with doses given I.V. —Metabolic: increased BUN —Skin: maculopapular and erythematous rashes, urticaria (hives), photosensitivity, increased pigmentation —Local: irritation after I.M. injection, thrombophlebitis.
4 Discuss patient guidelines for taking tetracycline.	The patient should follow these guidelines while taking tetracycline: —Take the drug exactly as prescribed, even after symptoms are gone. —Take each dose on an empty stomach with a full glass of water at least 1 hour before meals or 2 hours afterward. Take the last dose of the day at least 1 hour before bedtime to prevent irritation of the esophagus. —Avoid direct sunlight and ultraviolet light. Use a sunscreen to help prevent photosensitivity. Be aware that photosensitivity persists for some time after discontinuing the drug. —Do not expose tetracycline to light or heat. —For diabetics: Because tetracycline may cause false-negative readings of Clinistix or Tes-Tape, use a different product to test urine sugar levels.

THEOPHYLLINE (Elixophyllin, Slo-Phyllin, Theo-Dur)

Patient objectives	*Teaching plan content*
1 State the name of the medication, the dose prescribed, and the ordered frequency of administration.	This information should be obtained from the patient's physician.
2 Explain the use of theophylline.	Theophylline is used to treat respiratory diseases, such as bronchial asthma, chronic bronchitis, and emphysema, because of its ability to relax smooth muscle in the respiratory tract, thus enhancing breathing.
3 Identify potential side effects of theophylline.	Theophylline has the following side effects: —CNS: restlessness, dizziness, headache, insomnia, light-headedness, convulsions —CV: palpitations, sinus tachycardia, extrasystoles, flushing, marked hypotension, increased respiratory rate —GI: nausea, vomiting, anorexia, bitter aftertaste, dyspepsia, heavy feeling in stomach, diarrhea —Skin: urticaria (hives).
4 Discuss patient guidelines for taking theophylline.	The patient should follow these guidelines while taking theophylline: —Take the drug exactly as directed. —Take the medication with a full glass of water after meals to avoid GI distress. —Avoid over-the-counter medications that contain ephedrine in combination with theophylline salts, because excessive nervous system stimulation may occur. —Be aware that dizziness may occur at the start of therapy.

THYROGLOBULIN (Proloid)

Patient objectives	*Teaching plan content*
1 State the name of the medication, dose prescribed, and ordered frequency of administration.	This information should be obtained from the patient's physician.
2 Explain the use of thyroglobulin.	Thyroglobulin is used to replace thyroid hormone in the treatment of hypothyroidism.

3 Identify potential side effects of thyroglobulin.	Thyroglobulin has the following side effects: —CNS: hyperirritability, nervousness, insomnia, twitching, tremors, headache —CV: increased cardiac output, tachycardia, cardiac dysrhythmias, angina pectoris, increased blood pressure, cardiac decompensation and collapse —GI: diarrhea, abdominal cramps, vomiting —Other: weight loss, heat intolerance, hyperhidrosis (excessive sweating), menstrual irregularities; in infants and children, accelerated rate of bone maturation.
4 Discuss patient guidelines for taking thyroglobulin.	The patient should follow these guidelines while taking thyroglobulin: —Take the drug only as directed. Do not adjust the dose or stop taking it without the physician's approval. —Take it at the same time each day (preferably in the morning) to maintain constant hormone levels. —Call the physician at once if chest pain, palpitations, difficulty breathing, sweating, or nervousness occurs. Also, report any unusual bleeding or bruising. —Be aware that this drug will alter thyroid function test results. —For children: Be aware that, during the first few months of therapy, temporary partial hair loss may occur.

THYROID U.S.P. (DESSICATED) (S-P-T, Thyrar, Thyro-Teric)

Patient objectives	*Teaching plan content*
1 State the name of the medication, the dose prescribed, and the ordered frequency of administration.	This information should be obtained from the patient's physician.
2 Explain the use of thyroid USP.	Thyroid USP is used to replace thyroid hormone in the treatment of hypothyroidism.
3 Identify potential side effects of thyroid USP.	Thyroid USP has the following side effects: —CNS: hyperirritability, nervousness, insomnia, twitching, tremors, headache —CV: increased cardiac output, tachycardia, cardiac dysrhythmias, angina pectoris, increased blood pressure, cardiac decompensation and collapse —GI: diarrhea, abdominal cramps, vomiting —Other: weight loss, heat intolerance, hyperhidrosis (excessive sweating), menstrual irregularities; accelerated rate of bone maturation in infants and children.

4 Discuss patient guidelines for taking thyroid USP.	The patient should follow these guidelines while taking thyroid USP: —Take the drug only as directed. Do not adjust the dose or stop taking it without the physician's approval. —Take it at the same time each day (preferably in the morning) to maintain constant hormone levels. —Call the physician at once if chest pain, palpitations, difficulty breathing, sweating, or nervousness occurs. Also, report any unusual bleeding or bruising. —Be aware that this drug will alter thyroid function test results. —For children: Be aware that, during the first few months of therapy, temporary partial hair loss may occur.

TIMOLOL (Blocadren)

Patient objectives	*Teaching plan content*
1 State the name of the medication, the dose prescribed, and the ordered frequency of administration.	This information should be obtained from the patient's physician.
2 Explain the use of timolol.	Timolol is used to treat hypertension because of its ability to lower blood pressure. It may also be used after the acute phase of myocardial infarction to provide long-term prophylaxis.
3 Identify potential side effects of timolol.	Timolol has the following side effects: —CNS: fatigue, lethargy, vivid dreams —CV: bradycardia, hypotension, congestive heart failure, peripheral vascular disease —GI: nausea, vomiting, diarrhea —Metabolic: hypoglycemia without tachycardia —Skin: rash —Other: increased airway resistance, fever.
4 Discuss patient guidelines for taking timolol.	The patient should follow these guidelines while taking timolol: —Take the drug exactly as prescribed, even after symptoms are gone. Do not adjust the dose without consulting the physician. —Be aware that abrupt discontinuation can precipitate chest pain (angina) and/or myocardial infarction. —For diabetics: Because this drug masks the common signs of hypoglycemia, discuss with the physician the need for blood glucose self-monitoring.

TOLAZAMIDE (Tolinase)

Patient objectives	*Teaching plan content*
1 State the name of the medication, the dose prescribed, and the ordered frequency of administration.	This information should be obtained from the patient's physician.
2 Explain the use of tolazamide.	Tolazamide is used to treat Type II diabetes (uncontrolled by diet alone) because of its ability to lower blood sugar levels by stimulating the release of insulin from the pancreas.
3 Identify potential side effects of tolazamide.	Tolazamide has the following side effects: —Blood: bone marrow aplasia (underdevelopment of the bone marrow) —GI: nausea, vomiting —Metabolic: hypoglycemia —Skin: rash, urticaria (hives), facial flushing —Other: hypersensitivity reactions.
4 Discuss patient guidelines for taking tolazamide.	The patient should follow these guidelines while taking tolazamide: —Take the drug only as directed. Do not adjust the dose or stop taking it without the physician's approval. —Maintain the diabetic diet, as ordered. This drug does not replace dietary means to control blood sugar levels. —Be aware that hypoglycemia may occur. (See the "Diabetes Mellitus" teaching plan in Chapter 5, Endocrine Disorders, for further instructions.) —Avoid moderate to large intake of alcohol, as unpleasant side effects may occur with tolazamide. —Do not take over-the-counter medications in conjunction with tolazamide without first consulting the physician.

TOLBUTAMIDE (Mobenol, Novobutamide, Orinase, SK-Tolbutamide, Tolbutone)

Patient objectives	*Teaching plan content*
1 State the name of the medication, the dose prescribed, and the ordered frequency of administration.	This information should be obtained from the patient's physician.

2 Explain the use of tolbutamide.	Tolbutamide is used to treat Type II diabetes (uncontrolled by diet alone) because of its ability to lower blood sugar levels by stimulating the release of insulin from the pancreas.
3 Identify potential side effects of tolbutamide.	Tolbutamide has the following side effects: —Blood: bone marrow aplasia (underdevelopment of bone marrow) —GI: nausea, heartburn —Metabolic: hypoglycemia —Skin: rash, pruritus (itching), facial flushing —Other: hypersensitivity reactions.
4 Discuss patient guidelines for taking tolbutamide.	The patient should follow these guidelines while taking tolbutamide: —Take the drug only as directed. Do not adjust the dose or stop taking it without the physician's approval. —Maintain the diabetic diet, as ordered. This drug does not replace dietary means to control blood sugar levels. —Be aware that hypoglycemia may occur. (See the "Diabetes Mellitus" teaching plan in Chapter 5, Endocrine Disorders, for further instructions.) —Avoid moderate to large intake of alcohol, as unpleasant side effects may occur with tolbutamide. —Do not take over-the-counter medications in conjunction with tolbutamide without first consulting the physician.

TRIHEXYPHENIDYL HYDROCHLORIDE (Aparkane, Artane, Hexaphen, Novohexidyl, T.H.P., Trihexane, Trihexidyl)

Patient objectives	*Teaching plan content*
1 State the name of the medication, the dose prescribed, and the ordered frequency of administration.	This information should be obtained from the patient's physician.
2 Explain the use of trihexyphenidyl hydrochloride.	Trihexyphenidyl hydrochloride is used to reduce the rigidity, tremor, sluggish movement, and gait disturbances of Parkinson's disease.
3 Identify potential side effects of trihexyphenidyl hydrochloride.	Trihexyphenidyl hydrochloride has the following side effects: —CNS: nervousness, dizziness, headache, restlessness, agitation, hallucinations, euphoria, delusions, amnesia —CV: tachycardia

	—EENT: blurred vision, mydriasis (dilation of the pupil), increased intraocular pressure —GI: constipation, dry mouth, nausea —GU: urinary hesitancy or retention. Side effects are dose-related.
4 Discuss patient guidelines for taking trihexyphenidyl hydrochloride.	The patient should follow these guidelines while taking trihexyphenidyl hydrochloride: —Take the drug only as directed. Do not adjust the dose without the physician's approval. —Avoid activities that require alertness until the nervous system response is known. —Do not take the drug on an empty stomach; it causes nausea if taken before meals. —Relieve mouth dryness with cool drinks, ice chips, or sugarless gum or candy. —Report urinary hesitancy or retention immediately to the physician.

VERAPAMIL (Calan, Isoptin)

Patient objectives	*Teaching plan content*
1 State the name of the medication, dose prescribed, and ordered frequency of administration.	This information should be obtained from the patient's physician.
2 Explain the use of verapamil.	Verapamil reduces the oxygen demand of the heart and is used to manage angina pectoris. It is also used to regulate the rhythm of the heart.
3 Identify potential side effects of verapamil.	Verapamil has the following side effects: —CNS: dizziness, headache, fatigue —CV: transient hypotension, heart failure, bradycardia, AV block, ventricular asystole, peripheral edema —GI: constipation, nausea —Hepatic: elevated liver enzymes.
4 Discuss patient guidelines for taking verapamil.	The patient should follow these guidelines while taking verapamil: —Take the drug only as directed. Do not abruptly stop taking it or adjust the dose without the specific recommendation of the physician. —Notify the physician if swelling of the hands or feet or shortness of breath occurs. —Continue to take sublingual nitroglycerin, as ordered, when angina symptoms are acute.

WARFARIN SODIUM (Coufarin, Coumadin, Panwarfin, Warfilone Sodium, Warnerin)

Patient objectives	*Teaching plan content*
1 State the name of the medication, the dose prescribed, and the ordered frequency of administration.	This information should be obtained from the patient's physician.
2 Explain the use of warfarin sodium.	Warfarin sodium is a blood thinner that reduces the ability of blood to clot by acting on the liver to inhibit vitamin K–dependent production of several clotting factors.
3 Identify potential side effects of warfarin sodium.	Warfarin sodium has the following side effects: —Blood: hemorrhage with excessive dosage, leukopenia (decrease in white blood cells) —GI: paralytic ileus, intestinal obstruction (both resulting from hemorrhage), diarrhea, vomiting, cramps, nausea —GU: excessive uterine bleeding —Skin: dermatitis, urticaria (hives), rash, necrosis, alopecia (hair loss) —Other: fever.
4 Discuss patient guidelines for taking warfarin sodium.	The patient should follow these guidelines while taking warfarin sodium: —Always take warfarin sodium at the same time of day. Take it only as prescribed. Never skip a dose or take extra doses without first checking with the physician. —Carry a personal I.D. card that includes the following: a statement that an anticoagulant is being used, the name of the anticoagulant, the dose, and the frequency of administration. —Do not take any other drugs, including nonprescription drugs, without first asking the physician. —See the physician on a regular schedule, as periodic blood tests need to be performed to ensure safe dosage and proper control of the clotting factors. —Avoid eating larger-than-normal amounts of leafy green vegetables, because they contain vitamin K and, in large amounts, may decrease the effectiveness of the drug. —Use alcohol sparingly, because it can either increase or decrease the effect of this drug. —Avoid over-the-counter products containing aspirin or other salicylates, because they may interact with warfarin sodium and cause bleeding. —Use an electric razor when shaving to avoid scratching the skin, and brush teeth with a soft toothbrush.

Patient-Teaching Aid

HOW TO USE LYPRESSIN NASAL SPRAY

Dear Patient:
Frequent urination and thirst are signs of diabetes insipidus. Your physician has prescribed lypressin, a nasal spray that treats this condition.

You may regulate the dosage according to your needs. Spray the medication as directed in one or both nostrils. Take an extra dose at bedtime if you are urinating frequently at night. If the usual dosage is inadequate, use the medication more often; do not increase the number of sprays each time you use it.

Here is how to spray the medication most effectively:

1

Before you begin, read the medication label carefully, so you know the exact amount of medication to administer. Make sure you have tissues handy. Then, sit upright, with your head tilted back.

2

Now, place the tip of the squeeze bottle about ½″ (1 cm) inside your nostril. Point it straight up your nose, toward the inner corner of your eye. Do not angle the squeeze bottle downward, or the medication will run down your throat.

Without inhaling, squeeze the bottle once, quickly and firmly. Use just enough force to coat the inside of your nose with medication. Too much force may send the medicine into your sinuses and give you a headache. Then spray again if the instructions on the label order it. Repeat the procedure in the other nostril.

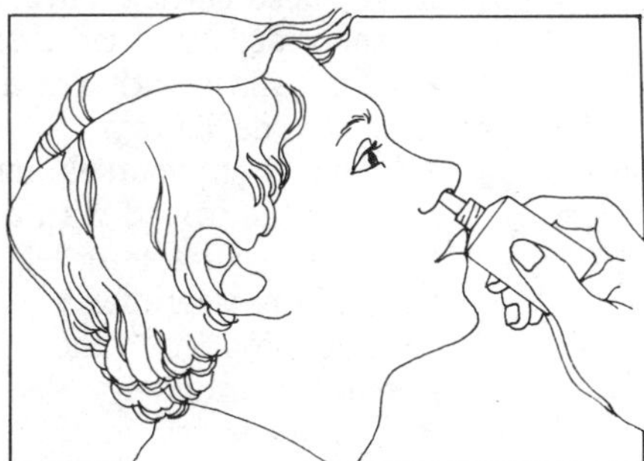

3

Keep your head tilted back for several minutes, so the medication has time to work. Avoid blowing your nose while you wait.

Patient-Teaching Aid

TAKING ANTICOAGULANT MEDICATION

Dear Patient:
The physician has ordered that you take a medication called ____________. This medication affects your blood's clotting mechanisms to keep clots from forming inside your blood vessels. Take it ________ times a day. While you are taking this medication, you may experience such side effects as:

____

____.

Because this medication reduces your blood's ability to clot, you must take special precautions to keep from bruising or cutting yourself. Also, you must be careful to avoid a bad reaction from combining this medication with other medications. To avoid any such problems, be sure to follow these guidelines:

- Wear a Medic Alert bracelet with the information that you are taking anticoagulants stamped on it.
- Take your medication at the same time each day, as prescribed.
- Keep all appointments for blood tests. You may have blood taken at home by a visiting nurse or at the hospital by laboratory personnel.
- Increase or decrease your medication only as directed by the physician.
- Prevent getting bruised by placing furniture out of pathways and by putting a rubber bath mat and safety rails in your bathtub.
- Never walk barefoot.
- Do not cut your toenails unless they grow very long. If they need cutting, have a family member, visiting nurse, or podiatrist cut them.
- Do not shave with a straight razor. Use an electric razor or a depilatory.
- If you do cut yourself, immediately apply pressure directly to the wound with a clean, dry dressing or cloth. If you cut your arm or leg, elevate it above heart level. Maintain pressure for 5 to 10 minutes. If the bleeding does not stop, go to the emergency department of a hospital immediately.
- If you have any dental work done, tell your dentist that you are taking an anticoagulant.
- Always check with your physician before taking any new medication. Other medications might react badly with your anticoagulant medication.
- Never take aspirin or over-the-counter preparations that contain aspirin. Read all labels carefully.

TAKING ANTICOAGULANT MEDICATION—*continued*

• Avoid alcoholic beverages. They may alter your blood clotting time. Because the effect varies from patient to patient, ask your physician for specific advice.

In addition, immediately report any of the following signs or symptoms to your physician:

• nosebleeds
• coughing up red to black mucus
• bruises that persist longer than usual or that increase in size
• bleeding gums
• blood in your urine or stool (which may be bright red or tarry)
• weariness
• dizziness, faintness
• anxiety and apprehension
• irritability
• confusion.

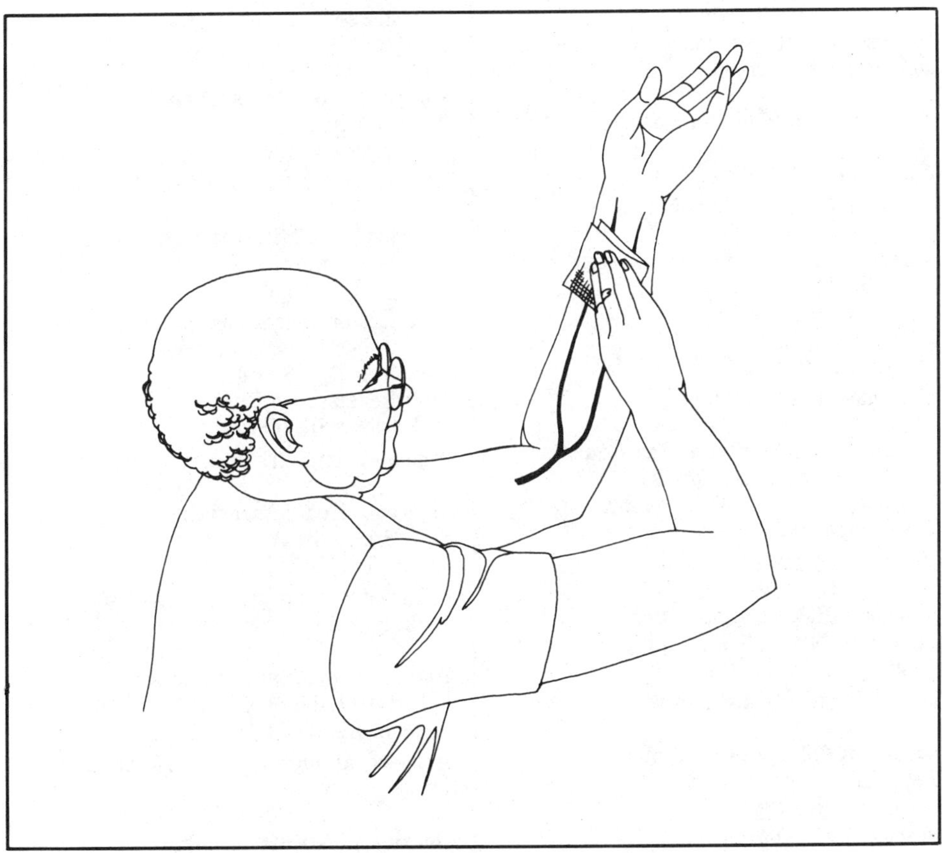

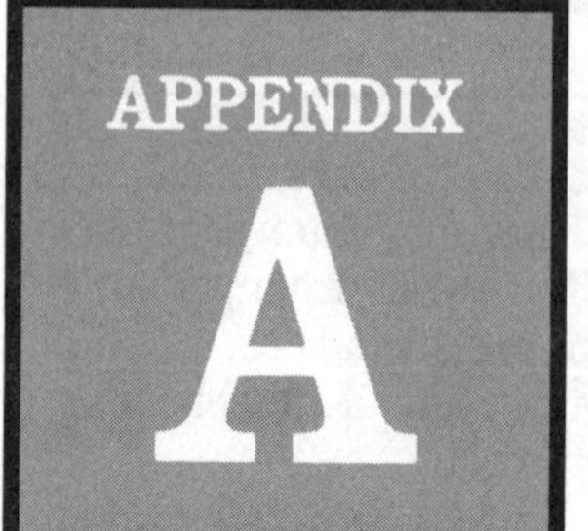

APPENDIX A Educational Resources

The following educational resources have been compiled for the use of both the health care professional and the patient. Some materials may be provided free; others may involve a charge. Inclusion in this list does not necessarily constitute the publisher's endorsement of any of the materials or organizations.

A

Abbott Laboratories
Scientificom Distribution Center
14th St. and Sarian
North Chicago, Ill. 60064
Multimedia on hypertension, gynecology, and weight control

Action on Smoking and Health
2013 H St.
Washington, D.C. 20006
Printed materials on smoking

American Association for Maternal and Child Health
c/o Harold J. Fishbein
233 Prospect, P-204
La Jolla, Calif. 92037
Materials on gynecology

American Association of Sex Educators, Counselors, and Therapists
11 Dupont Circle, N.W., Suite 220
Washington, D.C. 20036
Materials on sex education

American Bakers Association
1111 14th Street, N.W., Suite 300
Washington, D.C. 20005
Materials on nutrition and weight control

American College of Cardiology
9111 Old Georgetown Rd.
Bethesda, Md. 20814
Professional materials only

American College of Obstetrics and Gynecology
600 Maryland Ave., S.W., Suite 300
Washington, D.C. 20024
Pamphlets on cancer, obstetrics, and gynecology

American Diabetes Association
Two Park Ave.
New York, N.Y. 10016
Information on diabetic teaching

American Dry Milk Institute
130 North Franklin St.
Chicago, Ill. 60606
Materials on weight control and nutrition

American Egg Board
1460 Renaissance Dr.
Park Ridge, Ill. 60068
Pamphlets on nutrition and weight control

American Heart Association
7320 Greenville Ave.
Dallas, Tex. 75231
Multimedia on stroke, arteriosclerosis, smoking, rubella, diet, and heart problems

American Hospital Association
840 North Lake Shore Dr.
Chicago, Ill. 60611
Professional multimedia for patient education

American Institute of Baking
Consumer Service Department

1213 Bakers Way
Manhattan, Kan. 66502
Printed materials on nutrition and weight control

American Lung Association
1740 Broadway
New York, N.Y. 10019
Audiovisual and printed material on lung diseases, smoking, and air pollution

American Meat Institute
Department of Public Relations
P.O. Box 3556
Washington, D.C. 20007
Pamphlets on nutrition and weight control

American Medical Association
535 North Dearborn St.
Chicago, Ill. 60610
Pamphlets, posters, and teaching kits on multiple health topics

American Nurses' Association
2420 Pershing Rd.
Kansas City, Mo. 64108
Publications for the nurse on patient education

American Physical Therapy Association
1111 N. Fairfax St.
Alexandria, Va. 22314
Materials on rehabilitation

American Public Health Association
1015 15th St., N.W.
Washington, D.C. 20005
Educational materials for health workers

American Red Cross
17th and D Sts., N.W.
Washington, D.C. 20006
Materials on health and safety

American Social Health Association
260 Sheridan Ave., Suite 307
Palo Alto, Calif. 94306
Information on venereal disease and drug abuse

Ames Company
Division of Miles Laboratories, Inc.
1127 Myrtle St.
Elkhart, Ind. 46514
Multimedia on diabetes

Armour International Company
Consumer Services Department
Greyhound Towers
Phoenix, Ariz. 85077
Pamphlets on nutrition and weight control

Association for the Advancement of Health Education
1900 Association Dr.
Reston, Va. 22091
Materials on nutrition and weight control

Asthma & Allergy Foundation of America
1302 18th St., N.W., Suite 303
Washington, D.C. 20036
Information on respiratory diseases

Asthma Information
Cooper Laboratories, Inc.
110 East Hanover Ave.
Cedar Knolls, N.J. 07927
Information on respiratory diseases

Ayerst Laboratories
(Division of American Home Products Corporation)
685 Third Ave.
New York, N.Y. 10017
Materials on gynecology

B

Becton, Dickinson and Company
Mack Centre Dr.
Paramus, N.J. 07652
"Getting Started" Program on diabetes

Beecham-Massengill
Division of Beecham, Inc.
501 Fifth St.
Bristol, Tenn. 37620
Pamphlets on gynecology

Best Foods
(Division of CPC International, Inc.)
Consumer Service Department
International Plaza
Englewood Cliffs, N.J. 07632
Multimedia on nutrition and weight control

Boehringer Ingleheim Ltd.
90 East Ridge
Ridgefield, Conn. 06877
Materials on hypertension

Borden Chemical Division
Marketing Services
180 East Broad St.
Columbus, Ohio 43215
Materials on nutrition and weight control

Bristol Laboratories
(Division of Bristol-Myers Company)
Thompson Road, P.O. Box 657
Syracuse, N.Y. 13201
Materials on hypertension

C

California Prune Advisory Board
103 World Trade Center
San Francisco, Calif. 94111
Information on nutrition and weight control

Campbell Soup Company
Food Service Products Division
Campbell Place
Camden, N.J. 08101
Multimedia on nutrition and weight control

Carnation Company
Medical Marketing Department
5045 Wilshire Blvd.
Los Angeles, Calif. 90036
Information on nutrition and weight control

Centers for Disease Control
Bureau of Health Education
1600 Clifton Road, N.E.
Atlanta, Ga. 30033
Information on accident prevention and disease control

The Children's Hospital
700 Children's Dr.
Columbus, Ohio 43205
Pamphlets on diabetes

Children's Hospital of Los Angeles
4650 Sunset Blvd.
Los Angeles, Calif. 90054
Audiovisual material on hypertension

Ciba-Geigy Corporation
556 Morris Ave.
Summit, N.J. 07901
Multimedia on hypertension

Consumer and Foods Economic Institute
Room 325-A, Federal Building
Hyattsville, Md. 20782
Materials on nutrition

Consumers Union of the United States
256 Washington St.
Mount Vernon, N.Y. 10550
Materials on home health, dental care, and breast cancer

Core Communications in Health, Inc.
1916-38 Park Ave.
New York, N.Y. 10037
Multimedia on most medical-surgical problems

D

Davol, Incorporated
100 Sockanosset Crossroads
Cranston, R.I. 02920
Multimedia on ostomies

Del Monte Corporation
One Market Plaza
San Francisco, Calif. 94105
Information on nutrition

Department of Agriculture
Office of Information
14th St. and Independence Ave.
Washington, D.C. 20250
Materials on nutrition and farm safety

Diabetes and Arthritis Program
Building 10, Room 9N-222
Bethesda, Md. 20205
Materials on diabetes

Diabetes Education Center
4959 Escelsior Blvd.
Minneapolis, Minn. 55416
Multimedia on nutrition and weight control in diabetes

Division of Long-Term Care
Health Standards and Quality Bureau
Dogwood East Building
1849 Gwynn Oak Ave.
Baltimore, Md. 21207
General health information

Dorsey Laboratories
Division of Sandoz, Inc.
Post Office Box 83288
Lincoln, Neb. 68501
Information on respiratory diseases

E

Educational Television Department
Auburn University
Auburn, Ala. 36830
Materials on hypertension

Epilepsy Foundation of America
4351 Garden City Dr.
Landover, Md. 20785
Multimedia on epilepsy

Equitable Life Assurance Society of the United States
1285 Avenue of the Americas
New York, N.Y. 10019
Materials on nutrition and weight control

F

Fleischmann's Margarine
Division of Nabisco Brands, Inc.
Nabisco Brands Plaza
Parsippany, N.J. 07054
Pamphlets on heart disease and nutrition

Food and Agriculture Organizations of the United States
North American Regional Office
1776 F St., N.W.
Washington, D.C. 20437
Printed materials on nutrition and weight control

Food Council of America
1750 Pennsylvania Ave., N.W.
Washington, D.C. 20005
Materials on nutrition

Food and Drug Administration
Parklawn Building, 5600 Fishers Lane
Rockville, Md. 20857
Materials on safety

Food and Nutrition Information and Educational Materials Center
National Agricultural Library
Beltsville, Md. 20705
Printed materials on nutrition and weight control

G

General Foods Corporation
Consumer Service Department
250 North St.
White Plains, N.Y. 10625
Materials on nutrition

Green Giant Company
Home Services Department
200 S. 6th St.
Minneapolis, Minn. 55402
Information on nutrition

John F. Greer Company
530 East Twelfth St.
Oakland, Calif. 94606
Information on ostomies

H

Health Films Library
One West Wilson St., P.O. Box 309
Madison, Wis. 53701
Multimedia on cancer

Health Insurance Institute
1850 K St.
Washington, D.C. 20006
General health information

H.J. Heinz Co.
Consumer Relations
600 Grant St.
Pittsburgh, Pa. 15230
Pamphlets on nutrition

Hollister, Incorporated
2000 Hollister Dr.
Libertyville, Ill. 60048
Materials on ostomies

I

Institute of Allergy and Infectious Diseases
9000 Rockville Pike
Bethesda, Md. 20205
Materials on respiratory disease

Institutes for the Achievement of Human Potential
8801 Stenton Ave.
Philadelphia, Pa. 19118
Information on brain injury

International Apple Institute
Public Relations
P.O. Box 1137
6707 Old Dominion Dr.
McLean, Va. 22101
Information on nutrition

International Society of Endocrinology
9650 Rockville Pike
Bethesda, Md. 20014
Materials on endocrine disorders

K

Kaiser Permanente Health Center Audiovisual Workshop
280 West McCarther Blvd.
Oakland, Calif. 94611
Multimedia on arthritis, obstetrics, and gynecology

Kellogg Company
Department of Home Economic Services
235 Proter St.
Battle Creek, Mich. 49016
Materials on nutrition

Knox Gelatin, Incorporated
(Subsidiary of Thomas J. Lipton, Inc.)
800 Sylvan Ave.
Englewood Cliffs, N.J. 07632
Information on nutrition

Kraft Foods
Kraft Court
Glenview, Ill. 60025
Information on nutrition

L

Lawren Productions, Inc.
P.O. Box 1452
Burlingame, Calif. 94010
Multimedia on hypertension

Eli Lilly and Company
307 East McCarty St., P.O. Box 618
Indianapolis, Ind. 46285
Materials on diabetes

M

Martland Hospital Health Education Project
College of Medicine and Dentistry of New Jersey
100 Bergen St.
Newark, N.J. 07102
Audiovisual materials on health subjects

Mead Johnson Pharmaceutical Division
Division of Mead Johnson and Company
2400 West Pennsylvania St.
Evansville, Ind. 47721
Material on gynecology, respiratory diseases, nutrition, and weight control

Medfact, Incorporated
1112 Andrew, N.E.
Massilon, Ohio 44645
Multimedia on respiratory diseases, stroke, diabetes, heart disease, hypertension, and gynecology

Medic-Alert Foundation, International
1000 North Palm
Turlock, Calif. 95380
Medical identification

Merck Sharp & Dohme
(Division of Merck and Company, Inc.)
West Point, Pa. 19486
Pamphlets on nutrition and weight control

Mercy Medical Center
Patient Education Division
Mercy Drive
Dubuque, Iowa 52001
Audiovisuals on diabetes

Metropolitan Life Insurance Company
Health and Welfare Division
One Madison Ave.
New York, N.Y. 10010
Multimedia on hypertension

N

Nabisco Brands, Inc.
Nabisco Brands Plaza
Parsippany, N.J. 07054
Materials on nutrition

National Academy of Sciences
National Research Council, Food and Nutrition Board
2101 Constitution Ave., N.W.
Washington, D.C. 20418
Materials on nutrition and weight control

National Association of the Deaf
814 Thayer Ave.
Silver Spring, Md. 20910
Materials on hearing and hearing loss

National Council on the Aging
600 Maryland Ave., S.W.
Washington, D.C. 20024
Professional materials on the elderly

National Dairy Council
6300 North River Rd.
Rosemont, Ill. 60018
Materials on heart disease, nutrition, and weight control

National Heart, Lung, and Blood Institute
National Institutes of Health
Building 31, Room 5A52
Bethesda, Md. 20205
Multimedia on heart disease, hypertension, and stroke

National High Blood Pressure Education Program
Information Center
120-80 National Institutes of Health
Bethesda, Md. 20014
Information on hypertension

National Institute of Neurological and Communicative Disorders and Stroke
9000 Rockville Pike
Bethesda, Md. 20205
Pamphlets on stroke

National Interagency Council on Smoking and Health
American Cancer Society
90 Park Ave.
New York, N.Y. 10016
Pamphlets on smoking

National Kidney Foundation
Two Park Ave.
New York, N.Y. 10016
Printed material on kidney disease and organ-donor programs

National League for Nursing
Ten Columbus Circle
New York, N.Y. 10019
Information for the nurse on patient education

National Parkinson Foundation
1501 N.W. Ninth Ave.
Miami, Fla. 33136
Information on Parkinson's disease

National Retired Teachers Association
(Division of AARP)
1909 K St., N.W.
Washington, D.C. 20049
Multimedia on chronic diseases

National Society for Medical Research
1029 Vermont Ave., N.W., Suite 700
Washington, D.C. 20005
Materials on heart disease

Nutrition Foundation
888 17th St., N.W.
Washington, D.C. 20006
Materials on nutrition and weight control

Nutrition Section, Office of Clinical Services
Bureau of Community Health Services
5600 Fishers Lane
Rockville, Md. 20857
Printed materials on weight control and nutrition

O

Office of Consumer Affairs
621 Reporters Building
300 Seventh Ave., S.W.
Washington, D.C. 20201
General health information

Ortho Pharmaceutical Corporation
Route 202
Raritan, N.J. 08869
Materials on gynecology

P

Parkinson's Disease Foundation
William Black Medical Research Building
Columbia Presbyterian Medical Center
640 West 168th St.
New York N.Y. 10032
Information on Parkinson's disease

Pennwalt Pharmaceutical Division
Pennwalt Corporation
P.O. Box 1212
Rochester, N.Y. 14603
Materials on nutrition and weight control

Pet Incorporated
Office of Consumer Affairs
400 South Fourth St.
St. Louis, Mo. 63102
Pamphlets on nutrition

Pfizer Laboratories
(Division, Pfizer Inc.)
235 East 42nd St.
New York, N.Y. 10017
Materials on diabetes

Pharmaceutical Manufacturers Association
1155 Fifteenth St., N.W.
Washington, D.C. 20005
Materials on drugs from member drug companies

Pritchett and Hull
2122 Faulkner, N.E.
Atlanta, Ga. 30324
Multimedia on diabetes, respiratory diseases, and heart disease

Professional Research, Inc.
12960 Coral Tree Pl.
Los Angeles, Calif. 90066
Multimedia on stroke, hypertension, heart disease, and gynecology

The Prudential Insurance Company of America
P.O. Box 388
Fort Washington, Pa. 19034
Materials on weight control

Public Affairs Committee Film Library
381 Park Ave., South
New York, N.Y. 10016
Films and slides on diabetes

Public Health Service
200 Independence Ave., S.W.
Washington, D.C. 20201
Materials on general health

The Public Television Library
475 L'Enfant Plaza, S.W.
Washington, D.C. 20024
Videotaped materials on health

Q

Quaker Oats Company
Consumer Services
Merchandise Mart Plaza
Chicago, Ill. 60654
Pamphlets on nutrition

Quaker Oats Company
SVC Division
Home Economics Department
6815 E. 34th St.
Indianapolis, Ind. 46226
Information on nutrition

R

Ralston Purina Company
Nutrition Service
Checkerboard Square
St. Louis, Mo. 63164
Information on nutrition

Research Media, Inc.
14 Story St.
Cambridge, Mass. 02138
Multimedia on heart disease

Rice Council
9317 Richmond Ave., P.O. Box 22802
Houston, Tex. 77027
Information on nutrition

Riker Laboratories, Inc.
(Subsidiary of 3M Company)
19901 Nordhoff St.
Northridge, Calif. 91324
Materials on respiratory diseases

Roche Laboratories
(Division of Hoffman-La Roche Inc.)
340 Kingsland St.
Nutley, N.J. 07110
Materials on nutrition and weight control

S

Sister Kenny Institute
800 E. 28th St. at Chicago Ave.
Minneapolis, Minn. 55407
Multimedia on ostomies

Smith Kline and French Laboratories
(Division of SmithKline Beckman Corporation)
1500 Spring Garden St.
Box 7929
Philadelphia, Pa. 19101
Information on hypertension

Society for Nutrition Education
1736 Franklin St.
Oakland, Calif. 94612
Materials on food, pregnancy and nutrition, diets, and weight control

Squibb Corporation
P.O. Box 4000
Princeton, N.J. 08540
Materials on ostomies and diabetes

Albert Steiner Memorial Lung Clinic
Saint Joseph's Infirmary
56665 Peachtree Dunwoody
Atlanta, Ga. 30342
Information on respiratory diseases

Sunkist Growers, Inc.
Consumer Services
P.O. Box 7888
Van Nuys, Calif. 91409
Materials on nutrition

Swift and Company
Public Relations Department
1919 Swift Dr.
Oak Brook, Ill. 60521
Materials on nutrition

Syntex Laboratories
1344 Elmwood Ave.
Wilmette, Ill. 60091
Materials on nutrition and weight control

T

The Trainex Corporation
12601 Industry St., P.O. Box 116
Garden Grove, Calif. 92641
Multimedia on heart disease, hypertension, diabetes, respiratory disease, and ostomies

U

United Fresh Fruit and Vegetable Association
727 North Washington St.
Alexandria, Va. 22314
Information on nutrition

United Ostomy Association
2001 W. Beverly Blvd.
Los Angeles, Calif. 90057
Printed materials on ostomies

United States Pharmacopeial Convention, Inc.
Publication Department
12601 Twinbrook Pkwy.
Rockville, Md. 20852
Patient information on drugs and drug therapy; also professional patient-education materials

University of Illinois Medical Center
Public Information Office
840 S. Wood St.
Chicago, Ill. 60612
Videotapes on health information

University of Kansas
College of Health Sciences and Hospital
39th and Rainbow Sts.
Kansas City, Kan. 66103
Videotapes on health topics

University of North Carolina at Chapel Hill
Institute of Nutrition
Allied Health Sciences Building
311 Pittsboro St., 256-H
Chapel Hill, N.C. 27514
Multimedia on nutrition and weight control

University of Toronto
Division of Instructional Media Services
Eight Taddlecreek Rd.
Toronto, Ontario, Canada M5S-1A8
Videotapes on health topics

Upjohn Company
7000 Portage Rd.
Kalamazoo, Mich. 49001
Multimedia on diabetes, nutrition, weight control, and preventive medicine

V

Vidcom
4470 Chamblee-Dunwoody Rd.
Atlanta, Ga. 30338
Materials on respiratory disease

Video Communication, Inc.
Suite 904, Watergate Office Building
2600 Virginia Avenue, N.W.
Washington, D.C. 20037
Materials on hypertension

Vitamin Information Bureau, Inc.
383 Madison Ave.
New York, N.Y. 10017
Multimedia on nutrition and weight control

W

Warner Chilcott Laboratories
(Division Parke-Davis)
201 Tabor Rd.
Morris Plains, N.J. 07950
Information on heart disease

Wheat Flour Institute
Home Economics Department
1776 F St., N.W.
Washington, D.C. 20006
Materials on nutrition

Wyeth Laboratories
(Division of American Home Products Corporation)
P.O. Box 8299
Philadelphia, Pa. 19101
Information on gynecology

APPENDIX

B Preoperative & Postoperative Teaching

PREOPERATIVE TEACHING

Before any type of surgery or invasive procedure is performed, a patient must be informed of the nature of the procedure, its risks and benefits, what is expected of him before and after the procedure, and any options he might have. In most cases, a permit must be signed by the patient before the procedure is performed. This legal document is the responsibility of the physician; the nurse's responsibility is to teach the patient what he needs to know in order to make informed choices concerning the proposed procedure(s).

Prior to initiating teaching with the patient, it is helpful if the nurse contacts the physician to find out what procedure is planned and what special modifications, if any, will be made (for example, the use of a local versus a general anesthetic). When the nurse approaches the patient, she should begin by asking him what procedure the physician told him would be performed. His answer may reveal inaccuracies in his understanding or at least give her an idea of where to begin her teaching.

One of the roles of nurses is to encourage patients to be their own health care advocates and to question health care providers about the care being received. The nurse can encourage a patient to seek answers to his questions from physicians and nurses; to seek a second opinion, if he so desires; and to obtain the information necessary for him to make informed decisions concerning appropriate treatment.

Preoperative teaching includes both physical *and* psychological preparation. In addition to being taught about his specific treatment, a patient must be given the time and the media to express himself. He should be provided with paper and pencil to write down his questions, thoughts, or concerns and encouraged to express his fears and hopes about the procedure. Only misperceptions should be corrected.

Preoperative teaching includes information about what will happen before, during, and after the procedure. Communicating this information can be accomplished by discussion, demonstration, the use of pictures, or even having the patient talk to another patient who had the same procedure. Topics to be discussed include the following:

Topic	*Considerations*
1 **Preoperative medications**	—When will medication(s) be given, and by what route? —What is the purpose of the medication(s), and what restrictions will be placed on the patient after administration?
2 **Nutrition restrictions**	—Will the patient be NPO; if so, starting when? —May the patient have water?
3 **Preoperative treatments**	—GI (enemas or special mixtures to clean out the system): How much time and inconvenience will be involved in bowel evacuation? How much discomfort will be involved? Why is it necessary? —Skin preparation: What is the rationale for this? Where will it be performed, when, by whom, and what will it entail? How much of the body will be prepped? Is a shower required? —Starting an I.V.: When will this be done and by whom? How long will the I.V. be necessary? How often might it have to be changed? —Insertion of a urinary catheter: When will this be done and by whom? How much discomfort will be involved? How long will the catheter remain in place?
4 **Anesthesia**	—What kind of anesthetic will the patient get? How does it work? What precautions will be taken before and after its administration? Will he be awake for the procedure? Will he feel anything?
5 **Room change**	—If the patient will be recovering in a special room, such as an ICU, inform him of this, and, if possible, take him to see the unit before the procedure. Make sure he is aware of the routine noises and sights in that unit.

6 Preparation for postoperative treatment

—This is the time to prepare the patient for the skills he will be required to use after the surgical procedure. The patient should be taught the use of incentive spirometry, deep breathing, and supported coughing (chest splinting) as well as how to turn in bed or use a trapeze while he is free of pain.

—Also, prepare the patient at this time for the various routine tasks that will be performed and the equipment (such as tubes) that will be present after the procedure so that he will know that they are normal; for example, frequent monitoring of vital signs, function and nursing responsibility for various tubes and catheters, I.V.'s, and dietary restrictions. Include a discussion of the various consequences of the procedure that may be expected, such as bloody urine.

7 Personal business and psychological support

—Some patients need to write a will or discuss with you what they would like to happen "just in case something goes wrong." Listen without being judgmental, and then bring the discussion back to their preparation for the procedure.

—Assure the patient that he will not be alone before or during the procedure. Also assure him that his privacy will be respected and that he will be covered except for the operative site.

8 Significant others

—Can significant others stay at the hospital the night before the procedure? Can they visit the morning before the procedure? Can they accompany the patient to the procedure site? Where can they wait while the procedure is in progress, and will the physician come to talk to them immediately after the procedure? How can they assist in the preoperative and postoperative management of their loved one?

9 Valuables

—Discuss arrangements for valuables and/or prostheses. Does the patient understand why prostheses must be removed?

10 Hospital dress code for procedures

—Can nail polish be worn? Does the patient need to wear a hospital gown and/or surgical hat, and why?

11 Transportation

—How will the patient get to the procedure? Does he have a choice?

POSTOPERATIVE TEACHING

Because patients are often uncomfortable immediately after surgery, postoperative teaching should be short and to the point. Because of the anesthetic and medications in the patient's system, teaching may need to be repeated and reinforced many times. Teaching should include the following:

Topic	*Considerations*
1 Termination of the test or procedure	—Explain to the patient that the test or procedure is over. This may have to be repeated as the patient awakens.
2 Pain medication	—Explain the availability of pain medication, if applicable, and how often it can be administered. Develop a scale for measuring pain, such as 1 = mild pain and 10 = severe pain. This gives the patient some control in assessing his pain and determining his need for pain medication.
3 Reinforcement of information	—Once the physician has informed the patient what was done and the results of the procedure, the nurse should ensure that the patient understands what was done and its implications.
4 Psychological support	—The patient may project anger toward the health care providers for the pain, disfigurement, and grieving that he has gone through. This release is important for the patient's mental health, and the nurse can incorporate measures to enhance its expression in her nursing plan.

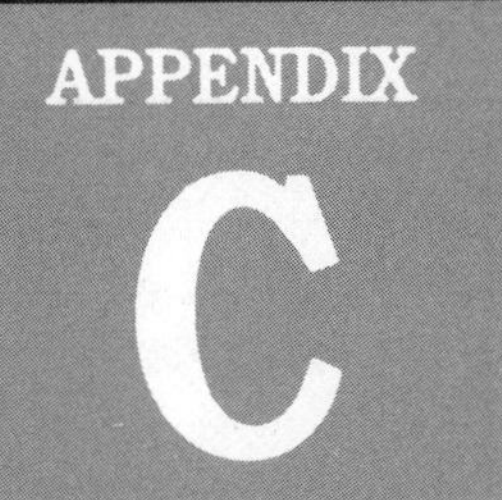

Patient Checklist Chart

This Patient-Teaching Checklist will assist you in your role as teacher. It has a fourfold purpose designed to help you:

- organize your teaching sessions
- record the content
- evaluate the effectiveness
- save time.

Copy it and use it to focus on specific learning objectives on a daily basis.

With this information at your fingertips, you can save much of your valuable time and be more effective in helping the patient maintain or regain good health.

PATIENT-TEACHING CHECKLIST FOR ____________

PATIENT OBJECTIVES	PRE-TEST RESULTS	SESSION I CONTENT	SESSION II CONTENT	POST-TEST RESULTS
	Date: ______	Date: ______	Date: ______	Date: ______
	Date: ______	Date: ______	Date: ______	Date: ______
	Date: ______	Date: ______	Date: ______	Date: ______

PATIENT-TEACHING CHECKLIST FOR ____________

PATIENT OBJECTIVES	PRE-TEST RESULTS	SESSION I CONTENT	SESSION II CONTENT	POST-TEST RESULTS
	Date: ______	Date: ______	Date: ______	Date: ______
	Date: ______	Date: ______	Date: ______	Date: ______
	Date: ______	Date: ______	Date: ______	Date: ______

APPENDIX D

Medication Administration

INTRODUCTION

Teaching your patient how to give himself his medication is essential before his discharge. Without this knowledge and skill, he can never achieve independence in his daily life. To assess his learning needs, determine the following:

—Has he ever given himself medication by the route prescribed?

- If yes, can he describe the procedure?
- If yes, can he demonstrate the procedure correctly?

—Does he have the manual dexterity to administer the medication at the present time?

—Has he ever administered medication in the prescribed route to anyone else?

—How does he feel about giving himself medication in the prescribed route?

Once you have determined your patient's learning needs, plan for ample time to explain the procedure, demonstrate the skill required, and have him return the demonstration until he performs it correctly and confidently. To further enhance his learning, provide him with the appropriate patient-teaching aids that follow. These aids can be used in the health care setting to provide step-by-step instructions as he is learning the skill required under your supervision; they can also provide him with written instructions on the procedure upon discharge. If necessary, arrange for follow-up supervision in the home.

Patient-Teaching Aid

TAKING YOUR ORAL MEDICATIONS

Dear Patient:
For your drug therapy to be effective, you must take your medications exactly as your physician directs, particularly when taking several medications at one time. Here are some helpful hints:

Label empty jars, extra prescription bottles (you can get these from your pharmacist), or envelopes with the times of day or the days of the week you must take medication. Use a separate container for each time. Each morning fill these containers with the appropriate dose of each medication.
NOTE: Some drugs may deteriorate when exposed to light. Before you remove drugs from their original containers, check with your pharmacist or physician.

Make a medication calendar. Use a calendar that has enough space to fill in the names of the drugs you need to take each day. Then put a check mark next to the name of the drug after you take each dose.

Make a chart. List:
- name of drug
- what it is for
- what it looks like (shape, color)
- directions for taking the drug
- special cautions or side effects
- time of day to take drug.

Hang this chart near your medicine cabinet.

Set your alarm clock or ask a relative or friend to remind you when to take your medications.

Patient-Teaching Aid

GIVING YOURSELF EYE DROPS

Dear Patient:

To relieve your eye infection or irritation, your physician has prescribed these eye drops: ______________________

____

Use them exactly as directed on the label. Here is how:

- Begin by washing your hands thoroughly.
- Hold the bottle up to the light and examine it. If the medication is discolored or contains sediment, discard it immediately and have the prescription refilled. If it looks OK, warm the medication to room temperature by holding the bottle between your hands for 2 minutes.
- Next, moisten a rayon ball or tissue with water, and clean all secretions from around your eyes. Use a fresh rayon ball or tissue for each eye, so you do not spread infection.
- Now, stand or sit before a mirror, or lie on your back, whichever is most comfortable for you. Squeeze the bulb of the eyedropper to fill the dropper with medication.
- Tilt your head slightly back and toward the eye you are treating. Pull down your lower eyelid. (Do not pull your upper eyelid, or you will put unnecessary pressure on your eye.)
- Position the dropper over the conjunctival sac you have exposed between your lower lid and the white of your eye. Steady your hand by resting two fingers against your cheek or nose.
- Look away from the dropper. Then squeeze the prescribed number of drops into the sac. Do not drop the medication directly onto your eyeball. Take care not to touch the dropper to your eye or eyelashes. Wipe away excess medication with a clean tissue.
- Repeat the procedure in the other eye, if the physician orders.
- Recap the medication. Store the bottle away from light and extreme heat.

IMPORTANT: Call your physician immediately if you notice any of these side effects: ______________________

____

And remember, never put any medication in your eyes unless the label reads FOR OPHTHALMIC USE or FOR USE IN THE EYES.

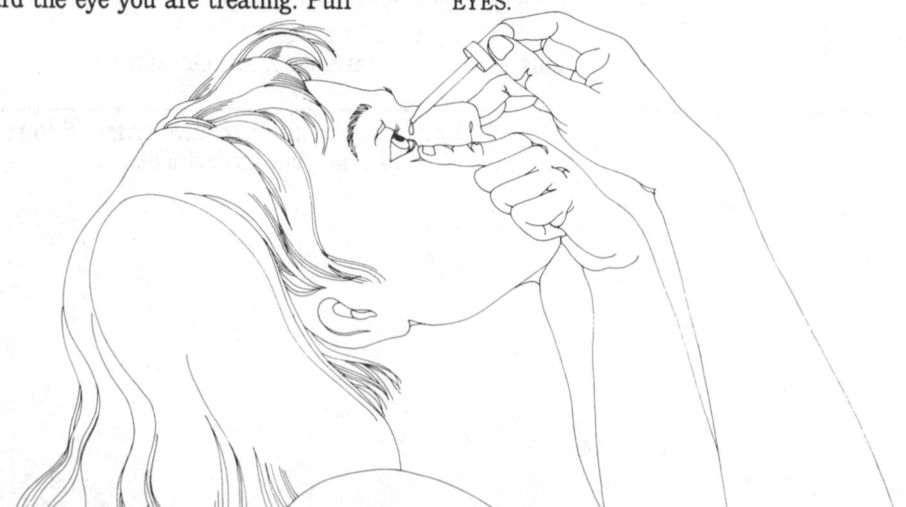

Patient-Teaching Aid

GIVING YOURSELF EARDROPS

Dear Patient:

To relieve your ear infection, your physician has prescribed these eardrops:

____

Use them exactly as directed on the label. Here is how:

• Begin by washing your hands thoroughly.

• Examine the medication. If it is discolored or has sediment in it, notify the physician and get your prescription refilled. If nothing is wrong with the medication, proceed to the next step.

• For your own comfort, warm the medication by holding the bottle between your hands for 2 minutes.

• Shake the bottle, if directed, and open it.

• Fill the dropper; then place the open bottle and dropper within easy reach.

• Lie on your side so the ear you are treating is exposed.

• Gently pull the top of your ear up and back, as shown below, to straighten the ear canal.

• Position the dropper above your ear, taking care not to touch your ear with it. Squeeze the dropper's bulb to release one drop.

• Wait until you feel the drop in your ear. Then, if directed, squeeze the bulb again. Repeat this step until you have administered the prescribed number of drops.

• To keep the drops in your ear, continue to lie on your side for about 10 minutes.

• If you wish, plug your ear with cotton moistened with ear drops. Do not plug your ear with dry cotton, unless the physician directs. Dry cotton will absorb the drops.

• If the physician directs, repeat the procedure for the other ear.

• Recap the bottle. Store your drops away from light and extreme heat.

IMPORTANT: Call your physician immediately if you have any of these side effects: ______________________________
____
____

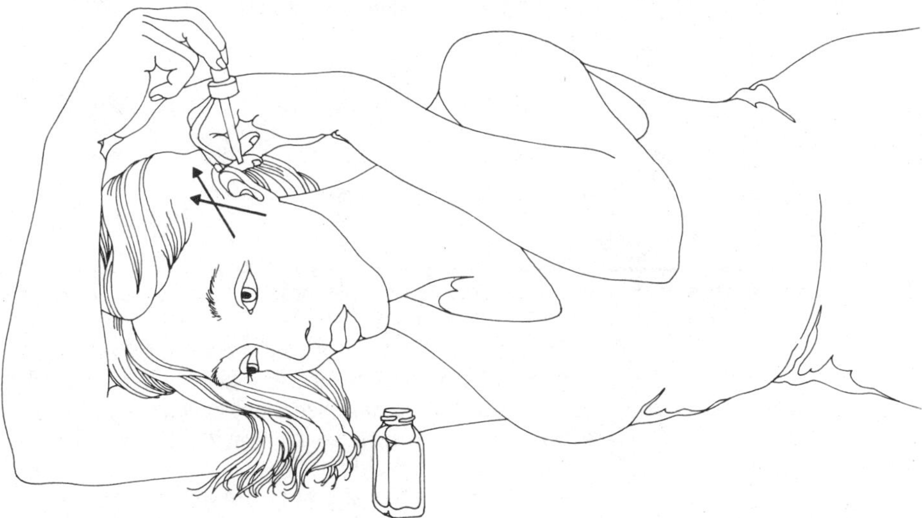

Patient-Teaching Aid

HOW TO USE NOSE DROPS

Dear Patient:
Your physician has prescribed nose drops for you to use at home. Here is what you will need to know:

To instill nose drops

- Before you use your nose drops, look at the container to make sure you have the right medication and to check the prescribed dosage.
- Position the dropper as shown in this illustration so the drops will flow down the back of your nose, not your throat.
- Squeeze the dropper bulb to instill the correct number of drops.
- Repeat the process in the other nostril, if indicated.
- Breathe through your mouth so you do not sniff the drops into your sinuses or aspirate them into your lungs.

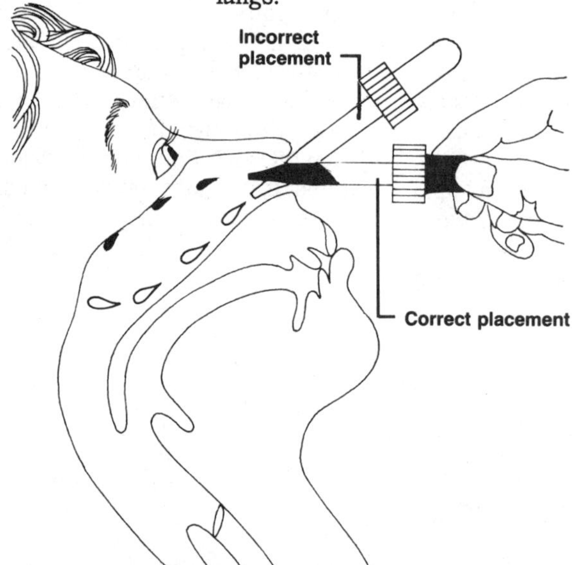

Precautions to take

- Follow your physician's orders exactly. Do not overuse your nose drops.
- Because nose drops are easily contaminated, do not buy more than you will use in a short time. Discard nose drops that contain sediment or look discolored.
- Do not share your nose drops with family members. Doing so may spread infection.
- Call your physician if you notice any side effects.

Patient-Teaching Aid

TAKING MEDICATION BY THE SUBLINGUAL OR BUCCAL ROUTE

Dear Patient:
Your physician has prescribed medications for you to take by the sublingual or buccal route. Taking your medication either way permits direct entry of the medication into your bloodstream, so it can take effect quickly. To take tablets via these routes, follow these instructions:

Sublingual route

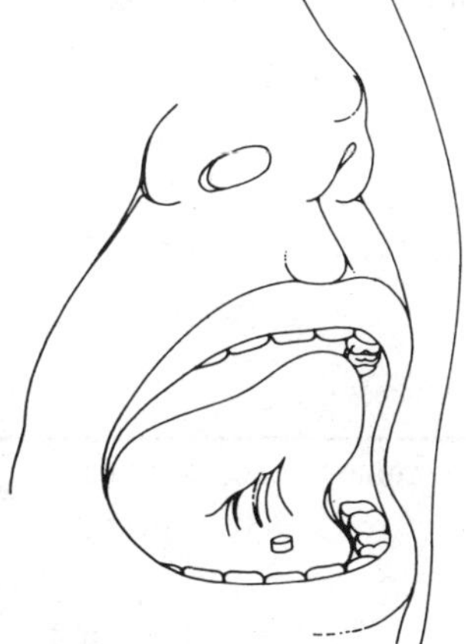

Place the tablet under your tongue, as shown at left. Hold it in place until it is absorbed.

Buccal route

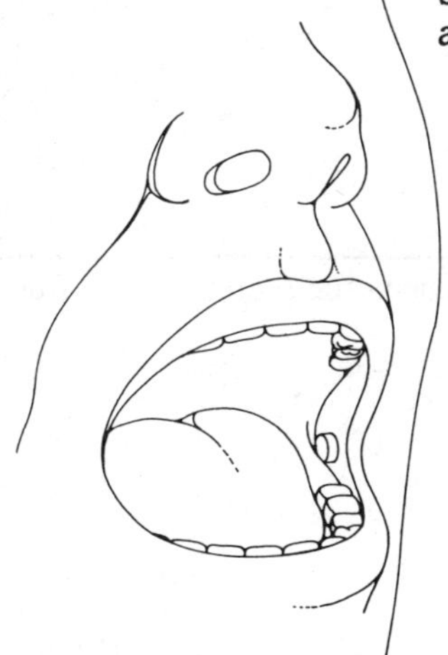

Place the tablet between your cheek and teeth, as shown at left. Close your mouth and hold the tablet against your cheek until it is absorbed.

IMPORTANT: In either case, do not swallow the tablet.

Patient-Teaching Aid

HOW TO USE A NASAL AEROSOL DEVICE (TURBINAIRE)

Dear Patient:
Your physician wants you to use a medicated aerosol spray to relieve nasal irritation. Here is how:

1

First, read the medication label so you know the exact amount of medication to administer. Then put together the spray device by placing the stem of the medication cartridge in the plastic nasal adapter, as shown here. (If you are inserting a refill cartridge, first remove the protective cap from the stem.)

2

Now gently blow your nose to remove excess mucus.

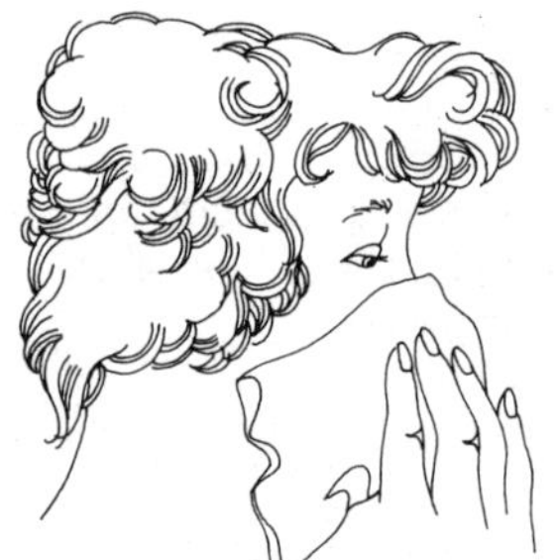

3

Shake the device well. Remove the protective cap from the adapter tip.

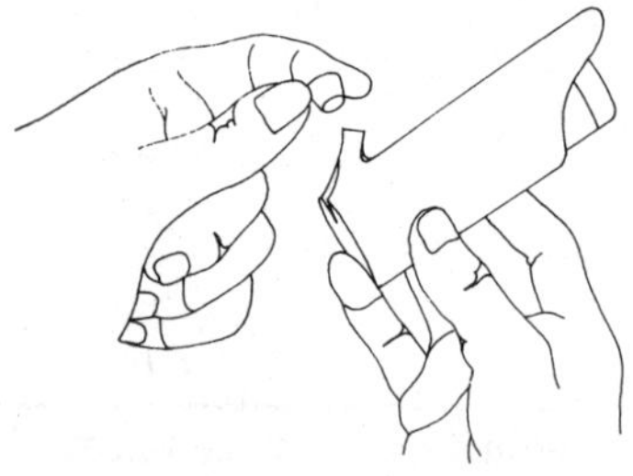

HOW TO USE A NASAL AEROSOL DEVICE (TURBINAIRE)—*continued*

4

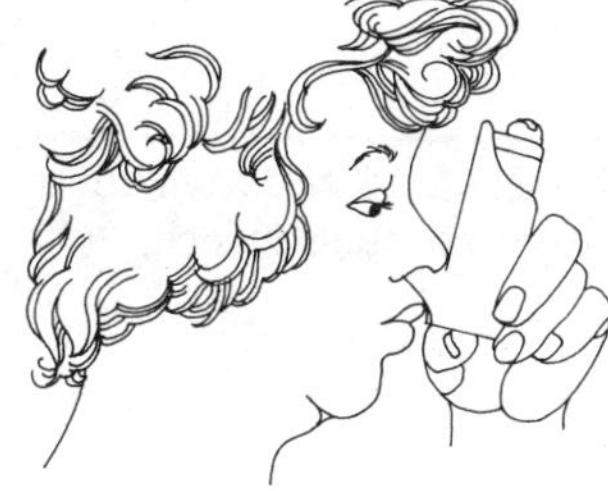

Now place the tip inside your nostril. Holding your breath, firmly press down once on the cartridge; then release it. Continue to hold your breath for several seconds afterward. Do not inhale the mist.

5

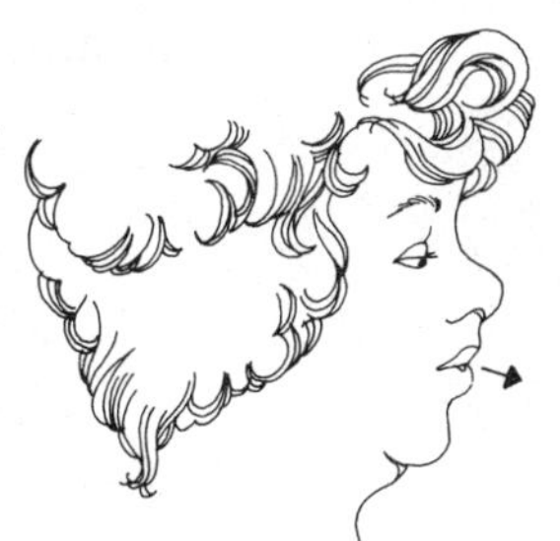

Remove the adapter tip from your nostril and exhale. If necessary, reinsert the adapter in the same nostril, and spray again. Then repeat this procedure in the other nostril, if ordered. IMPORTANT: Do not blow your nose for at least 2 minutes.

6

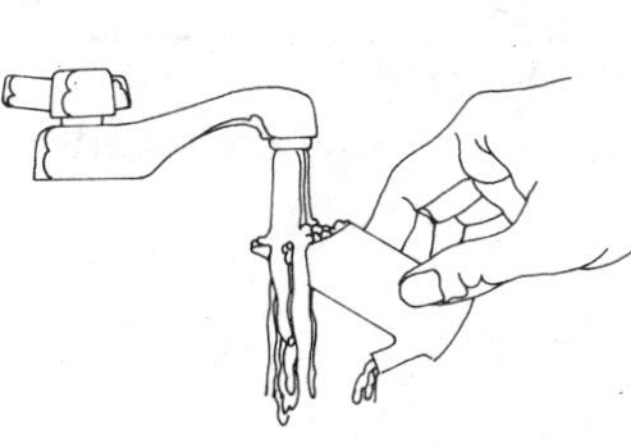

Replace the protective cap on the adapter tip. Then put the entire device in a plastic bag to keep it clean. Once a day, remove the medication cartridge and thoroughly rinse the plastic adapter with warm water. CAUTION: Follow the physician's directions exactly. Let him know at once if you feel increased nasal irritation, itching, or bleeding; increased nasal congestion; coughing; headache; or dizziness.

Patient-Teaching Aid

HOW TO USE A METERED-DOSE NEBULIZER

Dear Patient:
Inhaling the medication in this metered-dose nebulizer will help you breathe more easily. Use it exactly as your physician has ordered, at these times: ________.
Here is how:

1

First, remove the white mouthpiece and cap from the bottle. Then remove the cap from the mouthpiece.

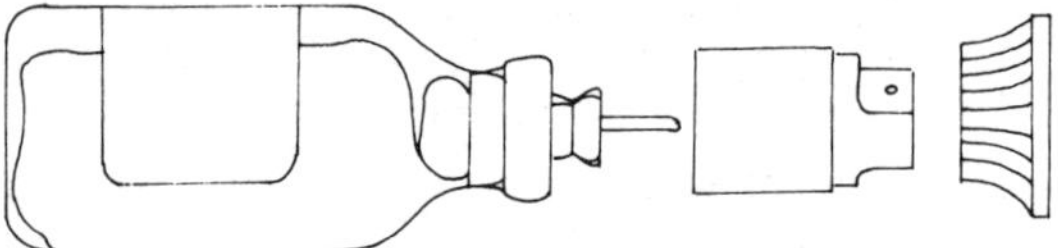

2

Turn the mouthpiece sideways. On one side of the flattened tip, you will see a small hole. Fit the metal stem on the bottle into the hole.

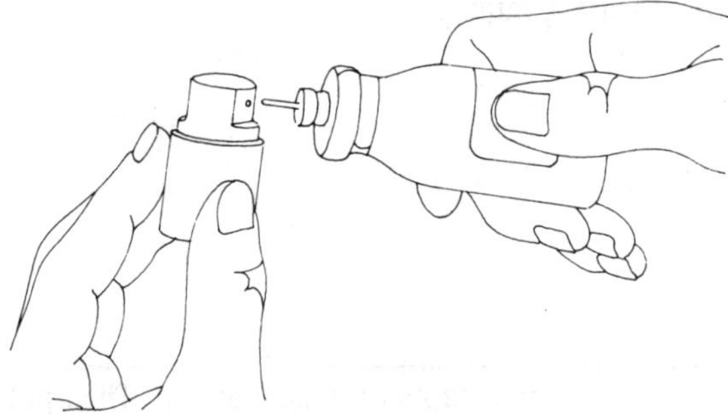

3

Now exhale. Hold the nebulizer upside down, as you see here, and close your lips loosely around the mouthpiece.

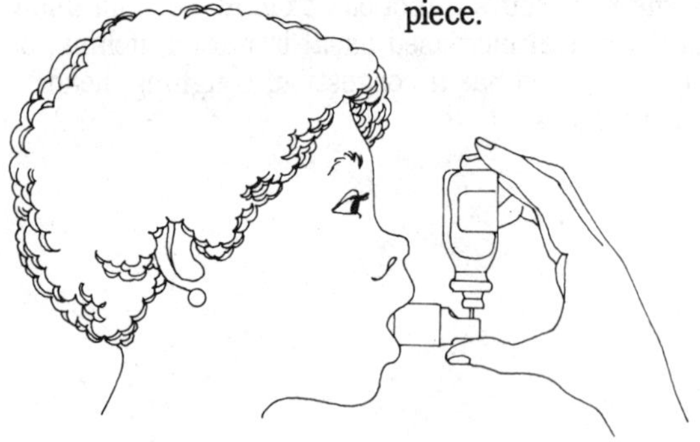

HOW TO USE A METERED-DOSE NEBULIZER—*continued*

4

Inhale slowly. As you do, firmly push the bottle against the mouthpiece—one time only—to release one dose of medication. Continue inhaling until your lungs feel full.

5

Take the mouthpiece away from your mouth, and hold your breath momentarily.

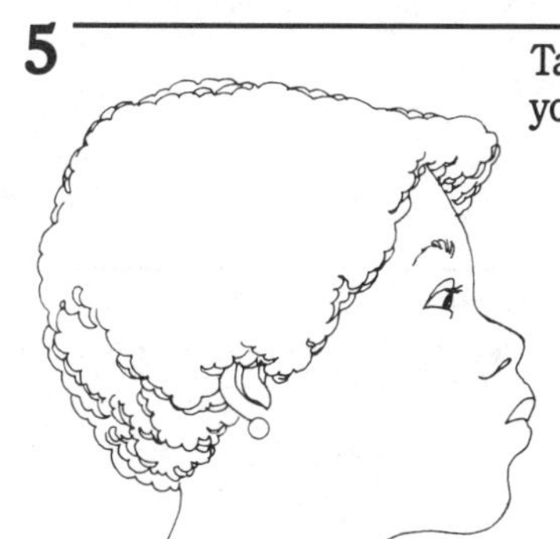

6

Then purse your lips and exhale slowly. If the physician directs, repeat the procedure.

IMPORTANT: Never overuse your nebulizer. Follow your physician's instructions exactly. Finally, rinse the mouthpiece with warm water.

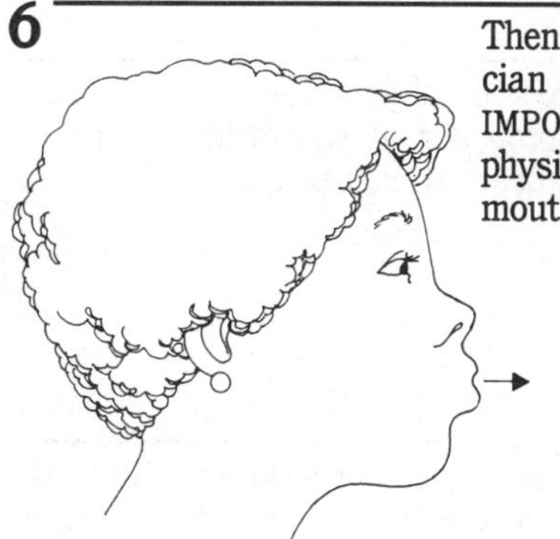

Patient-Teaching Aid

HOW TO USE A TURBO-INHALER

Dear Patient:
Inhaling the medication in this whirlybird inhalation device will help prevent asthma attacks. Use it exactly as your physician has ordered, at these times: ________

________.

CAUTION: Never use more than four capsules a day.

1

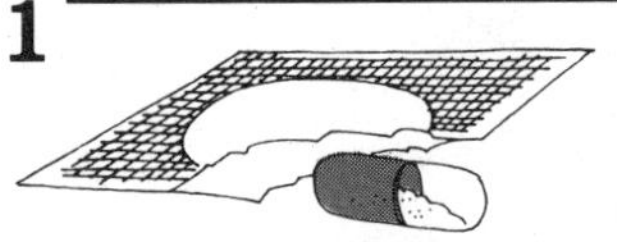

Before you begin, wash and dry your hands. Unwrap one capsule so it is ready to use.

2

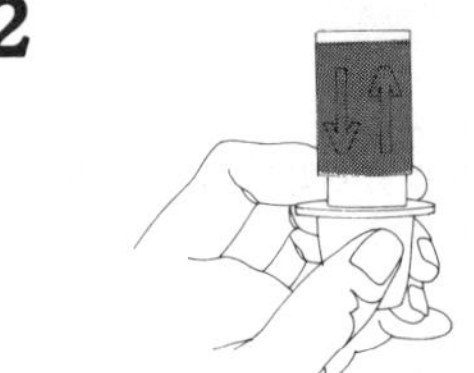

Then hold the device so the white mouthpiece is on the bottom, like this. Slide the gray sleeve all the way to the top.

3

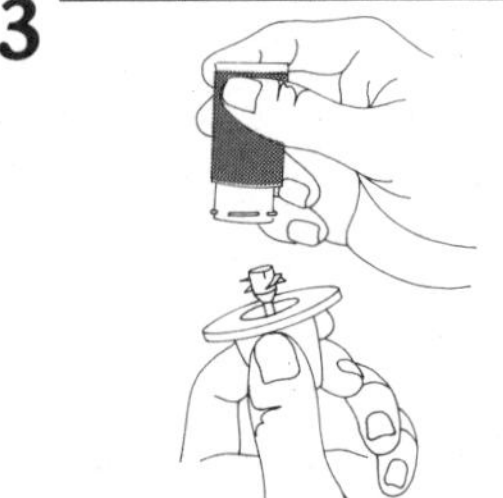

Open the mouthpiece by unscrewing its tip counter-clockwise. Inside, you will see a small propeller on a stem.

4

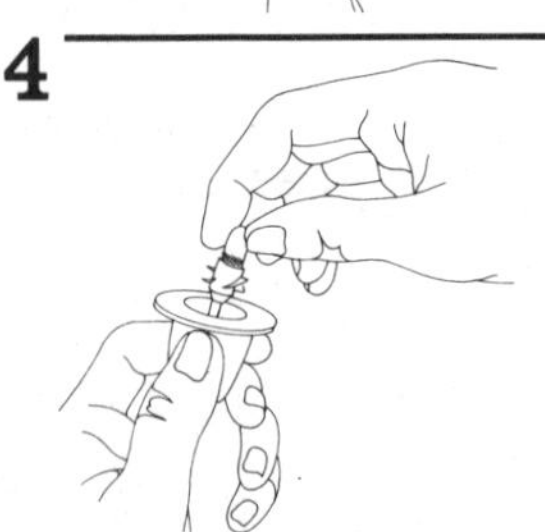

Firmly press the colored end of your medication capsule into the center of the propeller, as shown here. Avoid overhandling the capsule, or it may soften.

5

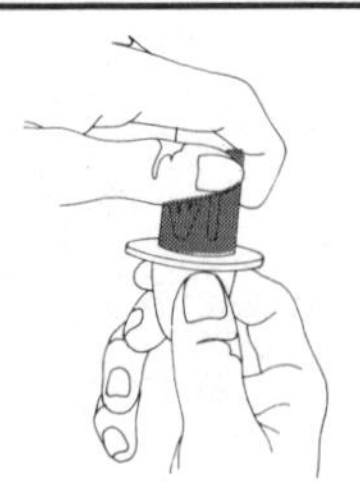

Now screw the device back together securely, and hold it with the mouthpiece at the bottom, as shown here. To puncture the capsule and release the medication, slide the gray sleeve all the way down. Then slide it up again. Do this step one time only.

HOW TO USE A TURBO-INHALER—*continued*

6

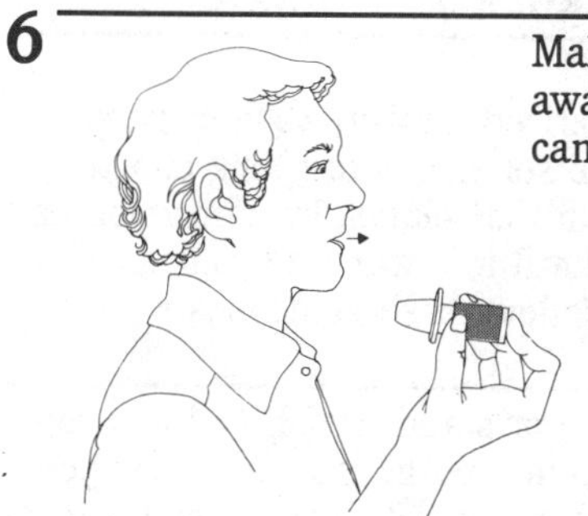

Make sure everything is secure. Then hold the device away from your mouth, and exhale as much air as you can.

7

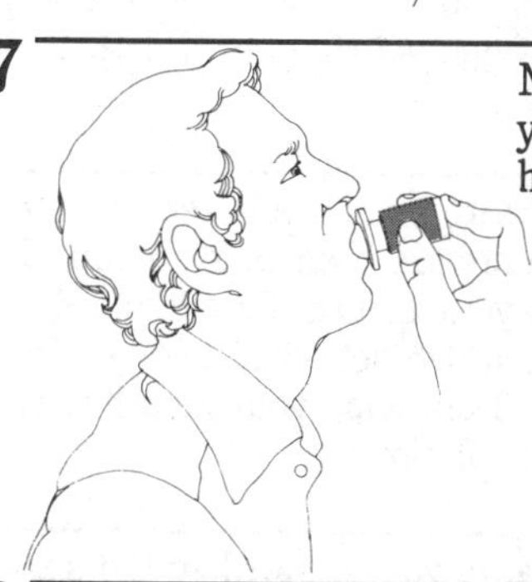

Now tilt your head backward. Place the mouthpiece in your mouth, and close your lips around it, as shown here. Quickly inhale once to fill your lungs.

8

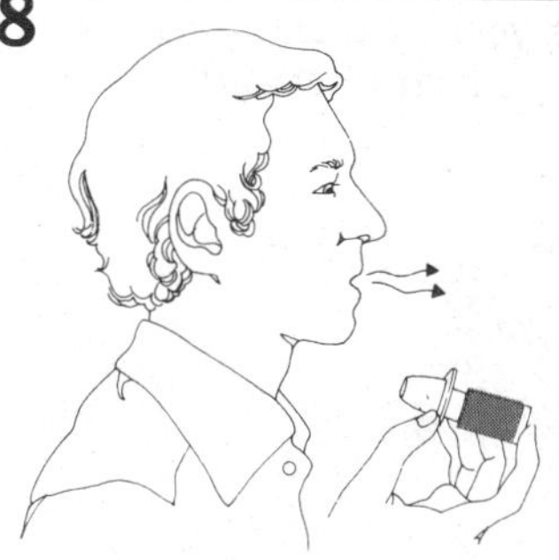

Hold your breath for several seconds. Then remove the device from your mouth, and exhale as much air as you can. Repeat steps 7 and 8 several times, until all the medication in the device is gone. Never exhale through the mouthpiece.

9

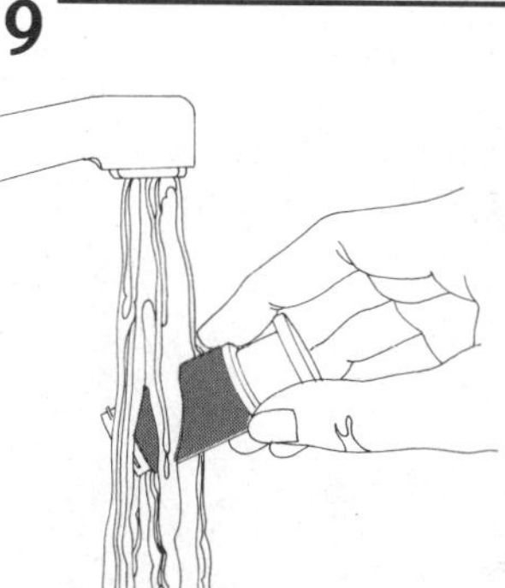

Discard the empty medication capsule. Then place the entire device in its metal can, and screw on the lid. At least once a week, remove the device from the can, take it apart, and rinse it thoroughly with warm water. Make sure it is completely dry before reassembling it. Keep the capsules from deteriorating too rapidly by leaving them wrapped until needed.

IMPORTANT: Follow your physician's instructions exactly. Notify him at once if you have throat or chest irritation, coughing or choking, nasal congestion, dizziness, headache, or nausea.

Patient-Teaching Aid

HOW TO ADMINISTER A MOUTHWASH OR GARGLE

Dear Patient:
Your physician has prescribed a mouthwash or gargle for you. First, gather the solution, a drinking cup, a basin, and tissues. Warm the solution by immersing its container in hot water until it is warm to your touch. Then, to administer it, follow these guidelines:

Mouthwash

Sit in an upright position or stand. Swish 1/8 to 1/4 cup of the solution around your mouth, especially over your teeth and gums. Do not swallow it. Instead, spit it into the basin. Use a tissue to wipe your mouth. Discard the used solution.

Gargle

Sit in an upright position, with your head erect or tilted back slightly. Take a deep breath, then take 1/8 cup of the solution and hold it in your mouth. Exhale slowly to create the gargling action. Do not aspirate the solution; spit it into the basin. Then wipe your mouth with a tissue. Discard the used solution.

NOTE: If your physician wants you to swallow the solution so it coats and soothes your irritated throat tissue, do not eat or drink for 1/2 hour afterward.

Patient-Teaching Aid

HOW TO APPLY A MEDICATED CREAM OR OINTMENT

Dear Patient:

To help treat your ________ condition, your physician wants you to apply ________ cream/ointment to your ________. The nurse has shown you the proper way to apply it. When you apply the medication yourself, follow the directions on the label, and observe these guidelines:

- Wash your hands thoroughly before beginning the procedure.
- Use warm water and soap to cleanse the skin of any old cream/ointment.
- When you uncap the container, place the cap so the grooved side is up.
- Apply the cream/ointment as directed.
- Do/do not cover the area with a loose/tight dressing.
- Notify the physician if you notice any of the following: a change in the amount, color, consistency, or odor of drainage; or increased swelling or redness.

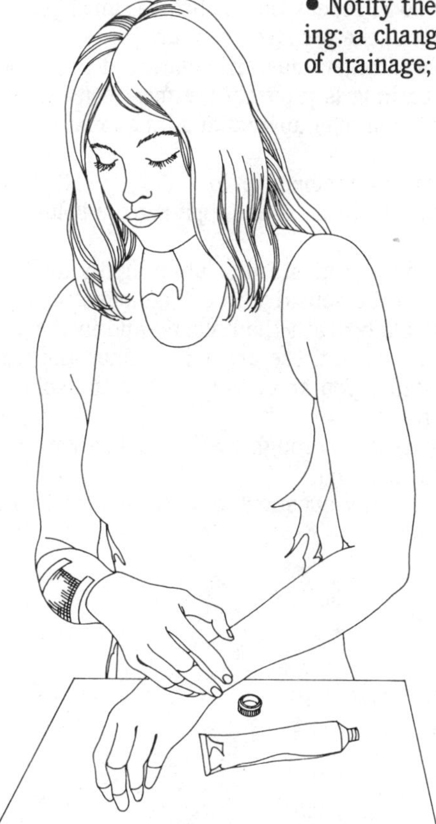

Patient-Teaching Aid

HOW TO APPLY NITROGEN MUSTARD TO THE SKIN

Dear Patient:

- Each small vial of nitrogen mustard contains 10 mg of powder. Transfer the contents to a 2-oz (60-ml) bottle. Add enough tap water to dissolve the powder, but do not fill the bottle.
- Add 1 to 3 teaspoons (5 to 15 ml) of an emulsified oil. This will help prevent your skin from becoming too dry.
- Fill the mixing bottle with water and shake well; the nitrogen mustard solution is then ready to use.
- Using your hands, apply the nitrogen mustard solution to your *entire body surface,* whether it shows any sign of disease or not. Be sure to include the skin on your scalp, eyelids, and groin, and between the toes. If you have any nitrogen mustard solution left after coating your entire body, repeat the application until you have used up all of the prepared mixture.
- You may apply nitrogen mustard solution at any time; however, after bathing is probably the most convenient time. Afterward, you may apply a soothing cream if you wish.
- To reduce irritation, remember to:
  —keep your eyes closed when applying the solution to your face.
  —apply the nitrogen mustard solution lightly and just one time to the sensitive intertriginous areas (under the arms, beneath the breasts, and in the groin), as the skin in these areas is thinner and may become irritated if you apply too much of the solution too vigorously.
  —wash your hands thoroughly after application to remove excess solution.
- Should you have any questions or problems, call your physician.

Patient-Teaching Aid

APPLYING A NITROGLYCERIN DISK

Dear Patient:

Your physician has prescribed nitroglycerin for your angina. Nitroglycerin relieves anginal pain by temporarily dilating (widening) veins and arteries. This brings more blood and oxygen to the heart when it needs it most. This way your heart does not have to work so hard.

The nitroglycerin your physician has prescribed comes in a disk. The disk consists of a gel-like substance attached to an adhesive bandage. (See the illustration below, which shows the different disk layers.) When applied to the skin, the disk allows nitroglycerin to be absorbed through the skin into the bloodstream. A single application lasts 24 hours.

Apply the disk to any convenient skin area—preferably on the upper arm or chest—without touching the gel or surrounding tape. Use a different site every day to avoid skin irritation. If necessary, you can shave an appropriate site. Avoid any area that may cause uneven absorption, such as skin folds, scars, and calluses, or any irritated or damaged skin areas. Also, do not apply the disk below the elbow or knee.

After application, wash your hands to remove any nitroglycerin that may have rubbed off.

Try not to get the disk wet when you shower. If the disk should leak or fall off, throw it away. Then clean the site, and apply a new disk at a different site.

To ensure 24-hour coverage, apply the nitroglycerin disk at the same time every day. Bedtime application is ideal, because body movement is at a minimum during the night. Also, to ensure continuous nitroglycerin therapy, apply a new disk about 30 minutes before removing the old one.

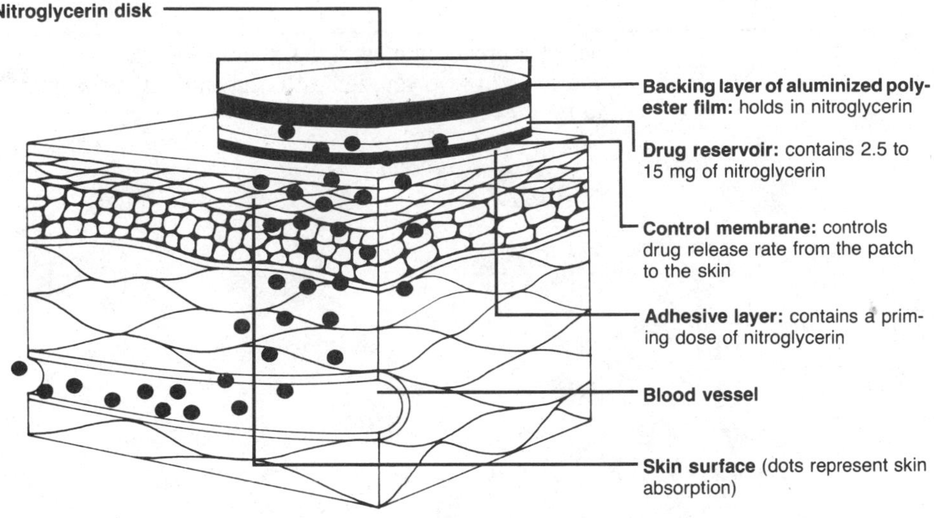

Patient-Teaching Aid

HOW TO GIVE YOURSELF A SUBCUTANEOUS INJECTION

Dear Patient:
This aid is meant to supplement, not replace, the instructions from your nurse. Use it as a written reminder of what the nurse has taught you. Before beginning the procedure, wash your hands thoroughly. Check the expiration date on your medication vial, and read the label to make sure the medication is the correct strength and type. Now follow these guidelines:

1

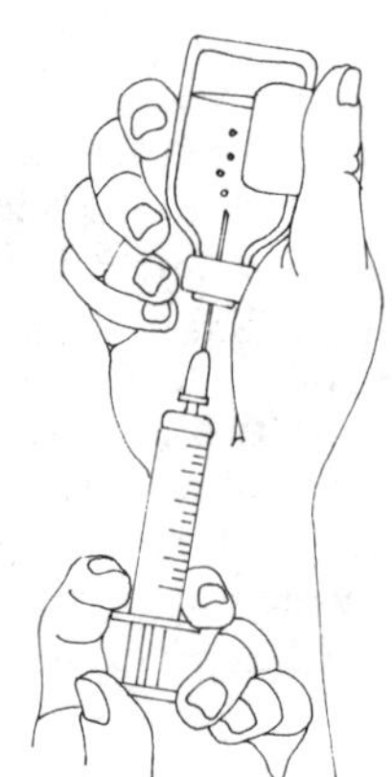

If the medication must be drawn into a syringe, use an alcohol swab to cleanse the rubber stopper on top of the vial. Inject an equal amount of air into the vial before you draw up the medication. This way, you avoid creating a vacuum in the vial and make withdrawing your medication easier.
NOTE: If you see air bubbles in the syringe after you fill it with your medication, tap the syringe lightly to remove them. Draw up more medication, if necessary.

2

Select a proper site, as illustrated in the diagrams. (If you need to give yourself an injection daily, remember to rotate the site.)

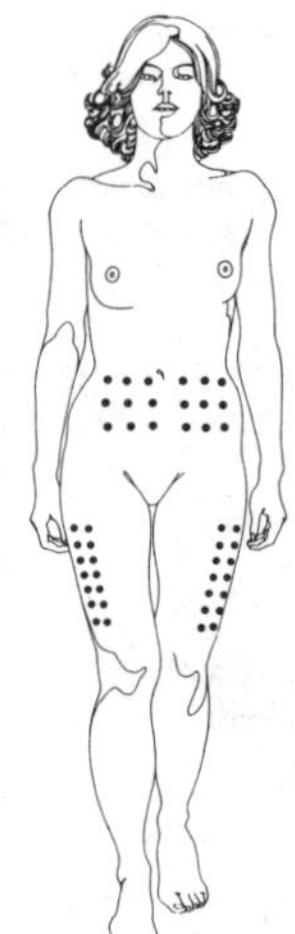

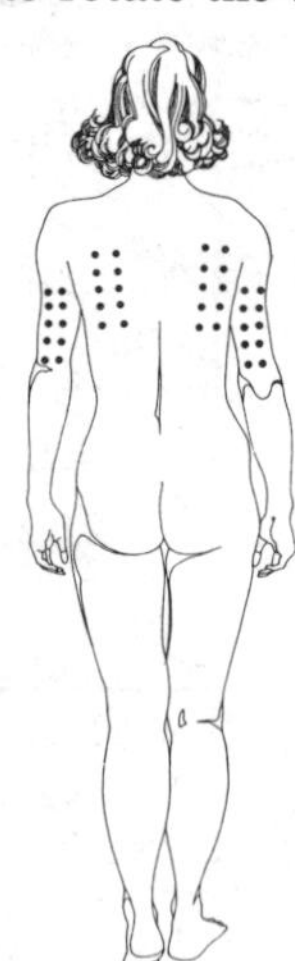

HOW TO GIVE YOURSELF A SUBCUTANEOUS INJECTION—*continued*

3

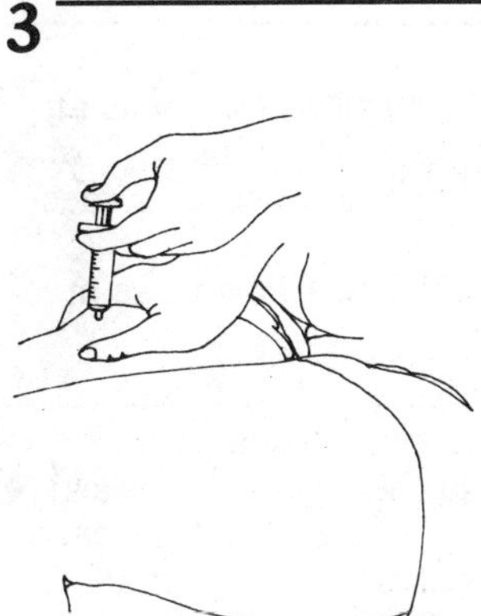

Pull the skin taut, and use an alcohol swab or a cotton ball soaked in alcohol to clean it in a circular motion. Now pinch the skin at the cleansed site between your thumb and forefinger. Quickly plunge the needle into the fat fold at a 90-degree angle, right up to its hub. As you hold the syringe with one hand, pull back on the plunger slightly with your other hand to check for blood backflow. If blood appears in the syringe, discard everything and start again. If no blood appears, slowly inject the medication.

4

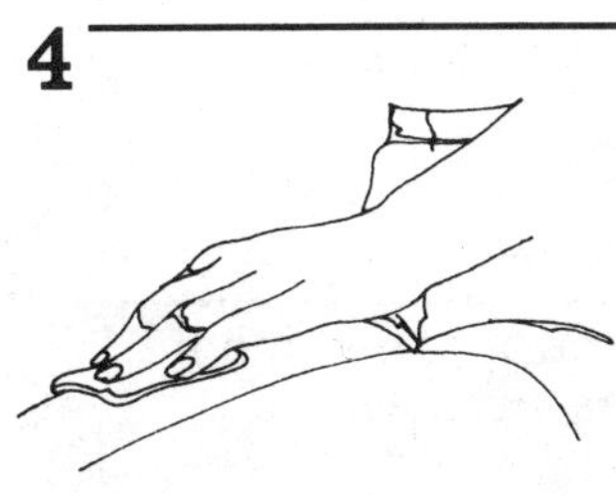

Place an alcohol swab over the site. Use the swab to press lightly on the site as you withdraw the needle. Snap the needle off the syringe. Dispose of the needle and syringe properly.

5

If you are administering heparin subcutaneously, follow the usual procedure as described above, except for these considerations:

- Use a ½″ 25G or 26G needle.
- Select an injection site on your abdomen just above the level of your anterior iliac spine, as shown. Remember, you must rotate injection sites. Study the illustration to determine which site to choose.
- Pinch a ½″ (1.3 cm) fold of tissue between your thumb and forefinger, and insert the needle into the fold at a 90-degree angle. Using this technique will minimize heparin's irritating qualities. Applying ice to the site before injecting may help too—but do not apply it until you check with your physician.
- Do not check for blood backflow. You could damage the tissue and cause a hematoma.
- Never massage the site after the injection. You could rupture the small blood vessels and cause a hematoma.

Patient-Teaching Aid

HOW TO USE NITROGLYCERIN OINTMENT

Dear Patient:
Your physician has prescribed your nitroglycerin as an ointment. In this form, nitroglycerin is continuously absorbed through the skin into the circulation; it is effective for about 4 hours.

To get the most from your therapy, follow these instructions carefully:

1

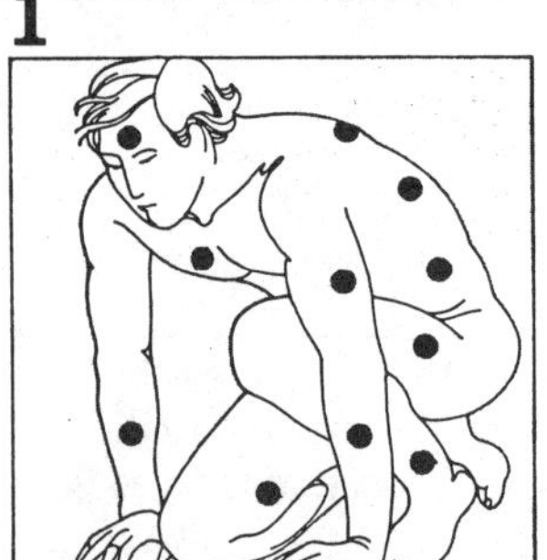

Apply ointment to a hairless or shaved skin area (chest, arm, thigh, abdomen, forehead, ankle, or back) to promote uniform absorption. Choose a new site each time you apply a dose to prevent minor skin irritations. Remove any traces of ointment left from a previous application.

2

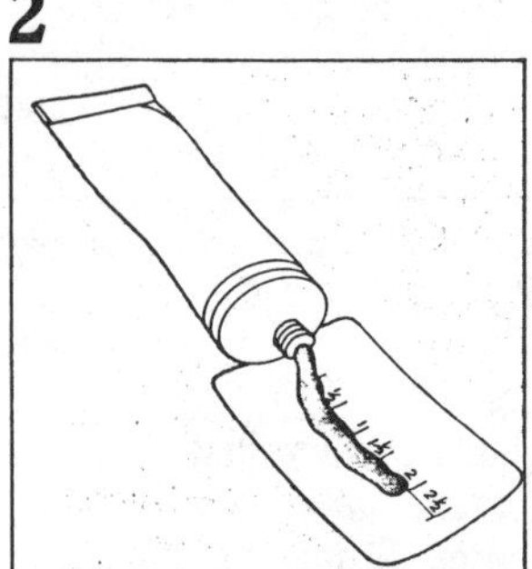

Use the ruled applicator paper that comes with the ointment to measure your dose accurately.

3

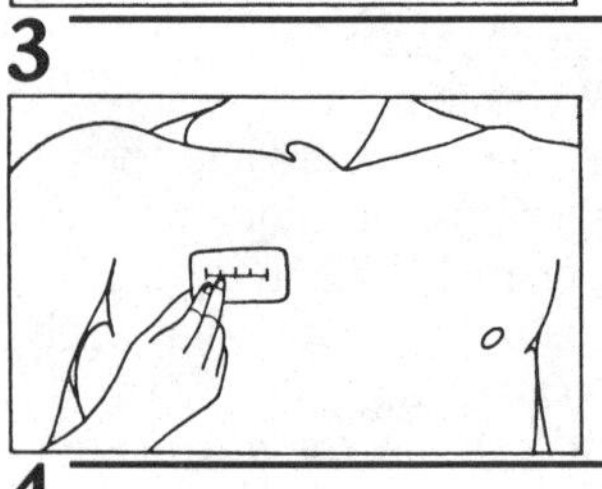

Use the applicator paper to apply the ointment in a thin, uniform layer over an area of about 3″ to 6″ (8 to 15 cm). Leave the applicator paper on the site.

4

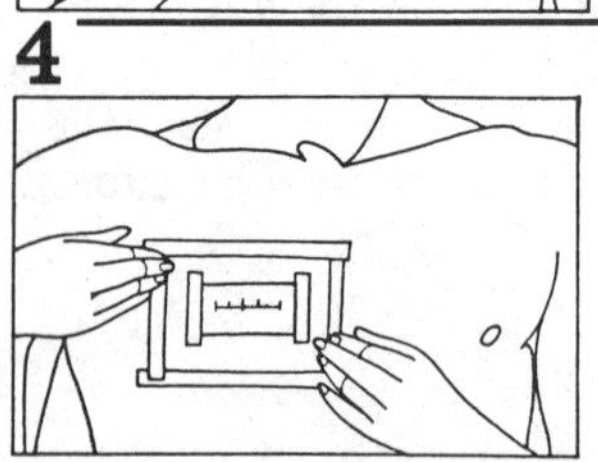

Cover the applicator paper with plastic wrap and secure it with tape. This will protect your clothing and ensure maximum absorption.

Call your physician immediately if you experience a headache, feel dizzy or faint, or notice any redness or irritation at the application site. He may want to adjust your dosage or check the application site.

Patient-Teaching Aid

HOW TO GIVE MEDICATION THROUGH YOUR GASTROSTOMY

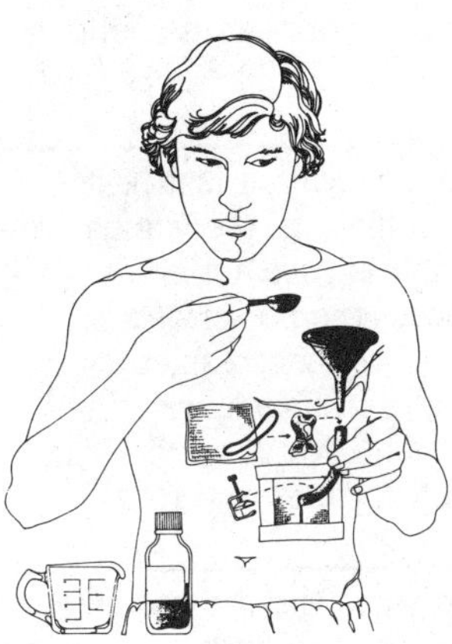

Dear Patient:

Your physician has placed a tube in the opening to your stomach, and the nurse has shown you how to use it. Here are some guidelines to help you when you return home (refer to the illustration at left):

- Be aware that medication must be in liquid form. To convert medication to liquid, obtain specific instructions from your pharmacist.
- To medicate yourself, sit down and attach a clean funnel or syringe (with the plunger or bulb removed) to the tube. Then unclamp the tube.
- Make sure the tube is not clogged by pouring about 2 tablespoons (30 ml) of water into the funnel. (If the water does not flow into your stomach, the tube is probably clogged. Stop the procedure, and call your physician immediately.)
- When you are certain that the tube is open, pour the medication into the funnel. Let it drip slowly into your stomach. Do not try to rush the procedure by forcing it.
- After the medication is completely in your stomach, clear the tube by pouring an additional 2 tablespoons of water into the funnel.
- Replace the clamp on the tube, and remove the funnel. (If you lose the clamp, fold the tube on top of itself and fasten it with a rubber band.)
- Cover the end of the tube with a gauze pad to keep it clean. Then wrap a rubber band around the pad to hold it in place.
- Stay seated upright for at least 30 minutes.
- Using warm water, wash the funnel thoroughly after every use.
- Examine the skin around the opening. Call your physician if the skin feels sore, looks red, or seems puffy. Also call your physician if you find your medication seeping from the insertion site or if you feel any discomfort in your stomach.

Patient-Teaching Aid

ADMINISTERING A VAGINAL MEDICATION

Dear Patient:
Your physician has prescribed a vaginal medication for you. To insert the medication into your vagina, follow these instructions:

1 Plan to administer the vaginal medication just before bedtime to ensure that it will remain in the vagina longer than if administered during daytime activities. Collect the equipment you will need: the prescribed medication (suppository, cream, ointment, tablet, or jelly), an applicator, gloves, water-soluble lubricating jelly, a bed-protector pad or towel, several cotton balls, soap, water, a hand mirror, and a paper towel.

2 Next, empty your bladder, and place the bed-protector pad or towel on the bed. Sit on the bed with your knees flexed and legs spread apart. After opening the medication wrapper or container, put on your gloves.

3 Using the hand mirror, carefully inspect your perineum. If you see signs of increased irritation, withhold the medication and notify the physician. He may select an alternate medication.

4 If you see discharge, soak several cotton balls in warm, soapy water. Working from front to back, clean the left side of the perineum, using a downward stroke. Discard the cotton ball. Using a fresh cotton ball, repeat the procedure on the right side and then the center of the perineum. Be sure to use a fresh cotton ball for each stroke. Continue as necessary until the perineum is cleansed.

ADMINISTERING A VAGINAL MEDICATION—*continued*

5 If you are administering a vaginal suppository, place the prescribed medication dose in the applicator. (Vaginal suppositories come in either diamond or teardrop shapes.)

6 To make insertion easier, lubricate the suppository and applicator tip with water or water-soluble lubricating jelly. The medication may feel cold. Then spread apart your labia with one hand, and insert the applicator into the vagina with your other hand. Advance the applicator about 2″ (5 cm), angling it slightly toward your sacrum.

7 Push the plunger to insert the suppository.
NOTE: You would administer a vaginal jelly, ointment, cream, or tablet in the same manner.

8 Remove the applicator and discard it, if it is disposable. If it is reusable, thoroughly wash it with soap and warm water, dry it with the paper towel, and return it to its container.

9 Remain lying down for about 30 minutes, so the medication will not run out of your vagina. Apply a perineal pad to avoid staining clothes and bed linens. Then check your vaginal mucosa for signs of allergic reaction. If the area seems unusually red or swollen, notify your physician immediately.

Patient-Teaching Aid

HOW TO APPLY A RECTAL OINTMENT

Dear Patient:
Your physician has prescribed a rectal ointment for your sore or inflamed rectal area. To apply a rectal ointment, follow these guidelines:

1 Begin by collecting the equipment you will need: a glove or 4″ × 4″ gauze pad if the ointment is to be applied externally; an applicator and water-soluble lubricant if it is to be applied internally.

2 Figure on using approximately 1″ (2.5 cm) of ointment. If the ointment is to be applied externally, sit on the toilet or lie down on your side on the bed. Wipe the ointment on the external rectal area, using a gloved hand or the 4″ × 4″ gauze pad. Place a 4″ × 4″ gauze pad between your buttocks to absorb excess ointment. Remove gloves, if used, and wash your hands.

3 If you are to place the ointment internally in the rectum, gauge how much pressure to use to obtain approximately 1″ of ointment by squeezing out the correct amount before you attach the tube to the applicator. Then attach the applicator to the tube, and coat the applicator tip with water-soluble lubricant.

4 Sit on the toilet, and expose the anus with one hand. Take several deep breaths through your mouth to relax your anal sphincter; then slowly insert the applicator into your anus.

5 When you have inserted the entire applicator, slowly squeeze the tube to eject the medication. Remove the applicator.

6 Place a folded 4″ × 4″ gauze pad between your buttocks to absorb any excess ointment. Disassemble the tube and applicator, and recap the tube. Clean the applicator thoroughly with warm water and soap, and dry. Wash your hands.

Patient-Teaching Aid

HOW TO INSERT A RECTAL SUPPOSITORY

Dear Patient:
Your physician has prescribed medication in the form of a rectal suppository. To administer a rectal suppository, follow these guidelines:

1. First, wash your hands and gather the equipment you will need: the suppository, a glove or finger cot (can be purchased in a pharmacy), and water-soluble lubricant. If the suppository is too soft, it will adhere to the wrapper. Remedy this by holding it under cold running water until it becomes firm, or place it in the refrigerator for several minutes.

2. Expose the rectal area by sitting on the edge of the toilet. Put on a glove or finger cot. Remove the suppository from the wrapper, and lubricate it with water-soluble lubricant.

3. With your ungloved hand, separate your buttocks. Take a deep breath, and with your gloved hand, gently insert the suppository through the rectal opening, tapered end first. Use your forefinger to direct it along the rectal wall. Continue to advance it 3″ (7.5 cm), or about the length of your finger; otherwise, it may be expelled. Take care not to push it into a fecal mass.

4. Stand up and hold your buttocks together until the urge to defecate subsides. Then cleanse the excess lubricant from the anus. Remove and dispose of your glove or finger cot, and wash your hands. Retain the suppository for at least 20 minutes; however, if the suppository is to relieve your constipation, defecate as soon as you feel the urge.

Patient-Teaching Aid

HOW TO GIVE YOURSELF AN INSULIN INJECTION

Dear Patient:
This aid is meant to supplement, not replace, the instructions from your nurse. Use it as a written reminder of what the nurse has taught you.

1 Before beginning the procedure, wash your hands thoroughly. Then remove the insulin from the refrigerator. Warm and mix it by rolling the vial between your palms. Check the expiration date, and read the label to make sure the medication is the correct strength and type. IMPORTANT: Never shake the vial.

Using an alcohol swab, cleanse the rubber stopper on top of the vial.

2 Select a proper site, remembering what you learned from the nurse about site rotation. Pull the skin taut, and use an alcohol swab or a cotton ball soaked in alcohol to clean it in a circular motion.

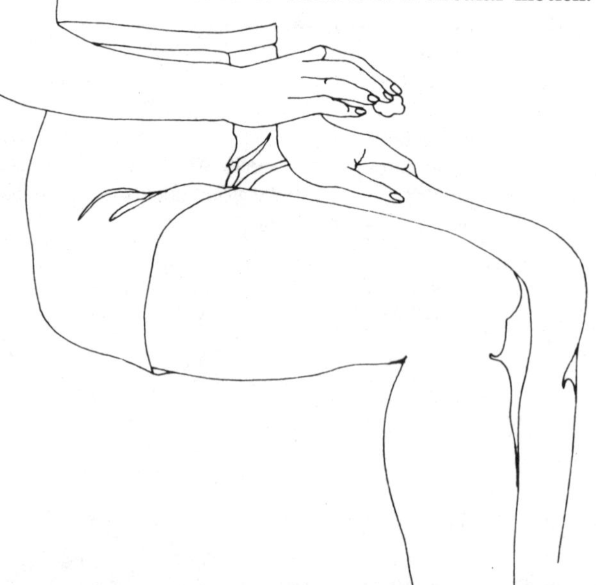

HOW TO GIVE YOURSELF AN INSULIN INJECTION—*continued*

3

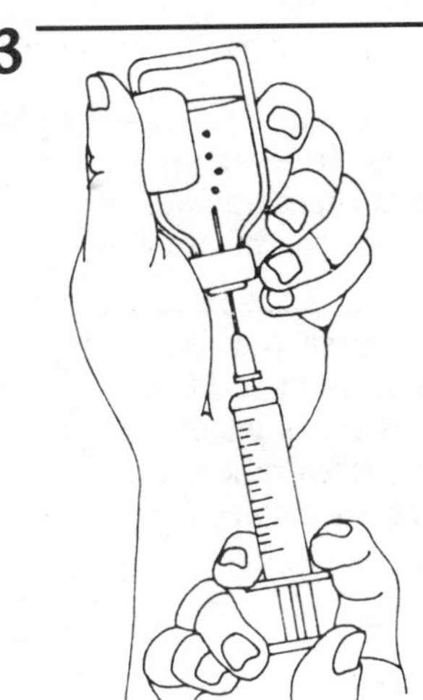

Inject an equal amount of air into the vial before you draw up the insulin. This way, you avoid creating a vacuum in the vial and make withdrawing your insulin easier.

NOTE: If you see air bubbles in the syringe after you fill it with insulin, tap the syringe lightly to remove them. Draw up more insulin, if necessary.

4

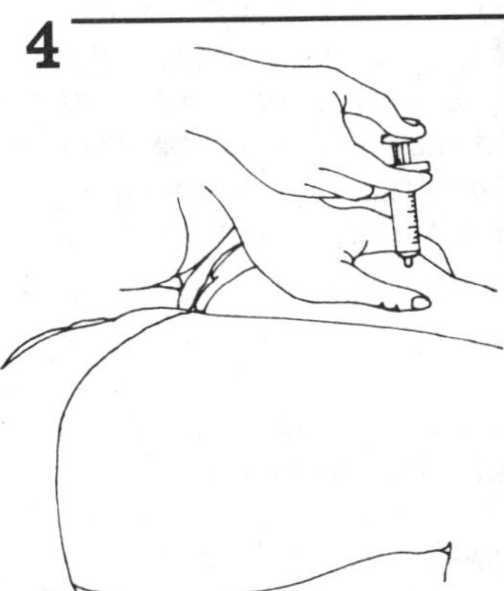

Now pinch the skin at the cleansed site between your thumb and forefinger. Quickly plunge the needle into the fat fold at a 90-degree angle, right up to its hub. As you hold the syringe with one hand, pull back on the plunger slightly with your other hand to check for blood backflow. If blood appears in the syringe, discard everything and start again. If no blood appears, inject the insulin slowly.

5

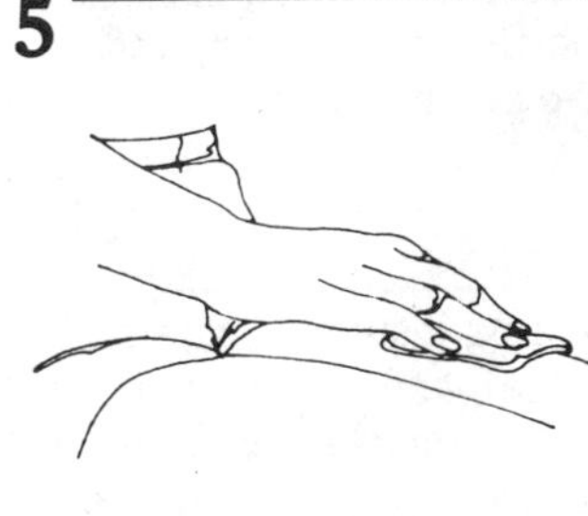

Place an alcohol swab over the site. Use the swab to press lightly on the site as you withdraw the needle. Snap the needle off the syringe. Dispose of the needle and syringe properly. The nurse will give you an aid that will show you how to rotate your injection sites correctly. (See *How to Give Yourself a Subcutaneous Injection*, pp. 536-537.) To help you remember, use a calendar to mark which site you plan to use each day.

IMPORTANT: If you travel, keep a bottle of insulin and a syringe with you at all times. The insulin does not need to be refrigerated if you keep it away from heat.

Patient-Teaching Aid

MIXING REGULAR AND LONG-ACTING INSULINS

Dear Patient:
Your physician has prescribed regular and long-acting insulins to control your diabetes. To avoid separate injections, you can mix these two types and administer them together. Here are the steps you must follow:

1

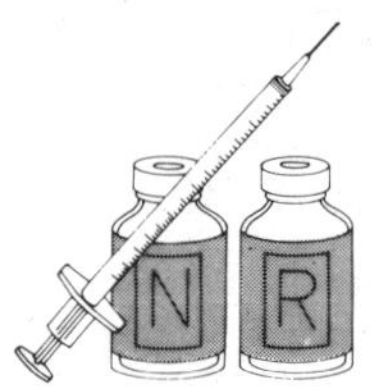

Check your equipment: Always wash your hands first, and prepare the mixture in a clean area. Make sure you have alcohol swabs, both types of insulin, and the proper syringe for the insulin concentration. Then warm each vial by rolling it gently between your palms.

2

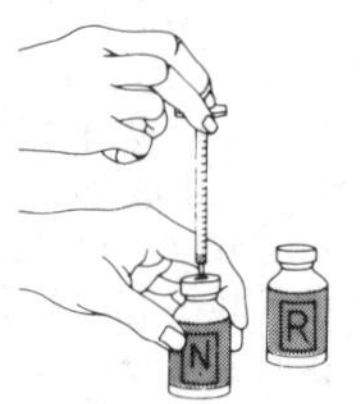

Put air into the vial marked N of long-acting insulin: Clean the rubber stopper of the vial with an alcohol swab. To put air into the syringe, pull the plunger back to the appropriate number of units of long-acting insulin. Then insert the needle into the top of the vial, making sure the point does not touch the insulin. Push in the plunger, and withdraw the syringe.

3

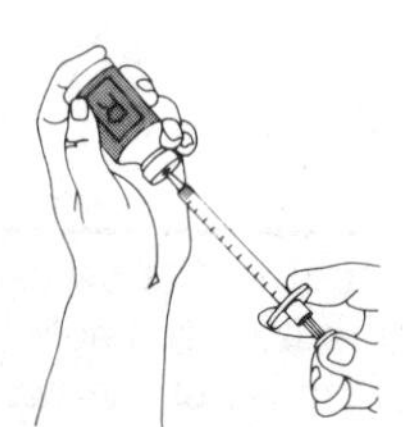

Withdraw your dose of regular insulin from vial marked R: Clean the rubber stopper of the regular insulin vial with an alcohol swab. Next, pull back the plunger to the necessary number of units of regular insulin, and inject air into the bottle. With the needle still in the bottle, turn the bottle upside down, and withdraw the proper dose of regular insulin.

4

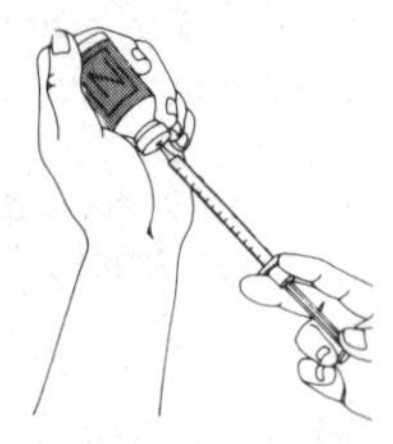

Withdraw your dose of long-acting insulin: Clean the top of the long-acting insulin vial, and insert the needle into it, without pushing down the plunger. Then invert the bottle, and withdraw the appropriate number of units. (Remember to pull the plunger back to the number of units needed for the *total* dose. For instance, if you have 10 units of regular insulin in the syringe and you need 20 units of long-acting insulin, pull the plunger back to 30 units.)

Patient-Teaching Aid

HOW TO USE AN ATOMIZER

Dear Patient:
To relieve your nasal congestion, your physician wants you to use an atomizer to spray medication into your nose. Here is how:

1

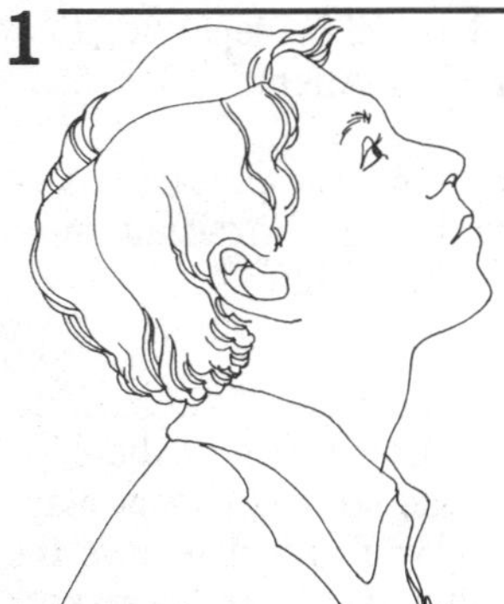

Before you begin, read the medication label carefully, so you know the exact amount of medication to administer. Make sure you have tissues handy. Then sit upright, with your head tilted back, as shown here.

If that position is uncomfortable for you, lie on your back instead. Place a pillow under your shoulders, so your head tilts back.

2

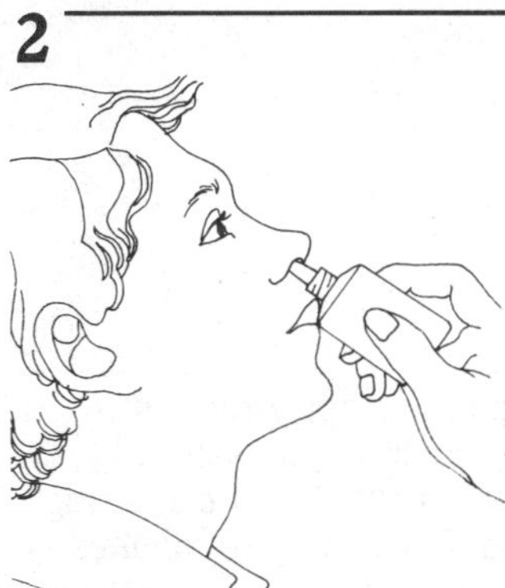

Now place the tip of the atomizer about ½″ (1 cm) inside your nostril. Point it straight up your nose, toward the inner corner of your eye. Do not angle the atomizer downward, or the medication will run down your throat.

Without inhaling, squeeze the atomizer once, quickly and firmly. Use just enough force to coat the inside of your nose with medication. Too much force may send the medicine into your sinuses, and give you a headache. Then spray again, if the instructions on the label order it. Repeat the procedure in the other nostril.

3

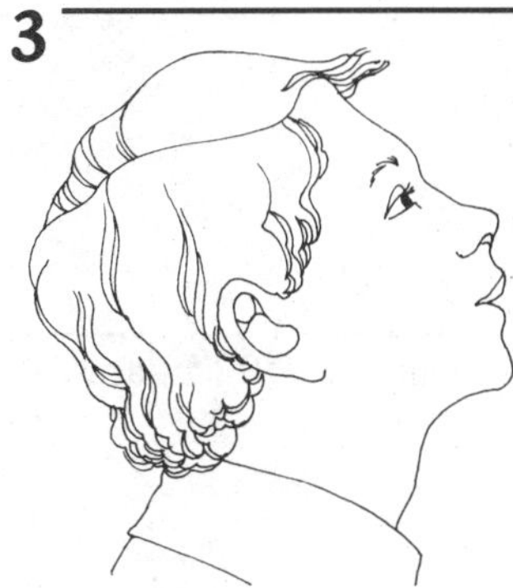

Keep your head tilted back for several minutes so the medication has time to work. Avoid blowing your nose while you wait. Never use your atomizer more often than the physician directs. Doing so may actually increase your congestion instead of relieve it.

Patient-Teaching Aid

HOW TO USE AN ANAPHYLAXIS KIT

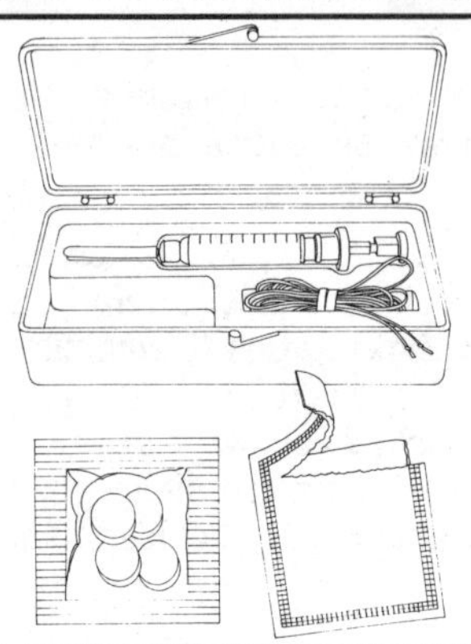

Dear Patient:
Because you risk having a severe reaction from an insect sting or other antigen, your physician has given you this emergency anaphylaxis kit. Everything you need to combat the allergic reaction is inside: a prefilled syringe containing two doses of epinephrine, alcohol swabs, a tourniquet, and Chlo-Amine (antihistamine) tablets.

If you are stung by an insect—despite precautions—use the kit as follows. Also, notify your physician immediately, or ask someone else to call him.

1

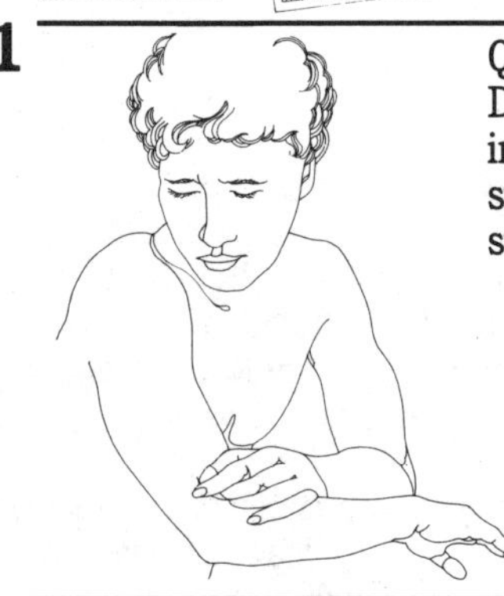

Quickly remove the insect's stinger if it is still there. Do not pinch, push, or squeeze the stinger, as you may imbed it farther into the skin. If you cannot remove the stinger quickly, do not keep trying. Go on to the next step immediately.

2

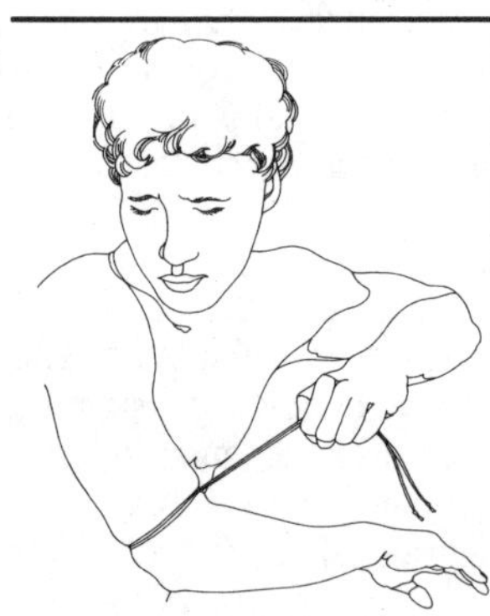

If you were stung on an arm or leg, apply the tourniquet between the sting and your heart, as shown here. Tighten the tourniquet by pulling the end of one string. Remember to release the tourniquet after 10 minutes by pulling on the metal ring.

3

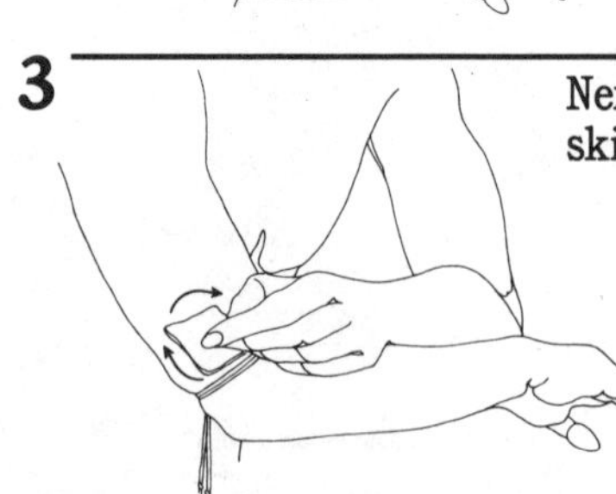

Next, use an alcohol swab to clean a 4″ (10 cm) area of skin above the tourniquet.

HOW TO USE AN ANAPHYLAXIS KIT—*continued*

4

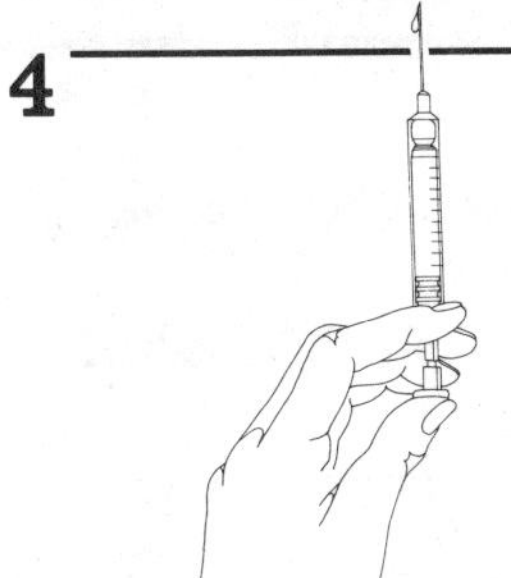

Then lift the prefilled syringe from the kit, and remove the needle cover. Hold the syringe with the needle pointing upward. Then expel the air from it by carefully pushing on the plunger, as shown here.

5

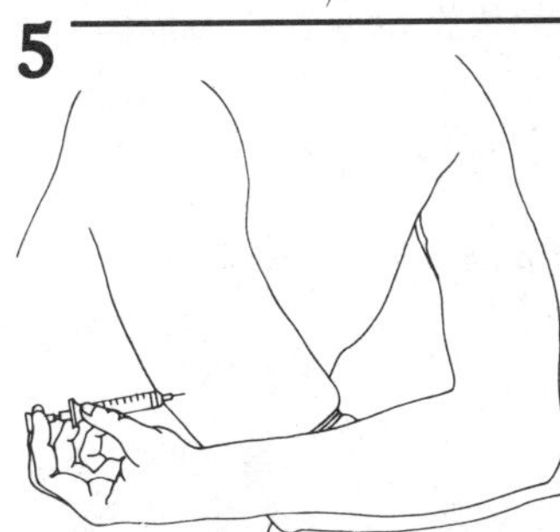

Now you are ready to inject the epinephrine. To do this properly, insert the entire needle straight down into the cleansed skin. Then pull back slightly on the plunger. If you see blood in the syringe, the needle is inside a blood vessel. Withdraw the needle, and reinsert it in another site.

6

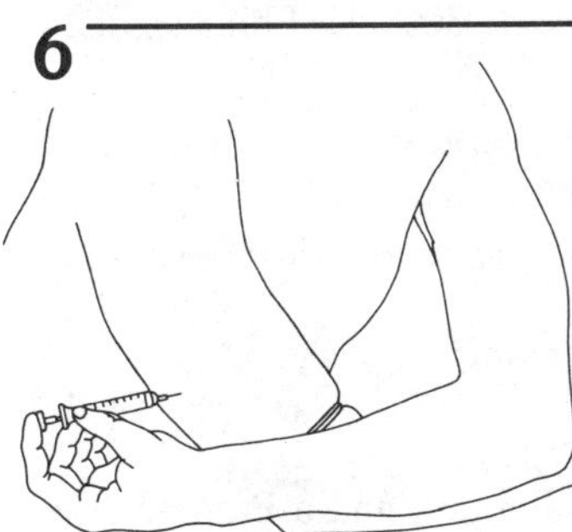

As soon as you are sure the needle is not in a blood vessel, push down on the plunger, and inject the epinephrine. Use the following guidelines for proper dosage: adults, and children over age 12—dosage range is 0.1 to 0.5 ml; children between ages 2 and 12—usual dose is 0.15 to 0.2 ml.

7

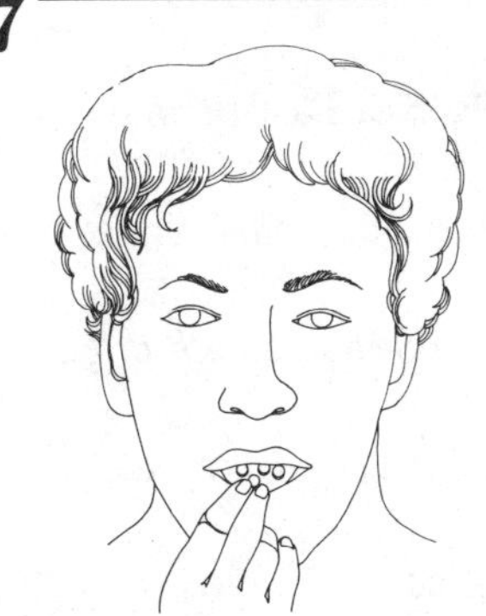

Withdraw the needle and syringe. Then chew and swallow the Chlo-Amine tablets. If you are over age 12, take four tablets; if you are under age 12, take two tablets.

Next, apply ice packs, if available, to the affected area. Avoid exertion, keep warm, and see a physician immediately.

IMPORTANT: If you do not notice an improvement within 10 minutes, give a second injection. To do this, rotate the rectangular plunger a quarter turn to the right, and line it up with the rectangular slot in the syringe. Do not depress the plunger until you are ready to administer the second injection. Then follow the same injection procedure as before.

Selected References

Barber, Triphy, and Langfitt, Dot E. *Teaching the Medical-Surgical Patient: Diagnostics and Procedures.* East Norwalk, Conn.: Appleton & Lange, 1983.

Barnhart, Edward R., ed. *Physicians' Desk Reference,* 41st ed. Oradell, N.J.: Medical Economics Books, 1987.

Bille, D.A. *Practical Approaches to Patient Teaching.* Boston: Little, Brown & Co., 1981.

Bloom, B., et al. *Taxonomy of Educational Objectives. Handbook I: Cognitive Domain.* White Plains, N.Y.: Longman Inc., 1977.

Brunner, Lillian, and Suddarth, Doris. *Textbook of Medical-Surgical Nursing,* 5th ed. Philadelphia: J.B. Lippincott Co., 1984.

Buckley, Kathleen, and Kulb, Nancy W., eds. *Handbook of Maternal-Newborn Nursing.* New York: John Wiley & Sons, 1983.

Cardiovascular Care Handbook. Springhouse, Pa.: Springhouse Corp., 1986.

Clark, Carolyn C. *Classroom Skills for Nurse Educators,* vol. 4. New York: Springer Publishing Co., 1978.

Clemente, Carmine D., ed. *Gray's Anatomy of the Human Body,* 30th ed. Philadelphia: Lea & Febiger, 1984.

Cushing, Maureen. "Legal Lessons on Patient Teaching," *American Journal of Nursing* 84(6):721-22, June 1984.

Czerwinski, Barbara. *Manual of Patient Education for Cardiopulmonary Dysfunctions.* St. Louis: C.V. Mosby Co., 1980.

Diagnostics, 2nd ed. Springhouse, Pa.: Springhouse Corp., 1986.

Diseases, 2nd ed. Springhouse, Pa.: Springhouse Corp., 1987.

D'Onofrio, C.N. "Evaluating Patient Education: Purposes, Politics, and a Proposal for Practitioners," in *Patient Education—An Inquiry into the State of the Art.* Edited by Squyres, W.D. New York: Springer Publishing Co., 1980.

Donovan, Marilee, and Richardson, S.G., eds. *Cancer Care Nursing.* East Norwalk, Conn.: Appleton & Lange, 1984.

Drug Information for the Health Care Provider, vol. 1. Rockville, Md.: United States Pharmacopeial Convention, Inc., 1985.

DuBrey, Rita. *Promoting Wellness in Nursing Practice: A Step-by-Step Approach in Patient Education.* St. Louis: C.V. Mosby Co., 1982.

Falvo, Donna R. *Effective Patient Education: A Guide to Increased Compliance.* Rockville, Md.: Aspen Systems Corp., 1984.

Freedman, Carol. *Teaching Patients.* San Diego: Courseware, Inc., 1978.

Given, Barbara, and Simmons, Sandra. *Gastroenterology in Clinical Nursing,* 4th ed. St. Louis: C.V. Mosby Co., 1984.

Griffith, H. Winter. *Instructions for Patients,* 3rd ed. Philadelphia: W.B. Saunders Co., 1982.

Health Assessment Handbook. Springhouse, Pa.: Springhouse Corp., 1985.

Isselbacher, Kurt, et al. *Harrison's Principles of Internal Medicine: Update Two,* 9th ed. New York: McGraw-Hill Book Co., 1982.

Karch, Amy. *Cardiac Care: A Guide for Patient Education.* East Norwalk, Conn.: Appleton & Lange, 1981.

Kernaghan, Salvinija. "Preadmission Preoperative Teaching: A Promising Option, but Easier Said than Done," *Promoting Health* 6(2):6-8, March/April 1985.

Luckmann, Joan, and Sorenson, Karen. *Medical-Surgical Nursing: A Psychophysiologic Approach,* 2nd ed. Philadelphia: W.B. Saunders Co., 1980.

Madnick, Myra E., ed. *Consumer Health Education: A Guide to Hospital-Based Programs.* Rockville, Md.: Aspen Systems Corp., 1980.

Massachusetts General Hospital Staff. *Massachusetts General Hospital Department of Nursing Teaching Guides for Patients with Neurologic Disorders.* Reston, Va.: Reston Publishing Co., 1984.

McConnell, Edwina, and Nimmerman, Mary F. *Care of Patients with Urologic Problems.* Philadelphia: J.B. Lippincott Co., 1982.

Medication Teaching Manual, 3rd ed. Washington, D.C.: American Society of Hospital Pharmacists, 1983.

Nursing87 Drug Handbook. Springhouse, Pa.: Springhouse Corp., 1987.

Nursing87 MediQuik Cards. Springhouse, Pa.: Springhouse Corp., 1987.

Olds, Sally B., et al. *Maternal-Newborn Nursing, A Family-Centered Approach,* 2nd ed. Reading, Mass.: Addison-Wesley Publishing Co., 1984.

Parker, Susan. *Pediatric Care: A Guide for Patient Education.* East Norwalk, Conn.: Appleton-Century-Crofts, 1982.

Rankin, Sally, and Duffy, Karen L. *Patient Education: Issues, Principles and Guidelines.* Philadelphia: J.B. Lippincott Co., 1983.

Redman, Barbara K. *The Process of Patient Teaching in Nursing,* 5th ed. St. Louis: C.V. Mosby Co., 1983.

Rivlin, Michel, et al. *Manual of Clinical Problems in Obstetrics and Gynecology with Annotated Key References.* Boston: Little, Brown & Co., 1982.

Robertson, Carolyn. "Clear the Exercise Hurdles for Your Diabetic Patient," *Nursing84* 14(10):58-64, October 1984.

Shamansky, Sherry L., et al. *Primary Health Care Handbook: Guidelines for Patient Education.* Boston: Little, Brown & Co., 1984.

Shipes, E. "Principles of Teaching," in *Principles of Ostomy Care.* Edited by Broadwell, D., and Jackson, B. St. Louis: C.V. Mosby Co., 1981.

Slusarczyk, Susan, and Hicks, Franklin. "Helping Your Patient to Live with a Permanent Pacemaker," *Nursing83* 13(4):58-64, April 1983.

Smith, Dorothy L. *Medication Guide for Patient Counseling,* 2nd ed. Philadelphia: Lea & Febiger, 1981.

Steiner, George, and Lawrence, Patricia A. *Educating Diabetic Patients.* New York: Springer Publishing Co., 1980.

Storlie, Frances. *Patient Teaching in Critical Care.* East Norwalk, Conn.: Appleton-Century-Crofts, 1975.

Veenker, C.H., "Evaluating Health Practice and Understanding," *Health Education* 16(2):80-82, February 1985.

Walsh, P.C., et al. *Campbell's Urology.* Philadelphia: W.B. Saunders Co., 1986.

Wintrobe, Maxwell M., et al. *Clinical Hematology,* 8th ed. Philadelphia: Lea & Febiger, 1981.

Woldum, Karyl, et al. *Patient Education: Foundations of Practice.* Rockville, Md.: Aspen Systems Corp., 1984.

Index

A

B

C

D

E

H

I

J

K

L

M

N

O

Q

R

S

T

U

V

W